High-risk Pregnancy

High-risk Pregnancy

Edited by

AA Calder MD, FRCOG, FRCP (Glas)

The Centre For Reproductive Biology
University of Edinburgh, UK

and

W Dunlop PhD, MBChB, FRCOG, FRCS (Ed)

Department of Obstetrics and Gynaecology
University of Newcastle upon Tyne, UK

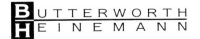

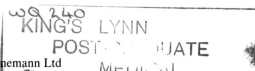
Butterworth-Heinemann Ltd
Linacre House, Jordan Hill, Oxford OX2 8DP

 PART OF REED INTERNATIONAL BOOKS

OXFORD   LONDON   BOSTON
MUNICH   NEW DELHI   SINGAPORE   SYDNEY
TOKYO   TORONTO   WELLINGTON

First published 1992

© Butterworth-Heinemann Ltd 1992

British Library Cataloguing in Publication Data
Calder, A.A.
   High-risk pregnancy.
   I. Title   II. Dunlop, W.
   618.3

ISBN 0 7506 1324 6

Library of Congress Cataloguing in Publication Data
High-risk pregnancy / edited by A.A. Calder and W. Dunlop.
      p.   cm.
   Includes bibliographical references and index.
   ISBN 0 7506 1324 6
   1. Pregnancy, Complications of.   I. Calder, A.A. (Andrew Alexander)
   II, Dunlop, W. (William, PhD).
   [DNLM: 1. Pregnancy Complications.   2. Risk Factors.   WQ 240 H6374]
   RG571.H44   1991
   618.3—dc20
   DNLM/DLC   91–29606
   for Library of Congress   CIP

Photoset, printed and bound in Great Britain by
Redwood Press, Melksham, Wiltshire

Contents

10 Prematurity   332
HL Halliday

11 Abnormalities of fetal growth   362
JP Neilson

12 Neurodevelopmental handicap: the obstetric perspective   387
David J Taylor

Contributors

SL Barron, MBBS, FRCS, FRCOG, Department of Obstetrics and Gynaecology, Princess Mary Maternity Hospital, Great North Road, Newcastle upon Tyne

Ian AD Bouchier, CBE, MD, FRCP, FRCPE, FRSE, FIBiol, FRSA, Department of Medicine, The Royal Infirmary, Edinburgh

Ray P Brettle, Department of Infectious Disease, City Hospital, Edinburgh

John Burn, BMedSci(Hons), MBBS, FRCP, Department of Human Genetics, University of Newcastle upon Tyne, 19 Claremont Place, Newcastle upon Tyne

AA Calder, MD, FRCOG, FRCP(Glas), Centre for Reproductive Biology, University of Edinburgh, 37 Chalmers Street, Edinburgh

JM Davison, BSc, MD, MSc, FRCOG, Department of Obstetrics and Gynaecology, Princess Mary Maternity Hospital, Great North Road, Newcastle upon Tyne

Michael de Swiet, MD, FRCP, Queen Charlotte's Hospital for Women, Goldhawk Road, London

W Dunlop, PhD, MBChB, FRCOG, FRCS(ed), Department of Obstetrics and Gynaecology, Princess Mary Maternity Hospital, Great North Road, Newcastle upon Tyne

James R Gray, MD, FRCP(C), Research Fellow, Department of Medicine, The Royal Infirmary, Edinburgh

IA Greer, MD, MRCP, MRCOG, Muirhead Professor, Department of Obstetrics and Gynaecology, University of Glasgow, Glasgow Royal Infirmary, Glasgow

HL Halliday, MD, FRCP, DCH, The Nuffield Department of Child Health, The Queen's University of Belfast, Institute of Clinical Science, Grosvenor Road, Belfast

M Hepburn, BSc, MD, MRCGP, MRCOG, Departments of Obstetrics and Gynaecology, and Social Policy and Social Work, University of Glasgow, Royal Maternity Hospital, Rottenrow, Glasgow

Frank D Johnstone, Department of Obstetrics and Gynaecology, Centre for Reproductive Biology, 37 Chalmers Street, Edinburgh

Elizabeth A Letsky, MBBS, FRCPath, Department of Haematology, Queen Charlotte's Hospital for Women, Goldhawk Road, London

MJA Maresh, BSc, MBBS, MRCOG, St Mary's Hospital for Women and Children, Whitworth Park, Manchester

Jacqueline Mok, Department of Paediatrics, City Hospital, Edinburgh

JP Neilson, BSc, MD, MRCOG, Department of Obstetrics and Gynaecology, University of Edinburgh, Centre for Reproductive Biology, 37 Chalmers Street, Edinburgh

MM Reid, BSc, MD, BS, FRCP, MRCPath, DCH, Department of Haematology, Royal Victoria Infirmary, Newcastle upon Tyne

David J Taylor, MD, FRCOG, Department of Obstetrics and Gynaecology, University of Dundee Medical School, Ninewells Hospital, Dundee

Stephen A Walkinshaw, BSc, MD, MRCOG, Fetal Centre, Liverpool Maternity Hospital, Oxford Street, Liverpool

Part One

Maternal Disorders

Chapter 1

Diabetes

MJA Maresh

Introduction

If one reviewed some of the most recent results from units providing special services for the pregnant woman with diabetes one could believe that the perinatal morbidity and mortality associated with the condition are hardly greater than those of the general population. However this is a false impression of the national situation in a particular country, as has been demonstrated by regional and national studies.

The management of the pregnant woman with diabetes remains a challenge. This is a high-risk problem from conception until well past delivery. There is little room for complacency and compromise. It is only the recognition of these facts and the high standards of care achieved that are producing better results.

The primary objective of management is to achieve normoglycaemia and an associated normal metabolic environment for the developing fetus; this is also in the long-term interests of maternal health. Normoglycaemia should be striven for in all cases, although it may not be achievable in all. It provides no absolute guarantee of a normal outcome, although it should result in one that is not very different from normal.

Such care is costly in terms of having an experienced multidisciplinary team with the time to devote to the problems. It also demands much of the mother and it is important that the mother should not be allowed to feel guilty if problems arise.

This chapter outlines the particular risks to the mother and the fetus and then presents a logical scheme of management based on prevention of these problems. Most discussion is focused on insulin-dependent diabetic women, although women with non-insulin dependent diabetes and some women with abnormal glucose tolerance are also in high-risk groups and are mentioned where appropriate.

Maternal risks

General

The metabolic alterations of pregnancy result in an increased insulin requirement and this may tip the women with prodromal insulin dependent diabetes into the actual condition. The incidence of this occurring has been estimated to be 12 per

100 000 deliveries (Buschard *et al.*, 1987). The vast majority of these will occur in late pregnancy as resistance to insulin becomes more marked. In addition, women with undiagnosed non-insulin-dependent diabetes may also occasionally deteriorate rapidly. Simple urine testing for glycosuria should at least alert one to the possibility of this developing. If missed, ketoacidosis may develop with high fetal and maternal risks. Studies highlighting these increased risks are reviewed by Cousins (1987). The prevalence of ketoacidosis in these studies was high (up to 24 per cent), but many were old. In the last review of maternal deaths in the UK 1985–1987 (Department of Health, 1991), neither of the two deaths in diabetic women were associated with ketoacidosis.

Ketonuria is more common in the pregnant than in the non-pregnant state, owing to the more rapid activation of lipolysis with short periods of fasting – the 'accelerated starvation' concept (Freinkel, 1965). This should not cause confusion with ketoacidosis, which presents in the pregnant state in the same way as in the non-pregnant with hyperglycaemia. Provided that the mother is measuring her blood glucose levels, additional insulin can be added before diuresis, dehydration and hyperosmolality supervene, with the result that ketoacidosis should be a preventable condition. Classically, infections will precipitate this condition, but more recently it has been induced iatrogenically by β-sympathomimetics and corticosteroids used in the management of preterm labour.

Retinopathy

Much of the confusion surrounding diabetic retinopathy in pregnancy relates to a failure to understand the basic natural history of the condition outside of pregnancy. After 15 years of diabetes there will almost always be evidence of background retinopathy. With further time, proliferative retinopathy may gradually develop. Accordingly, over a 9-month period of observation (e.g. a pregnancy) in a large series one would expect to find a number of cases developing proliferative retinopathy. The situation is further complicated by the observation that improvements in diabetic glucose control may cause an ischaemic retinopathy and that deteriorations in retinopathy may be more episodic than gradual in nature.

Most of the retinal changes described in diabetic pregnancy can be understood, bearing these facts in mind. Background retinopathy may develop for the first time during pregnancy (Horvat *et al.*, 1980). There may be worsening of the background retinopathy as shown by the development of soft exudates with improved metabolic control (Moloney and Drury, 1982). These changes – ischaemic retinopathy – usually resolve spontaneously and are not associated with proliferative retinopathy.

In pregnancy, proliferative retinopathy develops in a small number of diabetic women with background retinopathy. Series are small but numbers vary between none in ten (Price *et al.*, 1984), none in 11 (Jovanovic and Jovanovic, 1984), three in 19 (Dibble *et al.*, 1982), four in 33 (Moloney and Drury, 1982) and seven in 32 (Forrester, Towler and Pearson, 1989). Provided that proliferative retinopathy, whether new or pre-existing, is treated with laser therapy there appears to be no deterioration in visual acuity after pregnancy (Jovanovic and Jovanovic, 1984).

In conclusion, it appears that regular retinal surveillance during pregnancy and active treatment of proliferative disease results in pregnancy having no additional worsening effect on the progression of diabetic retinal disease. The whole subject has been reviewed recently by Forrester, Towler and Pearson (1989).

Nephropathy

Just as with retinopathy, it is important to consider that the natural history of nephropathy is a gradual deterioration of renal function with time. Kitzmiller *et al.* (1981) found no worsening of the condition during pregnancy in the majority of diabetic women. The subsequent decline in renal function appeared similar to that expected in a population of diabetic subjects with nephropathy. In their series, the lowest creatinine clearance in a subject in the first trimester was 24 ml/min and Steel, Johnstone and Smith (1989) had a good outcome in women where it was >40 ml/min. Accordingly, unless a woman is about to go into renal failure requiring therapy, termination of pregnancy is not usually considered. Even if she is close to failure, termination is not necessarily indicated because her condition may remain relatively stable over the pregnancy and dialysis remains a possibility. Although pregnancy after renal transplantation may not cause a problem, any associated complications such as vascular disease and hypertension may have risks to the mother and fetus. Regular attention to renal function should allow detection of early deterioration and thus minimize risks to mother and fetus.

Occasionally, a severe transient diabetic nephrotic syndrome may develop (Patterson, Lunan and MacCuish, 1985; Weinstock *et al.*, 1988). Differentiation from pre-eclampsia can be made only by renal biopsy, but this is not indicated on clinical grounds and delivery cannot usually be postponed for long. Although pregnancy in the diabetic woman with nephropathy may be successfully achieved, there is a higher incidence of obstetric and perinatal morbidity (see below).

In view of the progressive nature of the disease and its associated increased mortality, it is advisable for women wishing to have children to do so as soon as they feel that they are able. Delaying is likely to be complicated by a deterioration of renal function and development of hypertension and cardiovascular disease.

Fetal risks

Congenital malformations

Epidemiology
There is universal agreement that maternal diabetes is associated with a two- to fourfold increase in congenital malformations of the infant. Series from the UK (Lowy, Beard and Goldschmidt, 1986), USA (Simpson *et al.*, 1983; Mills *et al.*, 1988a) and Denmark (Molsted-Pedersen, 1980) are all in general agreement, with rates varying between 49 and 90/1000 contrasted with control populations of 20–30/1000. Slight variations between studies can be accounted for by: (a) methodological differences in assessing malformation, (b) the different populations studied, (c) variations in the severity of the diabetes and its control (see below) and (d) differing policies with regard to screening and termination of pregnancy.

This marked increase in congenital malformations when contrasted with the general population has become much more noticeable over the last 20 years as improved perinatal care has led to a dramatic reduction in perinatal mortality. Reports from major centres emphasize this point: our only perinatal death in a diabetic mother at St Mary's, Manchester, over the last 10 years was one neonatal death from multiple malformations (rate 5.9/1000) and figures from King's College,

London (Brudenell and Doddridge, 1989) are similar. However, this is not necessarily the national situation and in 1980 a UK survey of mothers with established diabetes revealed that only 30 per cent of perinatal deaths could be attributed to congenital malformations (Lowy, Beard and Goldschmidt, 1986).

There is no evidence for an increased incidence of malformations in infants born to mothers with gestational diabetes (Malins, 1979). This would be expected in view of the lack of metabolic disturbance found during embryogenesis in gestational diabetes.

Malformation patterns
Specific types of congenital malformations are seen in association with maternal diabetes.

1. Caudal regression syndrome (sacral agenesis) is estimated to be 200 times more common with maternal diabetes when contrasted with the general population (Kucera, 1971). In the UK survey there were three cases (4/1000) (Lowy, Beard and Goldschmidt, 1986).
2. Neural tube defects are also increased, in particular anencephaly, microcephaly and holoprosencephaly. Previous reports have estimated a rate of 19.5/1000 contrasted with a background rate of 1–2/1000 (Milunsky *et al.*, 1982). The exact risk is now difficult to determine, owing to the varying availability of antenatal diagnosis and the possibility of termination of pregnancy. For instance, in the UK survey no infants were born with anencephaly, whereas in the Diabetes in Early Pregnancy Study (Mills *et al.*, 1988a) the rate was 6/1000.
3. Cardiac abnormalities are also more common and figures as high as a fivefold increase have been quoted (40/1000) (Rowland, Hubbell and Nadas, 1973). In the UK survey the rate was not as high, with 15 infants having major anomalies (19.4/1000) which was estimated as a 2.6-fold increase. The commonest cardiac lesions found were transposition of the great vessels and ventricular septal defects.

There is less evidence to support other anomalies as being specifically increased, although Kucera (1971) noted an increase in urological disorders. Imperforate anus may also be increased, although this could be regarded as an aspect of the caudal regression syndrome.

Pathogenesis
An association between poor diabetic control and an increase in malformations has long been described (Pedersen, 1977). This has been made more clear by a number of studies where glycosylated haemoglobin was measured towards the end of the first trimester, thus giving an idea of overall diabetic control during embryogenesis (Leslie *et al.*, 1978; Miller *et al.*, 1981; Reid *et al.*, 1984; Ylinen *et al.*, 1984; Stubbs *et al.*, 1986). These studies have all shown that higher concentrations are associated with an increase in malformations. The Diabetes in Early Pregnancy Study (Mills *et al.*, 1988a) showed that women who were seen within 21 days of conception had a significantly lower risk of congenital malformations than those seen subsequently (49 versus 90/1000). It was not altogether surprising that no relationship was found between the degree of glycaemic control and congenital malformations in the 'early' group. Most of these women must have been well motivated and were moderately well controlled and few had the degree of elevation of glycosylated haemoglobin found in the studies mentioned above. Studies comparing women attending pre-

conceptionally for advice have also shown a decrease in congenital malformations when contrasted with those seen after the diagnosis of pregnancy (Steel *et al.*, 1990; Fuhrmann *et al.*, 1983).

An association between congenital malformations and the severity of diabetic vascular disease has also been known for many years (Molsted–Pederson, Tygstrup and Pedersen, 1964). However, the latest reports (Damm and Molsted-Pedersen, 1989) show a major reduction in malformations in the more severe groups (White's classes D and F), so that there was no longer a significant difference. This could not be accounted for by terminations of pregnancy. Indeed, in the 1982–1986 cohort of 258 women, the overall congenital malformation rate was not significantly raised above that in the controls (39 versus 28/1000) (Damm and Molsted-Pedersen, 1989).

Epidemiological considerations would suggest that high concentrations of glucose, or another metabolite that is disturbed when there is hyperglycaemia, may be responsible for this embryopathy. In the mouse and rat, malformations can be produced by inducing maternal diabetes and can then be prevented by introducing insulin at critical times during embryogenesis (Horii, Watanabe and Ingalls, 1966; Baker *et al.*, 1981; Eriksson *et al.*, 1982). Specific lesions seen include lumbosacral malformations, as seen in the human. In vitro, whole embryo culture techniques using rats also showed similar results (Cockroft and Coppola, 1977) although the glucose concentrations were very high (67–83 mmol/l). However, the fetus of the diabetic mother is exposed to more than one abnormal metabolite and Lewis, Akazawa and Freinkel (1983) demonstrated that ketonaemia could potentiate these effects at lower glucose concentrations. The exact mechanisms by which these metabolic changes cause teratogenesis remain speculative.

Hypoglycaemia has also been investigated to see if this is associated with congenital malformations. Studies in vivo and in vitro in rats have suggested an increase in congenital malformations and growth retardation when hypoglycaemia is induced (Buchanan, Schemmer and Freinkel, 1986; Akazawa *et al.*, 1987). However, whether transient maternal hypoglycaemia in the human is associated with fetal hypoglycaemia is uncertain, and the placental impermeability to insulin should protect it. To date there is no clinical evidence of an association with congenital malformations (Steel, Johnstone and Smith, 1989).

Spontaneous abortion

As congenital anomalies are more frequent in diabetic pregnancy, one would also anticipate a higher rate of spontaneous abortion than in a control population. In the past this has generally not been shown, although some of the studies have been poorly designed. The prospective uncontrolled studies of Miodovnik and associates have shown an overall 30 per cent spontaneous abortion rate (Miodovnik *et al.*, 1984), with rates increasing as disease worsened (White's classification). These workers also found an increased risk of abortion if periconceptional diabetic control was unsatisfactory. This was assessed by measuring glycosylated haemoglobin at 8–9 weeks (Miodovnik *et al.*, 1986), a measurement which should reflect diabetic control over the previous 8 weeks. These smaller uncontrolled studies have now been amplified by the Diabetes in Early Pregnancy Study (Mills *et al.*, 1988b) which included 386 insulin dependent diabetics and 432 controls recruited within 21 days of conception. Although there was no difference in abortion rates between the diabetics and the controls (16 per cent), those who aborted had higher fasting and postprandial glucose concentrations than those with continuing pregnancies. In addition, there was a relationship with increasing glycosylated haemoglobin. Women attending for preconception advice are likely to have different characteristics from those who do not; the former should thus have a lower rate of spontaneous abortion, as shown in the study by Dicker *et al*. (1988a).

Fetal growth disturbance

Early fetal growth disturbance

Disturbances of fetal growth in the first trimester are likely to have major effects on pregnancy survival and also may be associated with congenital abnormalities. Pedersen and Molsted-Pedersen (1979) described this phenomenon in diabetic pregnancy. They subsequently reported that, in women with reliable menstrual data, a fetal crown–rump length equivalent to 6 days less than expected was associated with an 18 per cent risk of malformation (Pedersen and Molsted-Pedersen, 1981). Furthermore, in women with more severe diabetes a similar discrepancy (White's classes D and F) was associated with a 27 per cent risk. The infants were followed up and had psychomotor assessment at 4 years of age (Petersen *et al*., 1988). Those who were 'growth delayed' appeared to have developmental delay in comparison with those who did not.

Other workers have tried to detect this phenomenon and failed (Whittaker, Aspillaga and Lind, 1983; Steel, Johnstone and Corrie, 1984; Cousins *et al*., 1988; Harper and Morrow, 1988). Their overall conclusions are that the apparent early growth delay simply reflects delayed ovulation. Until more data emerge, this remains the more likely explanation.

Later fetal growth disturbance

Excessive growth is regarded as a characteristic of the diabetic fetus. It puts the fetus at risk of a traumatic delivery or, alternatively, subjects it and its mother to the additional hazards of caesarean birth. It is also almost certainly associated with an increased risk of unexplained fetal death and neonatal morbidity (see below).

Typical series show a figure of about 25 per cent of infants born to diabetic mothers having birthweights above the 90th percentile (Beard and Maresh, 1989). It has been suggested recently that all infants are growth accelerated and that there is a general shift of the normal weight distribution from that of the whole hospital population (Bradley, Nicolaides and Brudenell, 1988). However, this study has been criticized because no attempt was made to obtain matching controls.

The increase in birthweight is secondary to increase in fat, muscle and organ size. The pathogenesis of these disorders is fetal hyperinsulinaemia. This theory was first put forward by Pederson (1954), who suggested that maternal hyperglycaemia leads to fetal hyperglycaemia, to pancreatic β-cell hyperplasia and fetal hyperinsulinaemia. The hypothesis has subsequently been reinforced by numerous workers and an extended, modified version is shown in Figure 1.1. Critical pieces of research supporting this were as follows:

1. The autopsy finding of fetal pancreatic β-cell hyperplasia in association with maternal diabetes (Cardell, 1953; Driscoll, Benirschke and Curtis, 1960; Naeye, 1965).
2. The presence of functional hyperinsulinaemia in the newborn infant of the mother (Baird and Farquhar, 1962).

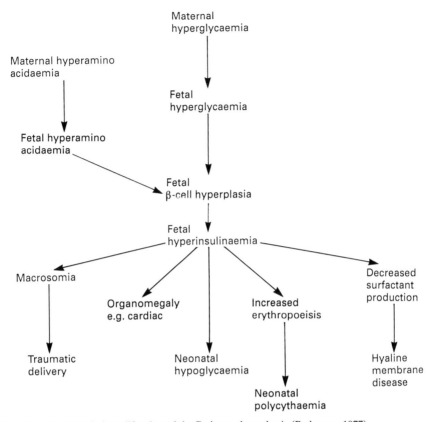

Figure 1.1.   An expanded modification of the Pedersen hypothesis (Pedersen, 1977)

3. An association between increased amniotic fluid C-peptide and insulin with the large-for-gestational-age infant of the diabetic mother (Falluca *et al.*, 1985). In addition, the relationship between amniotic fluid C-peptide and maternal hyperglycaemia (Persson *et al.*, 1986).

4. The association between maternal hyperglycaemia and elevated glycosylated haemoglobin with increased skinfold thickness in the newborn (Whitelaw, 1977; Stubbs, Leslie and John, 1981).

5. Increased bodyweight and enlarged heart and liver in the normoglycaemic hyperinsulinaemic rhesus monkey model (Susa and Schwartz, 1985).

6. The maximum tolerated insulin regimen of Roversi *et al.* (1979), suggesting that a normal birthweight distribution could be produced by rendering diabetic patients almost hypoglycaemic.

Although insulin can be detected in the fetus in the first trimester of pregnancy, it has generally been considered that the fetal pancreas does not respond to hyperglycaemia by hyperplasia until late in the second trimester. Recent work on fetal blood obtained from samples taken for karyotyping at about 20 weeks of pregnancy has suggested that fetal insulin levels may already be raised at this stage (RJ Bradley, 1988, personal communication). However, the major growth acceleration pattern does not appear before 26 weeks.

Glucose may not be the only stimulator of fetal growth. Branched-chain amino acids, which may be raised in the mother with only mild degrees of glucose intolerance (Metzger *et al.*, 1980), are also stimulators of pancreatic insulin secretion (Milner *et al.*, 1979). This may be a factor in fetal hyperinsulinaemia and could be one reason why there are continued reports of high-birthweight infants despite apparent good glucose control. Excessive fetal growth could also be caused by increased concentration of circulating somatomedins – insulin growth factors. Longitudinal studies, however, have not shown a correlation with birthweights (Lind and Whittaker, 1989).

Apart from the supply of nutrients and growth factors to the fetus, the other factor that can affect fetal growth is the utero-placental vascular supply. The association between low-birthweight babies and vascular disease (e.g. retinopathy, nephropathy) in diabetics could be due to the effect of the vascular disease on the uterine supply. Attempts to assess blood flow using the readily available Doppler techniques have shown conflicting results, especially in diabetic pregnancy. Although blood flow may be a limiting factor on fetal growth, it seems unlikely that it has a growth-promoting influence.

There is agreement that gestational diabetes is associated with increased birthweight; however, the controversy relates to the relevance of maternal obesity. In a controlled study of treated gestational diabetics, the excess in fetal weight was nearly all accounted for by the maternal obesity and the degree of diabetic control had an insignificant effect (Maresh *et al.*, 1989). Thus, although the large baby of the gestational diabetic will still be at risk of mortality or morbidity, this is more likely to result from a traumatic delivery than from defective maternal metabolism.

Unexplained fetal death

Major influences on the management of diabetic pregnancy have resulted from attempts to avoid unexplained fetal death *in utero*. These attempts are responsible for the high elective preterm delivery rate and caesarean section rate, with figures of 50 and 58 per cent respectively in the UK survey of 1979–1980 (Beard and Lowy, 1982). However, unexplained stillbirths still accounted for 50 per cent of the perinatal mortality in that survey and recent reports from major UK diabetic centres still show the occasional unexplained fetal death despite close monitoring (Bradley, Brudenell and Nicolaides, 1988; Tyrrell, 1988).

The classic case is a mature, normally formed, normal weight fetus in a pregnancy perhaps complicated by mild polyhydramnios and pre-eclampsia. The pathogenesis is almost certainly multifactorial, with the final event being an asphyxial death. A number of observations produce the asphyxial hypothesis outlined in Figure 1.2.

Uterine blood flow
Although Doppler blood flow measurements in diabetic pregnancy have produced conflicting results, the occurrence of worse outcome in women with known diabetic vascular disease (White's Classes F and R) suggests that uterine blood flow may be impaired in some pregnancies. Furthermore, although pre-eclampsia is not as common in diabetic pregnancy as is frequently claimed, it still occurs at least as frequently as in the general population (Cousins, 1987) and its associated spiral artery disorder will decrease uterine blood flow in some pregnancies.

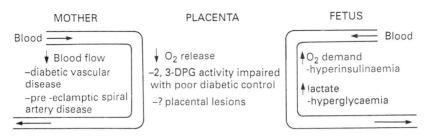

MOTHER   PLACENTA   FETUS

Blood ⟶   ⟵ Blood

↓ Blood flow   ↓ O₂ release   ↑ O₂ demand
–diabetic vascular   –2, 3-DPG activity impaired   -hyperinsulinaemia
disease   with poor diabetic control
–pre-eclamptic spiral   –? placental lesions   ↑ lactate
artery disease   -hyperglycaemia

Figure 1.2. An asphyxial hypothesis for the cause of the 'unexplained' stillbirth in the diabetic mother

Oxygen release

It has been observed that red blood cell 2,3-diphosphoglycerate (DPG) is increased in diabetic pregnancy and that the 2,3 DPG-induced change in oxygen affinity is impaired (Madsen and Ditzel, 1982). In this study, increases in glycosylated haemoglobin were associated with decreased oxygen release in the mother. Although these changes were slight and would, on their own, not have accounted for hypoxia *in utero*, all of the subjects were relatively well-controlled diabetics [HbA_{1c} (median) 7.8%, and HbA_{1c} (maximum) 9.9%]. Whether there is a significant deterioration with increasing glycosylation of haemoglobin is unknown. Ketoacidosis will also affect oxygen release, again decreasing tissue oxygenation.

Placental transfer of oxygen

There have been claims that oxygen transport by the placenta will be impaired in the diabetic, because of reduced transfer area resulting from infarction and from thickening of the basement membrane. In a recent review, Fox (1989) found little evidence to support this claim.

Fetal oxygen demand

That the incidence of unexplained death can be reduced by good diabetic control suggests that the hyperinsulinaemic fetus may be at particular risk. The organomegaly induced by the hyperinsulinaemia will result in an increased fetal demand for oxygen, as has been shown in animal experiments (Carson *et al.*, 1980). In addition, hypoglycaemia in fetal lambs causes a mild lactic acidosis (Shelley, Bassett and Milner, 1975). Although this on its own may not be significant, if combined with hypoxia it may have adverse consequences.

Support for this theory would be provided by evidence of chronic hypoxia in the fetus and, indeed, extramedullary haematopoiesis has been observed at fetal autopsy. However, early studies did not reveal increased cord erythropoietin concentrations in infants whose mothers had elevated glycosylated haemoglobin concentrations in the third trimester (Widness *et al.*, 1981) and further studies are awaited.

The theory is best illustrated by a case report. A poor clinic attender presented at 29 weeks of pregnancy with polyhydramnios and ultrasound evidence of excessive fetal growth. She agreed to hospitalization and serial measurements of fetal abdominal circumference were performed (Figure 1.3). Regular cardiotocographs were also arranged and when spontaneous and irregular contractions began at 37 weeks, late decelerations were observed. An emergency caesarean section was performed and a mildly asphyxiated baby (cord venous pH 7.18) was delivered, having passed meconium. Its birthweight was 2.58 kg (20th percentile). This 'near miss' suggests that an initially macrosomic fetus was influenced by growth-retarding factors (presumably uterine vascular disease) and that the addition of mild hypoxia induced by weak contractions was enough to cause acidosis.

Other complications of pregnancy

The claim that diabetic pregnancy is associated with increased risks of most complications does not hold when one considers women achieving good control and where the diagnosis is carefully made. The subject has been comprehensively reviewed by Cousins (1987). Hypertension is a good example: the overall incidence of hypertension is higher in diabetics who have had the disease longer or who already have complications (White's classes D, F and R), but this is accounted for by pre-existing hypertension rather than pregnancy-induced hypertension. Some will also have proteinuria from diabetic renal damage. The incidence of hypertension is less frequent if the diabetes is of shorter duration (White's classes B and C), being little different from that in control or gestational diabetic subjects. Thus, it is unlikely that the actual incidence of pregnancy-induced hypertension is significantly elevated in diabetic pregnancy.

Whether preterm labour is more common in the diabetic woman is again a confusing issue caused by a failure sometimes to differentiate between spontaneous labour and an iatrogenic preterm induction or caesarean section. For instance, in the

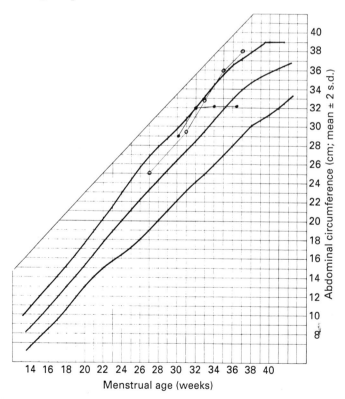

Figure 1.3.   Ultrasound abdominal circumference chart showing patterns of abnormal growth in diabetic pregnancy: ● superimposed growth retardation; ○ growth acceleration

UK survey of diabetic pregnancy (Beard and Lowy, 1982) 50 per cent of women were delivered before 38 weeks, but two-thirds of these deliveries resulted from obstetric intervention. Polyhydramnios clearly will also predispose to preterm labour, but in the absence of these factors there is little evidence to suggest an increased incidence of preterm delivery in the diabetic. If preterm labour occurs, attempts to suppress uterine contractions with β-sympathomimetic drugs may affect diabetic control because of their gluconeogenic effect. If this treatment is coupled with the use of steroids (to help fetal lung maturation), then diabetic control may be further compromised through their antagonistic effects on insulin action. Accordingly, these treatments should only be given after careful consideration. Their successful use in diabetic women was described by Steel and Parboosingh (1977) and subsequently by other authors (Borberg *et al.*, 1978; Barnett, Stubbs and Mander, 1980). The reports show that, provided that glucose control is monitored very closely (e.g. hourly), increased insulin can be given intravenously to counter the hyperglycaemia and prevent ketoacidosis. Large doses need to be given and an initial starting dose of 5 U/h of insulin appears appropriate. Clearly, this type of treatment cannot be continued for long periods as it is potentially dangerous to mother and fetus. This situation would therefore be an indication for assessing lung maturity by measurement of phosphatidylglycerol (see below).

Other complications such as pyelonephritis, claimed to be more common in diabetic pregnancy, have similarly been shown not to occur more frequently (Cousins, 1987).

Intrapartum risks

The fetus of the diabetic mother is at increased risk of the two major complications of labour – asphyxia and trauma. As mentioned above, there are a number of reasons why the fetus may be suffering from a mild degree of asphyxia during the antenatal period and this will be worsened in labour by hypoxia during contractions. If diabetic control is unsatisfactory during labour, there is more likelihood of an abnormal cardiotocograph, as hyperglycaemia is associated with patterns suggestive of asphyxia. Fetal acid–base balance therefore needs to be assessed. Kitzmiller *et al.* (1978) reported a 25 per cent incidence of late decelerations and scalp pH <7.25. Furthermore, hypoglycaemia has been reported to be associated with bradycardia (Langer and Cohen, 1984). Accordingly the successful outcome of labour demands meticulous diabetic control and careful fetal monitoring.

Trauma at delivery relates almost exclusively to shoulder dystocia, because the head of the macrosomic fetus is not significantly enlarged. Four out of 46 vaginal deliveries suffered this type of trauma in the series by Kitzmiller *et al.* (1978). However, in three recent reports where there has been a less interventional approach, there have been no incidents of significant trauma (Gillmer *et al.*, 1984; Murphy *et al.*, 1984; Drury, 1986). Careful attention to the progress of labour, both in the first and second stage, is mandatory to avoid this complication and in our Manchester series there was one case of shoulder dystocia where this did not occur. This problem also occurs in the gestational diabetic who is at risk, especially if obese. Finally, it must be remembered that asphyxia will predispose the fetus to intracranial haemorrhage; if instrumental delivery is required, therefore, and the head is not in a favourable position for delivery, a fetal blood sample should be taken from the scalp for acid–base determination.

Neonatal risks

Apart from the risks of trauma and asphyxia, the infant of the diabetic mother is at higher risk of a number of biochemical disturbances and of organ dysfunction. The majority of these are explained through the modified Pedersen hypothesis (Figure 1.1).

Respiratory dysfunction

The classic descriptions of neonatal respiratory distress syndrome can be partly explained by the previously high incidence of preterm deliveries and caesarean sections. That the problem is now less frequent with less intervention, would accord with this explanation. However, the claim that even if correction was made for gestation and mode of delivery, respiratory distress syndrome was still significantly increased in the diabetic (Robert *et al.*, 1976) led to much research in this field. There is a considerable amount of data to support the hypothesis that hyperinsulinaemia leads to inhibition of surfactant production and may also affect phosphatidylglycerol synthesis. The subject has been extensively reviewed by Bourbon and Farrell (1985). Transient tachypnoea of the newborn is also more common in the infant of the diabetic and this is likely to be related to lung fluid retention associated with the increase in delivery by caesarean section.

Hypertrophic cardiomyopathy

A transient cardiac hypertrophy has long been recognized in the infants of diabetic mothers; this is not present in the macrosomic infant of the non-diabetic. The experiments of Schwartz's group using the hyperinsulinaemic normoglycaemic rhesus monkey (Susa and Schwartz, 1985) suggest that hyperinsulinaemia is responsible for the hypertrophy. Thus once more, the efficacy of control of diabetes may help to explain the variation in the incidence of the condition, which has been claimed to be present in up to 30 per cent of cases, with 10 per cent having evidence of cardiac dysfunction (Leslie, Shen and Strauss, 1982).

The characteristic abnormality is an asymmetrical septal hypertrophy (Gutgesell *et al.*, 1976) which, if sufficiently severe, will produce subaortic stenosis, causing ventricular outflow obstruction. In comparison with the familial hypertrophic cardiomyopathy, fibre disarray is not a prominent feature and the condition resolves over the succeeding weeks or months (Halliday, 1981).

Hypoglycaemia

There is some controversy about what actually constitutes neonatal hypoglycaemia. Plasma glucose concentrations <2 mmol/l are not uncommon in the neonate and are usually asymptomatic. Symptoms that may precede hypoglycaemic convulsions include jitteriness, hypotonia and apnoea. In the absence of convulsions, there appear to be no long-term sequelae (Persson, Gentz and Stangenberg, 1979). Glucose concentrations in the neonate will be affected by diabetic control during pregnancy and labour. Neonatal glucose concentrations have been shown to correlate well with maternal glucose concentrations during the third trimester, as assessed by the glucose tolerance test in untreated gestational diabetics (Gillmer *et al.*, 1975) and glycosylated haemoglobin in insulin dependent diabetics (Ylinen, Raivio and Teramo, 1981). Neonatal hypoglycaemia has also been shown to correlate with increasing cord C-peptide concentrations, an indicator of fetal hyperinsulinaemia and fetal pancreatic hyperplasia. Other workers have confirmed these findings. This all fits in with the Pedersen hypothesis (Figure 1.1), that poor diabetic control leads to fetal hyperinsulinaemia and that, after delivery, persistent neonatal hyperinsulinaemia leads to neonatal hypoglycaemia. Accordingly, one would expect studies that investigate neonatal hypoglycaemia to show varying incidences of the condition, depending on the degree of diabetic control: whereas Roversi et al. (1979), with their very tightly controlled diabetic regimen, had only a 15 per cent incidence, Kitzmiller et al. (1978) reported a 47 per cent incidence.

Polycythaemia and jaundice

Polycythaemia appears to be more common in the infants of diabetic mothers. A venous haematocrit of 65 per cent or more was found in 29 per cent of infants of diabetic mothers, but in only 6 per cent of controls (Mimouni et al., 1986). In this series there was a correlation with neonatal hypoglycaemia, although not with maternal control. However, in gestational diabetes a relationship between neonatal polycythaemia and the severity of the diabetes has been demonstrated (Maresh et al., 1989). The mechanism appears to be increased erythropoietin production, and umbilical cord concentrations have been found to be higher in the babies of established diabetics than in those of gestational diabetics and of controls (Widness et al., 1981). Furthermore, the correlation with hyperinsulinaemia suggests that this again could be the stimulus for increased erythropoietin and erythropoiesis.

Polycythaemia with its associated hyperviscosity could result in a number of neonatal complications, such as necrotizing enterocolitis, renal vein thrombosis, worsening of respiratory dysfunction through poor pulmonary vascular perfusion and increased cardiac work. Increased destruction of red cells, possibly associated with relative liver immaturity or dysfunction, could account for the widely reported increased incidence of neonatal hyperbilirubinaemia, which cannot be explained by differences in gestational age. The condition has been reported in up to 53 per cent of cases (Ylinen, Raivio and Teramo, 1981), although findings of values exceeding 15 mg/dl in 19 per cent of neonates are more typical (Kitzmiller et al., 1978).

Hypocalcaemia and hypomagnesaemia

Hypocalcaemia has not always been investigated in reported series. The often-quoted incidence of hypocalcaemia occurring in over 50 per cent of neonates is based on a detailed study of ten infants of insulin-dependent diabetic mothers (Tsang et al., 1972). Two subsequent larger series have shown lower incidences – 22 per cent (Kitzmiller et al., 1978) and 5 per cent (Persson, Gentz and Stangenberg, 1979). Neonatal hypomagnesaemia has also been reported in about 50 per cent of neonates, in an uncontrolled study of 25 infants born to insulin-dependent diabetic mothers (Tsang et al., 1976); there was a relationship with maternal magnesium concentrations. Further studies have suggested that the concentration of magnesium in amniotic fluid is decreased during diabetic pregnancy (Mimouni et al., 1987). Reduced parathyroid hormone levels have been reported in diabetic pregnancy, whereas calcium concentrations are unchanged (Cruickshank et al., 1983).

It does appear that there is an inter-related disturbance in calcium and magnesium in the infant of the diabetic mother and that, like the other neonatal morbidities, this relates to the degree of diabetic control. While further information is awaited, hypocalcaemic fits in the neonate should be avoided by careful surveillance and treatment.

Management of diabetic pregnancy

Preconceptional care

Advice about pregnancy should begin in adolescence or whenever diabetes is diagnosed. Accordingly, all medical and paramedical workers should stress the need for
planning pregnancy when control is good, complications have been assessed and are
under control and the woman is in the right frame of mind for pregnancy. The
motivation required to remain normoglycaemic during pregnancy means that managing an unplanned and perhaps unwanted pregnancy may be difficult.

Different strategies have been attempted for achieving a satisfactory maternal
condition at conception. The establishment of preconceptional clinics, whether
general or specifically for diabetes, has not been very successful. Typically they are
attended by highly motivated women with less need for assistance, whereas they are
not used by the majority of diabetic mothers. The particular exception has been in
(East) Germany, where Fuhrmann et al. (1983) have been able to obtain a high
attendance rate. The most successful clinic in the United Kingdom has been the one
in Edinburgh, where the same physician runs the adolescent and pregnancy service
with the result that about 75 per cent of women have specific pre-pregnancy counselling (Steel, Johnstone and Smith, 1989). In Manchester we have developed another
strategy: we have capitalized on the tendency for diabetics to be cared for in diabetes
centres. We have a midwife who, apart from helping to look after the woman while
pregnant and training midwives in this field, spends much of her time attached to the
diabetes centre; there she can approach women in the reproductive age group
attending the centre. In the case of non-attenders who are registered, she can use the
age–sex register to seek them out at home.

Whoever is involved with pre-pregnancy counselling, whether it is the family
doctor or the health visitor, the physician or the specialized nurse, the obstetrician or
the specialized midwife, a number of specific areas need to be covered.

1. Capillary blood glucose testing should be instituted if this has not already been
    done, and frequent testing should be encouraged. Glycosylated haemoglobin
    should also be measured. The non-insulin-dependent diabetic woman on oral
    hypoglycaemics should be started on insulin before pregnancy, because ad-
    equate control will be difficult otherwise and control should not be lost by a
    change in treatment during pregnancy. When these measures show that nor-
    moglycaemia is being achieved, conception may be advised if no other contrain-
    dications have been detected.
2. The retina should be assessed and any proliferative retinopathy treated.
3. Renal function should be assessed. If proteinuria is not present, no further
    action is needed. If it is present and renal evaluation shows significant impair-
    ment, careful consideration needs to be taken before undertaking pregnancy
    (see later).
4. Body mass index should be assessed and, if it is outside the normal range,
    attempts should be made to correct it.
5. Smoking should be actively discouraged because of additional risks to the
    pregnancy if there is diabetic vascular disease (which may be undetected), over
    and above its effects on general health, pregnancy and diabetes.
6. Rubella immunity should be determined and immunization offered if
    appropriate.

7. A gynaecological examination may also be indicated. Apart from checking cervical cytology, inspection for vulval warts (to which the diabetic appears to be more prone) should be undertaken and treatment given before there is any exacerbation in pregnancy. Diabetic women are also more prone to menstrual irregularities and it is very frustrating if, when they are all ready for pregnancy, this causes subfertility. Appropriate treatment may be needed earlier, rather than later.

8. The woman should be given instructions about which member of the diabetic pregnancy team to contact when she is pregnant, and told that she should do this as soon as she feels that she may be pregnant.

Contraception

Although the combined oral contraceptive has theoretical disadvantages, its reliability in the young sexually active diabetic without obvious vascular disease makes it the preferred method. For those with vascular disease, the intrauterine contraceptive device is preferable. Suggestions that it may have a high failure rate in diabetic women have not been confirmed in a large study (Skouby and Molsted-Pedersen, 1982). The progesterone-only contraceptive pill is perhaps, the method of choice in the parous woman between pregnancies, but once the family is complete, sterilization is nearly always readily acceptable. Barrier methods have no contraindication and may also be encouraged.

Principles of diabetic care

Joint diabetic clinic
The optimal solution for care is to have a multidisciplinary team present together in one joint clinic. This can be justified only if sufficient numbers of women are cared for. As the average UK obstetrician will look after only about two cases of insulin-dependent diabetes a year, it is important that care is centralized to one obstetrician within each hospital. Furthermore, there is a need in a health region (e.g. 40 000–60 000 births per year) for there to be a tertiary referral centre for the most difficult cases.

There are a number of key members of the team apart from an experienced obstetrician and physician. A specialist diabetic nurse or midwife is required, particularly with the trend towards less hospitalization. She has a major role in ensuring successful home glucose monitoring and in teaching women how to adjust insulin dosage. She also needs time to be able to perform home visits. Midwifery skills are required, normal antenatal care must not be overlooked when managing a complicated pregnancy. A dietitian is required to help with dietary modification throughout pregnancy and postnatally, and also to initiate treatment in the gestational diabetic. Successful outcome comes from a close-knit, communicative team.

Achieving normoglycaemia
The major objective of treatment is to achieve normoglycaemia. This is 3.5–4.5 mmol/l and is rarely >5.5 mmol/l, except immediately after meals. These concentrations are lower than those that the insulin-dependent diabetic is used to; in trying to achieve them she may well have hypoglycaemic attacks, and so must be taught about this carefully and reassured strongly. She should do as many capillary blood glucose measurements as possible, to see whether normoglycaemia is being achieved with the changing insulin requirements of pregnancy. Although most blood testing

should be done preprandially, some postprandial measurements need to be done as well in order to avoid excessive glucose peaks. In addition, the occasional nocturnal measurement is recommended. Blood glucose determinations using measurement strips (Dextrostix, Ames Division, Slough; B-M stix, BCL, Lewes, E. Sussex), whether assessed visually or with meters, are usually satisfactory but need to be backed up by other assessments. Home capillary blood samples can be checked by collecting small samples into micro-collecting tubes or by impregnation of special paper; these can then be analysed quantitatively in the laboratory. These forms of double checking become more critical in the third trimester if there is any concern that the pregnancy is not progressing normally. In addition, glycosylated haemoglobin should be determined monthly. If control does not appear to be satisfactory, admission to hospital may be required and should not be considered as a failure by either the team or the woman. There is little time available and it is not satisfactory to send a woman away each week hoping that the next set of adjustments will work. Hospital admission, although having potential problems with regard to changes in diet and exercise patterns, does allow a full 24 h glucose profile to be determined in the laboratory (e.g. 3-hourly). It also allows plenty of time for teaching from the specialist nurse, midwife and dietitian, a benefit which may be very important for those women whose outpatient care has not been perfect. Attention to the woman's lifestyle is also important, as work or domestic stresses may account for problems with control.

Actual insulin regimens vary with the physician's preference. Typically a short- and a long-acting insulin needs to be given twice a day, although with the large array of pre-prepared combinations it may be possible to limit injections to two per day. However, this may not be sufficient for 24 h normoglycaemia, and adjustments such as introducing an extra dose of soluble insulin at midday or giving the evening long-acting component at bedtime may be required. Becoming more popular are the pen-type syringes, which are a very convenient way of administering doses of soluble insulin. They can be given preprandially and then a long-acting insulin given once a day (e.g. at night). Although it means four injections a day, the flexibility of the regimen and the ease of use of the pen make it attractive. Continuous subcutaneous insulin infusion (CSII) does not appear to have any advantage in pregnancy and needs the back up of a 24 h CSII service. It might have a role in the occasional diabetic woman who is difficult to control, but in Manchester we have not needed to use it in our last 100 consecutive cases. Non-insulin-dependent diabetic women need to be changed to insulin, because oral hypoglycaemic agents cannot usually achieve tight enough control.

The majority of gestational diabetics can be managed by dietary modification. This not only decreases postprandial hyperglycaemia, but also makes insulin action more efficient, as shown by a decrease in the insulin:glucose ratio (Maresh et al., 1985), thereby decreasing fasting glucose concentrations. The diet should be in the order of 1800 calories, low in fat and high in fibre. The very obese and those of low to normal weight will need appropriate adjustments. Assessment of dietary compliance can be gauged by weight gain: the obese woman should not be putting on weight. Current policy is to give insulin to those women who have elevated fasting glucose concentrations. If one takes a fasting level of 7 mmol/l, about 14 per cent of gestational diabetics will require insulin (Persson et al., 1985). However, many authorities favour introducing insulin if concentrations are persistently >6 mmol/l. A typical treatment regimen would be twice daily biphasic insulin (i.e. soluble and medium-acting combinations) starting with a total dose of about 20 units. This is steadily increased, as monitored by capillary blood testing. Although clinical and biochemical evidence of hypoglycaemia is not reported in published series, any woman requiring treatment should be transferred to the diabetic team. Insulin is not the answer for those who cannot keep to their diet, because the insulin will cause the food substrates to be laid down as more fat, thus increasing the peripheral resistance to insulin action.

Care during the first trimester

Many diabetic women know that they are pregnant at a very early stage because the placental hormones will interfere with insulin action. This factor, combined with nausea, may require urgent help to ensure that normoglycaemia is maintained during this crucial embryonic stage. Early ultrasound is justifiable to determine that the pregnancy is viable. If there is any concern about the quality of the diabetic control, admission to hospital is advisable. For the woman who has not had preconceptional management, admission offers an opportunity for a full assessment and education. This exercise is as important for the non-insulin dependent diabetic as it is for the insulin dependent. For those not admitted there must be time in the clinic to go through aspects which should have been discussed before, in particular the importance of normoglycaemia and dietary advice. For those who did attend before, a little repetition should do no harm.

Care during the second trimester

With pregnancy successfully established, the main objectives of the second trimester are continuing to achieve good diabetic control (see above) and to offer screening for congenital anomalies. If the glycosylated haemoglobin was significantly elevated (e.g. 10 per cent or more) at the end of the first trimester, even more care should be taken to exclude anomalies. Maternal serum alphafetoprotein screening for neural tube defects needs care in interpretation, in view of the observations of Wald *et al*. (1979) that values are a little lower in diabetic pregnancy, a fact confirmed by most repeat studies. There is no specific reason for offering amniocentesis and so the bulk of screening rests on ultrasound imaging at 18–20 weeks' gestation. This may be difficult in the presence of obesity. Apart from a general fetal overview, the following areas need particular attention:

1. The brain and spine.
2. The heart: although a four chamber view will suffice in most cases, a detailed cardiac scan should be obtained if control has not been good preconceptionally. This is not necessarily aimed at consideration of termination of pregnancy, but more for organizing perinatal management in advance if an abnormality is found.
3. Sacral agenesis may be suspected by the presence of an unusual sacral appearance and shortened femurs.

Routine antenatal care should not be forgotten. All standard pregnancy investigations should be reviewed and rhesus negative management instituted when appropriate, a factor sometimes overlooked in a complicated pregnancy.

Attention should be paid to any abnormalities of weight gain, blood pressure and urine testing. If proteinuria is present, renal evaluation (24 h protein and creatinine excretion) is indicated on a monthly basis. The retinae should also be reviewed. An ultrasound measurement of fetal head and abdominal circumference performed at 24–26 weeks' gestation will act as a baseline for assessing fetal growth in the remainder of the pregnancy.

Gestational diabetes
Gestational diabetes usually does not present until late in the second trimester or during the third; those presenting earlier are likely to be undiagnosed diabetics. Assuming that the fetuses of undiagnosed non-insulin dependent diabetics are at increased risk, as well as those of severe gestational diabetics, then screening for diabetes in pregnancy can be justified. Current screening tests have recently been reviewed (Maresh and Beard, 1989). In brief, there are only two methods that could be regarded as adequate. The first is the method of O'Sullivan *et al.* (1973), in which the woman is given a 50 g glucose load unfasted and, if the plasma glucose concentration is >7.7 mmol/l, then a full glucose tolerance test is performed. This is best done at 28 weeks of pregnancy and gives a sensitivity of 79 per cent. Restricting this to women over 25 years of age will considerably reduce the workload, while having minimal effect on sensitivity (74 per cent). The second method is that popularized in Denmark (Mortensen *et al.*, 1985), which uses the combination of three potential diabetic features (maternal obesity, previous overweight baby, and family history in a first-degree relative) combined with glycosuria and fasting blood glucose determination; this method gave a sensitivity of over 90 per cent. Jowett, Samanta and Burden (1987) applied this method and found a sensitivity of 92 per cent and a specificity of 49 per cent.

Care during the third trimester

This is the key time when good care and attention to detail can have such a major effect on the incidence of complications and perinatal outcome. Apart from maternal indices of maternal normoglycaemia (blood glucose profiles, glycosylated haemoglobin), the obstetrician has the additional markers of fetal macrosomia and polyhydramnios. Accordingly, continuity of obstetric care with careful palpation and measurement of fundal height is required.

Ultrasound
Clinical assessment must be supplemented by ultrasound. Head measurements appear to be no different in the fetus of the diabetic woman when compared with that of the non-diabetic. Measurement of the fetal abdominal circumference is a good index of fetal growth and should be performed, together with an assessment of amniotic fluid volume, every 2 weeks. Examples of abnormal growth patterns are shown in Figure 1.3. Cases of gestational diabetes should be assessed in the same way. If Doppler blood flow estimations are performed, results must be interpreted cautiously. Although an abnormal value should lead to further investigation (e.g. antenatal cardiotocograph, biophysical profile) a normal one should not lead to the assumption that an unexplained fetal death cannot occur within the next 3 days (Bradley, Brudenell and Nicolaides, 1988; Tyrrell, 1988).

Biochemical tests of placental function
Biochemical tests of placental function no longer appear to have a role in diabetic pregnancy (Dooley *et al.*, 1984; Stange *et al.*, 1985), having been supplanted by the biophysical methods mentioned here.

Antenatal cardiotocography
As asphyxia is the final precursor of unexplained fetal death, antenatal cardiotocography may be considered to be the best currently available indicator of impending demise. From what stage of gestation, and how often, should it be performed? A general rule would be two or three times weekly from 36 weeks onwards. However, there are a number of exceptions to this:

1. If diabetic control is poor: Teramo *et al.* (1983) found a significant association between poor diabetic control and abnormal cardiotocographs.
2. If there is maternal vascular disease. The uteroplacental blood supply may be affected and monitoring should be started at about 32 weeks.
3. If there is an abnormal growth pattern, whether excessive (indicative of fetal hyperinsulinaemia) or retarded (perhaps due to vascular disease) monitoring should be started when the pattern appears.

Cardiotocography is not necessary in the well-controlled gestational diabetic, but should be reserved for the minority who require insulin or where there is an abnormal growth pattern.

Biophysical profile
Full biophysical profile scoring of the fetus has been proposed as a routine in two recent series (Dicker *et al.*, 1988b; Johnson *et al.*, 1988). However, no evidence was presented to suggest that the addition of the three parameters not assessed in the above protocol (ultrasound detection of fetal breathing, movement and tone) has anything additional to offer. This is in accord with the earlier series of Golde *et al.* (1984). Accordingly, use of the biophysical profile is best reserved for evaluating the difficult pregnancy where there is already concern about the fetus.

Hospitalization
Although the initial objective may be out-patient care, this should not be sought at all costs and it may be preferable to admit intermittently for assessment if there are complications such as nephropathy, hypertension or abnormal growth patterns. The need to attend regularly for cardiotocographs may cause problems if the woman lives at a distance, unless telemetric cardiotocography is available. A certain amount of individualization of care is required under these circumstances, which can be achieved only if senior and experienced clinicians are directly involved.

Timing and route of delivery

These two areas, which are the main ones over which an obstetrician may be able to have some control, evoke the most controversy and differing policies were contrasted in a pair of recent reports (Drury, 1986; Molsted-Pedersen and Kuhl, 1986). Concern about possible unexplained stillbirth favours the early approach, with its increased risks of maternal morbidity from caesarean section and of perinatal morbidity associated with premature delivery. The UK survey of diabetic pregnancy in 1979–1980 (Beard and Lowy, 1982) showed a 58 per cent incidence of caesarean section and a 50 per cent incidence of delivery before 38 weeks. On the other hand, the conservative approach of awaiting spontaneous labour and aiming for vaginal delivery (Gillmer *et al.*, 1984; Murphy *et al.*, 1984; Drury, 1986) demands considerable commitment from the woman and those looking after her. If careful assessment and management by an experienced team do not occur with this approach, there will be increasing incidences of unexplained stillbirth and of traumatic delivery. The following description of the conservative approach gives examples of typical situations but cannot attempt to cover all eventualities: an individual approach is still required.

Assuming that the pregnancy is progressing satisfactorily in terms of diabetic control, maternal complications and fetal monitoring of condition, then the pregnancy should be allowed to continue and spontaneous labour awaited. For the diabetic woman with vascular disease, induction of labour may be considered at 38 weeks of pregnancy if the cervix is favourable; otherwise, admission to hospital may be simplest, so that close monitoring can be achieved. Uncomplicated mild hypertension should not necessarily require intervention.

The onset of late growth retardation should be managed by early recourse to delivery. Vaginal delivery is not necessarily contraindicated, as continuous intrapartum monitoring should be routinely used in all diabetics. Growth acceleration poses more of a problem because of the conflict between the risks of pulmonary immaturity if the baby is delivered too soon, and of possible traumatic delivery if the fetus grows too large. If the fetus clearly appears to be grossly macrosomic, caesarean section will be required. This is one of the few circumstances when amniocentesis should be undertaken and lecithin–sphingomyelin ratios and phosphatidylglycerol concentrations determined. If results are normal, caesarean section should be performed; if not, daily cardiotocographs should be arranged and the test repeated at weekly intervals. The other indications for using estimates of lung maturity are when an elective caesarean section is planned before 38 weeks of pregnancy and when delivery is considered and gestational age is uncertain. Milder cases of macrosomia may be considered suitable for vaginal delivery. Evaluation of the pelvis may be performed radiologically, the anteroposterior diameter being most important. Measurement of the fetal head is easy by ultrasound but measurement of the bisacromial diameter cannot be obtained. Accordingly, ultrasound prediction of shoulder dystocia has had to rely upon thoracic circumference measurements, which should be undertaken.

Other ultrasound measurements have been used to predict the fetus with birthweight in excess of the 90th percentile. These have been reviewed (Kitzmiller *et al.*, 1987) and appear to have no particular advantages over thoracic circumference or area. Computed tomographic radiography can provide actual shoulder measurements in nearly all cases, and this can be combined with pelvimetry. If available, this is the method of choice and does not put the fetus at excessive risk of radiological exposure (Kitzmiller *et al.*, 1987). This policy should also be adhered to when macrosomia is suspected in the obese gestational diabetic woman.

Intrapartum management

Because of the probable higher risk of intrapartum asphyxia, the diabetic woman should be advised not to delay coming into hospital if she thinks that she is in labour. During labour continuous fetal monitoring should be used, supplemented by pH measurement if indicated. Progress in labour should be assessed assiduously and although a primary uterine inertia pattern should be supplemented by oxytocin, its use in late labour to augment a secondary arrest pattern is best avoided. Provided that normoglycaemia is being obtained, labour can safely be allowed to continue while progress is being made. An experienced obstetrician should be available for delivery, particularly if macrosomia is suspected. Assessment and conduction of instrumental deliveries should again be done by an experienced obstetrician in view of the sinister possibility that delay in the second stage may be a forerunner of shoulder dystocia.

Normoglycaemia in labour can be achieved by various means. The most sensitive method is to use an intravenous infusion of glucose and insulin via a pump. Various methods have been described but one using 7.5 per cent glucose (50 g of 50 per cent added to 1 litre of 5 per cent over 8 hours) works well and is usually balanced by an insulin rate of 1–2 U/h (Beard and Maresh, 1989). Capillary blood glucose concentration should be assessed hourly using testing sticks, or preferably, a meter if the staff are used to it (or the woman or her partner can use her own). The glucose concentrations should be kept between 3.5 and 7.0 mmol/l by appropriate adjustments. If there appears to be a discrepancy between glucose measurements and expected values, urgent laboratory confirmation should be obtained. The usual problems are staff unfamiliarity with glucose measuring, the infusion pump being accidentally unplugged or oxytocin being given in a glucose solution rather than normal saline.

This regimen can be maintained for a long time, but if labour is prolonged (e.g. >12 h) consideration should be given to adding potassium chloride to the infusate (e.g. 20 mmol/l).

Management after delivery

After delivery, insulin and glucose infusions should be discontinued, as insulin sensitivity rapidly returns to non-pregnant levels with the delivery of the placenta. For those delivered by caesarean section, infusion may be continued for a further 24 h with the insulin dosage reduced in response to regular capillary glucose determinations. It is often simplest for the insulin-dependent diabetic to revert to her pre-pregnancy dosage, which can then be altered as required. The gestational diabetic treated with insulin should stop this therapy, but should have occasional capillary blood glucose testing on the postnatal ward to ensure that she is not grossly hyperglycaemic (which is rare). Arrangements should be made for her to have a glucose tolerance test (GTT) done after at least 6 weeks have elapsed. About 80–90 per cent are likely to have a normal GTT and should be encouraged to maintain ideal bodyweight in order to try to prevent the development of diabetes. Follow-up studies have indicated that over 50 per cent will have an abnormal GTT by 25 years (O'Sullivan, 1984); in another series, 29 per cent had an abnormal GTT and 6 per cent diabetes within 13 years (Stowers, 1984). This incidence might be preventable through diet (Sartor et al., 1980). For those with an abnormal GTT, continued attention to diet and follow-up by a specialist in diabetes is required.

Breast feeding should be encouraged, but because of increased nutritional demands an extra 50 g carbohydrate per day is advised (Whichelow and Doddridge, 1983). An alternative philosophy is to reduce insulin at this time (Davies et al., 1989).

Neonatal

The early detection of the complications mentioned previously, forms the basis of neonatal care. Improvements in antenatal care are decreasing these complications, allowing the philosophy of non-separation of the mother and baby to be extended to the diabetic. However the nursing of the baby on the normal ward must be vigilant. The baby should be fully examined at an early stage to look for any abnormalities (such as a cardiac anomaly) that might have been missed antenatally. Regular checks on respiratory rate should be maintained in order to detect transient tachypnoea of the newborn at an early stage. Early feeding should be encouraged and regular capillary heel-prick testing for the detection of hypoglycaemia should be performed, starting at 1–2 h of life. These tests should be continued at 4-hourly intervals for at least the first 24 h and, if values <1 mmol/l are obtained, intravenous glucose should be started. It is advisable to check for polycythaemia and hypocalcaemia, particularly if diabetic control has not been perfect. If the haematocrit exceeds 70 per cent, exchange transfusion is recommended. Once the first 48 h have been negotiated without incident, further problems are unlikely.

Conclusions

The successful management of pregnancy in the diabetic woman demands high levels of care from preconception to the puerperium. This is best achieved by the centralization of women to experienced multidisciplinary teams who are achieving results approaching that for normal pregnancy. The quest for normoglycaemia, combined with detailed antenatal investigation, requires much of the woman, but brings its rewards.

References

Akazawa, SK, Akazawa, A, Hashimoto, M *et al*. (1987) Effects of hypoglycaemia on early embryogenesis in rat embryo organ culture. *Diabetologia*, **30**, 791–796

Baird, JD and Farquhar, JW (1962) Insulin-secreting capacity in newborn infants of normal and diabetic women. *Lancet*, **i**, 71–74

Baker, L, Egler, JM, Klein, SH and Goldman, AS (1981) Meticulous control of diabetes during organogenesis prevents congenital lumbosacral defects in rats. *Diabetes*, **30**, 955–959

Barnett, AH, Stubbs, SM and Mander, AM (1980) Management of premature labour in diabetic pregnancy. *Diabetologia*, **18**, 365–368

Beard, RW and Lowy, C (1982) The British survey of diabetic pregnancies. *British Journal of Obstetrics and Gynaecology*, **89**, 783–786

Beard, RW and Maresh, M (1989) Diabetes. In *Medical Disorders in Obstetric Practice* (edited by M de Swiet) pp. 584–632. Oxford: Blackwell

Borberg, G, Gillmer, MDG, Beard, RW and Oakley, NW (1978) Metabolic effects of beta-sympathomimetic drugs and dexamethasone in normal and diabetic pregnancy. *British Journal of Obstetrics and Gynaecology*, **85**, 184–189

Bourbon, JR and Farrell, PM (1985) Fetal lung development in the diabetic pregnancy. *Pediatric Research*, **19**, 253–267

Bradley, RJ, Brudenell, JM and Nicolaides, KH (1988) Chronic fetal hypoxia in diabetic pregnancy. *British Medical Journal*, **296**, 790

Bradley, RJ, Nicolaides, KH and Brudenell, JM (1988) Are all infants of diabetic mothers 'macrosomic'? *British Medical Journal*, **297**, 1583–1584

Brudenell, JM and Doddridge, M, Eds (1989) *Diabetic Pregnancy*, p. 90. London: Churchill Livingstone

Buchanan, TA, Schemmer, JK and Freinkel, N (1986) Embryotoxic effects of brief maternal insulin-hypoglycaemia during organogenesis in the rat. *Journal of Clinical Investigation*, **78**, 643–649

Buschard, K, Buch, I, Molsted-Pedersen, L, *et al*. (1987) Increased incidence of true type I diabetes acquired during pregnancy. *British Medical Journal*, **294**, 275–279

Cardell, BA (1953) Hypertrophy and hyperplasia of the pancreatic islets in new born infants. *Journal of Pathology and Bacteriology*, **66**, 335–338

Carson, BS, Philipps, AF, Simmons, MA, *et al.* (1980) Effects of a sustained insulin infusion upon glucose uptake and oxygenation of the ovine fetus. *Pediatric Research*, **14**, 147–152

Cockroft, DL and Coppola, PT (1977) Teratogenic effects of excess glucose on head-fold rat embryos in culture. *Teratology*, **16**, 141–146

Cousins, L (1987) Pregnancy complications among diabetic women: review 1965–1985. *Obstetrical and Gynecological Survey*, **42**, 140–149

Cousins, L, Key, TC, Schorzman, L and Moore, TR (1988) Ultrasonographic measurement of early fetal growth in insulin-treated diabetic pregnancies. *American Journal of Obstetrics and Gynecology*, **159**, 1186–1190

Cruikshank, DP, Pitkin, RM, Varner, MW *et al.* (1983) Calcium metabolism in diabetic mother, fetus and newborn infant. *American Journal of Obstetrics and Gynecology*, **145**, 1010–1016

Damm, P and Molsted-Pederson, L (1989) Significant decrease in congenital malformations in newborn infants of an unselected population in diabetic women. *American Journal of Obstetrics and Gynecology*, **161**, 1163–1167

Davies, HA, Clark, JDA, Dalton, KJ and Edwards, OM (1989) Insulin requirements of diabetic women who breast feed. *British Medical Journal*, **298**, 1357–1358

Department of Health (1989) *Report on Confidential Enquiries into Maternal Deaths in the United Kingdom 1985–1987*. London: HMSO

Dibble, CM, Kochenour, NK, Worley, RJ, *et al.* (1982) Effect of pregnancy on diabetic retinopathy. *Obstetrics and Gynecology*, **59**, 699–704

Dicker, D, Feldberg, D, Samuel, N, *et al.* (1988a) Spontaneous abortion in patients with insulin-dependent diabetes mellitus: the effect of preconceptional diabetic control. *American Journal of Obstetrics and Gynecology*, **158**, 1161–1164

Dicker, D, Feldberg, D, Yeshaya, A *et al.* (1988b) Fetal surveillance in insulin-dependent diabetic pregnancy: predictive value of the biophysical profile. *American Journal of Obstetrics and Gynecology*, **159**, 800–804

Dooley, SL, Depp., R, Socol, ML, *et al.* (1984) Urinary estriols in diabetic pregnancy: a reappraisal. *Obstetrics and Gynecology*, **64**, 469–475

Driscoll, SG, Benirschke, K and Curtis, GW (1960) Neonatal deaths among infants of diabetic mothers. *American Journal of Diseases in Children*, **100**, 818–830

Drury, MI (1986) Management of the pregnant diabetic patient – are the pundits right? *Diabetologia*, **29**, 10–12

Eriksson, U, Dahlstrom, E, Larsson, KS and Hellerstrom, C (1982) Increased incidence of congenital malformations in the offspring of diabetic rats and their prevention by maternal insulin therapy. *Diabetes*, **31**, 1–6

Falluca, F, Gargiulo, P, Troili, F, *et al.* (1985) Amniotic fluid insulin, C peptide concentrations and fetal morbidity in infants of diabetic mothers. *American Journal of Obstetrics and Gynecology*, **153**, 534–540

Forrester, JV, Towler, HMA and Pearson, DWM (1989) Pregnancy and diabetic retinopathy. In *Carbohydrate Metabolism in Pregnancy and the Newborn*, *(Aberdeen 1988)*, edited by HW Sutherland, JM Stowers and DWM Pearson, pp. 189–200. London: Springer-Verlag

Fox, H (1989) The placenta in diabetes mellitus. In *Carbohydrate Metabolism in Pregnancy and the Newborn*, *(Aberdeen 1988)* (edited by HW Sutherland, JM Stowers and DWM Pearson) pp. 109–117. London: Springer-Verlag

Freinkel, N (1965) Effects of the conceptus on the maternal metabolism during pregnancy. In *On the Nature and Treatment of Diabetics* (edited by NBA Liebel and GA Wrenshall) pp. 679–691. Amsterdam: Excerpta Medical Foundation

Fuhrmann, K, Reiher, H, Semmler, K, *et al.* (1983) Prevention of congenital malformations in infants of insulin-dependent diabetic mothers. *Diabetes Care*, **6**, 219–223

Gillmer, MDG, Beard, RW, Brooke, FM and Oakley, NW (1975) Carbohydrate metabolism in pregnancy. *British Medical Journal*, **3**, 399–404

Gillmer, MDG, Holmes, SM, Moore, MP, *et al.* (1984) Diabetes in pregnancy – obstetric management 1983. In *Carbohydrate Metabolism in Pregnancy and the Newborn (Aberdeen 1983)* (edited by HW Sutherland and JM Stowers) pp. 102–118. Edinburgh: Churchill Livingstone

Golde, SH, Montoro, M, Good-Anderson, B, *et al.* (1984) The role of nonstress tests, fetal biophysical profile, and contraction stress tests in the outpatient management of insulin-requiring diabetic pregnancies. *Obstetrics and Gynecology*, **148**, 269–273

Gutgesell, HP, Mullins, CE, Gillette, PC, *et al.* (1976) Transient hypertrophic subaortic stenosis in infants of diabetic mothers. *Journal of Pediatrics*, **89**, 120–125

Halliday, HL (1981) Hypertrophic cardiomyopathy in infants of poorly-controlled diabetic mothers. *Archives of Disease in Childhood*, **56**, 258–263

Harper, MA, and Morrow, RJ (1988) Early growth delay in diabetic pregnancy. *British Medical Journal*, **296**, 1005–1006

Horii, K, Watanabe, G and Ingalls, T (1966) Experimental diabetes in pregnant mice. *Diabetes*, **15**, 194–204

Horvat, M, Maclean, H, Goldberg, L and Crock, GW (1980) Diabetic retinopathy in pregnancy: a 12 year prospective survey. *British Journal of Ophthalmology*, **64**, 398–403

Johnson, JM, Lange, IR, Harman, CR, *et al.* (1988) Biophysical profile scoring in the management of the diabetic pregnancy. *Obstetrics and Gynecology*, **72**, 841–846

Jovanovic, R and Jovanovic, L (1984) Obstetric management when normoglycaemia is maintained in diabetic pregnant women with vascular compromise. *American Journal of Obstetrics and Gynecology*, **149**, 617–623

Jowett, NI, Samanta, AK and Burden, AC (1987) Screening for diabetes in pregnancy: is a random blood glucose enough? *Diabetic Medicine*, **4**, 160–163

Kitzmiller, JL, Cloherty, JP, Younger, MD, *et al.* (1978) Diabetic pregnancy and perinatal morbidity. *American Journal of Obstetrics and Gynecology*, **131**, 560–580

Kitzmiller, JL, Brown, ER, Phillipe, M, *et al.* (1981) Diabetic nephropathy and perinatal outcome. *American Journal of Obstetrics and Gynecology*, **141**, 741–751

Kitzmiller, JL, Mall, JC, Gin, GD, *et al.* (1987) Measurement of fetal shoulder width with computed tomography in diabetic women. *Obstetrics and Gynecology*, **70**, 941–945

Kucera, J (1971) Rate and type of congenital anomalies among offspring in diabetic women. *Journal of Reproductive Medicine*, **7**, 61–70

Langer, O and Cohen, WR (1984) Persistent fetal bradycardia during maternal hypoglycaemia. *American Journal of Obstetrics and Gynecology*, **149**, 688–690

Leslie, J, Shen, SC and Strauss, L (1982) Hypertrophic cardiomyopathy in a midtrimester fetus born to a diabetic mother. *Journal of Pediatrics*, **100**, 631–632

Leslie, RDG, Pyke, DA, John, PN and White, JM (1978) Haemoglobin A$_1$ in diabetic pregnancy. *Lancet*, **ii**, 958–959

Lewis, NJ, Akazawa, S and Freinkel, N (1983) Teratogenesis from beta-hydroxybutyrate during organogenesis in rat embryo organ culture and enhancement by subteratogenic glucose. *Diabetes*, **32**, suppl. 1, 11A

Lind, T and Whittaker, PG (1989) The placenta as an endocrine regulator. In *Fetal Growth* (edited by F Sharp, RB Fraser and RDG Millner) pp. 53–67. London: Royal College of Obstetricians and Gynaecologists

Lowy, C, Beard, RW and Goldschmidt, J (1986) Congenital malformations in babies of diabetic mothers. *Diabetic Medicine*, **3**, 458–462

Madsen, H and Ditzel, J (1982) Changes in red blood cell oxygen transport in diabetic pregnancy. *American Journal of Obstetrics and Gynecology*, **143**, 421–424

Malins, J. (1979) Fetal anomalies related to carbohydrate metabolism. The epidemiological approach. In *Carbohydrate Metabolism in Pregnancy and the Newborn (Aberdeen, 1978)* (edited by HW Sutherland and JM Stowers) pp. 229–263. Berlin: Springer-Verlag

Maresh, M and Beard, RW (1989) Screening and management of gestational diabetes mellitus. In *Carbohydrate Metabolism in Pregnancy and the Newborn (Aberdeen, 1988)* (edited by HW Sutherland, JM Stowers and DWM Pearson) pp. 201–208. London: Springer-Verlag

Maresh, MJA, Gillmer, MDG, Beard, RW, *et al.* (1985) The effect of diet and insulin on metabolic profiles of women with gestational diabetes mellitus. *Diabetes*, **34**, suppl 2, 88–93

Maresh, M, Beard, RW, Bray, CS, *et al.* (1989) Factors predisposing to and outcomes of gestational diabetes. *Obstetrics and Gynecology*, **74**, 342–346

Metzger, BE, Phelps, RL, Freinkel, N and Navickas, IA (1980) Effects of gestational diabetes on diurnal profiles of plasma glucose, lipids and individual amino acids. *Diabetes Care*, **3**, 402–409

Miller, E, Hare, JW, Cloherty, JP, et al. (1981) Elevated maternal haemoglobin A_{1c} in early pregnancy and major congenital anomalies in infants of diabetic mothers. New England Journal of Medicine, **304**, 1331–1334

Mills, JL, Knopp, RH, Simpson, JL, et al. (1988a) Lack of relation of increased malformation rates in infants of diabetic mothers to glycemic control during organogenesis. New England Journal of Medicine, **318**, 671–676

Mills, JL, Simpson, JL, Driscoll, SG, et al. (1988b) Incidence of spontaneous abortion among normal women and insulin–dependent diabetic women whose pregnancies were identified within 21 days of conception. New England Journal of Medicine, **319**, 1617–1623

Milner, RDG, Gasparo, M de, Milner, GR and Wirdnam, PK (1979) Amino acids and development of the beta cell. In Carbohydrate Metabolism in Pregnancy and the Newborn (Aberdeen, 1978) (edited by HW Sutherland and JM Stowers) pp. 132–151. Berlin: Springer-Verlag

Milunsky, A, Alpert, E, Kitzmiller, JL, et al. (1982) Prenatal diagnosis of neural tube defects. VIII. The importance of serum alpha-fetoprotein screening in diabetic pregnant women. American Journal of Obstetrics and Gynecology, **142**, 1030–1032

Mimouni, F, Miodovnik, M, Siddiqi, TA, et al. (1986) Neonatal polycythemia in infants of insulin-dependent diabetic mothers. Obstetrics and Gynecology, **68**, 370–372

Mimouni, F, Miodovnik, M, Tsang, RC, et al. (1987) Decreased amniotic fluid magnesium concentration in diabetic pregnancy. Obstetrics and Gynecology, **69**, 12–15

Miodovnik, M, Lavin, JP, Knowles, HC, et al. (1984) Spontaneous abortion among insulin-dependent diabetic women. American Journal of Obstetrics and Gynecology, **150**, 372–376

Miodovnik, M, Mimouni, F, Tsang, RC, et al. (1986) Glycemic control and spontaneous abortion in insulin-dependent diabetic women. Obstetrics and Gynecology, **68**, 366–369

Moloney, JBM and Drury, MI (1982) The effect of pregnancy on the natural course of diabetic retinopathy. American Journal of Ophthalmology, **93**, 745–756

Molsted-Pedersen, L (1980) Pregnancy and diabetes, a survey. Acta Endocrinologica, **suppl 238**, 13–19

Molsted-Pedersen, L and Kuhl, C (1986) Obstetrical management in diabetic pregnancy: the Copenhagen experience. Diabetologia, **29**, 13–16

Molsted-Pedersen, L, Tygstrup, I and Pedersen, J (1964) Congenital malformations in newborn infants of diabetic women. Correlation with maternal diabetic vascular complications. Lancet, **i**, 1124–1126

Mortensen, HB, Molsted-Pedersen, L, Kuhl, C and Backer, P (1985) A screening procedure for diabetes in pregnancy. Diabète et Métabolisme, **11**, 249–253

Murphy, J, Peters, J, Morris, P, Hayes, TM and Pearson, JF (1984) Conservative management of pregnancy in diabetic women. British Medical Journal, **288**, 1203–1205

Naeye, RL (1965) Infants of diabetic mothers: a quantitative morphologic study. Pediatrics, **35**, 980–988

O'Sullivan, JB (1984) Subsequent morbidity among gestational diabetic women. In Carbohydrate Metabolism in Pregnancy and the Newborn (Aberdeen, 1983) (edited by HW Sutherland and JM Stowers) pp. 174–180. Edinburgh: Churchill Livingstone

O'Sullivan, JB, Mahan, CM, Charles, D and Dandrow, RV (1973) Screening criteria for high risk gestational diabetic patients. American Journal of Obstetrics and Gynecology, **116**, 895–900

Patterson, KR, Lunan, CB and MacCuish, AC (1985) Severe transient nephrotic syndrome in diabetic pregnancy. British Medical Journal, **291**, 1612

Pedersen, J (1954) Weight and length at birth of infants of diabetic mothers. Acta Endocrinologica, **16**, 330–342

Pedersen, J. (1977) The Pregnant Diabetic and Her Newborn – Problems and Management, 2nd edn. Copenhagen: Munksgaard

Pedersen, JF and Molsted-Pedersen, L (1979) Early growth retardation in diabetic pregnancy. British Medical Journal, **1**, 18–19

Pedersen, JF and Molsted-Pedersen, L (1981) Early fetal growth delay detected by ultrasound marks increased risk of congenital malformation in diabetic pregnancy. British Medical Journal, **283**, 269–271

Persson, B, Gentz, J and Stangenberg, M (1979) Neonatal problems. In Carbohydrate Metabolism in Pregnancy and the Newborn (Aberdeen, 1978) (edited by HW Sutherland and JM Stowers) pp. 376–391. Berlin: Springer–Verlag

Persson, B, Stangenberg, M, Hansson, U and Nordlander, E (1985) Gestational diabetes mellitus (GDM): comparative evaluation of two treatment regimens, diet versus insulin and diet. *Diabetes*, **34**, suppl. 2, 101–105

Persson, B, Pschera, H, Lunell, NO, *et al.* (1986) Amino acid concentrations in maternal plasma and amniotic fluid in relation to fetal insulin secretion during the last trimester of pregnancy in gestational and type I diabetic women and women with small-for-gestational age infants. *American Journal of Perinatology*, **3**, 98–103

Petersen, MB, Pedersen, SA, Greisen, G, *et al.* (1988) Early growth delay in diabetic pregnancy: relation to psychomotor development at age 4. *British Medical Journal*, **296**, 598–600

Price, JH, Hadden, DR, Archer, DB and Harley, JMcDG (1984) Diabetic retinopathy in pregnancy. *British Journal of Obstetrics and Gynaecology*, **91**, 11–17

Reid, M, Hadden, D, Harley, JMG, *et al.* (1984) Fetal malformations in diabetics with high haemoglobin A_{1c} in early pregnancy. *British Medical Journal*, **289**, 1001

Robert, MF, Neff, RK, Hubbell, JP, *et al.* (1976) Association between maternal diabetes and the respiratory-distress syndrome in the newborn. *New England Journal of Medicine*, **294**, 357–360

Roversi, GD, Gargiulo, M, Nicolini, U *et al.* (1979) A new approach to the treatment of diabetic pregnant women: 479 cases (1963–75). *American Journal of Obstetrics and Gynecology*, **135**, 567–576

Rowland, TW, Hubbell, JP and Nadas, AS (1973) Congenital heart disease in infants of diabetic mothers. *Journal of Pediatrics*, **83**, 815–820

Sartor, G, Schersten, B, Carlstrom, S, *et al.* (1980) Ten year follow-up of subjects with impaired glucose tolerance. *Diabetes*, **29**, 41–49

Shelley, HJ, Bassett, JM and Milner, RDG (1975) Control of carbohydrate metabolism in the fetus and newborn. *British Medical Bulletin*, **31**, 37–43

Simpson, JL, Elias, S, Martin, AO, *et al.* (1983) Diabetes in pregnancy, Northwestern University series (1977–1981). 1. Prospective study of anomalies in offspring of mothers with diabetes mellitus. *American Journal of Obstetrics and Gynecology*, **146**, 263–270

Skouby, SO and Molsted-Pedersen, L (1982) Intrauterine contraceptive devices for diabetics. *Lancet*, **i**, 968

Stange, L, Stangenberg, M, Carlstrom, K and Persson, B (1985) Surveillance of the diabetic pregnancy with antepartum fetal nonstress testing and urinary estriol excretion. *Gynaecological and Obstetric Investigations*, **20**, 141–148

Steel, JM and Parboosingh, J (1977) Insulin requirements in pregnant diabetics with premature labour controlled by ritodrine. *British Medical Journal*, **1**, 880

Steel, JM, Johnstone, FD and Corrie, JET (1984) Early assessment of gestation in diabetics. *Lancet*, **ii**, 975–976

Steel, JM, Johnstone, FD and Smith, AF (1989) Pre-pregnancy preparation. In *Carbohydrate Metabolism in Pregnancy and the Newborn (Aberdeen, 1988)* (edited by HW Sutherland, JM Stowers and DWM Pearson) pp. 129–139. London: Springer-Verlag

Steel, JM, Johnstone, FD, Hepburn, DA and Smith, AF (1990) Can pregnancy care of diabetic women reduce the risk of abnormal babies? *British Medical Journal*, **301**, 1070–1074

Stowers, JM (1984) Follow up of gestational diabetic mothers treated thereafter. In *Carbohydrate Metabolism in Pregnancy and the Newborn (Aberdeen, 1983)* (edited by HW Sutherland and JM Stowers) pp. 181–183. Edinburgh: Churchill Livingstone

Stubbs, SM, Leslie, RDG and John, PN (1981) Fetal macrosomia and maternal diabetic control in pregnancy. *British Medical Journal*, **282**, 439–440

Stubbs, SM, Doddridge, MC, John, PN, *et al.* (1986) Haemoglobin A_1 and congenital malformation. *Diabetic Medicine*, **4**, 156–159

Susa, JB and Schwartz, R (1985) Effects of hyperinsulinaemia in the primate fetus. *Diabetes*, **34**, suppl 2, 36–41

Teramo, K, Ammala, P, Ylinen, K and Raivio, KO (1983) Pathologic fetal heart rate associated with poor metabolic control in diabetic pregnancies. *Obstetrics and Gynecology*, **61**, 559–565

Tsang, RC, Kleinman, LI, Sutherland, JM and Light, IJ (1972) Hypocalcemia in infants of diabetic mothers. *Journal of Pediatrics*, **80**, 384–395

Tsang, RC, Strub, R, Brown, DR, *et al.* (1976) Hypomagnesemia in infants of diabetic mothers: perinatal studies. *Journal of Pediatrics*, **89**, 115–119

Tyrrell, SN (1988) Doppler studies in diabetic pregnancy. *British Medical Journal*, **296**, 428

Wald, NJ, Cuckle, HS, Boreham, J, *et al*. (1979) Maternal serum alpha-fetoprotein and diabetes mellitus. *British Journal of Obstetrics and Gynaecology*, **86**, 101–105

Weinstock, RS, Kopecky, RT, Jones, DB and Sunderji, S. (1988) Rapid development of nephrotic syndrome, hypertension and haemolytic anaemia early in pregnancy in patients with IDDM. *Diabetic Care*, **11**, 416–421

Whichelow, MJ and Doddridge, MC (1983) Lactation in diabetic women. *British Medical Journal*, **287**, 649–650

Whittaker, PG, Aspillaga, MO and Lind, T (1983) Accurate assessment of early gestational age in normal and diabetic women by serum human placental lactogen concentration. *Lancet*, **ii**, 304–306

Whitelaw, A (1977) Subcutaneous fat in newborn infants of diabetic mothers: an indication of quality of diabetic control. *Lancet*, **i**, 15–18

Widnes, JA, Susa, JB, Garcia, JF, *et al*. (1981) Increased erythropoiesis and elevated erythropoietin in infants born to diabetic mothers and in hyperinsulinaemic rhesus fetuses. *Journal of Clinical Investigation*, **67**, 637–642

Ylinen, K, Raivio, K and Teramo, K (1981) Haemoglobin A_{1c} predicts the perinatal outcome in insulin-dependent diabetic pregnancies. *British Journal of Obstetrics and Gynaecology*, **88**, 961–967

Ylinen, K, Aula, P, Stenman, U-H. *et al*. (1984) Risk of minor and major fetal malformations in diabetics with high haemoglobin A_{1c} values in early pregnancy. *British Medical Journal*, **289**, 345–346

Chapter 2

Hypertension

IA Greer

Introduction

The major hypertensive disorder of pregnancy is pregnancy-induced hypertension. This remains the leading cause of maternal death in the United Kingdom today. To class pregnancy-induced hypertension as a hypertensive disorder is perhaps a gross understatement and oversimplification for it is much more: it is a multisystem disorder that can affect virtually every organ and system in the body, with hypertension representing only the tip of the iceberg that makes up an extensive and poorly understood disease process. The 'tip of the iceberg' may even be submerged so that, unless spotted by a wary lookout, the danger may not be seen until it is too late. Failure of the obstetrician to look beyond hypertension and appreciate the multisystem effects and alternative presentations of this disease represents a major source of mortality and morbidity for women suffering from pregnancy-induced hypertension. These problems are, perhaps, compounded by difficulties in classifying hypertensive disorders of pregnancy. Such classifications depend almost exclusively on the presence of hypertension and proteinuria, which are but two manifestations of what is likely to be a variety of underlying disease processes. The use of these diagnostic criteria must not blind the obstetrician to the wider spectrum of manifestations of the multisystem disorder which is pregnancy-induced hypertension.

Definitions and classification

The classification of hypertension in pregnancy is a difficult and confusing area. These difficulties stem from the variety of conditions which make up the hypertensive disorders of pregnancy, from our lack of knowledge as to the aetiology of these conditions and from a lack of agreement on their nomenclature and classification. In addition, the true diagnosis and therefore the classification may be evident only retrospectively, several weeks or even months after the pregnancy is completed. Although this may be satisfactory for the epidemiologist, it is wholly unsatisfactory for the clinician faced with the problem during pregnancy. In this situation, some form of classification is essential to make diagnosis consistent, to help quantify the risk to mother and fetus and to guide decisions regarding the patient's management. Furthermore, this lack of agreed classification and nomenclature has hampered research in this area, preventing comparisons between centres and between countries.

Essentially, there are three possible varieties of hypertension that can occur in pregnancy. First, there are women who have hypertensive problems antedating the pregnancy. These women have chronic hypertension and usually this will be essential hypertension, which often has an inherited component but has no well-defined underlying pathology, although some women with chronic hypertension will have an underlying problem such as renal disease. Secondly, there are women who are normotensive before pregnancy and in early pregnancy and who then during pregnancy develop hypertension which remits within a few months of delivery. These women have pregnancy-induced hypertension (PIH). Thirdly, and rarely, hypertension in pregnancy may represent the coincidental development of a new medical cause of hypertension occurring in pregnancy, such as phaeochromocytoma or Conn's syndrome. Most classification systems will reflect these three situations. Perhaps the simplest way to classify these disorders is on the basis of two features – hypertension and proteinuria – as in the classification of the International Society for the Study of Hypertension in Pregnancy (Davey and MacGillivray, 1988). Within the group labelled pregnancy-induced hypertension the terminology is also somewhat confusing. Pre-eclampsia is a term that is often loosely applied to these patients; however, pre-eclampsia means different things to different people and can lead to further confusion. Traditionally, it is associated with three classic clinical findings, namely hypertension, proteinuria and oedema. As proteinuria is really a measure of disease severity (MacGillivray, 1961) and oedema is regularly a feature of normal pregnancy (Thomson, Hytten and Billewicz, 1967) this term should be reserved for severe (proteinuric) pregnancy-induced hypertension alone. Gestational hypertension without proteinuria can be termed mild/moderate PIH.

Diagnostic criteria

Blood pressure

Normal pregnancy is associated with a number of alterations in the cardiovascular system, which start to occur in early pregnancy. Blood pressure starts to fall in the first trimester, reaches a nadir in mid-pregnancy and then slowly rises during the third trimester to levels compatible with those in the non-pregnant state (MacGillivray, Rose and Rowe, 1969). Cardiac output increases by around 40 per cent in the first trimester and this is maintained through pregnancy (Lees *et al.*, 1967a), although it is reduced in the third trimester when measured in the supine position, owing to diminished venous return which is obstructed by the gravid uterus (Lees *et al.*, 1967b; Ueland *et al.*, 1969). As blood pressure is determined by cardiac output and peripheral resistance, the decrease in blood pressure must be due to a fall in the latter. These changes occur in early pregnancy. They must therefore reflect a change in systemic vascular resistance, as the uteroplacental circulation is not sufficiently large to account for such a reduction in peripheral resistance at this stage of pregnancy. In PIH the increase in blood pressure is the result of an increase in systemic vascular resistance (Ginsburg and Duncan, 1967) in the face of an unchanged cardiac output occurring in the second half of pregnancy. Thus blood pressure is really a 'second-hand' measure of one of the manifestations of PIH, namely vasoconstriction. Despite this, blood pressure is the mainstay of the diagnosis of pregnancy-induced hypertension. Within the population it is continuously distributed and the dividing line between normal and abnormal is somewhat arbitrary and artificial. The accepted dividing line is a diastolic blood pressure of 90 mmHg after 20 weeks of pregnancy

(Butler and Bonham, 1963). There is some justification for this as the perinatal mortality rate has been shown to increase when maternal diastolic blood pressure exceeds 90 mmHg (Butler and Alberman, 1969; Page and Christianson, 1976). This cut-off also corresponds to statistical descriptions of the distribution of blood pressure in the population. A diastolic pressure of 90 mmHg is 3SD above the mean for mid pregnancy, 2SD above the mean for 34 weeks gestation but, owing to the physiological rise in blood pressure towards term (MacGillivray, Rose and Rowe, 1969), is only 1.5 SD above the mean at term. Consequently this level is unsatisfactory in late pregnancy, leading to overdiagnosis of the problem and, frequently, unnecessary intervention. This threshold will also exclude some women with a substantial rise in blood pressure but whose diastolic pressure does not exceed 90 mmHg and will include some women with mild chronic hypertension who have a minimal rise in blood pressure (Redman and Jeffries, 1988). The systolic pressure is much more variable than the diastolic pressure and has been shown not to contribute to the diagnostic or prognostic significance of hypertension occurring in pregnancy (Davey and MacGillivray, 1988) and therefore is not widely used in classification or diagnosis. To circumvent the problems of a threshold definition, increases in systolic and diastolic blood pressures of 30 and 15 mmHg respectively have been employed as alternative diagnostic criteria for hypertension by the American College of Obstetricians and Gynecologists (Hughes, 1972). This increment is probably too modest, as the average diastolic increment in normal pregnancy is around 10–12 mmHg (Chesley, 1976; MacGillivray, Rose and Rowe, 1969). Recently, Redman and Jeffries (1988) have proposed that both a threshold level and an increment be used together as this will improve the diagnosis when compared with either measurement alone. They suggest that to diagnose the problem the patient should have a blood pressure of <90 mmHg in the first 20 weeks of pregnancy with a subsequent rise of at least 25 mmHg and a maximum reading of at least 90 mmHg. It should also be noted that blood pressure can fluctuate quite widely both in the non-pregnant and pregnant individual and that a diurnal variation also exists with the highest pressures being recorded in the afternoon and early evening, and the lowest pressures being obtained between midnight and 4 a.m. (Seligman, 1971; Redman, Beilin and Bonnar, 1976a; Murnaghan, Mitchell and Ruff, 1980; Sawyer *et al.*, 1981; Murnaghan, 1987). This nocturnal fall can be lost or even reversed in patients with PIH (Redman, Beilin and Bonnar, 1976a; Murnaghan, Mitchell and Ruff, 1980). Thus, multiple measures of blood pressure should be made to obtain a true assessment of the situation. It is also customary in pregnancy to use Korotkoff phase IV as the measure of diastolic pressure as disappearance of the sounds (Korotkoff phase V) may not occur in pregnancy.

Proteinuria

Proteinuria is much easier to quantify than hypertension. It is an indicator of disease severity. Its presence is associated with a substantial increase in the perinatal mortality rate (MacGillivray, 1958; Naeye and Friedman, 1979) and the degree of proteinuria has also been shown to correlate with the perinatal mortality rate and incidence of growth retardation (Tervila, Groecke and Timonen, 1973). In women who become eclamptic, the presence of proteinuria is even more strongly associated with perinatal mortality (Nelson, 1955). The accepted threshold for significant proteinuria in pregnancy is 0.3 g per 24 h (Davey and MacGillivray, 1987). Although 'dipstick' testing is used to screen for proteinuria in the clinical situation, it is best to quantify proteinuria with a formal 24 h collection as there is considerable variability in urinary protein excretion in successive 4 h periods (Chesley, 1939). Random urine samples assessed by 'dipstick' may produce false-positive results due to contamination of the urine by vaginal discharge or by chlorhexidine preparations, and positive readings may also be obtained if the urine is highly alkaline or very concentrated (specific gravity ⩾1.030). False-negative results may occur if the urine is very dilute (specific gravity <1.010). These problems can largely be overcome by testing with multiple reagent dipsticks such as the Multistix-S G (Ames), which will test for specific gravity and pH so that the tester may be alerted to potential inaccuracies related to the degree of dilution and pH of the urine (Davey and MacGillivray, 1987). Using such test sticks a trace of protein corresponds to approximately 0.1 g/l; 1+ to 0.3 g/l; 2+ to 1.0 g/l; 3+ to 3.0 g/l and 4+ to 10.0 g/l (Davey and MacGillivray, 1987). Clearly then, ⩾2+ of protein on dipstick testing is significant, and 1+, being borderline, requires repeated testing and a 24 h collection to provide accurate quantification. Davey and MacGillivray (1987) have also suggested that proteinuria should be classed as severe if there are ⩾3 g protein in a 24 h collection. Although proteinuria is indicative of severe disease, the absence of proteinuria does not preclude a severe form of PIH. Eclampsia, which is perhaps the most severe form of this problem, can occur without proteinuria (Sibai *et al.*, 1981) and the patient may be severely hypertensive with diastolic blood pressures persistently in excess of 110 mmHg without proteinuria. In addition, proteinuria occurring in the absence of significant hypertension can still be attributable to pre-eclampsia and denotes a severe form of the disease which may be associated with major growth retardation.

Other diagnostic features

Oedema is included in the classic definition of pre-eclampsia and is used as a diagnostic feature in several classification systems of hypertension in pregnancy. Pathological oedema, perhaps most notable in the face, occurs in 85 per cent of women with pre-eclampsia and is associated with a rapid increase in weight (Thomson, Hytten and Billewiz, 1967). However, severe pre-eclampsia and eclampsia can occur without oedema (Sibai *et al.*, 1981) and the perinatal mortality rate has been shown to be higher in pre-eclampsia without oedema than in pre-eclampsia with oedema (Vosburgh, 1976). Significant oedema can also be found in 80 per cent of normal pregnancies (Robertson, 1971). In a prospective study of oedema in pregnancy the incidence of hypertension did not differ between those with and without oedema (Robertson, 1971). As oedema is difficult to assess objectively, some observers have utilized rapid weight gain in pregnancy to identify patients with developing pre-eclampsia. However, rapid weight gain can occur without pre-eclampsia and in one series of eclamptics only 10 per cent had rapid weight gain (Chesley, 1978). From the foregoing discussion it is clear that, although oedema is often a feature of PIH and pre-eclampsia, it is of no value as a diagnostic sign.

Hyperuricaemia is, diagnostically, a most useful feature of PIH (Lancet and Fisher, 1956). It occurs in advance of proteinuria and is of value in distinguishing women with PIH from those with chronic hypertension alone (Redman, Beilin and Bonnar, 1976b). Redman *et al.* (1976a) showed that elevated plasma urate associated with hypertension was linked to a substantial increase in perinatal mortality compared with pregnancies with the same degree of hypertension but with normal plasma urate levels. Again, however, elevated plasma urate is not totally specific to PIH and it should be noted that values normally increase during pregnancy as documented by Redman (1989), who showed that 2SD above the mean of the plasma urate concentrations at 16, 28, 32 and 36 weeks was 0.28, 0.29, 0.34 and 0.39 µmol/l, respectively.

The platelet count also tends to fall in pre-eclampsia and is often an early feature occurring in the second trimester (Redman, Bonnar and Beilin, 1978). Because of the wide range of platelet counts in normal pregnancy, the platelet count is not of great diagnostic value in PIH unless combined with other features, although serial counts will be more helpful. It is also an inconsistent feature of the disease, with only around 30 per cent of a series of eclamptic women having absolute thrombocytopenia ($<150 \times 10^9$/l) (Pritchard, Cunningham and Mason, 1976).

Clinical classification

From the foregoing discussion it is apparent that hypertensive disorders in pregnancy are difficult to diagnose and classify, reflecting the problem inherent in the use of signs of the condition(s) to define the problem. This point is well made by Redman (1987): 'a disease can never be defined by its clinical signs, however elaborately they are specified' . . . 'pre-eclampsia cannot be defined without an understanding of its cause or causes'.

Despite this problem, the clinician when faced with a hypertensive patient must make a diagnosis in order to make management decisions based on the prognostic implications of the underlying problem, and also to conduct meaningful research within the area. It must be accepted that the diagnosis made during pregnancy may be erroneous and that this may be apparent only after the pregnancy is completed, so that the clinician must act on the basis of all the information available to him during the pregnancy and make a provisional diagnosis.

Essentially there are only a few diagnostic groups which the clinician must consider and these are reviewed below. This classification corresponds broadly with the classification of Davey and MacGillivray (1988). The nomenclature used for these groupings is employed throughout this chapter.

Chronic hypertension

Chronic hypertension is usually diagnosed by an elevated blood pressure occurring in the first or early second trimester with a diastolic pressure of 90 mmHg being an appropriate threshold. As blood pressure still undergoes the physiological fall in the first half of pregnancy in chronic hypertension, this problem can easily be missed if the patient is not seen until later in pregnancy. This can lead to diagnostic confusion when her blood pressure rises physiologically in the late second and third trimester. Plasma urate measurements may be of value in this situation distinguishing chronic hypertensives not previously recognized from those with PIH.

Pregnancy-induced hypertension (PIH)

This can be diagnosed in women who are normotensive in the first 20 weeks of pregnancy and who then develop hypertension (see above) in the second half of pregnancy. When this occurs without proteinuria, it is classed as mild/moderate PIH; if it occurs in association with significant proteinuria, then it should be considered as severe PIH or pre-eclampsia. As proteinuria is not a constant feature of severe disease, persistent elevation of diastolic blood pressure to >110 mmHg should also be considered as severe PIH (Davey and MacGillivray, 1988). A patient with chronic hypertension may develop superimposed PIH, which can be distinguished by a rising urate and the development of proteinuria.

Eclampsia

Eclampsia may appear as part of the continuum of pre-eclampsia, the inevitable consequence of disease progression. However, it may also arise *de novo* antenatally, during labour or in the early puerperium with apparent absence of any recognized prodrome (Campbell and Templeton, 1980; Villar and Sibai, 1988) in around 15–20 per cent of patients. It is characterized by grand mal seizures which are not attributable to epilepsy or to any other convulsive problem. It usually occurs during the second half of pregnancy or in the first weeks of the puerperium; it is more common around term (Templeton and Campbell, 1977). Approximately 50 per cent of cases occur before labour, 25 per cent during labour and 25 per cent in the puerperium (Villar and Sibai, 1988). Post-partum eclampsia usually occurs within the first 48 h but may occur up to 2–3 weeks later (Sibai, Schneider and Morrison, 1980; Watson *et al.*, 1983; Villar and Sibai, 1988). Eclampsia is usually associated with hypertension, but this need not be severe and, indeed, may only be a relative rise in blood pressure which does not reach the threshold for absolute hypertension. Proteinuria is also a common feature but again is absent in between 20 and 40 per cent (Porapakkham, 1979; Villar and Sibai, 1988). The patient may be asymptomatic or have prodromal symptoms which most commonly are headaches, epigastric pain and visual disturbance (Sibai, El-Nazer and Gonzalez-Ruiz, 1986). Hyperuricaemia, deranged liver function tests, thrombocytopenia and coagulation disturbances may also occur. From the foregoing discussion, it is clear that the potentially eclamptic patient may be difficult to diagnose before seizures occur. An awareness of the diversity of possible presentations should help to alert the clinician and trigger appropriate investigation. In particular, symptomatic patients with headache, epigastric pain and vomiting in pregnancy should be considered to have fulminating pre-eclampsia until proved otherwise. Hypertension and proteinuria must also be treated seriously. Routine biochemical testing including plasma urate and liver function tests, a platelet count and blood film should help to resolve the diagnosis and allow suitable therapeutic measures to be taken.

Epidemiology of hypertension in pregnancy

Risk factors and associations

Severe PIH has traditionally been regarded as a disease of primigravidae, with MacGillivray (1958) showing that the risk of severe disease was 15 times greater in a first than in a second pregnancy. This study suggested that a previous pregnancy was protective with regard to the development of proteinuric pre-eclampsia. Milder forms of the disease are also more common in primigravidae. This relationship to previous pregnancies has recently been examined more closely by Campbell and MacGillivray (1985), who showed that whereas a first trimester abortion (either spontaneous or induced) did not protect against pre-eclampsia in a second pregnancy, a late spontaneous abortion did significantly reduce the risk of pre-eclampsia in a subsequent pregnancy, to 1.7 per cent (Campbell and MacGillivray, 1985). If

the first pregnancy ended after 37 weeks' gestation without any hypertensive complication, the incidence of pre-eclampsia in the second pregnancy was reduced to 0.7
per cent. However, if the first pregnancy was complicated by proteinuric pre-
eclampsia, the incidence in the second pregnancy was similar to that in the first. If this
first pregnancy was also complicated by a low-birthweight baby ($<2.5\,kg$), the
incidence of pre-eclampsia in a second pregnancy increased to 11.9 per cent (Campbell and MacGillivray, 1985). These figures should be set against an incidence of
proteinuric pre-eclampsia of 6.1 per cent in a first pregnancy. Thus, it can be seen
that while the incidence of proteinuric pre-eclampsia is reduced overall to 1.9 per
cent in a second pregnancy, this is modified by the presence of hypertensive complications, length of gestation at delivery and birthweight during the first pregnancy
(Campbell and MacGillivray, 1985).

An association also exists between maternal age and PIH with the incidence rising
sharply after age 35 (Butler and Alberman, 1969). This increase may be related to an
increased prevalence of underlying chronic hypertension which increases the risk of
PIH or may be misdiagnosed as PIH. There does not appear to be any association
with social class (Baird, 1967) nor with increased maternal weight (Lowe, 1961)
although overweight women are more likely to have chronic hypertension. Diabetic
women are also at increased risk of PIH. This risk is difficult to quantify accurately,
as diabetics are predisposed to chronic hypertension and diabetic nephropathy, so
confounding the diagnosis of PIH. However, in a recent UK survey of diabetic
pregnancy the incidence of PIH was 12 per cent both in established and gestational
diabetics (Howy and Baird, 1982). Interestingly, cigarette smoking appears to
reduce the incidence of PIH (Duffus and MacGillivray, 1968; Andrews and
McGarry, 1972) (although smokers are at greater risk of having infants that are small
for gestational age). Fetal factors are also associated with an increased risk of PIH:
these include twin pregnancies (MacGillivray, 1958), hydrops fetalis (Scott, 1952),
hydatidiform moles (Scott, 1952), triploidy and trisomy 13 (Boyd, Lindenbaum and
Redman, 1987).

Genetics of PIH

It is clear that susceptibility to PIH is associated with an inherited component,
although the precise genetic basis is not clear (Adams and Finlayson, 1961; Chesley,
Cosgrove and Annitto, 1961; Chesley, Annitto and Cosgrove, 1968). On the basis of
a large family study using eclampsia as the index condition, Chesley and Cooper
(1986) showed that the disorder was heritable and that their data were compatible
with a single gene model, in keeping with the previous suggestion that a single
maternal autosomal recessive gene could be responsible (Cooper and Liston, 1979).
A second study, however, suggested that a fetal genetic component also contributed
(Cooper et al., 1988). As an association between eclampsia and miscarriage was
found in this study, there may be a genetic basis for disturbance of the normal
feto–maternal interaction in the placental bed and this may point to an immune
mechanism.

Several studies have implicated the major histocompatibility complex in the
genetic mechanism of PIH (Redman et al., 1978; Redman, 1986; Kilpatrick, 1987;
Kilpatrick et al., 1987). An increased incidence of HLA DR4 has been noted in
pre-eclamptic women and their babies (Kilpatrick et al., 1987). More recently
observations have been extended to the sisters of women with proteinuric PIH
(Kilpatrick et al., 1989). This study revealed that the sisters had a higher incidence of

PIH than the maternity hospital population and that the frequency of HLA DR4 was increased in the sisters who developed PIH compared with sisters with normotensive pregnancy. In addition, those affected had a higher incidence of sharing of HLA DR4 with their spouses (Kilpatrick *et al.*, 1989). The association with HLA DR4 suggests either an abnormal immune response related to the HLA DR4 gene or a genetic linkage between HLA DR4 and the putative PIH susceptibility gene. The genetic data from this study were consistent with the proposal that a fetal component to susceptibility was involved (Cooper *et al.*, 1988). The data of Kilpatrick *et al.* (1989) were also consistent with the involvement of a single recessive gene shared by mother and fetus. It is likely, then, that future research will concentrate on genetic linkage studies around the HLA complex on chromosome 6, although the association between PIH and trisomy 13 would also make chromosome 13 worthy of analysis. The importance of all this is not just in elucidating the aetiology of PIH, for if a single gene cause can be isolated then molecular biology may allow screening couples for risk of PIH. Identification of women at high risk of PIH has not hitherto been very successful, especially in primigravidae. The development of a screening technique would allow potential preventive therapy to be instituted.

Maternal outcome

The overall incidence of proteinuric PIH is around 3 per cent whereas the incidence of eclampsia is around 0.1 per cent (Campbell and MacGillivray, 1985). The incidence of mild/moderate PIH is difficult to establish because of the difficulties in diagnosis and classification previously discussed. However, the incidence does not appear to have changed significantly over the last 30 years or so, having remained around 20 per cent (Campbell and MacGillivray, 1985; Hall and Campbell, 1987), although this figure is almost certainly boosted by the diagnostic chaos of hypertension in pregnancy and the inclusion of chronic hypertensives. In contrast to this, we have very accurate data on the incidence of deaths from pre-eclampsia and eclampsia in the United Kingdom today, owing to the thorough and careful Reports on Confidential Enquiries into Maternal Deaths in England and Wales. Over the last 30 years or so there has been a substantial fall in the number of deaths attributable to this condition (Figure 2.1); nevertheless, it remains the major cause of maternal death in the UK today (Department of Health, 1989). The commonest mode of death is cerebral haemorrhage. Cerebral oedema, cerebral infarction, pulmonary oedema and hepatic necrosis are also primary causes of death, although liver damage, disseminated intravascular coagulation (DIC) and fluid overload are also associated with many of the deaths and are likely to be significant contributory factors. In addition to those deaths directly attributable to hypertensive complications of pregnancy, a number of deaths also occur which, although directly attributable to other causes such as pulmonary thromboembolism, are associated with hypertensive complications.

There does not appear to be any association between PIH and hypertension in later life. Three studies in this area show that women with pregnancies complicated by PIH and eclampsia have a prevalence of hypertension in later life similar to that of the general population (Bryans, 1966; Chesley, Annitto and Cosgrove, 1976; Fisher *et al.*, 1981). The data of Sibai, El-Nazer and Gonzalez-Ruiz (1986) however, suggest that, on follow-up for >10 years, there is an increase in subsequent chronic hypertension in women who have had 'pre-eclampsia–eclampsia' and that this is most marked where the hypertensive problem arises before 30 weeks' gestation or when there are recurrent pregnancy hypertension problems. As both early onset disease and recurrent disease are associated with an increased prevalence of chronic hypertension or renal problems, it is likely that the findings of this study, at least in part, reflect this association. In a study from Australia, Ihle, Long and Oats (1987) followed up women with early (<37 weeks' gestation) and late onset PIH (the groups were mixed in content with regard to the presence of proteinuric PIH with 44 per cent having proteinuria in the early onset group and 15 per cent in the late-onset group) to look for evidence of underlying renal disease. In the early-onset group, 65 per cent had underlying renal disease which was usually a glomerular nephropathy, and 25 per cent had essential hypertension. The figures for the late-onset group were 17 per cent and 18 per cent, respectively. The figures for primigravid and multiparous patients were broadly comparable. In women who have had normotensive pregnancies, the prevalence of hypertension in later life is much lower than that in the general population (Adams and MacGillivray, 1961; Fisher *et al.*, 1981). Women with a mild degree of hypertension in pregnancy appear to have an increased risk of subsequent hypertension, perhaps because underlying chronic hypertension is unmasked by pregnancy. Women with recurrent hypertensive problems in several pregnancies also have an increased risk of later hypertensive problems, as they often have an underlying chronic hypertensive problem with superimposed PIH (Chesley, Annitto and Cosgrove, 1976; Sibai, El-Nazar and Gonzalez-Ruiz, 1986).

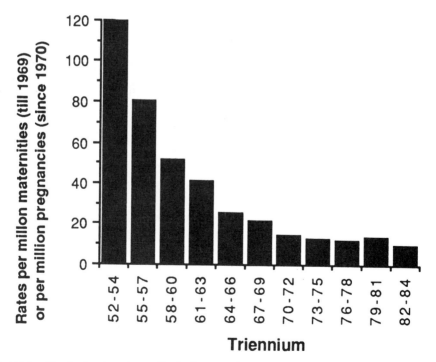

Figure 2.1.   Graph of maternal mortality for hypertensive disease in pregnancy in England and Wales 1952–1984. (Source: *Confidential Enquiries into Maternal Deaths in England and Wales*)

Fetal outcome

Severe (proteinuric) PIH and eclampsia are associated with a poor fetal outcome due to growth retardation, intrauterine asphyxia and iatrogenic prematurity. The perinatal death rate in eclamptic women has been estimated at between 136/1000 (Templeton and Campbell, 1977) and 213/1000 (Wightman, Hibbard and Rosen, 1978). The British Births Survey of 1970 (Chamberlain *et al.*, 1978) showed a perinatal mortality rate in severe PIH (and eclampsia) of 33.7/1000 compared with the rate of 19.2/1000 in normotensive pregnancies. The perinatal mortality rate was not increased in mild/moderate PIH and was reduced to 15.6/1000 in chronic hypertension. However, when chronic hypertension was complicated by superimposed pre-eclampsia, the rate rose to 30.7/1000. Similar figures have been found in studies from Aberdeen (MacGillivray, 1983). Severe PIH is also associated with intrauterine growth retardation (IUGR) (Moore and Redman, 1983) although mild/moderate PIH is not (Baird, Thomson and Billewicz, 1957; Low and Galbraith, 1974). There is also an association between severe PIH and neurodevelopmental disability (Taylor, 1988). Additionally, the fetus is at increased risk from abruption, which is approximately three times as common in severe disease as in normal pregnancy (Sibai, El-Nazar and Gonzalez-Ruiz, 1986).

Pathology of PIH

Pathology of the placental bed

In normal pregnancy, a series of physiological changes occurs in the spiral arteries of the placental bed as they are invaded by the cytotrophoblast (Brosens, Robertson and Dixon, 1967; Robertson and Khong, 1987). This cytotrophoblastic invasion occurs in two stages. In the first trimester the cytotrophoblast penetrates the decidual spiral arteries and migrates down these vessels. This endovascular trophoblast invades the vessel wall, removing the endothelium, internal elastic lamina and muscular coat of the vessel, which are largely replaced by fibrinoid material. By the end of the first trimester virtually every spiral artery in the decidua basalis will have undergone these physiological changes (Brosens and Dixon, 1966). In the early part of the second trimester a second wave of cytotrophoblast invasion occurs and the endovascular trophoblast similarly transforms the myometrial segments of the spiral arteries and sometimes even the distal segments of the radial arteries (Pijnenborg *et al.*, 1980, 1981, 1983). These physiological changes convert the vessels from muscular end-arteries to wide-mouthed sinusoids, so transforming the vascular supply from a high-pressure/low-flow system to a low-pressure/high-flow system (Moll, Kinzel and Hoberger, 1975) to meet the needs of the fetus and placenta. In addition, loss of the endothelium and muscular layers renders the vessels unable to respond to vasomotor stimuli.

In PIH the trophoblast invasion is somehow impaired: only about one-half to two-thirds of the decidual spiral arteries undergo these physiological changes (Khong *et al.*, 1986). Furthermore, the conversion of the myometrial portions of the spiral arteries fails to occur, even in vessels where the decidual segments have undergone physiological change (Brosens, Robertson and Dixon, 1972; Gerretsen, Huisjes and Elema, 1981; Sheppard and Bonnar, 1981) (Figure 2.2). These findings imply that the primary invasion of trophoblast is partially impaired and that the second wave fails to occur or is inhibited. This qualitative and quantitative restriction

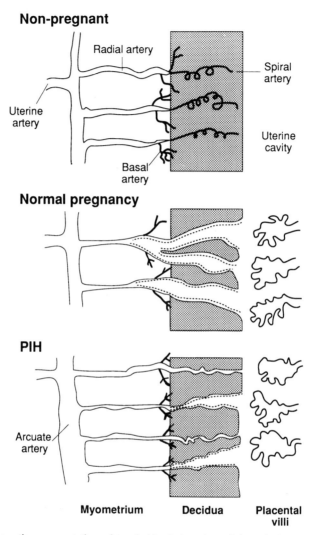

Figure 2.2. Schematic representation of trophoblastic invasion of the spiral arteries. Broken lines indicate trophoblast lining the vessels

of physiological change results in reduced placental blood flow (Robertson and Khong, 1987) which will become more threatening as the pregnancy advances and the demands of the conceptus increase. Additionally, as the vessels maintain their muscular coats, they remain sensitive to vasomotor stimuli.

PIH is also associated with a typical, although non-specific, vascular lesion termed 'acute atherosis' (Sexton *et al.*, 1950; Zeek and Assali, 1950; Labarrere, 1988), which can be seen in the intramyometrial segments of the spiral arteries in the placental bed, the basal arteries and the decidua parietalis, but not in the intradecidual vessels of the placental bed, which have undergone physiological change. This was first noted by Hertig in 1945 and was subsequently termed acute atherosis because of the presence of foam cells in the damaged vessel wall. Acute atherosis is a necrotizing arteriopathy characterized by fibrinoid necrosis, accumulation of lipid-laden macrophages and damaged cells, fibroblast proliferation and a mononuclear cell perivascular infiltrate (Labarrere, 1988). In the early stages this lesion is characterized by endothelial damage, insudation of plasma constituents into the vessel wall, cell proliferation and medial necrosis of the lipid-containing muscle cells (de Wolf, Robertson and Brosens, 1975). The lipid released is subsequently taken up by the macrophages which accumulate in the vessel wall. More recently, Shanklin and Sibai (1989) have shown that endothelial damage can be seen ultrastructurally in the decidua at sites outside the placental bed throughout the materno–fetal boundary. In addition they showed more direct correlation with the degree of maternal hypertension, although other workers have shown a correlation with plasma urate (McFadyen et al., 1986), highlighting the value of urate in predicting severity in PIH.

Failure of trophoblast invasion and acute atherosis are not specific to PIH, for these lesions can also be seen in normotensive intrauterine growth retardation (Sheppard and Bonnar, 1976, 1981; de Wolf, Brosens and Renaer, 1980). This does not necessarily mean that these disorders share a common aetiology, although it would appear that both are associated with defective trophoblastic–maternal interactions. It has been suggested that, in view of some evidence of IgM and complement deposition in these lesions and the perivascular mononuclear infiltrate, this lesion may be triggered by a maternal immune reaction against the trophoblast (Labarrere, 1988).

These abnormalities in the maternal placenta are likely to produce ischaemia of the fetal placenta, so explaining the changes that are seen there. These include placental infarcts, patchy necrosis and intracellular damage of the syncytiotrophoblast, an increase in villous cytotrophoblastic cells and an obliterative endarteritis of the fetal stem arteries (Fox, 1988). The latter change is responsible for the increased vascular resistance which is readily demonstrated by Doppler assessment of the umbilical artery, where absent or impaired end-diastolic flow can be seen in some pregnancies complicated by severe PIH.

The kidney

A number of pathological changes, which tend to parallel the clinical situation in terms of severity, occur in the kidney in PIH (Spargo, McCartney and Winemiller, 1959; Pollak and Nettles, 1960; Thomson et al., 1972; Sheehan and Lynch, 1973). The glomeruli enlarge and sometimes bulge and protrude into the proximal tubule, owing to swelling and vacuolation of the cytoplasm of the glomerular endothelial cells in the capillary loops. This swelling narrows the lumen. These glomerular changes were termed 'glomerular endotheliosis' by Spargo, McCartney and Winemiller (1959). Although the mechanism behind this is obscure, it is apparent that the primary change occurs in the endothelial cells. The epithelium of the glomerulus, including its foot processes, is essentially normal except for a few intracytoplasmic hyaline droplets. The mesangium, however, widens with an increase in mesangial matrix and expansion of the mesangial cell cytoplasmic foot processes. These processes can grow round the capillary between the endothelium and the basement membrane (Altcheck, Albright and Sommers, 1968; Seymour et al., 1976; Tribe et al., 1979).

This interposition is associated with deposition of mesangial matrix in the area between the basement membrane and the endothelium. These changes may be mistaken for thickening of the basement membrane – which does, in fact, appear normal (Fox, 1987). Deposits of IgM and fibrin may also be found, but there is no evidence of any other immunoglobulin or complement deposition (Fox, 1987). Although these findings are characteristic of PIH, they are not specific to it, as similar changes can be seen in placental abruption (Robson, 1976); they may be related to low-grade DIC and fibrin deposition, which can occur in both conditions. There is no major tubular damage in PIH although dilatation and epithelial thinning of the proximal tubules and hyaline deposition, related to protein reabsorption, have been noted (Sheehan and Lynch, 1973), as has tubular necrosis (Pollak and Nettles, 1960). The renal damage of PIH can be severe enough to produce acute renal failure, either by tubular or cortical necrosis (Lindheimer and Katz, 1986).

Functionally, the glomerular damage is manifest by reduced glomerular filtration rate and renal plasma flow, which are significantly lower than values found in normal pregnancy (Chesley, 1978) where both of these measurements normally increase (Davison and Hytten, 1974; Dunlop, 1981; Ezimokhai et al., 1981; Sims and Krantz, 1985). Although creatinine clearance is reduced, the serum creatinine does not usually increase noticeably in PIH because of the geometric relationship between clearance and serum creatinine.

Perhaps the most obvious clinical sign of glomerular dysfunction is proteinuria which, as discussed above, is a measure of disease severity, being associated with poor maternal and fetal outcomes (Butler and Bonham, 1963; Naeye and Friedman, 1979). The proteinuria is moderately non-selective in terms of molecular size (Robson, 1976; McEwan, 1968, 1969; MacLean, 1972). Although glomerular dysfunction is the underlying cause of proteinuria, the precise mechanism is not clear and could be related to loss of the strong negative charges that normally repel proteins from the basement membrane.

Whereas glomerular dysfunction is manifest as proteinuria, tubular dysfunction is associated with hyperuricaemia (Chesley and Williams, 1945). This reduction in uric acid clearance precedes the proteinuria indicative of glomerular damage in PIH and the fall in glomerular filtration rate (Gallery and Gyory, 1979). Redman et al. (1976a) showed that serum urate is a better predictor of perinatal outcome than blood pressure; it also correlates well with the renal biopsy appearances (Pollak and Nettles, 1960).

In normal pregnancy an increase in plasma volume occurs (Hytten and Paintin, 1963), whereas in PIH the plasma volume is significantly lower and is accompanied by haemoconcentration. This reduction antedates the onset of hypertension (Gallery, Hunyor and Gyory, 1979). It is not clear whether the hypertension is secondary to the reduced plasma volume or whether the reduced plasma volume is secondary to the hypertension. However, the work of Gallery, Hunyor and Gyory (1979), showing that the reduction in intravascular volume precedes the hypertension, and the haemodynamic studies of Groenendijk, Trimbas and Wallenburg (1984), would seem to favour the former view. The reduced plasma volume is also accompanied by sodium retention (Chesley, Valenti and Rein, 1958; Brown et al., 1988), and hypoalbuminaemia (Studd, Blainey and Bailey, 1970) with a subsequent reduction in intravascular osmotic pressure (Benedetti and Carlson, 1979). These changes may, at least in part, account for the capillary leakage and oedema that occur in PIH although there also may be a component of endothelial dysfunction. Although oedema is far from being a constant feature of PIH (as previously discussed), it is interesting that non-oedematous PIH ('dry pre-eclampsia') is associated with a poorer outcome than when oedema is present (Chesley, 1978).

The liver

The main hepatic lesions seen in PIH are lake haemorrhages, periportal fibrin deposition within the lake haemorrhages, and areas of infarction and necrosis (Sheehan and Lynch, 1973). Thrombosis of the capillaries of the portal tract and of small branches of the hepatic arteries is also seen. The haemorrhages probably arise in the arteries of the portal tract, which show evidence of vascular damage similar to that seen in other sites in the disease. These changes can be seen in 60 per cent of women dying of PIH. The pathogenesis of the hepatic lesions is obscure but is probably related to activation of the coagulation system, endothelial damage and vasoconstriction. The lesions are not specific to PIH, as similar changes can be seen in antepartum and postpartum haemorrhages (MacGillivray, 1983).

The pathological changes in the liver are associated with biochemical evidence of dysfunction and damage. This is manifest by increased activity of liver enzymes including SGOT/SGPT (Borglin, 1959; Theisen et al., 1961) and γ-glutamyl transferase, and also by elevated bilirubin levels, which may result in clinical jaundice. These problems may progress to hepatic failure or even subcapsular haematoma and hepatic rupture, which are associated with maternal death in PIH. Clinically, these changes may produce vomiting and epigastric pain and tenderness. Although such symptoms are usually indicative of a fulminating disease process, they may be absent and screening for hepatic dysfunction should be performed in women with the disorder. The mechanism behind epigastric pain and tenderness may be stretching of Glisson's capsule or possibly ischaemic pancreatitis, as evidence of pancreatic injury has been noted in severe disease (Haukland et al., 1987). Deranged liver function tests are not uncommon, with 21 per cent of 355 patients studied by Romero et al. (1988) having elevated levels of SGOT; this frequency is similar to that seen in other studies (Borglin, 1959; Theisen, 1961). Elevated SGOT is associated with severe disease and with an increased risk of premature delivery and intrauterine growth retardation (Romero et al., 1988). As the neonatal complications are independent of the severity of hypertension and the presence of proteinuria, hepatic dysfunction is likely to represent an independent risk factor for both mother and fetus (Romero et al., 1988).

The brain and nervous system

The brain can be involved in the pathological process of PIH with eclampsia being one of the most extreme clinical manifestations of this involvement. The pathological features that can occur include cerebral oedema, cerebral haemorrhage, petechial haemorrhages, thrombotic lesions and fibrinoid necrosis (Hibbard, 1973; Sheehan and Lynch, 1973; Lopes-Llera, Linores and Horta, 1976). These changes are thought to be attributable to vascular damage. Cerebral oedema is not a constant feature but may be seen on computerized tomography (CT) scanning of the brain in eclamptic patients (Naheedy et al., 1985; Richards, Graham and Bullock, 1988). The latter study showed cerebral oedema to be present on CT scanning in 27 of 43 women with neurological complications secondary to pre-eclampsia–eclampsia and this correlated with the duration of intermittent seizures. The authors suggest that oedema is not, therefore, the primary cause of the symptoms and signs of eclampsia, nor the cause of the seizures, but is a secondary feature occurring following seizures.

Cardiovascular and renin–angiotensin systems

In contrast to the normal pregnant situation, a contracted plasma volume occurs in PIH (Gallery, Hunyor and Gyory, 1979). This is associated with an increase in systemic vascular resistance, a reduction in cardiac output and reduced cardiac preload (Wallenburg, 1988). The key component of this process is likely to be vasoconstriction. How this vasoconstriction is mediated is not entirely clear, but it is not secondary to increased autonomic activity. This suggests that humoral factors and vascular sensitivity may be responsible. In normal pregnancy there are substantial changes in the renin–angiotensin system (Figure 2.3). Plasma concentrations of renin (PRC), renin substrate and angiotensin II (AII) all increase throughout gestation, reaching a peak around term when they are about four times greater than non-pregnant levels (Weir *et al.*, 1975; Skinner, Lumbers and Symonds, 1972; Oats *et al.*, 1981). Following delivery, concentrations of active renin and AII fall within 2 h of delivery, a change which is in keeping with the half-life of renin in the circulation. Subsequently, there is a rebound to levels greater than those in the non-pregnant situation (Jadoul, Broughton Pipkin and Lamming, 1982), a change which is compatible with the removal of an inhibitory influence on renal renin production. The increase in renin in pregnancy appears to have an extra-renal source: the myometrium, decidua, placenta and fetal membranes can produce renin (Symonds, Stanley and Skinner, 1968; Poisner *et al.*, 1981; Warren, Craven and Symonds, 1982; Johnson *et al.*, 1984) that is indistinguishable immunologically and enzymatically from renal renin (Acker *et al.*, 1982); renin substrate can also be produced from these sites. Immunohistochemically, renin granules can be found in clusters of cells round the spiral arteries in the myometrium close to the endometrium (Johnson *et al.*, 1984) and it is possible that they may function in a manner similar to that of the juxtaglomerular apparatus in the kidney. Thus, it appears that a complete renin–angiotensin system is present in the intrauterine tissues. This intrauterine system may, just as in the kidney, have a role in the regulation and control of local blood flow.

Despite this substantial increase in the activity of the renin–angiotensin system in normal pregnancy, it appears to remain under control mechanisms similar to those in the non-pregnant individual, with activation and suppression occurring following sodium deprivation and loading, respectively (Becker *et al.*, 1978; Bay and Ferris, 1979) and increased activity on standing after lying (Lindheimer, Del Greco and Ehrlich, 1973). Although plasma aldosterone concentration also increases in pregnancy, it does not correlate with changes in the renin–angiotensin system and these systems may be dissociated, with aldosterone being controlled more by sodium status (Karlberg, Ryden and Wichman, 1984; Brown, Broughton Pipkin and Symonds, 1988).

Despite the increased circulating levels of AII in pregnancy, blood pressure falls. This reflects the well-documented vascular insensitivity to AII seen in normal pregnancy, which is maximal in the second trimester then slowly returns towards the normal non-pregnant situation (Abdul-Karim and Assali, 1961; Talledo, Chesley and Zuspan, 1968; Gant *et al.*, 1973). Although this insensitivity may be related in part to progestogens, which can blunt the renal effects of AII in the non-pregnant state and the pressor effects in late pregnancy (Chesley and Tepper, 1967; Everett *et al.*, 1978b), possibly by suppressing AII receptors, it is most likely to be related to the production of vasodilator prostaglandins, stimulated by AII from the vessel wall (Gimbrone and Alexander, 1975). Inhibitors of prostaglandin synthesis potentiate

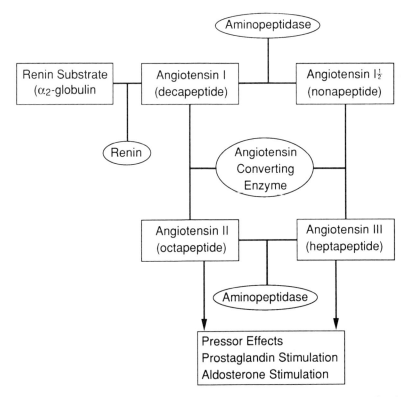

Figure 2.3. Simplified schematic diagram of renin–angiotensin system. Renin substrate (angiotensino-gen), an α_2-globulin, is converted by the action of renin (of renal or uterine origin) to the decapeptide angiotensin I. Angiotensin I (AI) has minimal biological activity and is rapidly converted to angiotensin II, an octapeptide, by the action of angiotensin converting enzyme (ACE). Angiotensin II has a short half-life of ≈ 2 min and is broken down by aminopeptides to angiotensin III, which is an effective stimulator of aldosterone with less pressor effect than angiotensin II. As angiotensin III can be formed from angiotensin I1/2, it is possible that the pressor effects and aldosterone-stimulatory effects can be dissociated. NB: Renin can be measured as plasma renin concentration (PRC) or plasma renin activity (PRA). PRC is assessed by incubating plasma in the presence of excess substrate and ACE and angiotensinase inhibitors and measuring the AI generated; it reflects the amount of renin and its activators and inhibitors in the plasma. PRA is assessed by incubating plasma in the presence of ACE and angiotensinase inhibitors and measuring the AI generated; it measures renin substrate, renin and renin activators and inhibitors in the plasma

the vasoconstrictor effects of AII in the umbilical artery *in vitro*, whereas PGE$_2$ and PGF$_{2\alpha}$ attenuate it (Bjoro, 1985). This effect can also be seen *in vivo* in the human, with indomethacin enhancing pressor effects (Jaspers, De Jong and Mulder, 1981) and PGE$_2$ and PGI$_2$ infusions blunting the pressor response further in human pregnancy (Broughton Pipkin *et al.*, 1982; Broughton Pipkin, Morrison and O'Brien, 1984). These data suggest that the attenuation of the pressor effects of AII in normal pregnancies is attributable to the stimulation of vasodilator prostaglandins by AII to maintain local blood flow, just as in the renal circulation. This system may also play a part in the local control of uteroplacental flow. Thus activation of the intrauterine renin–angiotensin system and subsequent prostaglandin production will result in local vasodilatation despite the increase in pressor agents. This hypothesis is supported by studies showing that AII infusions into the uterus in monkeys increase both prostaglandin production and blood flow, an effect that can be abolished with inhibitors of prostaglandin synthesis such as indomethacin (Franklin *et al.*, 1974; Speroff, Haning and Levin, 1977). Conversely, angiotensin-converting enzyme inhibitors reduce both uterine prostaglandin production and blood flow (Ferris and Weir, 1983) (these substances are therefore contraindicated for the treatment of PIH). Thus the increased activity of the renin–angiotensin system in normal pregnancy may have an important physiological role in maintaining and controlling uteroplacental blood flow.

Additionally, the systemic pressor effects of AII may be blunted by atrial natriuretic peptide (ANP), which is increased in normal pregnancy (Fievet *et al.*, 1988). This substance is known to reduce the constrictor effects of AII and to inhibit the secretion of renin and aldosterone (Atlas and Laragh, 1986), although there is evidence to suggest that ANP does not suppress aldosterone during pregnancy as it does in the non-pregnant (Fievet *et al.*, 1988).

Owing to methodological problems and the study of groups varying in disease severity, there have been problems in determining what changes occur in the renin–angiotensin system in PIH. However, the changes appear to fall into two patterns depending on disease severity. In late-onset non-proteinuric PIH there is an increase in plasma renin activity (Gallery *et al.*, 1980b; Fievet *et al.*, 1985) whereas AII may be unchanged or increased (Symonds, Broughton Pipkin and Craven, 1975; Symonds and Broughton Pipkin, 1978). In early-onset proteinuric PIH, plasma renin activity, AII and aldosterone are reduced (Weir *et al.*, 1973; Karlberg, Ryden and Wichman, 1984; Fievet *et al.*, 1985). In contrast to the suppression of the renin–angiotensin system in severe PIH, ANP is increased (Elias *et al.*, 1988; Fievet *et al.*, 1988; Hirai *et al.*, 1988; Miyamoto *et al.*, 1988; Sumioki *et al.*, 1989), indicating that PIH is not an ANP-deficiency state. Increased ANP may be a compensatory mechanism for the increased blood pressure, a hypothesis supported by the direct correlation that exists between blood pressure and plasma ANP levels in normal and hypertensive pregnancies (Fievet *et al.*, 1988). The control of ANP release in PIH is not clear: it is usually stimulated by volume expansion and an increase in atrial pressure; however, PIH is associated with a contracted plasma volume. Alternative mechanisms (or sources) for its release must be sought. Regardless of its control mechanism, the increased ANP levels in PIH may be important in suppressing the renin–angiotensin system and ameliorating the hypertension, as seen in early-onset proteinuric disease.

The pressor response to AII returns to non-pregnant levels in PIH and this antedates the development of the disease (Gant *et al.*, 1973). This increase in the AII pressor response is the basis of the angiotensin sensitivity test, which has been employed successfully in the late second trimester to identify women with a high risk of subsequently developing PIH. This test has a high false-positive rate (around 50 per cent) but a low false-negative rate. Although it is impracticable as a screening test for the identification of women with the disease within the general obstetric population, it has been successfully employed as a research tool to identify a population at high risk of developing the disease, in order to examine potential prophylaxis (Wallenburg *et al.*, 1986).

The increased sensitivity to AII can be seen in isolated resistance vessels of women with the disease (Aalkjaer *et al.*, 1984) and may be due to increased AII receptors (Baker, Broughton Pipkin and Symonds, 1989) and reduced production of vasodilator prostaglandins, such as PGI_2, in PIH. AII has been shown to stimulate less PGI_2 release from umbilical arteries *in vitro* in PIH than in normotensive pregnancy

(Bjoro, Stokke and Stray-Pedersen, 1987) and deficient PGI_2 production is a feature of PIH (see below). Perhaps one of the most important recent developments in this area is the study by Baker, Broughton Pipkin and Symonds (1989) showing an increase in AII-binding sites on platelets in women with PIH compared with normal pregnancy. Should this binding phenomenon antedate the development of the disease in parallel with the increased sensitivity to AII seen in the angiotensin sensitivity test, this would represent a major advance in the identification of women at risk. Such a test could be applied on a wide scale, with just a peripheral blood sample being required, in comparison to the invasive and impractical angiotensin sensitivity test. The identification and validation of such a large-scale test has assumed enormous importance now that potential prophylaxis in the form of anti-platelet therapy is available (see below). The application of such prophylaxis has hitherto been hampered by our inability to identify easily those women, and in particular those primigravidae, at risk of PIH.

Having established what changes occur in the renin–angiotensin system in PIH, it is important to try to determine how these fit into the pathophysiological process of PIH. The best theory would appear to be that proposed by Broughton Pipkin and Symonds (1986). They compare the changes which occur in the renin–angiotensin system with regard to renal perfusion, to those which occur in the uteroplacental bed with its intrinsic renin–angiotensin system. In the kidney when perfusion is impaired, the juxtaglomerular apparatus releases renin, which in turn stimulates AII production, resulting in peripheral vasoconstriction and increased arterial pressure to improve renal perfusion. The increased AII in the renal vascular bed stimulates the release of vasodilatory prostaglandins. Thus, increased perfusion pressure and systemic vasoconstriction occur simultaneously with intrarenal vasodilation, so protecting the renal vasculature from the vasoconstrictor effects of AII (Aiken and Vane, 1973).

In PIH the critical lesion is failure of trophoblast invasion into the maternal vasculature (see above), which will lead to reduced flow and tissue ischaemia. In experimental animals, reduction of flow is associated with stimulation of the renin–angiotensin system, hypertension and proteinuria (Abitbol et al., 1977), whereas AII and angiotensin converting enzyme inhibitors will respectively enhance and reduce prostaglandin production and blood flow (Franklin et al., 1974; Ferris and Weir, 1983). Broughton Pipkin and Symonds (1986) therefore suggest that, in late-onset non-proteinuric PIH, significant ischaemia attributable to failure of trophoblast invasion occurs late in pregnancy. The impaired perfusion is sensed by the renin secreting cells round the spiral arteries (the uterine equivalent of the juxtaglomerular apparatus), renin is released and AI and AII production occurs. This results in increased levels of these substances, vasoconstriction and increased blood pressure to enhance uteroplacental perfusion pressure. In the uteroplacental bed the AII stimulates the release of vasodilator prostaglandins from the endothelium, thus protecting the local circulation and maintaining flow. Activation of the renin–angiotensin system may therefore be a compensatory mechanism to maintain adequate uteroplacental perfusion. This is in keeping with the established relatively good prognosis for such patients and contrasts with early onset proteinuric PIH. In this situation there is reduced perfusion of the uteroplacental bed, which again stimulates the renin–angiotensin system to increase blood pressure in an attempt to improve perfusion; however, as these patients are deficient in the production of vasodilator prostaglandins there is no compensatory vasodilatation in the utero-placental or renal vascular beds to protect them. Thus, further damage can occur, which may result in placental insufficiency and proteinuria with a poorer prognosis than late-onset non-proteinuric disease. As the compensatory mechanism of prostaglandin production is impaired, less AII is required to provoke a vasoconstrictor effect. If there is negative feedback on the renin–angiotensin system by increased blood pressure *per se* and by increased ANP, then renin and AII may be reduced in keeping with the findings in severe early onset PIH. Despite this reduction, the lack of prostaglandin production means that lower AII concentration could still exert considerable pressor effects.

Pathophysiological mechanisms of PIH

The precise aetiology and pathophysiological mechanism of pre-eclampsia remain an enigma. So many hypotheses have been advanced over the years that in 1916 Paul Zweifel called it 'the disease of theories'. More recently, it has become apparent that more and more biological cascades are triggered leading MacGillivray (1981) to term it 'the disease of the cascades'. However, as far back as 1694, Francois Mauriceau, the celebrated French accoucheur, made three important observations about the disease: first, that it was a disease of primigravidae; secondly, that it resolved following delivery; and thirdly that it was due to 'an excess of heated blood rising from the uterus'. It could be argued that our knowledge about the problem has advanced little over the intervening three centuries. The third notion, that the problem is due to an excess of heated blood rising from the uterus, may at first sight seem rather quaint; however, it is clear that the disease originates within the uterus. The concept of 'heated blood' suggests a degree of 'friction' between the blood and the vessel wall to generate the heat. This 'friction' may arise from interaction between the endothelium and the blood components – the coagulation system, the platelets and the neutrophils – all of which can interact to produce the vascular damage and dysfunction that is common to all of the pathological features of PIH. These components are now examined in turn.

The coagulation and fibrinolytic systems in PIH

Deposition of fibrin has long been known to be a feature of the pathological vascular damage of PIH (Schmorl, 1893; Govan, 1954) suggesting that the coagulation system is activated. This is unlikely to be a primary phenomenon, and is more likely to be secondary to vascular damage; none the less it will still contribute to this damage, promoting a positive feedback loop. There is a degree of physiological activation of the coagulation system in normal pregnancy, and it may be that PIH represents an exaggerated form of this process.

The routine tests for coagulation defects are essentially normal in PIH unless complicated by full-blown DIC. The prothrombin time and activated partial thromboplastin time, measures of the extrinsic and intrinsic pathways of coagulation respectively, appear to be normal (Morris *et al.*, 1964; Imrie and Raper, 1977), despite one report of shortened prothrombin time in PIH (Lox, Dorsett and Hampton, 1983). The thrombin time is slightly prolonged (Pritchard, Cunningham and Mason, 1976). Although these gross tests of coagulation show no consistent change, this does not imply that coagulation activation is not occurring, as these tests are relatively insensitive. There is evidence of fibrinogen breakdown in the form of elevated fibrinopeptide A levels in severe PIH (Douglas *et al.*, 1982; Borok *et al.*,

1984). Fibrinopeptide A is a sensitive, readily accessible indicator of coagulation activation, being cleaved from fibrinogen by the action of thrombin. Fibrinogen concentration itself also increases in PIH compared with normal pregnancy (Howie, Prentice and McNicol, 1971; Inglis *et al.*, 1982; Lox, Dorsett and Hampton, 1983; Spencer *et al.*, 1983) but this may simply be an acute phase reactant increasing in response to the disease in general.

Factor VIII changes significantly in PIH. There is an increase in factor VIII coagulant (factor VIIIc) activity (Howie, Prentice and McNicol, 1971; Howie *et al.*, 1976; Lox, Dorsett and Hampton, 1983; Spencer *et al.*, 1983) but a greater incidence occurs in von Willebrand's factor antigen (previously termed factor VIII related antigen) giving an increase in the ratio between the activities of von Willebrand's factor and factor VIII coagulant (Redman *et al.*, 1977b; Thornton and Bonnar, 1977). This was initially thought to reflect consumption of factor VIIIc after activation, but it is now known that these two substances are distinct entities which join together in the circulation to form a macromolecular complex. Factor VIII coagulant is produced by the liver and von Willebrand's factor is synthesized by the vascular endothelium; the increase in von Willebrand's factor may therefore simply reflect endothelial damage, as it is released by the endothelium in response to damage.

There are no major changes in the majority of individual coagulation factors with factors, II, V, VII (Morris *et al.*, 1964), X, XI and XII (Condie, 1976a) showing no significant difference between normal and pre-eclamptic patients. Again, reports have not been totally consistent, with Lox, Dorsett and Hampton (1983) showing an increase in factors II, V, VII and X and Oian *et al.* (1985) showing a reduction in factor VII. In a prospective study, Condie (1976b) showed that there was a slight increase in factor XII and a slight reduction in factors X and XI in women who went on to develop PIH. The endogenous inhibitor of coagulation, antithrombin III (ATIII), is reduced in PIH in keeping with the low-grade DIC that occurs in this disorder (Howie, Prentice and McNicol, 1971; Spencer *et al.*, 1983; Weiner *et al.*, 1985), and reduced ATIII correlates with disease severity (Weiner and Brandt, 1982). Another endogenous inhibitor of the coagulation cascade, Protein C, is also reduced in severe disease (Aznar *et al.*, 1986). These data suggest that usually only minimal coagulation activation occurs in PIH, although occasionally this may progress to full-blown DIC in severe disease.

Activation of the coagulation cascade is usually associated with activation of the fibrinolytic system. The majority of studies in this area have reported increased levels of fibrinogen–fibrin degradation products both in urine and in serum (Bonnar *et al.*, 1969; Howie, Prentice and McNicol, 1971) and soluble fibrinogen-fibrin complexes are also increased (McKillop *et al.*, 1976; Edgar *et al.*, 1977). The activity of plasminogen activators initially appeared to be normal or slightly reduced in preeclampsia compared to normal pregnancy (Morris *et al.*, 1964; Bonnar, McNicol and Douglas, 1971; Howie, Prentice and McNicol, 1971). Recently, however, more precise assays of plasminogen activators and their inhibitors have become available. These show that plasma plasminogen activator remains unchanged, whereas tissue plasminogen activator concentration in plasma increases (Estelles *et al.*, 1987), possibly owing to stimulation of, or damage to, the endothelium where it is produced. The increase in plasminogen activator is accompanied by an increase in plasminogen activator inhibitors 1 and 2 (Estelles *et al.*, 1987). This feature had previously been noted as a reduction in urokinase activity by Howie, Prentice and McNicol (1971). Plasminogen activator inhibitor 2 is produced only from the placenta and is not found in plasma from non-pregnant subjects. The increase in this placentally-derived plasminogen activator inhibitor seen in PIH may again reflect placental vascular damage and would predispose to local thrombosis by local inhibition of fibrinolysis in the abnormal vessels of the placental bed. Again, however, all studies have not been consistent: de Boer *et al.* (1988) have shown an increase in total plasminogen activator inhibitor in PIH, with a reduction in the placentally derived inhibitor component compared with normal. They have also shown that low levels of placental plasminogen activator inhibitor were associated with poor fetal outcome and therefore might simply be a measure of placental function.

Other evidence of fibrinolytic activation is the increase in fibrinopeptide β1-42 levels in patients with PIH. This peptide reflects plasmin degradation of fibrin I, which is a soluble intermediate between fibrinogen and the polymerizing fibrin II (Borok *et al.*, 1984). This study also measured levels of the peptides cleaved from fibrinogen by the action of thrombin and so could determine the balance between fibrinolysis and coagulation. The results suggested that, in patients with severe disease, fibrinolysis was more pronounced than fibrin formation. Plasminogen (Spencer *et al.*, 1983) and the inhibitor of plasmin, α_2 antiplasmin (Oian *et al.*, 1985) have also been found to be reduced, in keeping with fibrinolytic activation. This increase in fibrinolysis may be a response to intravascular coagulation but may be impaired owing to the intravascular concomitant increase in inhibitors of plasminogen activation.

Platelets

Platelets have a pivotal role in the pathophysiology of PIH. When platelets are activated, as on contact with the subendothelium, they aggregate. Aggregation is a series of morphological and functional changes. The platelets first undergo a shape-change reaction, whereby they form pseudopodia and link together before forming a large aggregate. In parallel with this aggregation, functional changes occur: the platelet degranulates, releasing granule contents such as ADP and serotonin, and also synthesizes and releases thromboxane A_2 (TxA_2); these substances promote further aggregation and vasoconstriction, so amplifying the response. Such a response is essential for haemostasis but, in disease states such as PIH platelet aggregation can produce vascular damage and obstruction, by both physical and biochemical means, leading to tissue ischaemia and further damage.

TxA_2 is the major product of arachidonic acid metabolism in platelets (Figure 2.4). It is a potent vasoconstrictor and platelet-aggregating agent (Hamberg, Svensson and Samuelsson, 1975). As it has a short half-life it is normally measured as its stable hydration product TxB_2. The effects of TxA_2 are normally counterbalanced by prostacyclin (PGI_2). This is a potent vasodilator and anti-platelet agent, which is the major product of arachidonic acid metabolism in vascular endothelium. It has an important role in protecting the endothelium and limiting damage by inhibiting platelet aggregation and stimulating vasodilatation. These two substances, PGI_2 and TxA_2, function as local hormones and are important in the control of the platelet–endothelial interaction. They oppose each other through the regulation of platelet adenylate cyclase (Tateson, Moncada and Vane, 1977), which controls cAMP production and thereby platelet free calcium concentration; cAMP thus acts as the intermediary, linking receptor occupancy with cellular response. Pro-aggregatory substances such as thromboxane A_2 inhibit adenylate cyclase, allowing free calcium to rise, whereas platelet-inhibitory prostaglandins such as prostacyclin stimulate adenylate cyclase, thus increasing cAMP, reducing free calcium and thereby inhibiting platelet activation.

There is now considerable evidence implicating platelets in the pathophysiology of PIH. The circulating platelet count is reduced in PIH (Trudinger, 1976; Redman, Bonnar and Beilin, 1978) reflecting a reduced platelet life-span (Rakoczi et al., 1979). An inverse relationship between platelet count and fibrinogen–fibrin degradation products (FDPs) has been noted, suggesting that the fall in platelet count is due to the increased platelet consumption seen in the low-grade DIC that occurs in PIH (Howie, Prentice and McNicol, 1971). The platelet-specific protein β-thromboglobulin has also been found to be increased in PIH (Redman et al., 1977a; Douglas et al., 1982; Socol et al., 1985) and this is a marker of platelet activation in vivo. Furthermore, β-thromboglobulin has been shown to correlate with proteinuria and serum creatinine (Socol et al., 1985), linking platelet activation with renal microvascular damage in PIH.

The platelet count of 5-hydroxytryptamine is reduced in PIH (Whigham et al., 1978). This vasoactive amine is released when platelets aggregate, and its loss indicates platelet aggregation and stimulation of the platelet release reaction in vivo. Low platelet 5-hydroxytryptamine levels have also been associated with loss of platelet responsiveness to various aggregating agents (Whigham et al., 1978). The explanation suggested for these findings is that platelets are activated in the microcirculation of the placenta, kidney and liver, release their products such as β-thromboglobulin and 5-hydroxytryptamine and then re-enter the circulation in an 'exhausted' state, unable to respond normally to aggregating agents and having lower levels of 5-hydroxytryptamine (Howie, 1977). In support of this hypothesis, it had previously been noted that placentae from patients with PIH had high levels of 5-hydroxytryptamine (Senior et al., 1963), possibly of platelet origin. This platelet

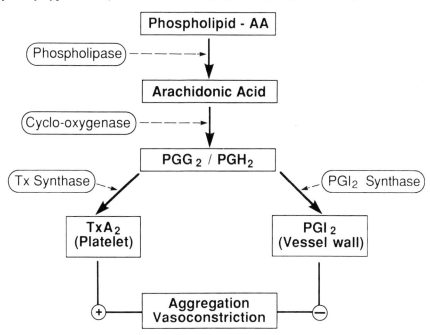

Figure 2.4.   Biosynthetic pathway for thromboxane (TxA$_2$) and prostacyclin (PGI$_2$)

exhaustion phenomenon has also been noted in molar pregnancy complicated by severe PIH, where anti-platelet therapy corrected the hypofunctional platelet response (Greer et al., 1987). A relative macrothrombocytosis is also seen in PIH and this is due to an increased entry of large, young platelets into the circulation (Giles and Inglis, 1981), which is in keeping with accelerated platelet consumption.

Platelets have also been shown to be less sensitive to the anti-aggregatory effects of prostacyclin in PIH (Briel, Kieback and Lippert, 1984), and this may contribute to the platelet consumption seen in this disease, especially as deficiency of prostacyclin production may coexist (Downing, Shepherd and Lewis, 1980; Remuzzi et al., 1980; Goodman et al., 1982), as discussed below. Increased platelet thromboxane A_2 production has been shown to occur in vitro in PIH complicated by intrauterine growth retardation (Wallenburg and Rotmans, 1982) and may also contribute to the pathogenesis of PIH. More recently, a whole-blood platelet aggregation technique has been used to study platelet reactivity in PIH (Greer et al., 1988a). This technique leaves platelets in their natural milieu surrounded by red cells and white cells, which may themselves influence aggregation, and thus may be a more physiological technique than traditional turbidometric techniques using platelet-rich plasma. This study showed that under these conditions platelet reactivity was enhanced in women with PIH, compared with normal pregnant and non-pregnant women. The role of platelets in the pathophysiology of PIH is also emphasized by the recent success of anti-platelet therapy in the treatment of pregnancies at high risk of the disease (Beaufils et al., 1985; Wallenburg et al., 1986).

All these changes in the coagulation system and platelet function in PIH, support the concept that DIC occurs in this condition. A 'coagulation index' of serum FDPs, platelet count and plasma factor VIII has been shown to correlate with a 'clinical index' of disease severity (Howie et al., 1976) and this highlights the association of DIC with PIH.

Prostacyclin and the vascular endothelium in PIH

This increase in platelet reactivity leads us to ask the question: what underlies the enhanced platelet reactivity seen in PIH? Normally, the activity of platelets is limited by the vascular endothelium. The endothelium is not merely an inert container for circulating blood, it has a wide range of functions. It plays a part in the control not only of haemostasis and thrombosis, but also of vascular tone. It can generate PGI_2, which can inhibit the activation of platelets and neutrophils (Boxer et al., 1980; Weksler and Jaffe, 1986), and substances such as tissue plasminogen activator which act to prevent or limit vascular damage. Conversely, the endothelium can render itself thrombogenic by secreting von Willebrand's factor, platelet activating factor and plasminogen activator inhibitor, which promote local coagulation and repair at the site of injury. The endothelium contributes to the regulation of vascular tone by release of PGI_2 and the recently characterized endothelium-derived relaxing factor (Palmer, Ferrige and Moncada, 1987; Moncada, Radomski and Palmer, 1988). The release of these two substances appears to be coupled (de Nucci et al., 1988) and stimulated by agents such as thrombin (Moncada, Radomski and Palmer, 1988). In the normal situation, the endothelium, platelets and neutrophils interact homeostatically. It has long been appreciated that denudation of the endothelium results in thrombosis (Baumgartner, 1973), but endothelial dysfunction may have similar effects and could transform the endothelium from a non-thrombogenic to a thrombogenic surface. There is now considerable evidence linking endothelial dysfunction to PIH.

Prostacyclin is a potent vasodilator, inhibitor of platelet aggregation (Moncada *et al.*, 1976) and stimulator of renin secretion (Patrono *et al.*, 1982). The pathological features of PIH are virtually a mirror image of these, as it is associated with vasoconstriction, platelet consumption and low renin secretion (Brown *et al.*, 1965). Furthermore, women with PIH are very sensitive to exogenous angiotensin II infusions, compared with normal pregnant women (Talledo, Chesley and Zuspan, 1968; Gant *et al.*, 1973). This insensitivity to angiotensin II seen in normal pregnancy can be abolished if women are treated with a cyclo-oxygenase inhibitor such as indomethacin (Everett *et al.*, 1978a), and enhanced by prostacyclin infusion (Broughton Pipkin, Morrison and O'Brien, 1984) or PGE_2 infusion (Broughton Pipkin *et al.*, 1982). These experiments suggest that in normal pregnancy angiotensin II may be balanced by the action of vasodepressor prostaglandins such as prostacyclin. A deficiency of prostacyclin might therefore result in the sensitivity to angiotensin II seen in PIH, and many investigators have now studied prostacyclin in this condition.

Maternal vascular prostacyclin production has been shown to be reduced in PIH (Bussolino *et al.*, 1980). Plasma prostacyclin metabolites have also been shown to be significantly lower in patients with PIH, especially those with severe disease, compared with normal pregnancy (Greer, 1985) and these results were confirmed in a prospective longitudinal study of prostacyclin metabolites (Greer *et al.*, 1985d). These findings are in agreement with those of other workers studying both plasma (Moodley, Norman and Reddi, 1984) and urinary (Goodman *et al.*, 1982) prostacyclin metabolites. On the other side of the equation, platelet thromboxane A_2 production is increased in PIH (Wallenburg and Rotmans, 1982) and placentae taken from pregnancies complicated by PIH have been shown to produce more thromboxane A_2 and less prostacyclin than those from normal pregnancies (Walsh, 1985). The resulting imbalance between prostacyclin and thromboxane is likely to contribute to the enhanced platelet reactivity and vascular damage seen in PIH.

Turning to the fetal side of PIH, studies have shown that production of prostacyclin from placenta and cord is reduced in PIH (Remuzzi *et al.*, 1979; Downing, Shepherd and Lewis, 1980; Walsh, Behr and Allen, 1985) and umbilical artery reactivity to serotonin *in vitro* is increased in PIH (Johnstone *et al.*, 1987). Makila, Viinikka and Ylikorkala (1984) have proposed that prostacyclin deficiency in pregnancy is specific to PIH, as they documented reduced prostacyclin production from umbilical artery in pregnancies complicated by PIH, but not in pregnancies complicated by chronic hypertension or intrauterine growth retardation. This, however, is at variance with other studies which have shown deficient prostacyclin production from placental cells (Jogee, Myatt and Elder, 1983) and from umbilical artery (Stuart *et al.*, 1981) to be a feature of intrauterine growth retardation. More recently, attention has focused on the ability of vascular endothelium to increase prostacyclin production following a physiological stimulus. In the past, most studies have used vascular rings or tissue homogenates; such methods will extensively traumatize the tissue and expose the subendothelium. A model has been developed to study prostacyclin production *in vitro* by the pulsatile perfusion of intact umbilical artery (McLaren *et al.*, 1986). Umbilical arteries from pregnancies with PIH were studied with this model (McLaren *et al.*, 1987) to assess their response to a stimulant of prostacyclin production. The results showed that the ability of the vascular endothelium to produce PGI_2 in response to a physiological stimulus is absent or substantially diminished in PIH. As umbilical artery lacks any innervation, it may depend on humoral control of blood flow by prostanoids (Tuvemo, 1980) to maintain the low-pressure/high-flow feto–placental circulation. Failure of the artery to produce prostacyclin in response to physiological stimulation may result in a high umbilical artery resistance due to vasoconstriction and low blood flow, especially when faced with the pathological challenge of increased thromboxane production in PIH. In addition, the deficiency of prostacyclin and resulting prostanoid imbalance may allow vascular damage to occur unchecked. The mechanism behind deficient prostacyclin production is obscure but it may be due to reduced activity of the enzyme systems required for prostacyclin production. These enzymes could be inactivated by free radicals or proteolytic enzymes, which might be elevated in PIH, making the PGI_2 deficiency a feature of endothelial damage and dysfunction. Other markers of endothelial damage and dysfunction, such as elevated levels of fibrinectin (Saleh et al., 1988), increased concentrations of von Willebrand's factor and plasminogen activator inhibitors can be found in PIH. These data, of course, prompt the question; what causes the endothelial damage in PIH?

Neutrophils in PIH

Neutrophils have been implicated in the pathophysiology of such vascular damage in the non-pregnant as myocardial infarction, and neutrophil depletion will attenuate such vascular injury. When neutrophils are activated, they release a variety of substances capable of mediating vascular damage: these include the contents of neutrophil granules such as elastase and other proteases which can destroy the integrity of the endothelial cells, vascular basement membrane and subendothelial matrix (Harlan, 1987). In addition, toxic oxygen species can result in membrane lipid peroxidation, lysis of endothelial cells, disruption of the endothelium and increased vascular permeability and reactivity (Harlan, 1987). Leukotrienes are also synthesized and released following neutrophil activation and they, too, will increase vascular permeability, induce vasoconstriction, and promote further neutrophil activation and adherence (Bray, 1983). A recent study using human neutrophil elastase as a measure of neutrophil activation in vivo, has shown that neutrophil activation occurs in PIH (Greer et al., 1989a). As neutrophil activation was found in both mild/moderate and severe disease, the authors suggested that neutrophil activation might be an early part of the disease process.

Neutrophil activation may contribute to the vascular lesions seen in PIH, such as those noted in the placental bed (Robertson and Khong, 1987). Neutrophil elastase can cause substantial tissue damage as its substrates include not only elastin, but also collagen, fibrinogen, complement and proteoglycans (Janoff, 1985). Release of elastase is accompanied by other neutrophil granule constituents: these include cationic proteins which increase vascular permeability (Janoff and Zweifach, 1964), and the previously mentioned acid and neutral proteases, which can destroy vascular basement membrane (Harlan, 1987). The reactive oxygen species that are also released by activated neutrophils are potent mediators of cell injury, producing membrane lipid peroxidation, lysis of endothelial cells, cell retraction, increased vascular permeability and vasoconstriction (Sacks et al., 1978). In addition, leukotriene generation by neutrophils will amplify the response by increasing adherence to vascular tissue and will also promote increased vascular permeability (Bray, 1983; Harlan, 1987). When neutrophils adhere to endothelium, a 'protected microenvironment' (Harlan, 1987) obtains at the interface between neutrophil and endothelial cell so that neutrophil granule proteases can degrade the vascular tissue while being inaccessible to plasma protease inhibitors such as α_1 antitrypsin and α_2 macroglobulin. Thus, it can be seen that activated neutrophils may contribute directly to the vascular damage seen in PIH, as well as interacting with the platelet, coagulation and complement systems that are activated in PIH. The activation of neutrophils in PIH is likely to be a secondary phenomenon, possibly triggered by immunological mechanisms which have been implicated in the aetiology of this disorder (Stirrat, 1987) or simply secondary to vascular damage *per se*; none the less, it may be an important contributor to the pathogenesis of this disease.

It is of interest that neutrophil granule enzymes (Miller *et al.*, 1985), reactive oxygen species (Ager and Gordon, 1984) and leukotrienes (Pologe *et al.*, 1984) have been shown to stimulate prostacyclin release from endothelial cells. This seems paradoxical, as PIH is associated with a deficiency of prostacyclin production, which is thought to contribute to the platelet consumption and vasoconstriction of PIH, as discussed above. However, the stimulation of prostacyclin release in response to these stimuli is likely to be a transient protective response to the initial damage. It is known that at low concentrations reactive oxygen species can stimulate cyclooxygenase, which is essential for prostacyclin production, but will inhibit both this enzyme and prostacyclin synthase at higher levels (Warso and Lands, 1983). Furthermore, high concentrations of reactive oxygen species can reorientate the arachidonic acid pathway in the cell away from the production of the cytoprotective and vasodilator agent prostacyclin towards thromboxane A_2 (Warso and Lands, 1983), a potent stimulator of platelet aggregation and vasoconstriction. As discussed above, thromboxane A_2 production is also known to be increased in PIH (Wallenberg and Rotmans, 1982). Thus, neutrophil activation may account for the necrotizing arteriopathy seen in PIH which hitherto has been poorly explained, and also for several other features of the disease, such as prostacyclin deficiency and enhanced thromboxane production. Such neutrophil activation is not confined to PIH: increased neutrophil activation has also been noted in diabetic pregnancy, compared with non-pregnant diabetics (Greer *et al.*, 1989b). It has also been shown that serum from women with PIH has a greater cytotoxic effect on cultured endothelial cells than has serum from normal pregnancies (Rodgers, Taylor and Roberts, 1988). Although the nature of this factor is not clear, the authors suggested that, as this effect diminishes following delivery, it might be released from the placenta in PIH but equally well might be related to neutrophil activation. There is also evidence of a serum factor in PIH that can increase vascular reactivity to AII *in vitro* (Tulenko *et al.*, 1987).

Summary of the pathophysiological mechanisms in PIH

From the foregoing discussion, it is clear that endothelial damage and dysfunction is a common feature in all the pathological features of PIH, whether in the uteroplacental bed or renal microcirculation. The biochemical evidence of endothelial damage includes elevated levels of von Willebrand factor and fibrinectin, which are released when endothelial cell injury occurs, and reduced PGI_2 production. Functionally, the vessels have an exaggerated response to angiotensin II and there is increased capillary permeability. Many of these features can be shown to antedate the disease process. Endothelial damage and dysfunction will stimulate activation of platelets and the coagulation system, which will promote further vascular damage. Neutrophils can also be activated by dysfunctional endothelium. Activation of platelets and the coagulation system can cause endothelial damage directly, and also

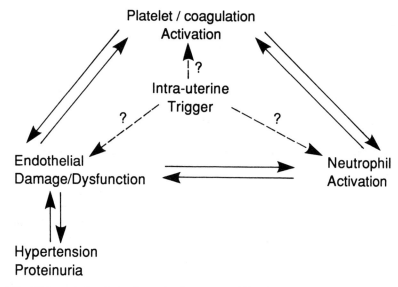

Figure 2.5. Vicious circle of platelet activation, neutrophil activation and endothelial damage and dysfunction in PIH

indirectly by activation of neutrophils. If neutrophils are activated, they will produce endothelial damage directly and also indirectly, by platelet activation. Thus, endothelial damage, the platelets and coagulation system, and neutrophils can all interact. Once one of these systems is triggered, a positive feedback loop will obtain to promote vascular damage (Figure 2.5). What triggers the initiation of this vicious circle is not clear, but it certainly originates in the uterus and most likely the placenta or uteroplacental bed, as this appears to be where the primary lesion occurs. The aetiology of the failure of trophoblast invasion also remains uncertain but the process leads to tissue ischaemia. This in turn will activate the vicious circle described above, to produce widespread endothelial damage and dysfunction. The mediator linking uteroplacental ischaemia to widespread systemic endothelial damage is not yet established. It is also obscure which facet of the vicious circle – endothelial damage, neutrophil activation or platelet activation – is triggered first. This does not mean, however, that treatment is not possible; it facilitates this, as we can focus on interrupting this positive feedback loop. Possible mechanisms to interrupt it are by treating the patient with an endothelial protectant, an anti-neutrophil agent or an anti-platelet agent. However, only the last possibility is practicable at the present time.

Anti-platelet therapy in the treatment and prevention of PIH

The above studies do not provide conclusive evidence of a cause-and-effect relationship for deficient PGI_2 production and enhanced platelet reactivity in PIH; endothelial damage and PGI_2 deficiency are more likely to be secondary phenomena in the disease. PGI_2 functions as a local protective hormone in the platelet–endothelial interaction. When platelet activation occurs, PGI_2 production is also stimulated, so that platelet aggregation and vascular damage are limited. Deficient PGI_2 production from the dysfunctional endothelium in this situation, might contribute to the pathogenesis of the vascular damage by allowing platelet activation to occur unchecked. In order to compensate for this PGI_2 deficiency, it is logical to study agents that have anti-platelet and vasodilator properties, in order to determine whether they are of any benefit to the disease process.

Prostacyclin infusion

Perhaps the most obvious choice is to replace the deficient PGI_2 by an exogenous infusion of PGI_2, which is now available as a therapeutic agent. This has been shown to be of benefit in peripheral vascular disease and Raynaud's phenomenon (Belch et al., 1983a, b). It has also been used in PIH (Belch et al., 1985; Greer and Belch, 1986), where it has been shown to lower blood pressure, reduce platelet consumption and increase urinary output in oliguric patients in the short term. However, relatively large amounts of prostacyclin were required and dose-related side effects, including flushing, headache, nausea and vomiting, were severe enough to limit the dose that could be given. In addition, tachyphylaxis rapidly developed, with loss of blood pressure control even on the maximum tolerated dose. In this situation the use of anti-hypertensive agents such as labetalol helped temporarily to restore blood pressure control. A further problem with PGI_2 infusion is that, owing to its short half-life, continuous intravenous infusions are required. These findings emphasize that prostacyclin deficiency is not the prime cause of PIH, as replacement of PGI_2 merely controls some of the features of the disease in the short term. If PGI_2 is not effective then other therapeutic possibilities must be explored.

Aspirin

Aspirin is the most practicable and effective agent available at present for clinical use as anti-platelet therapy. It has been used successfully as an anti-platelet agent in the non-pregnant situation where it has been effective in the secondary prevention of myocardial infarction and transient ischaemic attacks. More recently it has been used successfully in the prevention of PIH and IUGR. The biggest problem with regard to its use is perhaps that of identifying patients at risk who will require such therapy. This is especially true in PIH, where those with the most severe disease are often primigravidae. It acts by irreversibly inhibiting cyclo-oxygenase, which is required for prostaglandin and thromboxane production; it therefore reduces thromboxane generation and platelet activation.

There is, however, an aspirin dilemma (Greer et al., 1986a). The beneficial effects of aspirin may be offset by a similar inhibitory effect on vascular prostacyclin production, as cyclo-oxygenase is required for the production of both substances (Figure 2.6). Clearly, this is undesirable in PIH. However, low-dose aspirin may selectively block thromboxane production. Oral administration of low-dose aspirin is thought to produce pharmacologically active drug concentrations in the portal circulation and not in the systemic circulation, as aspirin is extensively metabolized by the liver. As platelet cyclo-oxygenase is irreversibly inhibited by aspirin, effective inhibition of platelet function would result from exposure to aspirin as the platelet passes through the portal circulation, while systemic vascular prostacyclin production might remain unaffected owing to lower concentrations in the systemic circulation. In addition, the nucleated vascular endothelial cells, unlike anucleate platelets, can synthesize new protein and therefore are able to replace any inactivated enzyme in a matter of hours (Heavey et al., 1985), thus maintaining prostacyclin production. The efficacy of low-dose aspirin in reducing TxA_2 production has largely been demonstrated in the non-pregnant, with doses as low as 20 mg a day reducing TxA_2 production by up to 95 per cent (Toivanen, Ylikorkala and Viinikka, 1984; Sinzinger, Virgolini and Peskar, 1989). However, it appears unlikely that any dose of aspirin can produce maximal inhibition of platelet TxA_2 production without affecting PGI_2 production to some extent, although there appears to be a high degree of relative sparing of PGI_2 production with low-dose aspirin (Fitzgerald *et al.*, 1983, 1987; Spitz *et al.*, 1988).

Perhaps the biggest concern regarding the use of aspirin in pregnancy is that of aspirin reaching the fetus and impairing haemostasis or closing the ductus arteriosus, especially around delivery. Stuart *et al.* (1982) have documented haemostatic problems in neonates whose mothers received aspirin up to 5 days before delivery. However, all of these women ingested large doses of aspirin (5–10 g). Ritter *et al.* (1987) have studied the effects of 37.5 mg aspirin administered for 2 weeks before the expected date of delivery in pregnant women. They found that this dose of aspirin, although significantly lowering maternal TxA_2 production, had no significant effect on TxA_2 production from neonatal blood or on PGI_2 production by the umbilical artery *in vitro*. This differential effect is likely to reflect the extensive first-pass metabolism of aspirin in the liver. The effects of chronic aspirin therapy (with 60 mg of aspirin a day) on neonatal platelet function have also been studied: no significant effect on neonatal platelet function was found (Louden *et al.*, 1989). Sibai *et al.* (1989) have also shown that chronic maternal therapy with aspirin in the range 20–80 mg/day has no effect on neonatal platelet function or on the ductus arteriosus. Thus, it would appear that low-dose aspirin, in the dose range employed in the clinical studies described below, has a selective effect on maternal platelet function,

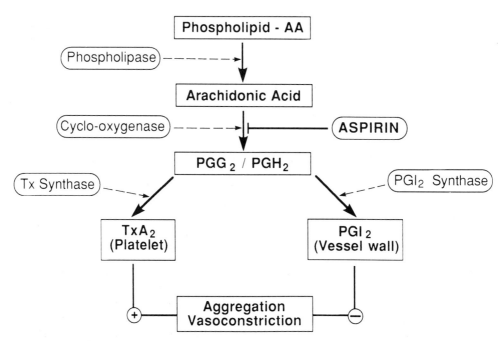

Figure 2.6.   Biosynthetic pathway for thromboxane (TxA_2) and prostacyclin (PGI_2). Effect of aspirin

Table 2.1.   Clinical studies of aspirin in pregnancies at risk of developing PIH

Study	Outcome measure	Active group	Placebo or control group	Significance
Beaufils et al. (1985)	Development of pre-eclampsia	0/48	6/45	p<0.01
	Fetal/neonatal loss	0/48	5/45	p<0.02
	Severe IUGR (live births)	0/48	4/45	p<0.05
	Mean duration of pregnancy (weeks)	38.6	36.5	p<0.001
Wallenburg et al. (1986)	Hypertensive complications	2/21	12/23	p<0.01
	Severe IUGR (<2.3 centile)	0/21	3/23	n.s.
Schiff et al. (1989)	Development of PIH	4/34	11/31	p = 0.024
	Development of pre-eclampsia	1/34	7/31	p = 0.019
	Mean adjusted birthweight centile	43.9	38.6	p<0.01
	Mean gestation at delivery (days)	278	261	p<0.001
Benigni et al. (1989)	Number developing PIH	0/17	3/16	n.s.
	Mean birthweight (g)	2922	2264	p<0.05
	No <10th centile	2/17	6/16	n.s.
	Mean duration of pregnancy (weeks)	39	35	p<0.01

sparing fetal platelet function and PGI_2 production. It is also reassuring that there is no obvious effect on the ductus arteriosus.

There have now been several studies examining the clinical efficacy of low-dose aspirin in the prevention of PIH. The first was that of Beaufils et al. (1985). They randomized 102 women at high risk of pre-eclampsia to receive either no therapy or 150 mg aspirin in combination with 300 mg dipyridamole daily. The patients were selected on the basis of their past medical and obstetric histories, such as essential hypertension or a series of complicated pregnancies. Ninety-nine of the women were parous. Owing to spontaneous abortion and patients being lost to follow-up, only 93 patients were included in the analysis. There was a significant reduction in complications in the treated group in terms of development of pre-eclampsia and perinatal outcome, as shown in Table 2.1. There were no side effects except headache associated with dipyridamole therapy, and no haemorrhagic complications were encountered. This study, however, had relatively small numbers and the groups were unbalanced with regard to several entry variables of prognostic significance, which could bring the results into question. In addition, it tested two drugs (aspirin and dipyridamole) in combination, although there is no evidence to suggest that dipyridamole will enhance the clinical effect of aspirin alone. Finally, 150 mg/day of aspirin was employed, substantially more than is required to produce effective inhibition of platelet TxA_2 production.

Shortly after this study, Wallenburg et al. (1986) (Table 2.1) published their exciting findings on low-dose aspirin therapy. They selected 46 primigravid women at risk of PIH for randomization into a double-blind placebo-controlled study of aspirin (60 mg/day) versus placebo. The selection was based on screening 207 women with angiotensin II infusions. Those who were sensitive to AII at 28 weeks' gestation, and therefore at risk of developing PIH, were recruited to the study. Forty-four women were included in the analysis. Although there was a significant reduction in the development of hypertensive complications, there was no significant effect on gestation at delivery or number of growth-retarded infants, although there was a tendency to lower incidences of these conditions in the treatment group.

In the study by Schiff et al. (1989) patients were selected on the basis of the 'roll over test' (Gant et al., 1974), although the predictive value of this test is disputed (Phelen et al., 1977). The test involves measuring blood pressure in the left lateral position; the patient then rolls on to her back, and after a few minutes the blood pressure measurement is repeated. An increase in diastolic BP of >15 mmHg after 'rolling over' is considered positive. After screening 791 women, 65 with positive tests were randomized to receive aspirin 100 mg/day or placebo in a prospective double-blind manner. The patients were of mixed parity. There was a significant reduction in hypertensive complications, an increase in gestation time at delivery, and an increase in adjusted birthweight centiles compared with the placebo group (Table 2.1). There were no maternal side effects and no maternal or neonatal haemorrhagic effects. Benigni et al. (1989) studied the effects of 60 mg aspirin or placebo in 33 women judged to be at risk of PIH on the basis of past obstetric history or past medical history, such as chronic hypertension. Treatment was started from the 12th week single blind. The treatment group had significantly higher birthweights and longer gestations than the placebo group but no other differences were noted. This study also examined urinary TxB_2 and 6-keto-$PGF_{1\alpha}$ levels following treatment. Although aspirin significantly and substantially reduced TxB_2, there was no effect on PGI_2 production as assessed by its metabolites in urine, indicating that a selective effect on platelets was occurring while sparing the endothelium. Again, no haemorrhagic complications were found in the newborn infants but there was a significant reduction in serum TxB_2 in the neonates in the treatment group, albeit not as great a reduction as occurred in the mothers. However, this suggests that, even with a dose as low as 60 mg aspirin/day, the fetus is still exposed to some active aspirin.

The potential efficacy of anti-platelet therapy with low-dose aspirin is not limited to PIH: pregnancies at risk of IUGR appear also to benefit from such therapy (Wallenburg and Rotmans, 1987; Trudinger et al., 1988). In addition, pregnancies at risk of IUGR and fetal loss because of maternal lupus erythematosus also appear to benefit (Elder et al., 1988). This is not surprising, as all these disorders are associated with vascular damage in the placental bed.

The studies on low-dose aspirin for the prevention of PIH are certainly encouraging, but do they merit the widespread introduction of such prophylaxis? The answer is not yet established as the numbers in all studies were small, and the randomization was based on past history, the controversial 'roll over test' or the AII sensitivity test, which is impracticable for widespread clinical use. The results are currently, therefore, far from conclusive. Furthermore, the majority of patients with severe disease will be primigravidae who clearly are not usually identifiable from past history. It is important, therefore, to determine whether such therapy is effective in the wider clinical setting where it could be readily and successfully employed in any obstetric unit. To this end, the Collaborative Low-Dose Aspirin Study in Pregnancy (CLASP) has been undertaken. This large double-blind placebo-controlled study should provide reliable evidence of low-dose aspirin efficacy, safety and long-term effects on the children of these pregnancies. Finally, as identification of patients, especially primigravidae, is a major problem, the report from Symonds' group (Baker, Broughton Pipkin and Symonds, 1989), that platelet AII receptors may identify women at high risk of PIH, is an exciting new development. This relatively simple test could be widely employed, with a positive result used as an indication for low-dose aspirin therapy. Until the results of large-scale studies such as CLASP are known and effective objective techniques for identification of patients at risk are available, the obstetrician must weigh up the available evidence for the benefits (and potential hazards) of aspirin against the patient's risk of significant clinical problems and treat the patient as seems appropriate.

Anti-hypertensive therapy and anti-platelet effects

Some physiologists would regard platelets as circulating smooth muscle cells, with contractile responses of their cytoskeleton related to Ca^{2+} availability. Anti-hypertensive agents are increasingly being used in the treatment of PIH. These agents will relax vascular smooth muscle. This led us to investigate the hypothesis that anti-hypertensive agents might influence platelet function. We have studied the effects of seven adrenoceptor antagonists on platelet aggregation in platelet-rich plasma *in vitro*. The drugs had differing receptor specificities, membrane-stabilizing activity, intrinsic sympathomimetic activity and lipid solubility. Labetalol ($\alpha_1\beta_1\beta_2$-blocker), pindolol ($\beta_1\beta_2$-blocker) with intrinsic sympathomimetic activity and propranolol ($\beta_1\beta_2$-blocker) inhibit platelet aggregation in a dose-dependent manner (Greer *et al.*, 1985a, e). This effect is independent of any α- or β-adrenoceptor blocking property, as atenolol (β_1-blocker), metoprolol (β_1-blocker), timolol (β_1-blocker) and prazosin (α_1-blocker) are without effect. This inhibitory effect appears to be related to the lipid solubility and membrane-stabilizing effects, as these properties are common to all three effective agents. These three drugs also inhibit thromboxane production in platelet-rich plasma and whole blood (Greer *et al.*, 1985e, f) and this appears to be due to inhibition of phospholipase A_2 activity (Greer *et al.*, 1985e).

Since these agents inhibit TxA_2 production, they might also inhibit prostacyclin production, which also depends on arachidonic acid being released from the cell membrane. However, labetalol, pindolol and propranolol have little effect on vascular prostacyclin production (Greer, McLaren and Forbes, 1990). This suggests that there may be some degree of selectivity between the effects of these agents on platelets and the vessel wall. In addition these drugs act synergistically with both exogenous prostacyclin and prostacyclin derived from umbilical arterial tissue to inhibit platelet aggregation *in vitro* (Greer, McLaren and Forbes, 1990). Such a synergistic effect might allow these drugs to compensate for PGI_2 deficiency by potentiating the effects of the residual PGI_2 produced. This ancillary effect may be of value when these agents are employed as anti-hypertensive therapy in PIH. There is also evidence suggesting that labetalol has platelet-protective effects *in vivo*. The platelet count has been shown to increase in women with severe disease after one week's therapy with labetalol (Greer *et al.*, 1985c) and platelet aggregation can be reduced *in vitro* (Greer *et al.*, 1987). Sibai *et al.* (1987) found no change in platelet count in women treated with labetalol compared with those who were not, but the initial platelet count was not suppressed in these women, suggesting that platelet consumption might not have been a significant feature in the patients studied.

These effects are not confined to the adrenoceptor antagonists, however, and calcium-channel-blocking agents have a similar effect on platelet aggregation *in vitro* (Greer *et al.*, 1986b) and platelet consumption *in vivo* (Rubin, Butters and McCabe, 1988). However, other studies with nifedipine have not noted an effect *in vivo* (Greer *et al.*, 1989c). The vasodilator hydralazine can also inhibit thromboxane production *in vitro* (Greer *et al.*, 1988b). As adrenoceptor antagonists and aspirin can inhibit platelet function by inhibition of phospholipase and cyclo-oxygenase respectively, a combination of an adrenoceptor antagonist and a low dose of aspirin might act synergistically to inhibit platelet function. The effect of a low dose of labetalol and a low dose of aspirin on platelet aggregation to collagen was therefore studied *in vitro* (Greer *et al.*, 1985b) where the combination of labetalol and aspirin acted synergistically to produce significant and substantial inhibition of platelet aggregation. This synergism may be due to the sequential inhibition of phospholipases and cyclo-oxygenase, which are both required for thromboxane production; it is not confined to adrenoceptor antagonists, as the calcium-channel blocker nicardipine has similar synergistic effects with aspirin. Such a therapeutic strategy might be of value in PIH, combining the anti-hypertensive and anti-platelet properties of adrenoceptor antagonists or calcium channel blockers with the more potent anti-platelet properties of aspirin. It may also allow even lower doses of aspirin to be used, in order to avoid the unwanted effects of aspirin therapy. Whether or not the anti-platelet effects of such anti-hypertensive therapy is of any clinical value remains to be established, but there are at least good theoretical reasons to employ an anti-hypertensive agent with anti-platelet properties in the treatment of PIH.

Management of PIH

Assessment of mother and fetus

It is clearly important to make the diagnosis of PIH as discussed above, at all times being aware of the multiplicity of possible presentations of this disorder. The severity of the disease and rate of progression must also be assessed. This will necessitate not only a blood pressure profile and assessment of proteinuria, but also laboratory assessment. The minimum that should be obtained is a full blood and platelet count, together with biochemical assessment of urea and electrolytes and plasma urate. Liver function tests should also be checked and this can often be carried out simultaneously with the electrolytes in the multiple analysis systems now available in most biochemistry departments. Those patients with fulminating disease will also require a coagulation screen.

The fetus should also be assessed as appropriate for its gestation and the clinical problem. Ultrasound assessment of growth will be required in pregnancies where growth retardation is suspected. Regular assessment of fetal well-being by fetal heart rate monitoring or biophysical profile is also required. Doppler ultrasound assessment of the umbilical artery flow velocity waveform may also be helpful in identifying fetuses at high risk of compromise (Cameron *et al.*, 1988; Haddad *et al.*, 1989), although in view of the progressive nature of the disease process in PIH, a normal flow velocity waveform is unlikely to provide any long-term prediction of fetal outcome.

The initial assessment can often be carried out in a day assessment unit (Walker, 1987), especially in those patients with mild/moderate hypertension detected at the routine antenatal clinic. The results of such an assessment will influence the subsequent management: those who are symptomatic or severely hypertensive clearly require immediate admission and treatment, as do those with significant proteinuria or evidence of gross systemic disturbances; patients with simple mild/moderate hypertension can often be monitored as outpatients. The frequency and type of monitoring tests require to be tailored to the patient's needs, as determined from the severity of the disease and presence of growth retardation. These investigations will also provide information as to the rate of progression of the disease. Thus, fully armed with information regarding the maternal and fetal condition, the obstetrician can institute management decisions. These will include when (if the subject is not already an inpatient) to admit her to hospital, how frequently maternal and fetal monitoring is required, whether anti-hypertensive therapy is required, and when and by what route delivery should be carried out.

The aim of treatment is to protect the mother and fetus from the consequences of hypertension and to prolong the pregnancy to avoid the problems of prematurity. This will require a constant evaluation and weighing up of the risks to mother and fetus of continuing the pregnancy against those of delivery, to optimize the situation for both patients.

Anti-hypertensive therapy

PIH is a curable form of hypertension; delivery will remove the disease. The philosophy of treatment is to protect the mother from the effects of hypertension, such as cerebrovascular haemorrhage and eclampsia in severe disease, and to attempt to reduce the disease progression and prolong the pregnancy where this is desirable, so reducing the risks of iatrogenic prematurity. The earlier in pregnancy the patient presents, the greater the justification in attempting conservative management, even in those with severe hypertension.

Traditionally, pre-eclampsia was treated by bed rest and sedation. Theoretically bed rest was used to try to reduce blood pressure, increase cardiac output (Ueland et al., 1969) and increase sodium excretion (Redd, Mosey and Langford, 1968). However, it may result in reduced cardiac output, due to the pressure of the gravid uterus on the great vessels (Lees et al., 1967b), and lower uteroplacental blood flow (Abitbol, 1977), which could be detrimental. There are only two controlled studies of bed rest in the literature: the first showed no benefit from bed rest in non-proteinuric hypertension (Mathews, 1977) whereas the second showed some benefit in severe proteinuric disease with intrauterine growth retardation (Mathews, Agarwal and Shuttleworth, 1982). Thus, although bed rest may be of some value in severe disease, the efficacy of bed rest in mild/moderate disease is not proven. There is no evidence to support the use of chronic sedation in the management of PIH, although it is obviously logical to employ anti-convulsants, some of which will have sedative properties, in the treatment of impending eclampsia.

The value of anti-hypertensive therapy in controlling disease progression is also far from clear. There is no doubt that anti-hypertensive treatment is essential in those with severe hypertension. However, the value of such therapy in mild/moderate disease is not universally accepted as the patient is in little immediate danger from her blood pressure per se and, if a drug is of no value, then the pregnant patient should avoid such unnecessary exposure with its risks of side effects. There is some evidence to suggest, however, that treatment of mild/moderate disease may be of benefit in reducing disease progression and hospital admissions (Walker, 1987). Thus, there is a compelling case for the use of anti-hypertensive therapy in severe disease but in mild/moderate disease the obstetrician must assess the available evidence and judge whether the benefits of treatment outweigh any potential risks or hazards in each case. The efficacy and side effects of the commonly employed agents are discussed below. It is my practice to treat those patients with mild/moderate early-onset (<36 weeks' gestation) disease. Where delivery is imminent there is little to be gained by such therapy. The benefits of this practice are not firmly established, but it may delay or reduce induction of labour or operative delivery, reduce anxiety for both mother and obstetrician, reduce the need for hospital admission and possibly reduce the incidence of progression to proteinuric disease, as discussed below, while having little in the way of obvious adverse effects.

When employing anti-hypertensive therapy in PIH a stepwise approach is required. It is often difficult to predict how a patient will respond to a particular agent in terms of blood pressure control. In addition, the patient's requirements may increase with disease progression and the rate of progression can vary from hours to weeks. Some patients with severe disease may respond well to minimal therapy, whereas some with mild/moderate disease may progress rapidly. Such a stepwise approach appears to be suitable for chronic hypertension as well as mild/moderate and severe PIH. The treatment then should consist of first-line, second-line and third-line agents: first-line therapy basically is either methyldopa or an adrenoceptor antagonist such as labetalol, atenolol or oxprenolol; second-line therapy usually takes the form of a vasodilator such as hydralazine, or more recently, nifedipine; third-line therapy will be either an adrenoceptor antagonist or methyldopa, depending on which of these agents was employed as first-line therapy. There is no ideal drug in any of these categories and, again, the obstetrician must decide which drug best suits the patient's needs. My own practice is to start therapy with labetolol 200 mg three times daily increasing to 300 mg four times daily as required. If blood pressure is not controlled, nifedipine is added in a dose of 10–20 mg two to four times a day. Usually such therapy is sufficient and if blood pressure is not adequately controlled on the combination of labetalol and nifedipine, the disease is usually sufficiently advanced to warrant delivery. However, occasionally a third-line agent is required and in this situation methyldopa is added, with the dose range being from 0.5 to 2.0 g/day. Where an adrenoceptor antagonist is felt to be contraindicated, the methyldopa is used as first-line therapy with an initial dosage of 250 mg twice daily. It should be stressed that the use of nifedipine in pregnancy is not yet firmly established (see below).

Methyldopa

Methyldopa is undoubtedly the most extensively studied drug in the treatment of hypertension in pregnancy. The first controlled trial of its use looked at the combination of methyldopa (0.5–2.0 g/day) and bendrofluazide (5–10 mg/day) versus no therapy (Leather et al., 1968). This study suggested that treatment resulted in reduced pregnancy losses (i.e. midtrimester abortions and perinatal deaths), increased birthweight and longer gestation, especially when hypertension occurred in the first half of pregnancy.

The study by Redman and colleagues (Redman et al., 1976b; Redman, Beilin and Bonnar, 1977) assessed 242 patients randomized to receive methyldopa (initial dose 0.75–1.0 g/day) or no therapy. The criteria for entry were blood pressure >140/90 mmHg before 28 weeks' gestation, or >150/95 mmHg after 28 weeks' gestation. In both subgroups such an elevation in blood pressure was found on two separate occasions at least 24 h apart. There was a significant difference in the pregnancy loss rate between the groups, with only one loss (a stillbirth) in the 117 patients in the treatment group versus nine losses (four midtrimester abortions, three stillbirths and two neonatal deaths) in the control group. The one loss in the treatment group was associated with a significant fetal abnormality, although severe pre-eclampsia also occurred. Of the five perinatal deaths in the control group, three were associated with severe pre-eclampsia, one with a small-for-gestation-age infant and intrauterine death without pre-eclampsia, and one with congenital abnormality and birth asphyxia. Overall, there was no obvious effect of treatment on fetal growth or birthweight, although in the late-onset (>28 weeks' gestation) group, gestation was significantly more advanced at delivery. Treatment also significantly reduced the frequency of severe hypertension occurring antenatally or in labour and the late-onset (>28 weeks' gestation) group spent less time in hospital than the control group. However, there was no effect on the incidence of development of proteinuria or pre-eclampsia.

One drawback to the use of methyldopa is the frequency of side effects. In the study by Redman, Beilin and Bonnar (1977), 14.5 per cent of the treatment group stopped methyldopa because of minor, but none the less troublesome, side effects. These included tiredness, loss of energy, dizziness, depression, flushes, headache, vomiting and palpitations; only the incidences of loss of energy and dizziness were significantly different between the treatment and control groups. One of the greatest strengths of this study was the long-term follow-up carried out on the children (Cockburn et al., 1982), confirming that there were no long-term adverse effects. Thus, methyldopa appears to be an effective agent for control of blood pressure and may improve fetal outcome. The relatively high incidence of side effects, however, detracts from its benefits.

Adrenoceptor antagonists

There is a wide range of adrenoceptor antagonists that have varying receptor specificities and varying degrees of intrinsic sympathomimetic activity. Only atenolol, labetolol and oxprenolol have been studied to any great extent in pregnancy, although others such as propranolol and pindolol have also been used. Adrenoceptor antagonists had a poor start in PIH as several anecdotal and uncontrolled reports suggested that they might have harmful side effects, such as depressed neonatal respiration (Tunstall, 1969), growth retardation (Pruyn, Phelan and Buchanan, 1979), neonatal hypoglycaemia (Habib and McArthy, 1977), and an increase in perinatal mortality (Lieberman et al., 1978). These complications, however, can all result from the disease process itself. Larger controlled or comparative studies have not shown significant differences in such complications between adrenoceptor-antagonist-treated and methyldopa-treated patients or untreated control groups (Rubin et al., 1983; Gallery, Ross and Gyory, 1985; Pickles, Symonds and Broughton Pipkin, 1989), but one large study has suggested a higher incidence of growth retardation in patients treated with labetalol compared with an untreated control group (Sibai et al., 1987). In the atenolol study carried out by Rubin et al. (1983), the infants were followed up after 1 year, and no harmful effects of treatment were found (Reynolds et al., 1984). Thus, at least in the short term, these agents appear to be safe for the fetus, although they have not yet been subject to the same long-term paediatric assessment as methyldopa.

There have been few placebo-controlled studies of anti-hypertensive therapy in pregnancy. Rubin et al. (1983) performed a prospective randomized placebo-controlled study of atenolol (a β_1 selective adrenoceptor antagonist) in the treatment of 120 women with mild/moderate hypertension in the third trimester. Atenolol treatment resulted in a significant fall in blood pressure, a significantly lower incidence of progression to proteinuric disease and a reduction in time spent in hospital. However there was no difference between the groups in birthweight, or in other measures of perinatal outcome. Perinatal mortality was low in this study, with only one death occurring in each group. It is of interest that the incidence of respiratory distress was higher in the control group. Bradycardia was noted in 37 per cent of neonates compared with 8 per cent of controls, but was not sufficiently troublesome to warrant treatment in any case. In contrast to the findings of studies on methyldopa, the drug was well tolerated, with only two patients in the treatment group (compared with one in the placebo group) withdrawing because of side effects. Although lassitude and breathlessness were reported more frequently in the atenolol-treated group, there was no significant difference between the groups regarding possible drug-related adverse effects. An additional report on this study showed that atenolol did not adversely affect fetal monitoring tests, in particular fetal heart-rate monitoring (Rubin *et al.*, 1984).

Metoprolol, another selective β_1-adrenoceptor antagonist, has also been assessed by placebo-controlled trial in 52 women (Wichman, Ryulden and Karlberg, 1984). Although blood pressure was reduced by metoprolol, there was no effect on progression to pre-eclampsia and there was a tendency for infants to be lighter in the metoprolol-treated group than in the placebo group.

Labetalol is a unique combined α_1, β_1, β_2-adrenoceptor antagonist. It has been subject to several controlled assessments although only one has been placebo controlled (Pickles, Symonds and Broughton Pipkin, 1989). In this study, data were analysed from 144 women with mild/moderate non-proteinuric disease with a starting dose of 100 mg three times daily increasing to 200 mg three times daily: labetalol significantly reduced blood pressure and this effect was sustained over several weeks. There were no perinatal deaths in the study, and there was no apparent beneficial or detrimental effect on fetal growth; however, the incidences of preterm delivery, respiratory distress syndrome and jaundice tended to be reduced in the labetalol group. An open randomized study of labetalol versus bed rest in 100 patients (Walker, 1987) showed that not only could labetalol control blood pressure, it could also significantly reduce disease progression in terms of the development of proteinuria or severe hypertension. A similar open study of labetalol and hospitalization versus hospitalization alone was conducted by Sibai *et al.* (1987). They studied 200 women with proteinuria and blood pressure readings between 140 and 160 mmHg systolic and 90–110 mmHg diastolic. There was a significant fall in blood pressure in the labetalol group. There was no difference in disease progression, length of gestation at delivery or degree of pregnancy prolongation between the groups. They found no improvement in perinatal outcome and the number of infants that were small for dates for their gestational age was significantly higher in the labetalol group. Thus, the reports on the effects of labetalol have not been consistent, although the study of Sibai *et al.* (1987) was on a group of patients with significant proteinuria, whose disease was therefore of greater severity than that of the patients reported by Walker (1987); clearly, no effect on development of proteinuria could be studied. These studies showed no detrimental effects on the neonate, in keeping with the study of MacPherson, Broughton Pipkin and Rutter (1986), which showed that babies born to women treated with labetalol had no adverse effects except for a mild non-problematic hypotensive effect.

These studies seem to support the view that treatment of mild/moderate (non-proteinuric) disease with anti-hypertensive agents may be beneficial. Fletcher and Bulpitt (1988), reviewing such studies, concluded that there was a clear case for anti-hypertensive therapy, and pointed out that improvements in neonatal care may have obscured some of the possible benefits in more recent studies. They performed pooled relative risk analyses on the studies they reviewed and found a relative risk of 0.37 [95 per cent confidence interval (CI) 0.17–0.80] for mortality (fetal, perinatal, neonatal) and 0.57 (95 per cent CI 0.29–1.12) for development of proteinuria or pre-eclampsia, to support their conclusions. They also noted that there was a tendency to lower birthweight in the treated groups, which could reflect either an effect of the treatment or improved survival of high-risk preterm infants.

The above discussion suggests that the disease should be treated with anti-hypertensive agents. Next, the choice of agent should be considered. It may be that, as Rubin (1987) suggested, the agent itself is not important but that the benefits may ensue simply from good blood pressure control. Several comparative studies have been performed. In particular, oxprenolol (a non-selective β-receptor antagonist with intrinsic sympathomimetic activity) and methyldopa have been compared in large controlled studies (Fidler *et al.*, 1983; Gallery, Ross and Gyory, 1985). Both agents appeared to be equally effective in controlling blood pressure but there was no difference in disease progression or perinatal outcome, although Gallery, Ross and Gyory (1985) showed that oxprenolol therapy was associated with a significantly higher number of infants of normal birthweight for gestation. However, this difference lost significance after 8 weeks' therapy. The authors have suggested that the early effect is attributable to oxprenolol producing peripheral vasodilatation and they suggest that, over time, the same effect can be achieved with long-term control of blood pressure, as seen in the methyldopa group.

Labetalol has been compared with methyldopa in the treatment of severe disease and was found to be as effective as, although not superior to, methyldopa (Redman, 1982). Again in severe disease, Michael (1986) compared intravenous labetalol and diazoxide immediately before delivery and found that labetalol appeared to produce better blood pressure control.

Lardoux *et al.* (1983) reported a comparative study of labetalol and atenolol and showed that both drugs effectively controlled blood pressure, with no significant adverse effects on mother or fetus. The results did suggest, however, that the atenolol group was associated with significantly lower birthweights. This was not a randomized study, so that the interpretation of these data is limited. Such an effect is not inconceivable, however, as labetalol and atenolol may have different effects upon blood flow. As labetalol has a direct α_1-adrenoceptor-blocking component it can produce peripheral vasodilatation. This may be useful in PIH that is associated with vasoconstriction, and might increase uteroplacental blood flow. However, studies on uteroplacental and fetal blood flow have shown (Lunell *et al.*, 1982; Jouppila *et al.*, 1986), that despite a significant fall in blood pressure there were no changes in fetal or placental flows. As atenolol is a β_1-cardioselective adrenoceptor antagonist, it has no direct vasodilator effect. As similar β_1-selective agents have been shown to reduce fetal tolerance to hypoxia in animals (Kjellmar *et al.*, 1984), Montan *et al.* (1987) assessed the effect of short-term atenolol therapy on fetal and placental blood flow using Doppler ultrasound. Although they found an increased pulsatility index in both the maternal arcuate arteries and fetal aorta, suggesting that an increase in vascular resistance was occurring, all values remained within the normal range. As there was no placebo-treated group it is difficult to draw firm conclusions from these findings.

Labetalol therefore offers some potential, although clinically unproven, advantages over atenolol by means of its vasodilator α_1-adrenoceptor antagonist activity.

In addition, labetalol has anti-platelet effects *in vitro* (Greer *et al.*, 1985a, e) and is synergistic with low-dose aspirin in inhibiting platelet aggregation *in vitro* (Greer *et al.*, 1985b). These effects may also be manifest *in vivo* (Greer *et al.*, 1985c, 1987) although again the clinical value of this is unconfirmed.

Thus, both methyldopa and adrenoceptor antagonists are suitable agents for the treatment of PIH. The adrenoceptor antagonists cause fewer subjective side effects than methyldopa. Within the adrenoceptor antagonist group, labetalol has several theoretical advantages over atenolol, although these are largely of unproven value in the clinical setting. Atenolol does, however, have a slower onset of action and a flatter dose–response curve than labetalol. The author therefore favours labetalol in view of its greater flexibility and potential beneficial effects. Ultimately, however, it is probably best for the clinician to use an accustomed agent to obtain good control of hypertension, which is the main objective.

Hydralazine

Hydralazine is established in the treatment of severe and acute hypertension, where it has been employed by intramuscular injection, intravenous boluses and continuous intravenous infusions. It is also used orally in the chronic situation as a second-line anti-hypertensive agent. It acts by inhibiting contraction of vascular smooth muscle, although the precise mechanism whereby this is achieved is not clear. It has a delay in onset of action of 20–30 minutes, even when given intravenously. It is associated with a tachycardia which is thought to be brought about by two mechanisms: a baroreceptor-mediated reflex tachycardia and prolonged stimulation of noradrenaline release (Lin *et al.*, 1983). The stimulation of noradrenaline release may account for symptoms, such as anxiety and restlessness as well as tachycardia, seen following hydralazine use. Headache is a significant side effect. This may be due to dilatation of the cerebral venous circulation leading to increased intracranial pressure and headache, before dilating the resistance vessels and increasing cerebral flow (Overgaard and Skinhoj, 1975). These side effects of hydralazine are unwelcome in the management of the severe pre-eclamptic, as the headache and noradrenaline-related effects may mimic the prodromal symptoms of eclampsia, so confusing the situation. Despite the fall in blood pressure and increased cardiac output that occurs, there is no evidence that hydralazine will improve uteroplacental perfusion (Lunell *et al.*, 1983; Jouppila *et al.*, 1985); indeed, noradrenaline release may reduce uteroplacental perfusion, as it has been shown to be a vasoconstrictor of this vascular bed in animal studies (Wallenburg and Hutchinson, 1979). These side effects can be reduced if hydralazine is used with methyldopa or an adrenoceptor antagonist which will inhibit the sympathetic effects and reflex tachycardia. In addition, it will potentiate the anti-hypertensive effects of these agents and is therefore a valuable second-line therapy in the chronic situation when administered orally. Hydralazine has been compared with labetalol (Walker, Greer and Calder, 1983; Mabie *et al.*, 1987). The study of Walker, Greer and Calder (1983) compared intramuscular hydralazine (10 mg) and oral labetalol (200 mg) in patients with acute hypertension (diastolic BP >105 mmHg): both agents produced a significant fall in blood pressure. However, those who received hydralazine had a higher incidence of side effects, namely tachycardia, headache and nausea, which did not occur with labetalol. Mabie *et al.* (1987) compared intravenous hydralazine and labetalol given as intermittent boluses in severe hypertension: both drugs effectively lowered blood pressure, with labetalol having a more rapid effect. Those patients receiving hydralazine again developed reflex tachycardia.

Hydralazine, although highly effective in reducing blood pressure, is far from ideal as a parenteral first-line anti-hypertensive in severe PIH, with its side effects liable to confuse the assessment of the situation. Labetalol is therefore becoming increasingly popular in this situation, with its faster onset of action and reduced side effects. Hydralazine, however, is an excellent second-line agent, where it will potentiate the effects of methyldopa and adrenoceptor antagonists with less noradrenaline-mediated side effects.

Calcium-channel-blocking agents

Calcium-channel-blocking agents such as nifedipine have recently become established as first- and second-line therapy in hypertension in the non-pregnant. These drugs are potent vasodilators with a rapid onset when given orally (or sublingually). They act by blocking calcium influx into smooth muscle cells, so interfering with excitation–contraction coupling (Braunwald, 1982). A useful attribute of these agents is that the degree of reduction in blood pressure they produce appears to be directly proportional to the pre-treatment pressure (Braunwald, 1982). The calcium-channel-blocking agent nitrendipine has been shown to reduce vascular sensitivity to angiotensin II infusions in pregnant sheep (Lawrence and Broughton Pipkin, 1986). These drugs also have inhibitory effects on platelet function *in vitro* and *in vivo* (Greer *et al.*, 1986b; Greer, 1987) and may therefore be of value in the treatment of PIH.

Both nifedipine (Walters and Redman, 1984) and nitrendipine (Allen *et al.*, 1987), which are dihydropyridine calcium antagonists, have been assessed in the acute treatment of hypertension in pregnancy where they were found to be effective in controlling blood pressure, with no major maternal or fetal adverse effects. Despite the vasodilator effect of these agents, there appear to be minimal problems with tachycardia. Transient facial flushing, headache and warm sweaty extremities appear to be the most common side effects.

Nifedipine has also been assessed as a second-line agent in PIH and essential hypertension (Constantine *et al.*, 1987; Greer *et al.*, 1989c). In the study by Constantine *et al.* (1987), nifedipine slow-release tablets were given in a dose of up to 120 mg/day as second-line therapy, where either atenolol or methyldopa was the first-line agent. The patients were mostly essential hypertensives. The study by Greer *et al.* (1989c) examined nifedipine in doses up to 80 mg/day as a second-line therapy in women with severe PIH who had been treated with labetalol as first-line therapy. In both studies it was found that nifedipine was an effective anti-hypertensive agent but there appeared to be no effect on disease progression, although Greer *et al.* (1989c) suggested that gestation might be prolonged simply by keeping the blood pressure under control. In both studies, maternal side effects were minimal and were similar to those noted by Walters and Redman (1984). Tachycardia in particular was not found to be a problem and this is likely to be related to pre-treatment with adrenoceptor antagonists. Although in these two studies of chronic nifedipine therapy there was no clear adverse effect on the fetus, the perinatal outcome was poor, with five small-for-gestational-age infants and one intrauterine death out of 17 patients reported by Greer *et al.* (1989c) and 13 small-for-gestational-age infants, two stillbirths and a neonatal death out of the 23 patients reported by Constantine *et al.* (1987). In view of the severity of the disease in the patients studied, the perinatal outcomes are more likely to be related to the disease process than the drug therapy. However, the possibility of a drug effect cannot be completely excluded and, therefore, although these agents are effective in controlling blood pressure, they should be used with caution in pregnancy until their safety is firmly established.

On this cautionary note, calcium-channel blockers have been reported to reduce uteroplacental blood flow in normotensive pregnant animals (Lirette, Holbrook and Katz, 1987) and hypoxaemia and acidosis have also been reported (Ducsay *et al.*, 1987). However, the normotensive situation differs substantially from PIH. In the former, the spiral arteries are converted to uteroplacental arteries by trophoblast invasion; in this process their muscular components are lost and a low-resistance/high-flow system is formed (see above). In PIH this change fails to occur and uteroplacental flow is reduced. Thus, while calcium-channel-blocking agents have little direct effect on the normal uteroplacental bed, they may be able to exert a direct vasodilatory effect in PIH because of the preservation of the muscular component of the arteries. As intervillous perfusion is pressure dependent in normal pregnancy and flow dependent in PIH, calcium-channel blockers may reduce flow in normotensive pregnancy and increase it in PIH. This, however, is speculative and further work is required to investigate the cardiovascular changes of these drugs in PIH to examine whether any beneficial or detrimental effect occurs on uteroplacental flow. Finally, it should be noted that nifedipine can be potentiated by magnesium sulphate, producing profound hypotension (Waisman *et al.*, 1988).

Fulminating pre-eclampsia

The fulminating pre-eclamptic woman requires intensive care in a labour ward equipped and staffed for such patients; management is best carried out by a team of an experienced obstetrician and anaesthetist. The patient must be rapidly assessed, as discussed above, treated and monitored. Monitoring, in addition to emergency biochemical tests, and assessment of coagulation status, will require automated blood pressure measurement, ideally by an arterial line, central venous pressure monitoring and hourly urine output measurement. Venous access is essential, but minimal fluids should be given to maintain access (around 60 ml/h) as these patients, although having a contracted intravascular volume, are overloaded with extracellular fluid. Excessive fluid administration such as dilute drug solutions can easily result in fluid overload and pulmonary oedema, especially if central venous monitoring is not employed. Prophylactic anticonvulsants should be administered as discussed in the section dealing with eclampsia. Blood pressure should be controlled. Hydralazine has been the main therapy employed in the past but labetalol is effective in this situation and has several advantages, including a more rapid onset and fewer side effects, as discussed above. It is best administered by continuous intravenous infusion with the dose titrated to control the patient's blood pressure. Diazoxide has been used in the past in this situation but has been associated with severe hypotension with cerebral damage. There is no longer any need for its use, as labetalol and hydralazine are better alternatives. Alternatives in the situation where good control is not obtained by labetalol or hydralazine include sodium nitropresside infusions. These are highly effective but, as the drug is potentially toxic to the fetus, it is best used following delivery or immediately pre-partum. Intravenous calcium channel blockers such as nicardipine, which has an intravenous preparation, may also prove useful but are as yet unexplored in this situation.

As PIH is associated with a contracted intravascular volume, the use of volume expansion therapy has been explored in severe disease in an attempt to lower blood pressure and increase renal and placental blood flow (Duncan, 1989). The mechanism underlying the hypotensive effect of volume expansion with plasma protein solutions is not clear and appears not to be related to plasma volume expansion *per se* (Gallery *et al.*, 1984). Although the successful use of volume expansion therapy has been documented (Belfort *et al.*, 1989), it is a potentially dangerous procedure as it may provoke circulatory overload and pulmonary oedema. If it is to be employed, then central monitoring with at least a central venous pressure line or preferably a Swan–Ganz catheter is mandatory to guide therapy. Volume expansion is usually combined with a vasodilator to facilitate the administration of volume expansion to an already contracted vascular compartment under high pressure. The usual haemodynamic status of women with severe PIH is an increased systemic vascular resistance, a hyperdynamic left ventricle and normal pulmonary vascular resistance (Clark and Cotton, 1988). Such a haemodynamic profile will usually be improved by volume expansion coupled with a vasodilator. If, however, the left ventricular function is depressed because of an excessive afterload and pulmonary artery pressures are increased, as sometimes occurs in PIH, then volume expansion can potentially worsen the situation. Similarly, if there is an increased pulmonary capillary permeability (diagnosed by pulmonary oedema on chest radiograph, with normal left ventricular function and pulmonary artery pressure) then, again, volume expansion with plasma protein solutions will exacerbate the pulmonary oedema by increasing the extravascular colloid osmotic pressure; hence the need for a Swan–Ganz catheter. Although beneficial in the short term, longer-term benefits from this form of therapy are not clear. It cannot, therefore, be considered an established and beneficial form of therapy. If it is to be employed it should be used only with experienced obstetric and anaesthetic personnel in an intensive care facility with central monitoring equipment.

Delivery must be expedited by the most suitable route, which will be decided by the obstetrician weighing up the relative risks of abdominal and vaginal delivery, taking into account both the maternal and fetal state and gestation. Epidural analgesia is ideal (in the absence of a coagulopathy) for both abdominal and vaginal deliveries. It will aid blood pressure control by reducing catecholamine release in response to pain, but should not be considered a primary treatment for hypertension. General anaesthesia can be hazardous in these patients: not only will they often have laryngeal oedema, making intubation difficult, but laryngoscopy may provoke extreme hypertension, risking cerebral complications. A controlled study (Ramanathan *et al.*, 1988a) has recently shown that this response can be ameliorated effectively by pre-treatment with intravenous labetalol.

If a coagulopathy complicates the situation, this is best corrected by delivery, combined with supportive measures with blood products such as platelet concentrate and fresh-frozen plasma, as required.

Management of eclampsia

The definition and diagnosis of eclampsia is discussed above. However it should again be noted that, although it is a rare problem in obstetrics in the UK, with an incidence of 0.036 per cent over the years 1978–86 reported in the Oxford area (Redman, 1988), it remains the leading cause of maternal death (Department of

Health, 1989). It can arise following PIH/pre-eclampsia or *de novo*. It may be asymptomatic or be preceded by the classic prodrome of headache, visual disturbance and epigastric pain. Hypertension and proteinuria may not previously have been noted. Indeed, hypertension may not be severe, and proteinuria can be absent in 20–40 per cent (Porapakkham, 1979; Villar and Sibai, 1988). Around 50 per cent of cases occur before labour, with 25 per cent occurring in the postpartum period. It is important, then, to be aware of all these possible presentations in order to provide prompt and adequate treatment, especially in view of the limited experience which obstetricians now have of this uncommon condition. Our inadequacies in diagnosis of patients at risk are highlighted by the finding that most women have their first seizure while in hospital. The differential diagnosis will include epilepsy, coincidental cerebrovascular accident, a space-occupying lesion, infection or metabolic disturbance, and such conditions may need to be considered and excluded, especially in patients with atypical or late-onset presentation.

Although pre-eclampsia is an indication for urgent delivery, it is important to control and prevent seizures, control blood pressure and assess the mother and fetus before delivery. This should include assessment of the maternal neurological, respiratory and cardiovascular systems, and also fetal well-being, to optimize the management and delivery. Laboratory assessments should be carried out. Full blood count is required to obtain a platelet count; the haematocrit may be increased in keeping with the reduced plasma volume. A blood film is required to detect the red cell fragmentation associated with possible microangiopathic haemolytic anaemia and a coagulation screen is required to assess the possibility of DIC complicating the disease process. Tests of arterial blood gases and biochemistry should be performed to assess respiratory, renal and liver functions. A chest radiograph may be required if pulmonary oedema is suspected and, occasionally, a CT brain scan may be indicated to exclude or diagnose intracranial pathology, although this is usually best delayed until the immediate problem is controlled and the patient delivered. An intravenous line and urinary catheter are essential and central venous monitoring is often required. The first priority, however, is to control seizures. Various anticonvulsants have been employed to arrest and prevent seizures but it is best to consider arrest and prevention as two separate functions as there is no single preparation which is ideal for both roles.

Diazepam and chlormethiazole

Diazepam is the drug of first choice for halting seizures. It should be given in repeated boluses of 10 mg intravenously (up to around 50 mg) until seizures are stopped. It can be given per rectum if venous access is impossible. It impairs the conscious level and, if high doses are used, can suppress respiration. It crosses the placenta and has effects on the fetus. It will suppress beat-to-beat variation on the cardiotocograph, and neonatal effects include respiratory depression, poor feeding, hypotonia and hypothermia (Owen, Irani and Blair, 1972; Scher, Hailey and Beard, 1972; Cree, Meyer and Hailey, 1973; Rowlatt, 1978). Although continuous diazepam infusions have been successfully used to prevent further seizures, these side effects mean that, whereas it is ideal for halting convulsions, it is not ideal for preventing seizures.

The use of chlormethiazole for eclampsia has been popularized in the UK following the report of Duffus, Tunstall and MacGillivray (1968) on its use in this situation. It is administered as a 0.8 per cent solution and is usually stored at 4°C. It is effective in stopping convulsions with a dose of around 40–100 ml intravenously. The dose is subsequently titrated to keep the patient drowsy but rousable, so preventing further seizures. The major maternal risk is respiratory depression or obstruction, and careful and continuous monitoring by a trained observer is essential. In addition, large volumes of fluid may be administered to gain control of seizures and there is a risk of fluid overload and pulmonary oedema, especially as these patients may have a contracted intravascular volume. In the neonate, respiratory depression can occur (Duffus et al., 1969). Again, as it is best to avoid sedative agents for prevention of seizures, chlormethiazole cannot be considered an ideal preparation. This is borne out by the risk of respiratory depression and fluid overload, which contribute to maternal deaths in this condition (Department of Health and Social Security, 1986). In addition, such an agent will hamper the neurological assessment of the patient, who may have significant intracerebral pathology.

Phenytoin

Phenytoin is one of the most commonly used anticonvulsants in non-pregnant patients and has recently been employed in the prevention of eclampsia (Slater et al., 1987; Ryan, Lange and Naugler, 1989). It has a rapid onset when administered intravenously and does not cause sedation at therapeutic levels. However, owing to rapid redistribution of the drug following administration, a large loading dose must be employed to obtain therapeutic levels. Several regimens have been employed. The first reported was that of Slater et al. (1987) who used an 18 mg/kg intravenous bolus as a loading dose, followed 12 h later by a 500 mg dose. Ryan, Lange and Naugler (1989) have recently compared a variety of dosing regimens. They suggest that the most effective in providing reliable therapeutic levels and minimizing side effects is an initial loading dose of 10 mg/kg followed by 5 mg/kg 2 h later, with maintenance therapy starting 12 h after the second dose. The initial maintenance dose is 200 mg three times daily given orally or intravenously but this requires to be adjusted according to plasma phenytoin levels, which should be checked 6 and 12 h after the second intravenous bolus, then daily as long as maintenance therapy continues. Assessment of levels should take into account the plasma albumin concentration, as phenytoin is protein bound and these patients are often hypo-albuminaemic. In addition, phenytoin clearance is increased in pregnancy (Winter and Tozer, 1986) and pregnant women require much higher doses to achieve therapeutic levels. After delivery, however, phenytoin clearance diminishes rapidly. Thus, if maintenance therapy is employed after delivery it is essential that plasma levels be monitored. Significant side effects are minimal: a burning sensation may be felt at the injection site; transient hypotension can occur but this appears to be related to the rate of the infusion rather than the total dose (Cranford et al., 1978). Cardiac arrhythmias have been reported with intravenous phenytoin, related to its membrane-stabilizing action; however, these are likely to occur only in patients with pre-existing cardiac problems (Cranford et al., 1978) such as ischaemic heart disease, or conduction problems, which are rare in the obstetric population. In the studies of Slater et al. (1987) and Ryan, Lange and Naugler (1989) no arrhythmias were encountered. Nevertheless, ECG, pulse and blood pressure monitoring should be employed during the infusion because of the small risk of cardiovascular collapse. Other transient side effects that may be encountered after loading are choreoathetosis, dizziness, visual upset, hyperacusis, tinnitus, nystagmus, nausea and vomiting, circumoral tingling and incoordination. Phenytoin can be administered in saline

(Slater *et al.*, 1987) but there is a small risk of precipitation and a filter should be used in the infusion line. As phenytoin can upset the production of vitamin K-dependent coagulation factors, the infants of such mothers should be treated with vitamin K. The papers of Slater *et al.* (1987) and Ryan, Lange and Naugler (1989) should be consulted by the reader before employing this agent. The regimen of Ryan, Lange and Naugler (1989) has been successfully employed in our unit for 2 years. It is impracticable (at least in one centre), owing to the rarity of eclampsia, to perform a controlled trial of secondary prophylaxis of eclamptic seizures with anticonvulsants, but phenytoin appears to be the most satisfactory agent for the prevention of seizures.

Magnesium sulphate

Although unpopular and little used in the UK, magnesium sulphate is widely used as an anticonvulsant in the United States where it has been found to be effective in controlling seizures (Pritchard and Pritchard, 1975). It does not cause maternal or neonatal depression. Although its precise mechanism of action is obscure, it appears to have a peripheral site of action at the neuromuscular junction (Ramanathan *et al.*, 1988b) and does not cross the intact blood–brain barrier (Donaldson, 1986). It does not appear to protect the patient from central seizure activity as recorded on electroencephalograms (Sibai *et al.*, 1984). The peripheral effects can be seen clinically, toxicity being associated with loss of patellar reflexes and, at higher magnesium levels, respiratory arrest, paralysis and cardiac arrest; the antidote for such toxicity is intravenous calcium gluconate. Neonatal hypermagnesaemia may also be seen after 24 h of therapy (Lipsitz, 1971).

Other therapy

In resistant cases where seizures are not controlled by anticonvulsants, the patient may require thiopentone, for general anaesthesia, and neuromuscular blocking agents. In parallel with whichever anticonvulsant is employed, parenteral anti-hypertensive therapy is also essential: usually intravenous labetalol or hydralazine will be employed, as discussed above. In addition, care should be taken with regard to fluid balance and monitoring of urinary output.

HELLP syndrome

Haemolysis, abnormalities of liver function and thrombocytopenia have long been recognized as complications of PIH. Such complications may exist without severe hypertension or gross coagulation disturbance. In 1982 Weinstein described 29 cases of severe pre-eclampsia or eclampsia complicated by microangiopathic haemolytic anaemia, elevated liver enzymes and low platelet count for which he derived the acronym HELLP: haemolysis (H), elevated liver enzymes (EL) and low platelets (LP). Weinstein (1982) argued that this was an entity distinct from pre-eclampsia *per se*, although part of the disease process. Others have suggested that it is simply three features of the disease that may appear together (Goodlin, 1976; MacKenna, Dover and Browne, 1983). It is difficult to believe that such a constellation of features is not simply part of the disease process of PIH. Although some workers have suggested that the thrombocytopenia and microangiopathic haemolytic anaemia cannot be attributable to DIC, as the coagulation tests (such as the prothrombin and kaolin cephalin clotting times) are normal, Greer, Cameron and Walker (1985) have argued that the phenomenon is really a reflection of low-grade DIC, which cannot be detected on these insensitive coagulation tests. Thus Weinstein's conclusions (Weinstein, 1982) may be based on the 'technical inadequacies' of these coagulation tests, for more sensitive measures of coagulation and fibrinolysis will be deranged, as discussed above. None the less, the classification of this syndrome is of value, as it draws the clinician's attention to the wider ramifications of the disease process of PIH, which may be present even when the blood pressure is not grossly elevated.

These patients, regardless of blood pressure, must be regarded as having severe PIH. The most common symptoms are epigastric or right hypochondrial pain, nausea and vomiting (Weinstein, 1982, 1985) and all pregnant women presenting with such symptoms should have PIH/HELLP syndrome excluded, regardless of blood pressure, as up to 50 per cent of such patients may be normotensive by conventional criteria.

To diagnose the problem, full blood count and a blood film are essential to measure platelet count and look for red cell fragmentation. Biochemical tests are required, to detect increased urate and elevated transaminases; bilirubin levels are often mildly elevated. A full coagulation screen should be performed, as such patients may have, or develop, gross DIC. In clinical practice this problem is frequently misdiagnosed as viral hepatitis, cholestasis of pregnancy, cholecystitis, hyperemesis, or acute fatty liver of pregnancy.

The management of such patients usually requires urgent delivery in the maternal interest although conservative management may be possible (MacKenna, Dover and Browne, 1983). Blood pressure control and careful maternal and fetal monitoring are required and supportive therapy for coagulation disorders may be necessary.

Chronic and secondary hypertension

Essential hypertension

Essential hypertension is a diagnosis of exclusion: hypertension without a recognized cause. The diagnosis can be made only after adequate investigation excluding renal disease, phaeochromocytoma, Conn's syndrome, Cushing's syndrome and coarctation of the aorta, and can usually be carried out completely only after pregnancy. The patient may, however, have had these diagnoses excluded before pregnancy or may present with significant hypertension in the first half of pregnancy, which is likely to indicate an underlying chronic hypertensive problem. The presence of essential hypertension will increase the risks of superimposed PIH (by around fivefold) (Butler and Bonham, 1963) and of growth retardation, although in the absence of superimposed PIH these women usually have a normal outcome. The severity of hypertension in the first half of pregnancy appears to correlate with outcome in terms of fetal loss and growth retardation (Chesley and Annito, 1947; Page and Christianson, 1976). Women with chronic hypertension are likely to develop recurrent superimposed PIH in future pregnancies and this can be increasingly severe; in contrast, the primigravida with 'pure PIH' and no underlying problem has a much-reduced risk of developing severe PIH in future pregnancies.

The patient with essential hypertension may have an exaggerated physiological fall in blood pressure during the first half of pregnancy (Chesley, 1978); the diagnosis may, therefore, be missed. On the other hand, during the second half of pregnancy, an exaggerated increase in blood pressure may occur with the risk of confusing the diagnosis with PIH. Plasma urate is usually a good discriminator in this situation.

In the patient who presents with a chronically elevated blood pressure (diastolic BP >90 mmHg) in the first half of pregnancy, an underlying chronic hypertensive problem is present and this is usually essential hypertension. A full medical history should be taken: in particular, any history of renal problems should be sought and a physical examination performed. Investigations should include a blood pressure profile, MSU for bacteriological tests, urinalysis, full blood count, and assessment of urea, creatinine and electrolytes and urinary catecholamine levels. Further investigations will depend on the results of these initial tests and may include renin and aldosterone levels, intravenous urogram, renal angiogram, renal biopsy and a dexamethasone suppression test. Clearly, many of these investigations cannot be performed until the pregnancy is completed and these women should be reviewed following delivery, to make a firm diagnosis. In the absence of positive investigations during the pregnancy, these patients will be provisionally labelled as having essential hypertension.

Treatment of essential hypertension with anti-hypertensive agents will reduce exacerbations of hypertension and may reduce fetal loss (Leather et al., 1968; Redman et al., 1976b; Redman, Beilin and Bonnar, 1977). If the patient has mild essential hypertension, she may be able to stop anti-hypertensive therapy before pregnancy; regular observations can be made of blood pressure during pregnancy, and treatment started when appropriate. Patients with moderate to severe hypertension should continue treatment, as the commonly used anti-hypertensive agents do not pose any teratogenic risk. If the patient is receiving diuretic therapy, this should be stopped as it may increase the plasma urate (confusing the diagnosis) and reduce the plasma volume (Sibai, Grossman and Grossman, 1984). It is probably best to prescribe an anti-hypertensive agent that has been extensively used in pregnancy: although methyldopa is the most widely studied agent, the adrenoceptor antagonists, labetalol, atenolol and oxprenolol, are also suitable as first-line agents. If blood pressure is not adequately controlled, then a second-line agent can be added: hydralazine is perhaps the most commonly employed agent, although, increasingly, calcium-channel-blocking agents such as nifedipine are being employed, especially when superimposed PIH occurs (Constantine et al., 1987; Greer et al., 1989c). Although nifedipine is certainly effective in controlling blood pressure, it has not been sufficiently widely used to exclude adverse effects completely in pregnancy, nor has it been subject to any controlled trial. If a third-line agent is required, then methyldopa or an adrenoceptor antagonist can be used, depending on the chosen first-line agent. Angiotensin-converting enzyme inhibitors are contraindicated, as they are associated with fetal loss in animals (Broughton Pipkin, Turner and Symonds, 1980) and growth retardation in humans, possibly owing to the role of the renin–angiotensin system in the regulation of uteroplacental blood flow (see above). When the patient with a very high blood pressure and chronic underlying hypertension is encountered in early pregnancy, there is no need to rush in with parenteral anti-hypertensive therapy, as the blood pressure problem is likely to have been longstanding, with autoregulatory mechanisms compensating with regard to organ flow such as cerebral perfusion. A stepwise approach with oral therapy can be used unless there is a hypertensive crisis. Finally, as discussed above, in view of the risk of superimposed PIH, these patients may benefit from prophylactic therapy in the form of low-dose aspirin.

Phaeochromocytoma

Phaeochromocytoma is a rare but important cause of hypertension in pregnancy: it is associated with a higher maternal mortality rate, although this has fallen in recent years with improved treatment (Schenker and Granat, 1982; Harper *et al.*, 1989). When it occurs in pregnancy, it may mimic PIH (Badui *et al.*, 1982), so confusing the diagnosis. Hypertensive crises can be provoked by delivery, anaesthesia and mechanical effects on the adrenal gland by the gravid uterus, or even fetal movements. As well as the problems of hypertension, it is associated with IUGR and fetal loss, possibly owing to reduced placental perfusion. Although appropriate treatment has substantially benefited the mother, it has not had the same impact on fetal outcome (Schenker and Granat, 1982; Harper *et al.*, 1989). Phaeochromocytoma is usually symptomatic, with paroxysmal headaches, palpitations and increased perspiration being classic. Arrhythmias, postural hypotension, cardiovascular collapse and hyperglycaemia can also occur. It should be noted, however, that symptoms do not always occur and that hypertension need not always be present.

Clearly, it is important to be alert to the possibility of this diagnosis. Patients with severe, intermittent or atypical hypertensive problems should be investigated. In view of the association with neurofibromatosis and multiple endocrine neoplasia syndrome (type II), patients with these conditions should be considered at high risk. The diagnosis will require a 24 h urine collection for estimation of urinary catecholamines: this has been recommended as a screening test in all women with hypertension in pregnancy in view of the difficulty in diagnosing phaeochromocytoma (Schenker and Chowers, 1971). Initial treatment is by α- and β-adrenoceptor blockade. Tumour localization may be carried out by ultrasound, computerized tomography, arteriography and selective venous sampling, but may have to be delayed until the puerperium, in some cases. Surgical removal may be carried out during pregnancy until around 24 weeks; thereafter, it should be delayed until the fetus is mature; delivery can then be carried out by elective caesarean section followed by tumour removal. In view of the risk of recurrence, careful follow-up is required.

Conn's syndrome and Cushing's syndrome

Primary aldosteronism (Conn's syndrome) is a very rare cause of secondary hypertension in pregnancy. It is characterized by a hypokalaemic alkalosis and hypertension; diagnosis may be difficult as aldosterone normally increases in pregnancy. Successful pregnancies are possible but anti-hypertensive therapy and treatment of hypokalaemia will be required.

There are very few reports of Cushing's syndrome in pregnancy (de Swiet, 1989) as these women are usually infertile, so that it is unusual for it to make its primary presentation during pregnancy. When it does occur, the patient may have clinical diagnostic features and this diagnosis can be confirmed by employing the dexamethasone suppression test and by measuring plasma cortisol levels, which show loss of the diurnal rhythm; measurement of ACTH levels may also be helpful. As the majority of cases in pregnancy are associated with a pituitary origin, skull radiography and perimetry will be required. The condition should be localized to the pituitary or adrenal, and appropriate treatment arranged – pituitary surgery or radiotherapy, or adrenal exploration. The fetal outcome is poor in this condition, with a high incidence of fetal loss.

Renal disease

The contribution of renal disease to hypertension in pregnancy is dealt with in Chapter 5.

Conclusions

PIH is a multisystem disorder characterized by vascular damage and dysfunction. These pathological changes are associated with activation of platelets, neutrophils and the coagulation and fibrinolytic systems. The precise aetiology of these disturbances remains enigmatic; however, it is clear that there is a genetic component, possibly manifest as a defective immunological interaction between mother and fetus, and resulting in defective trophoblast invasion and placental ischaemia. This ischaemia triggers the pathological changes noted in this disease which are amplified as vascular damage that occurs in the placental bed. Current therapy focuses on controlling blood pressure, monitoring mother and fetus and optimizing the timing and mode of delivery. Anti-hypertensive therapy will control high blood pressure, which is just one manifestation of the disease process, and is not aimed at interrupting the actual pathophysiological mechanisms of the disease, although there is some evidence to suggest that such treatment may retard the disease process. Perhaps the best hope for intervention is anti-platelet therapy with low-dose aspirin, which can reduce the development of the disease. Although such treatment appears to be effective, its application is hampered by our inability to identify accurately primigravidae at high risk of PIH. Thus, if we wish to make significant inroads into the primary prevention of this disease, we must develop an effective screening test to identify those at risk in advance of the frank development of clinical signs. In the mean time, we must focus on early identification, assessment and treatment of women with the disease. Early recognition presupposes not only vigilance with regard to blood pressure and proteinuria but also an appreciation of the alternative presentations and variety of the disease processes that constitute this enigmatic condition.

References

Aalkjaer, C, Johannesen, P, Pedersen, EB, *et al*. (1984) Morphology and angiotensin II responsiveness of isolated resistance vessels from patients with pre-eclampsia. *Scandinavian Journal of Clinical Investigation*, **44**, Suppl 169, 57

Abdul-Karim, RE and Assali, NS (1961) Pressor response to angiotonin in pregnant and non-pregnant women. *American Journal of Obstetrics and Gynecology*, **82**, 246

Abitbol, MM (1977) Aortic compression and uterine blood flow during pregnancy. *Obstetrics and Gynecology*, **50**, 562–570

Abitbol, MM, Ober, WB, Gallow, GR, *et al*. (1977) Experimental toxemia of pregnancy in the monkey, with a preliminary report on renin and aldosterone. *American Journal of Pathology*, **86**, 573

Acker, GM, Galen, FX, Devaux, C *et al*. (1982) Human chorionic cells in primary culture: a model for renin biosynthesis. *Journal of Clinical Endocrinology and Metabolism*, **55**, 902

Adams, EM and Finlayson, A (1961) Familial aspects of pre-eclampsia and hypertension in pregnancy. *Lancet*, **ii**, 1375–1378

Adams, EM and MacGillivray, I (1961) Long term effects of pre-eclampsia on blood pressure. *Lancet*, **ii**, 1373–1375

Ager, A and Gordon, JL (1984) Differential effects of hydrogen peroxide on indices of endothelial cell function. *Journal of Experimental Medicine*, **159**, 592–603

Aiken, JW and Vane, JR (1973) Intrarenal prostaglandin release attenuates the renal vasoconstrictor activity of angiotensin. *Journal of Pharmacology and Experimental Therapeutics*, **184**, 678

Allen, J, Maigaard, S, Formon, A *et al.* (1987) Acute effects of nitrendipine in pregnancy-induced hypertension. *British Journal of Obstetrics and Gynaecology*, **94**, 222–226

Altchek, A, Albright, NL and Sommers, SC (1968) The renal pathology of toxemia of pregnancy. *Obstetrics and Gynaecology*, **31**, 595–607

Andrews, J and McGarry, JM (1972) A community study of smoking in pregnancy. *Journal of Obstetrics and Gynaecology of the British Commonwealth*, **79**, 1057

Atlas, SA and Laragh, JH (1986) Atrial natriuretic peptide – a new factor in hormonal control of blood pressure and electrolyte homeostasis. *Annual Review of Medicine*, **37**, 397–414

Aznar, J, Gilabert, J, Estelles, A and Espana, F (1986) Fibrinolytic activity and protein C in pre-eclampsia. *Thrombosis and Haemostasis*, **55**, 314

Badui, E, Mancilla, R, Szymanski, JJ *et al.* (1982) Diverse clinical manifestations of phaeochromocytomas. *Angiology*, **33**, 173–182

Baird, D (1967) Epidemiological aspects of hypertensive pregnancy. *Clinics in Obstetrics and Gynaecology*, **4**, 531–548

Baird, D, Thomson, AM and Billewicz, WF (1957) Birthweight and placental weights in pre-eclampsia. *Journal of Obstetrics and Gynaecology of the British Commonwealth*, **64**, 370

Baker, PN, Broughton Pipkin, F and Symonds, EM (1989) Platelet angiotensin II binding sites in hypertension in pregnancy. *Lancet*, **ii**, 1151

Baumgartner, HR (1973) The role of blood flow in platelet adhesion, fibrin deposition, and formation of mural thrombi. *Microvascular Research*, **5**, 167–179

Bay, WH and Ferris, TF (1979) Factors controlling plasma renin and aldosterone during pregnancy. *Hypertension*, **1**, 410

Beaufils, M, Uzan, S, Donsimoni, R and Colau, JC (1985) Prevention of pre-eclampsia by early anti-platelet therapy. *Lancet*, **i**, 840–842

Becker, RA, Hayashi, RH, Franks, RC and Speroff, L (1978) Effects of positional change and sodium balance on the renin–angiotensin–aldosterone system big renin and prostaglandins in normal pregnancy. *Journal of Clinical Endocrinology and Metabolism*, **46**, 467

Belch, JJF, McKay, A, McArdle, B *et al.* (1983a) Epoprostenol (prostacyclin) and severe arterial disease. A double blind trial. *Lancet*, **i**, 315–317

Belch, JJF, Newman, P, Drury, JK *et al.* (1983b) Intermittent epoprostenol (prostacyclin) infusion in patients with Raynaud's syndrome. A double blind controlled trial. *Lancet*, **i**, 313–315

Belch, JJF, Thorburn, J, Greer, IA *et al.* (1985) Intravenous prostacyclin in the management of pregnancies complicated by severe hypertension. *Clinical and Experimental Hypertension*, **B4**, 75–86

Belfort, M, Uys, P, Dommisse, J and Davey, DA (1989) Haemodynamic changes in gestational proteinuric hypertension: the effects of rapid volume expansion and vasodilator therapy. *British Journal of Obstetrics and Gynaecology*, **90**, 634–641

Benedetti, TJ and Carlson, RW (1979) Studies of colloid osmotic pressure in pregnancy induced hypertension. *American Journal of Obstetrics and Gynecology*, **135**, 308–311

Benigni, A, Gregorini, G, Frusca, T *et al.* (1989) Effect of low dose aspirin on fetal and maternal generation of thromboxane by platelets in women at risk for pregnancy induced hypertension. *New England Journal of Medicine*, **321**, 357–362

Bjoro, K (1985) Effects of angiotensin I and II and their interactions with some prostanoids in perfused human umbilical arteries. *Prostaglandins*, **30**, 989

Bjoro, K, Stokke, KT and Stray-Pedersen, S (1987) Fetal angiotensin induced prostanoid production is altered in pregnancy-induced hypertension. *Clinical and Experimental Hypertension*, **B6**, 86

de Boer, K, Lecander, I, ten Cate, JW *et al.* (1988) Placental-type plasminogen activator inhibitor in pre-eclampsia. *American Journal of Obstetrics and Gynecology*, **158**, 518–522

Bonnar, J, McNicol, GP and Douglas, AS (1971) Coagulation and fibrinolytic systems in pre-eclampsia. *British Medical Journal*, **2**, 12–16

Bonnar, J, Davison, JF, Pidgeon, CF *et al.* (1969) Fibrin degradation products in normal and abnormal pregnancy and parturition. *British Medical Journal*, **3**, 137–140

Borglin, NE (1959) Serum glutamic-oxalacetic transaminase (SGO-T) and serum glutamic-pyruvic transaminase (SGP-T) in toxemia of pregnancy. *Journal of Clinical Endocrinology*, **19**, 425

Borok, Z, Weitz, J, Owen, M *et al*. (1984) Fibrinogen proteolysis and platelet-granule release in preeclampsia/eclampsia. *Blood*, **63**, 523–531

Boxer, CA, Allen, JM, Schmidt, T *et al*. (1980) Inhibition of polymorphonuclear leukocyte adherence by prostacyclin. *Journal of Laboratory and Clinical Medicine*, **95**, 672–678

Boyd, PA, Lindenbaum, RH and Redman, CWG (1987) Pre-eclampsia and trisomy 13: a possible association. *Lancet*, **ii**, 425–427

Braunwald, E (1982) Mechanism of action of calcium-channel-blocking agents. *New England Journal of Medicine*, **307**, 1618–1627

Bray, MA (1983) The pharmacology and pathophysiology of leukotriene B4. *British Medical Bulletin*, **39**, 249–254

Briel, RC, Kieback, DG and Lippert, TH (1984) Platelet sensitivity to a prostacyclin analogue in normal and pathological pregnancy. *Prostaglandins, Leukotrienes and Medicine*, **13**, 335–340

Brosens, I and Dixon, HG (1966) The anatomy of the maternal side of the placenta. *Journal of Obstetrics and Gynaecology of the British Commonwealth*, **73**, 357–363

Brosens, I, Robertson, WB and Dixon, HG (1967) The physiological response to the vessels of the placental bed to normal pregnancy. *Journal of Pathology and Bacteriology*, **93**, 569–579

Brosens, I, Robertson, WB and Dixon, HG (1972) The role of the spiral arteries in the pathogenesis of pre-eclampsia. *Obstetric and Gynecological Annals*, **1**, 177–191

Broughton Pipkin, F and Symonds, EM (1986) Prostaglandins and pregnancy-induced hypertension. In: *Prostaglandins and Their Inhibitors in Clinical Obstetrics and Gynaecology* (edited by M Bydgeman, G Berger and L Keith), p. 337. Lancaster: MTP Press

Broughton Pipkin, F, Morrison, R and O'Brien, PMS (1984) Effects of prostacyclin on the pressor response to angiotensin II in human pregnancy. *European Journal of Clinical Investigation*, **14**, 3

Broughton Pipkin, F, Turner, SR and Symonds, EM (1980) Possible risk with captopril in pregnancy: some animal data. *Lancet*, **i**, 1256

Broughton Pipkin, F, Hunter, JC, Turner, SR and O'Brien, PMS (1982) Prostaglandin E$_2$ attenuates the pressor response to angiotensin II in pregnant, but not non-pregnant humans. *American Journal of Obstetrics and Gynecology*, **142**, 168

Brown, JJ, Davies, DL, Doak, PB *et al*. (1965) Plasma renin concentration in hypertensive disease of pregnancy. *Lancet*, **ii**, 1219

Brown, MA, Broughton Pipkin, F and Symonds, EM (1988) The effects of intravenous angiotensin II upon blood pressure and sodium and urate excretion in human pregnancy. *Journal of Hypertension*, **6**, 457–464

Brown, MA, Gallery, EDM, Ross, MR and Esber, RP (1988) Sodium excretion in normal and hypertensive pregnancy: a prospective study. *American Journal of Obstetrics and Gynecology*, **159**, 297–307

Bryans, CI (1966) The remote prognosis in toxaemia of pregnancy. *Clinics in Obstetrics and Gynecology*, **9**, 973

Bussolino, F, Benedetto, C, Massobrio, M and Comussi, G (1980) Maternal vascular prostacyclin activity in pre-eclampsia. *Lancet*, **ii**, 702

Butler, NR and Alberman, ED (1969) *Perinatal Problems: Second Report of the 1958 British Perinatal Mortality Survey*. Edinburgh: E and S Livingstone

Butler, NR and Bonham, DG (1963) *Perinatal Mortality*, pp. 86–100. Edinburgh: E and S Livingstone

Cameron, AD, Nicholson, SF, Nimrod, CA *et al*. (1988) Doppler waveforms in the fetal aorta and umbilical artery in patients with hypertension in pregnancy. *American Journal of Obstetrics and Gynecology*, **158**, 339–345

Campbell, DM and MacGillivray, I (1985) Pre-eclampsia in second pregnancy. *British Journal of Obstetrics and Gynaecology*, **92**, 131–140

Campbell, DM and Templeton, AA (1980) Is eclampsia preventable? In: *Pregnancy Hypertension* (edited by J Bonnar, I MacGillivray and EM Symonds) p. 483. Baltimore: University Park Press

Chamberlain, G, Phillipp, E, Howlett, B and Masters, K (1978) *British Births 1970: Volume 2: Obstetric Care*, pp. 80–107. London: William Heinemann Medical Books Limited

Chesley, LC (1939) The variability of proteinuria in the hypertensive complications of pregnancy. *Journal of Clinical Investigation*, **18**, 617

Chesley, LC (1976) Blood pressure, oedema and proteinuria in pregnancy. *Prognosis of Clinical and Biological Research*, **7**, 249–268

Chesley, LC (1978) *Hypertensive Disorders in Pregnancy*. New York: Appleton-Century-Crofts

Chesley, LC and Annitto, JE (1947) Pregnancy in the patient with hypertensive disease. *American Journal of Obstetrics and Gynecology*, **53**, 372

Chesley, LC and Cooper, DW (1986) Genetics of hypertension in pregnancy: possible single gene control of pre-eclampsia and eclampsia in the descendants of eclamptic women. *British Journal of Obstetrics and Gynaecology*, **93**, 898–908

Chesley, LC and Tepper, IH (1967) Effects of progesterone and estrogen on the sensitivity to angiotensin II. *Journal of Clinical Endocrinology and Metabolism*, **27**, 576

Chesley, LC and Williams, LO (1945) Renal glomerular and tubular functions in relation to the hyperuricemia of pre-eclampsia and eclampsia. *American Journal of Obstetrics and Gynecology*, **50**, 367

Chesley, LC, Annitto, JE and Cosgrove, RA (1968) The familial factor of toxemia of pregnancy. *Obstetrics and Gynecology*, **32**, 303–331

Chesley, LC, Annitto, JE and Cosgrove, RA (1976) The remote prognosis of eclamptic women: sixth periodic report. *American Journal of Obstetrics and Gynecology*, **124**, 446–459

Chesley, LC, Cosgrove, RA and Annitto, JE (1961) Pregnancy in the sisters and daughters of eclamptic women. *Pathology and Microbiology*, **24**, 622–666

Chesley, LC, Valenti, C and Rein, H (1958) Excretion of sodium loads by non-pregnant and pregnant, hypertensive and pre-eclamptic women. *Metabolism*, **7**, 575–588

Clark, SL and Cotton, DB (1988) Clinical indications for pulmonary artery catheterisation in the patient with severe preeclampsia. *American Journal of Obstetrics and Gynecology*, **158**, 453–458

Cockburn, J, Moar, VA, Ounsted, M and Redman, CWG (1982) Final report of study on hypertension during pregnancy: the effects of specific treatment on the growth and development of the children. *Lancet*, **i**, 647–649

Condie, RG (1976a) Components of the haemostatic mechanism at birth in pre-eclampsia with particular reference to fetal growth retardation. *British Journal of Obstetrics and Gynaecology*, **83**, 943–947

Condie, RG (1976b) A serial study of coagulation factors XII, XI and X in normal pregnancy and in pregnancy complicated by pre-eclampsia. *British Journal of Obstetrics and Gynaecology*, **83**, 636–639

Constantine, G, Beevers, DG, Reynolds, AL and Luesley, DM (1987) Nifedipine as a second line antihypertensive drug in pregnancy. *British Journal of Obstetrics and Gynaecology*, **94**, 1136–1142

Cooper, DW and Liston, WA (1979) Genetic control of severe pre-eclampsia. *Journal of Medical Genetics*, **16**, 409–416

Cooper, DW, Hill, JA, Chesley, LC and Iverson Bryans, C (1988) Genetic control of susceptibility to eclampsia and miscarriage. *British Journal of Obstetrics and Gynaecology*, **95**, 644–653

Cranford, RE, Leppik, IE, Patrick, B *et al.* (1978) Intravenous phenytoin: clinical and pharmacokinetic aspects. *Neurology*, **28**, 874–880

Cree, JE, Meyer, J and Hailey, DM (1973) Diazepam in labour: its metabolism and effects on the clinical condition and thermogenesis of the newborn. *British Medical Journal*, **4**, 251–255

Davey, DA and MacGillivray, I (1987) In *The Classification and Definition of the Hypertensive Disorders of Pregnancy* (edited by F Sharp and EM Symonds) pp. 401–408. New York: Perinatology Press

Davey, DA and MacGillivray, I (1988) The classification and definition of the hypertensive disorders of pregnancy. *American Journal of Obstetrics and Gynecology*, **158**, 892–898

Davison, JM and Hytten, FE (1974) Glomerular filtration during and after pregnancy. *Journal of Obstetrics and Gynaecology of the British Commonwealth*, **81**, 588

Department of Health (1989) *Report on Confidential Enquiries into Maternal Deaths in England and Wales 1982–84*. London: HMSO

Department of Health and Social Security (1986) *Report on Confidential Enquiries into Maternal Deaths in England and Wales 1979–1981*. London: HMSO

de Swiet, M (ed.) (1989) Diseases of the pituitary and adrenal glands. In *Medical Disorders in Obstetric Practice*, pp. 660–689. London: Blackwell Scientific

Donaldson, JO (1986) Does magnesium sulphate treat eclamptic convulsions? *Clinics in Neuropharmacology*, **9**, 37–45

Douglas, JT, Shah, M, Lowe, DGO *et al.* (1982) Plasma fibrinopeptide A and beta-thromboglobulin in pre-eclampsia and pregnancy hypertension. *Thrombosis and Haemostasis*, **47**, 54–55

Downing, I, Shepherd, GL and Lewis, PJ (1980) Reduced prostacyclin production in pre-eclampsia. *Lancet*, **ii**, 1374

Ducsay, CA, Thompson, JS, Wu, AT and Novy, MJ (1987) Effects of calcium entry blocker (nicardipine) tocolysis in rhesus macaques: fetal plasma concentration and cardiorespiratory change. *American Journal of Obstetrics and Gynecology*, **157**, 1482–1486

Duffus, GM and MacGillivray, I (1968) The incidence of pre-eclamptic toxaemia in smokers and non-smokers. *Lancet*, **i**, 994–995

Duffus, GM, Tunstall, ME and MacGillivray, I (1968) Intravenous chlormethiazole in pre-eclamptic toxaemia in labour. *Lancet*, **i**, 335–337

Duffus, GM, Tunstall, ME, Condie, RG and MacGillivray, I (1969) Chlormethiazole in the prevention of eclampsia and the reduction of perinatal mortality. *Journal of Obstetrics and Gynaecology of the British Commonwealth*, **76**, 645–651

Duncan, SLB (1989) Does volume expansion in pre-eclampsia help or hinder. *British Journal of Obstetrics and Gynaecology*, **96**, 631–633

Dunlop, W (1981) Serial changes in renal haemodynamics during normal human pregnancy. *British Journal of Obstetrics and Gynaecology*, **88**, 1

Edgar, W, McKillop, C, Howie, PW and Prentice, CRM (1977) Composition of soluble fibrin complexes in pre-eclampsia. *Thrombosis Research*, **10**, 567–574

Elder, MG, de Swiet, M, Robertson, A *et al.* (1988) Low dose aspirin in pregnancy. *Lancet*, **i**, 410

Elias, AN, Vaziri, ND, Pandian, MR *et al.* (1988) Atrial natriuretic peptide and arginine vasopressin in pregnancy and pregnancy-induced hypertension. *Nephron*, **49**, 140–143

Estelles, A, Gilabert, J, Espana, F *et al.* (1987) Fibrinolysis in pre-eclampsia. *Fibrinolysis*, **1**, 209–214

Everett, RB, Worley, RJ, MacDonald, PC and Gant, NF (1978a) Oral administration of theophylline to modify pressor responsiveness to angiotensin II in women with pregnancy-induced hypertension. *American Journal of Obstetrics and Gynecology*, **132**, 359–362

Everett, RB, Worley, RJ, MacDonald, PC and Gant, NF (1978b) Modification of vascular responsiveness to angiotensin II in pregnant women by intravenously infused 5-dihydro-progesterone. *American Journal of Obstetrics and Gynecology*, **131**, 352–357

Ezimokhai, M, Davison, JM, Phillips, PR and Dunlop, W (1981) Non postural serial changes in renal function during the third trimester of normal pregnancy. *British Journal of Obstetrics and Gynaecology*, **88**, 465–470

Ferris, TF and Weir, EK (1983) Effect of captopril on uterine blood flow and prostaglandin E synthesis in the pregnant rabbit. *Journal of Clinical Investigation*, **71**, 809

Fidler, J, Smith, V, Fayers, P and de Swiet, M (1983) Randomised controlled comparative study of methyldopa and oxprenolol for the treatment of hypertension in pregnancy. *British Medical Journal*, **286**, 1927–1930

Fievet, P, Pleskov, L, Desailly, I *et al.* (1985) Plasma renin activity, blood uric acid and plasma volume in pregnancy-induced hypertension *Nephron*, **40**, 429

Fievet, P, Fournier, A, de Bold, A *et al.* (1988) Atrial natriuretic factor in pregnancy-induced hypertension and pre-eclampsia. *American Journal of Hypertension*, **1**, 16–21

Fisher, KA, Luger, A, Spargo, BH and Lindheimer, MD (1981) Hypertension in pregnancy, clinical-pathological correlations and remote prognosis. *Medicine*, **60**, 267

Fitzgerald, DJ, Mayo, G, Catella, F (1987) Increased thromboxane biosynthesis in normal pregnancy is mainly derived from platelets. *American Journal of Obstetrics and Gynecology*, **157**, 325–330

Fitzgerald, GA, Oats, JA, Hawiger, J *et al.* (1983) Endogenous biosynthesis of prostacyclin and thromboxane and platelet function during chronic administration of aspirin in man. *Journal of Clinical Investigation*, **71**, 676–688

Fletcher, AE and Bulpitt, CJ (1988) A review of clinical trials in pregnancy hypertension. In *Handbook of Hypertension Volume 10: Hypertension in Pregnancy* (edited by PC Rubin) pp. 186–201. Amsterdam: Elsevier Science

Fox, H (1987) Histopathology of pre-eclampsia and eclampsia. In *Hypertension in Pregnancy* (edited by F Sharp and EM Symonds) pp. 119–130. New York: Perinatology Press

Fox, H (1988) The placenta in pregnancy hypertension. In *Handbook of Hypertension Volume 10: Hypertension in Pregnancy* (edited by PC Rubin) pp. 16–37. Amsterdam: Elsevier Science

Franklin, GO, Dowd, AJ, Caldwell, VB and Speroff, L (1974) The effects of angiotensin II intravenous infusion on plasma renin and prostaglandins A, E and F levels in the uterine vein of the pregnant monkey. *Prostaglandins*, **6**, 271

Gallery, EDM and Gyory, AZ (1979) Glomerular and proximal tubular function in pregnancy associated hypertension. A prospective study. *European Journal of Obstetrics, Gynaecology and Reproductive Biology*, **9**, 8

Gallery, EDM, Hunyor, SN and Gyory, AZ (1979) Plasma volume contraction: a significant factor in both pregnancy-associated hypertension (pre-eclampsia) and chronic hypertension in pregnancy. *Quarterly Journal of Medicine*, **48**, 593–602

Gallery, EDM, Mitchell, MDM and Redman, CWG (1984) Fall in blood pressure in response to volume expansion in pregnancy associated hypertension (pre-eclampsia): why does it occur? *Journal of Hypertension*, **2**, 177–182

Gallery, EDM, Ross, MR and Gyory, AZ (1985) Anti-hypertensive treatment in pregnancy: analysis of different responses to oxprenolol and methyldopa. *British Medical Journal*, **291**, 563–566

Gallery, EDM, Stokes, GS, Gyory, AZ *et al.* (1980b) Plasma renin activity in normal human pregnancy and in pregnancy-associated hypertension, with reference to cryoactivation. *Clinical Science*, **59**, 49

Gant, NF, Daley, GL, Chand, S *et al.* (1973) A study of angiotensin II pressor response throughout primigravid pregnancy. *Journal of Clinical Investigation*, **52**, 2682–2689

Gant, NF, Chand, S, Worley, RJ *et al.* (1974) A clinical test useful for predicting the development of acute hypertension in pregnancy. *American Journal of Obstetrics and Gynecology*, **120**, 1–7

Gerretsen, G, Huisjes, HJ and Elema, JD (1981) Morphological changes of the spiral arteries in the placental bed in relation to pre-eclampsia and fetal growth retardation. *British Journal of Obstetrics and Gynaecology*, **88**, 876–881

Giles, G and Inglis, TCM (1981) Thrombocytopenia and macrothrombocytosis in gestational hypertension. *British Journal of Obstetrics and Gynaecology*, **88**, 1115–1119

Gimbrone, MA and Alexander, RW (1975) Angiotensin II stimulation of prostaglandin production in cultured human vascular endothelium. *Science*, **189**, 219–220

Ginsburg, J and Duncan, SLB (1967) Peripheral circulation in hypertensive pregnancy. *Cardiovascular Research*, **1**, 356–361

Goodlin, RC (1976) Severe pre-eclampsia – another great imitator. *American Journal of Obstetrics and Gynecology*, **125**, 747–753

Goodman, RP, Killam, AP, Brash, AR and Branch, RA (1982) Prostacyclin production during pregnancy: comparison of production during normal pregnancy and pregnancy complicated by hypertension. *American Journal of Obstetrics and Gynecology*, **142**, 817–822

Govan, ADT (1954) Renal changes in eclampsia. *Journal of Pathology and Bacteriology*, **67**, 311–322

Greer, IA (1985) The effect of anti-hypertensive agents on platelets, prostacyclin and thromboxane and observations on prostacyclin and thromboxane in normal and hypertensive pregnancy. *MD Thesis*, University of Glasgow, Scotland, UK

Greer, IA (1987) Platelet function and calcium channel blocking agents. *Journal of Clinical Pharmacy and Therapeutics*, **12**, 213–222

Greer, IA and Belch, JJF (1986) Prostacyclin in pregnancy induced hypertension, Raynaud's phenomenon and haemolytic uraemic syndrome. In *Current Clinical Concepts, Prostacyclin Past Present and Future* (edited by EB Williams) pp. 37–45. Kent: MCS

Greer, IA, Cameron, AD and Walker, JJ (1985) HELLP syndrome: pathologic entity or technical inadequacy? *American Journal of Obstetrics and Gynecology*, **152**, 113–114

Greer, IA, McLaren, M and Forbes, CD (1990) Synergistic inhibitory effects of adrenoceptor antagonists and prostacyclin and umbilical artery derived prostacyclin like activity on platelet aggregation. *European Journal of Obstetrics Gynecology and Reproductive Biology*, **35**, 109–118

Greer, IA, Walker, JJ, Calder, AA and Forbes, CD (1985a) Inhibition of platelet aggregation in whole blood by adrenoceptor antagonists. *Thrombosis Research*, **40**, 631–643

Greer, IA, Walker, JJ, Calder, AA and Forbes, CD (1985b) Aspirin with an adrenergic or a calcium channel blocking agent as new combination therapy for arterial thrombosis. *Lancet*, **i**, 351–352

Greer, IA, Walker, JJ, Calder, AA and Forbes, CD (1985c) Influence of treatment on platelet consumption and thromboxane in pregnancy induce hypertension. *Archives of Gynecology*, **237**, 109

Greer, IA, Walker, JJ, Cameron, AD *et al.* (1985d) A prospective longitudinal study of immunoreactive prostacyclin and thromboxane metabolites in normal and hypertensive pregnancies. *Clinical and Experimental Hypertension*, **B4**, 167–182

Greer, IA, Walker, JJ, McLaren, M *et al.* (1985) A comparative study of the effects of adrenoceptor antagonists on platelet aggregation and thromboxane generation. *Thrombosis and Haemostasis*, **54**, 480–484

Greer, IA, Walker, JJ, McLaren, M *et al.* (1985f) Inhibition of thromboxane and prostacyclin production in whole blood by adrenoceptor antagonists. *Prostaglandins, Leukotrienes and Medicine*, **19**, 209–217

Greer, IA, Walker, JJ, Forbes, CD and Calder, AA (1986a) The low dose aspirin controversy solved at last? *British Medical Journal*, **391**, 1277–1278

Greer, IA, Walker, JJ, McLaren, M *et al.* (1986b) Inhibition of whole blood platelet aggregation by nicardipine and synergism with prostacyclin in-vitro. *Thrombosis Research*, **41**, 509–518

Greer, IA, Walker, JJ, Forbes, CD and Calder, AA (1987) Platelet function in pregnancy induced hypertension following treatment with labetalol and low dose aspirin. *Thrombosis Research*, **46**, 667–612

Greer, IA, Calder, AA, Walker, JJ *et al.* (1988a) Increased platelet reactivity in pregnancy-induced hypertension and uncomplicated diabetic pregnancy: an indication for antiplatelet therapy? *British Journal of Obstetrics and Gynaecology*, **95**, 1204–1208

Greer, IA, Walker, JJ, McLaren, M *et al.* (1988b) The effect of endralazine and hydralazine on platelet thromboxane production *in vitro. Clinical and Experimental Hypertension*, **B6**, 375–386

Greer, IA, Haddad, NG, Dawes, J, Johnstone, FD and Calder, AA (1989a) Neutrophil activation in pregnancy induced hypertension. *British Journal of Obstetrics and Gynaecology*, **96**, 978–982

Greer, IA, Haddad, NG, Dawes, J, Johnstone, TA, Johnstone, FD and Steel, JM (1989b) Increased neutrophil activation in diabetic pregnancy and non-pregnant diabetic women. *Obstetrics and Gynecology*, **74**, 878–881

Greer, IA, Walker, JJ, Bjornsson, S and Calder, AA (1989c) Second line therapy with nifedipine in severe pregnancy induced hypertension. *Clinical and Experimental Hypertension*, **B8**, 277–292

Groenendijk, R, Trimbas, JBMJ and Wallenburg, HCS (1984) Hemodynamic measurements in pre-eclampsia: preliminary observations. *American Journal of Obstetrics and Gynaecology*, **150**, 232–236

Habib, A and McArthy, JS (1977) Effects on the neonate of propranolol therapy in pregnancy. *Journal of Pediatrics*, **91**, 808–811

Haddad, NG, Johnstone, FD, Chambers, SE *et al.* (1989) Umbilical artery Doppler flow velocity waveform analysis and the outcome of hypertensive pregnancies. *Journal of Obstetrics and Gynaecology*, **9**, 9–13

Hall, MH and Campbell, DM (1987) Geographical epidemiology of hypertension in pregnancy. In *Hypertension in Pregnancy* (edited by F Sharp and EM Symonds) pp. 33–46. New York: Perinatology Press

Hamberg, M, Svensson, J and Samuelsson, B (1975) Thromboxanes: a new group of biologically active compounds derived from prostaglandin endoperoxides. *Proceedings of the National Academy of Sciences (USA)*, **72**, 2994–2998

Harlan, JD (1987) Neutrophil-mediated vascular injury. *Acta Medica Scandinavica (Suppl)*, **715**, 123–129

Harper, MA, Murnaghan, GA, Kennedy, L *et al.* (1989) Phaeochromocytoma in pregnancy. Five cases and a review of the literature. *British Journal of Obstetrics and Gynaecology*, **96**, 594–606

Haukland, HH, Florholmen, J, Oian, P *et al.* (1987) The effect of severe pre-eclampsia on the pancreas. *British Journal of Obstetrics and Gynaecology*, **94**, 765–767

Heavey, DJ, Barrown, SE, Hickling, NE and Ritter, JM (1985) Aspirin causes short-lived inhibition of bradykinin-stimulated prostacyclin production in man. *Nature*, **318**, 186–188

Hertig, AT (1945) Vascular pathology in the hypertensive albuminuric toxemias of pregnancy. *Clinics*, **4**, 602–613

Hibbard, LT (1973) Maternal mortality due to acute toxaemia. *Obstetrics and Gynecology*, **42**, 263–270

Hirai, N, Yanaihara, T, Nakayama, R *et al.* (1988) Plasma levels of atrial natriuretic peptide during normal pregnancy and in pregnancy complicated by hypertension. *American Journal of Obstetrics and Gynecology*, **159**, 27–31

Howie, PW (1977) The haemostatic mechanisms of pre-eclampsia. *Clinics in Obstetrics and Gynaecology*, **4**, 595–609

Howie, PW, Prentice, CRM and McNicol, GP (1971) Coagulation, fibrinolysis and platelet function in pre-eclampsia, essential hypertension and placental insufficiency. *Journal of Obstetrics and Gynaecology of the British Commonwealth*, **78**, 992–1003

Howie, PW, Begg, CB, Purdie, DW and Prentice, CRM (1976) Use of coagulation tests to predict the clinical progress of pre-eclampsia. *Lancet*, **ii**, 323–325

Howy, C and Baird, RW (1982) *Report to the Meeting on the Results of the UK Survey of Diabetic Pregnancies*. London: Royal College of Obstetricians and Gynaecologists

Hughes, EC (ed.) (1972) *Obstetric–Gynecologic Terminology*, pp. 422–423. Philadelphia: FA Davis

Hytten, FE and Paintin, DB (1963) Increases in plasma volume during normal pregnancy. *Journal of Obstetrics and Gynaecology of the British Commonwealth*, **70**, 402–407

Ihle, BU, Long, P and Oats, J (1987) Early onset pre-eclampsia: recognition of underlying renal disease. *British Medical Journal*, **294**, 79–81

Imrie, AH and Raper, CG (1977) Severe intravascular coagulation preceding severe eclampsia. *British Journal of Obstetrics and Gynaecology*, **84**, 71–72

Inglis, TCM, Stuart, AJ, George, AJ and Davies, AJ (1982) Haemostatic and rheological changes in normal pregnancy and pre-eclampsia. *British Journal of Haematology*, **50**, 461–465

Jadoul, FAC, Broughton Pipkin, F and Lamming, GD (1982) Changes in the renin-aldosterone system in normotensive primigravidae in the four days after normal spontaneous delivery. *British Journal of Obstetrics and Gynaecology*, **89**, 633

Janoff, A (1985) Elastase in tissue injury. *Annual Reviews of Medicine*, **36**, 207–216

Janoff, A and Zweifach, BW (1964) Production of inflammatory changes in the microcirculation by cationic proteins extracted from lysomes. *Journal of Experimental Medicine*, **120**, 747–764

Jaspers, WJM, De Jong, PA and Mulder, AW (1981) Angiotensin II sensitivity and prostaglandin synthetase inhibition in pregnancy. *European Journal of Obstetrics Gynecology and Reproductive Biology*, **11**, 379

Jogee, M, Myatt, L and Elder, MG (1983) Decreased prostacyclin production by placental cells in culture from pregnancies complicated by fetal growth retardation. *British Journal of Obstetrics and Gynaecology*, **90**, 247–250

Johnson, J, Johnson, IR, Ronan, JE and Craven, DJ (1984) The site of renin in the human uterus. *Histopathology*, **8**, 273

Johnstone, FD, Ugaily-Thulesius, L, Thulesius, O and Nasrat, AN (1987) Umbilical artery reactivity and ultrastructural changes in pregnancy induced hypertension and other complicated pregnancies. *Clinical Physiology*, **7**, 493–502

Jouppila, P, Kirkinen, P, Koivula, A and Ylikorkala, O (1985) Effects of dihydralazine infusion on the fetoplacental blood flow and maternal prostanoids. *Obstetrics and Gynecology*, **65**, 115–118

Jouppila, P, Kirkinen, P, Koivula, A and Ylikorkala, O (1986) Labetalol does not alter the placental and fetal blood flow or maternal prostanoids in pre-eclampsia. *British Journal of Obstetrics and Gynaecology*, **93**, 543–547

Karlberg, BE, Ryden, G and Wichman, K (1984) Changes in the renin–angiotensin–aldosterone and kallikrein–kinin systems during normal and hypertensive pregnancy. *Acta Obstetrica Gynaecologica Scandinavica (Suppl)*, **118**, 17

Khong, TY, de Wolf, F, Robertson, WB and Brosens, I (1986) Inadequate maternal vascular response to placentation in pregnancies complicated by pre-eclampsia and by small-for-gestational-age infants. *British Journal of Obstetrics and Gynaecology*, **93**, 1049–1059

Kilpatrick, DC (1987) Immune mechanisms and pre-eclampsia. *Lancet*, **ii**, 1460–1461

Kilpatrick, DC, Liston, WA, Jazwinska, EC and Smart, GE (1987) Histocompatibility studies in pre-eclampsia. *Tissue Antigens*, **29**, 232–236

Kilpatrick, DC, Liston, WA, Gibson, F and Livingstone, J (1989) Association between susceptibility to pre-eclampsia within families and HLA DR4. *Lancet*, **ii**, 1063–1065

Kjellmar, I, Dagbhartsson, A, Hrbek, A *et al.* (1984) Maternal beta-adrenoceptor blockade reduces fetal tolerance to asphyxia. *Acta Obstetrica and Gynaecologica Scandinavica (suppl)*, **118**, 75–80

Labarrere, CA (1988) Acute atherosis. A histopathological hallmark of immune aggression. *Placenta*, **9**, 95–108

Lancet, M and Fisher, IL (1956) The value of blood uric acid levels in toxaemia of pregnancy. *Journal of Obstetrics and Gynaecology of the British Commonwealth*, **63**, 116–119

Lardoux, H, Gerard, J, Blazquez, G and Flouvat, B (1983) Which beta-blocker in pregnancy induced hypertension. *Lancet*, **ii**, 1194

Lawrence, MR and Broughton Pipkin, F (1986) Effects of nitrendipine on cardiovascular parameters in conscious pregnant sheep. *Abstracts of the 5th International Congress of the International Society for the Study of Hypertension in Pregnancy*, Nottingham

Leather, HM, Baker, P, Humphreys, DM and Chadd, MA (1968) A controlled trial of hypotensive agents in hypertension in pregnancy. *Lancet*, **ii**, 488

Lees, MM, Scott, DB, Kerr, MG and Taylor, SH (1967a) The circulatory effects of recumbent postural change in late pregnancy. *Clinical Science*, **32**, 453–465

Lees, MM, Taylor, SH, Scott, DB and Kerr, MG (1967b) A study of cardiac output at rest throughout pregnancy. *Journal of Obstetrics and Gynaecology of the British Commonwealth*, **74**, 319–327

Lieberman, BA, Stirrat, GM, Dohen, SL *et al.* (1978) The possible adverse effect of propranolol on the fetus in pregnancy complicated by severe hypertension. *British Journal of Obstetrics and Gynaecology*, **85**, 678–683

Lin, MS, McNay, JL, Shepherd, AMM, Musgrave, GE and Keeton, TK (1983) Increased plasma norepinephrine accompanies persistent tachycardia after hydralazine. *Hypertension*, **5**, 257–263

Lindheimer, MD and Katz, AI (1986) The kidney in pregnancy. In *The Kidney* (edited by BM Brenner and FC Rector) pp. 1253–1295. Philadelphia: WB Saunders

Lindheimer, MD, Del Greco, F and Ehrlich, EN (1973) Postural effects on Na and steroid excretion and serum renin activity during pregnancy. *Journal of Applied Physiology*, **35**, 343

Lipsitz, PJ (1971) The clinical and biochemical effects of excess magnesium in the newborn. *Pediatrics*, **47**, 501–509

Lirette, M, Holbrook, RH and Katz, M (1987) Cardiovascular and uterine blood flow changes during nicardipine tocolysis in the rabbit. *Obstetrics and Gynecology*, **69**, 79–82

Lopez-Llera, M, Linores, GR and Horta, JLH (1976) Maternal mortality rates in pre-eclampsia. *American Journal of Obstetrics and Gynecology*, **124**, 149–155

Louden, KA, Heptinstall, S, Broughton Pipkin, F *et al.* (1989) The effect of low-dose aspirin on platelet reactivity on pregnancy, PIH and neonates. *Clinical and Experimental Hypertension*, **B8**, 398

Low, JA and Galbraith, RS (1974) Pregnancy characteristics of intrauterine growth retardation. *Obstetrics and Gynecology*, **44**, 122

Lowe, CR (1961) Toxemia and pre-pregnancy weight. *Journal of Obstetrics and Gynaecology of the British Commonwealth*, **68**, 622–627

Lox, CD, Dorsett, MM and Hampton, RM (1983) Observations on clotting activity during pre-eclampsia. *Clinical and Experimental Hypertension in Pregnancy*, **B2**, 179–190

Lubbe, WF (1984) Hypertension in pregnancy. *Drug*, **28**, 170–188

Lunell, NO, Nylund, L, Lewander, R and Sarby, B (1982) Acute effect of an anti-hypertensive drug, labetalol, on uteroplacental blood flow. *British Journal of Obstetrics and Gynaecology*, **89**, 640–644

Lunell, NO, Lewander, R, Nylund, L *et al.* (1983) Acute effect of dihydralazine on uteroplacental blood flow in hypertension during pregnancy. *Gynaecologic and Obstetric Investigation*, **16**, 274–282

Mabie, WC, Gonzalez, AR, Sibai, BM and Amon, E (1987) A comparative trial of labetalol and hydralazine in the acute management of severe hypertension complicating pregnancy. *Obstetrics and Gynecology*, **70**, 328–333

McEwan, HP (1968) Investigation of proteinuria in pregnancy by immunoelectrophoresis. *British Journal of Obstetrics and Gynaecology*, **75**, 289–294

McEwan, HP (1969) Investigation of proteinuria associated with hypertension in pregnancy. *British Journal of Obstetrics and Gynaecology*, **76**, 809–812

McFadyen, IR, Greenhouse, P, Price, AB and Geirsson, RT (1986) The relation between plasma urate and placental bed vascular adaptation to pregnancy. *British Journal of Obstetrics and Gynaecology*, **93**, 482–487

MacGillivray, I (1958) Some observations on the incidence of pre-eclampsia. *Journal of Obstetrics and Gynaecology of the British Commonwealth*, **65**, 536

MacGillivray, I (1961) Hypertension in pregnancy and its consequences. *Journal of Obstetrics and Gynaecology of the British Commonwealth*, **68**, 557–569

MacGillivray, I (1981) Aetiology of pre-eclampsia. *British Journal of Hospital Medicine*, **26**, 110–119

MacGillivray, I (1983) *Pre-eclampsia. The Hypertensive Disease of Pregnancy*. London: WB Saunders

MacGillivray, I, Rose, GA and Rowe, D (1969) Blood pressure survey in pregnancy. *Clinical Science*, **37**, 395

MacKenna, J, Dover, NL and Browne, RG (1983) Pre-eclampsia associated with hemolysis, elevated liver enzymes and low platelets – an obstetric emergency. *Obstetrics and Gynecology*, **62**, 751–754

McKillop, C, Howie, PW, Forbes, CD and Prentice, CRM (1976) Soluble fibrinogen/fibrin complexes in pre-eclampsia. *Lancet*, **i**, 56–58

McLaren, M, Greer, IA, Walker, JJ and Forbes, CD (1986) Umbilical artery perfusion: a method to measure prostacyclin production *in vitro*. *Progress in Lipid Research*, **25**, 311–315

McLaren, M, Greer, IA, Walker, JJ and Forbes, CD (1987) Reduced prostacyclin production by umbilical arteries from pregnancy complicated by severe pregnancy induced hypertension. *Clinical and Experimental Hypertension*, **B6**, 365–374

MacLean, PR, Paterson, WG, Smart, GE *et al.* (1972) Proteinuria in toxaemia and abruptio placentae. *Journal of Obstetrics and Gynaecology of the British Commonwealth*, **79**, 321–326

MacPherson, M, Broughton Pipkin, F and Rutter, M (1986) The effect of labetalol on the newborn infant. *British Journal of Obstetrics and Gynaecology*, **93**, 539–543

Makila, VM, Viinikka, L and Ylikorkala, O (1984) Evidence that prostacyclin deficiency is a specific feature in pre-eclampsia. *American Journal of Obstetrics and Gynecology*, **148**, 772–774

Mathews, DD (1977) A randomised controlled trial of bed rest and sedation or normal activity and non-sedation in the management of non-albuminuric hypertension in late pregnancy. *British Journal of Obstetrics and Gynaecology*, **84**, 108–112

Mathews, DD, Agarwal, V and Shuttleworth, TP (1982) A randomised controlled trial of complete bed rest versus ambulation in the management of proteinuric hypertension during pregnancy. *British Journal of Obstetrics and Gynaecology*, **89**, 128–131

Michael, CA (1986) Intravenous labetalol and intravenous diazoxide in severe hypertension complicating pregnancy. *Australian and New Zealand Journal of Obstetrics and Gynaecology*, **26**, 26

Miller, DK, Sandowski, S, Soderman, DD and Kuel, FR Jr. (1985) Endothelial cell prostacyclin production induced by activated neutrophils. *Journal of Biological Chemistry*, **260**, 1006–1014

Miyamoto, S, Shimokawa, H, Sumioki, H *et al.* (1988) Circadian rhythm of plasma atrial natriuretic peptide, aldosterone, and blood pressure during the third trimester in normal and pre-eclamptic pregnancies. *American Journal of Obstetrics and Gynecology*, **158**, 393–399

Moll, W, Kinzel, W and Hoberger, J (1975) Haemodynamic implications of haemochorial placentations. *European Journal of Obstetrics and Gynaecology*, **5**, 67–74

Moncada, S, Radomski, MW and Palmer, RMJ (1988) Endothelium derived relaxing factor. Identification as nitric oxide and role in the control of vascular tone and platelet function. *Biochemical Pharmacology*, **37**, 2495–2501

Moncada, S, Gryglewski, RJ, Bunting, S and Vane, JR (1976) An enzyme isolated from arteries transforms prostaglandin endoperoxides to an unstable substance that inhibits platelet aggregation. *Nature*, **263**, 663–665

Montan, S, Liedholm, H, Lingman, G *et al.* (1987) Fetal and uteroplacental haemodynamics during short term atenolol treatment of hypertension. *British Journal of Obstetrics and Gynaecology*, **94**, 312–317

Moodley, J, Norman, RJ and Reddi, K (1984) Central venous concentrations of immunoreactive prostaglandins E, F, and 6-keto-prostaglandin F_1 in eclampsia. *British Medical Journal*, **288**, 1487–1489

Moore, MP and Redman, CWG (1983) Case control study of severe pre-eclampsia of early onset. *British Medical Journal*, **287**, 580

Morris, RH, Vassalli, P, Beller, FK and McCluskey, RT (1964) Immunofluorescent studies of renal biopsies in the diagnosis of toxaemia of pregnancy. *Obstetrics and Gynecology*, **24**, 32–46

Murnaghan, GA (1987) Methods of measuring blood pressure and blood pressure variability. In *Hypertension in Pregnancy* (edited by F Sharp and EM Symonds), pp. 19–28. New York: Perinatology Press

Murnaghan, GA, Mitchell, RH and Ruff, S (1980) Circadian variation of blood pressure in pregnancy. In *Pregnancy Hypertension* (edited by J Bonnar, I MacGillivray and EM Symonds) pp. 107–112. Lancaster: MTP

Naeye, RL and Friedman, EA (1979) Causes of perinatal death associated with gestational hypertension and proteinuria. *American Journal of Obstetrics and Gynecology*, **113**, 8–10

Naheedy, MH, Biller, J, Schiffer, M *et al.* (1985) Toxemia of pregnancy: cerebral findings. *Journal of Computer Assisted Tomography*, **9**, 497

Nelson, TR (1955) A clinical study of hypertension. *Journal of Obstetrics and Gynaecology of the British Empire*, **62**, 48–57

de Nucci, G, Gryglewski, RJ, Warner, TD and Vane, JR (1988) Receptor mediated release of endothelium derived relaxing factor and prostacyclin from bovine aortic endothelial cells is coupled. *Proceedings of the National Academy of Sciences (USA)*, **85**, 2334–2338

Oats, JN, Broughton Pipkin, F, Symonds, EM and Craven, DJ (1981) A prospective study of plasma angiotensin converting enzyme in normotensive primigravidae and their infants. *British Journal of Obstetrics and Gynaecology*, **88**, 1204

Oian, P, Omsjo, I, Maltau, JM and Osterud, B (1985) Increased sensitivity to thromboplastin synthesis in blood monocytes from pre-eclamptic patients. *British Journal of Obstetrics and Gynaecology*, **92**, 511–517

Overgaard, J and Skinhoj, E (1975) A paradoxical cerebral hemodynamic effect of hydralazine. *Stroke*, **6**, 402–404

Owen, JR, Irani, SF and Blair, AW (1972) Effects of diazepam administered to mothers during labour on temperature regulation in the neonate. *Archives of Disease in Childhood*, **47**, 107–110

Page, EW and Christianson, R (1976) The impact of mean arterial pressure in the middle trimester upon the outcome of pregnancy. *American Journal of Obstetrics and Gynecology*, **125**, 740–746

Palmer, RMJ, Ferrige, AG and Moncada, S (1987) Nitric oxide release accounts for the biological activity of endothelium derived relaxing factor. *Nature*, **327**, 524–526

Patrono, C, Pugliese, F, Ciabattoni, G *et al.* (1982) Evidence for a direct stimulatory effect of prostacyclin on renin release in man. *Journal of Clinical Investigation*, **69**, 231–239

Phelen, JP, Everidge, GJ, Wilder, TL and Newman, C (1977) Is the supine pressor test an adequate means of predicting acute hypertension in pregnancy? *American Journal of Obstetrics and Gynecology*, **128**, 173–176

Pickles, CJ, Symonds, EM and Broughton Pipkin, F (1989) The fetal outcome in a randomised double blind controlled trial of labetalol versus placebo in pregnancy-induced hypertension. *British Journal of Obstetrics and Gynaecology*, **96**, 38–43

Pijnenborg, R, Dixon, HG, Robertson, WB and Brosens, I (1980) Trophoblast invasion of human decidua from 8 to 18 weeks of pregnancy. *Placenta*, **1**, 3–19

Pijnenborg, R, Bland, JM, Robertson, WB *et al.* (1981) The pattern of interstitial trophoblastic invasion of the myometrium in early human pregnancy. *Placenta*, **2**, 303–316

Pijnenborg, R, Bland, JM, Robertson, WB and Brosens, I (1983) Uteroplacental arterial changes related to interstitial trophoblast migration in early human pregnancy. *Placenta*, **4**, 397–414

Poisner, AM, Wood, GW, Poisner, R and Inagami, T (1981) Localisation of renin in trophoblasts in human chorion laeve at term pregnancy. *Endocrinology*, **109**, 1150

Pollak, VE and Nettles, JB (1960) The kidney in toxemia of pregnancy: a clinical and pathologic study based on renal biopsies. *Medicine*, **39**, 469–526

Pologe, LG, Cramer, EV, Pawlowski, NA *et al.* (1984) Stimulation of human endothelial cell prostacyclin synthesis by select leukotrienes. *Journal of Experimental Medicine*, **160**, 1043–1053

Porapakkham, S (1979) An epidemiologic study of eclampsia. *Obstetrics and Gynecology*, **54**, 26–30

Pritchard, JA and Pritchard, SA (1975) Standardised treatment of 154 cases of eclampsia. *American Journal of Obstetrics and Gynecology*, **123**, 543

Pritchard, JA, Cunningham, FG and Mason, RA (1976) Coagulation changes in eclampsia: their frequency and pathogenesis. *American Journal of Obstetrics and Gynecology*, **124**, 855–864

Pruyn, SC, Phelan, JP and Buchanan, GC (1979) Longterm propranolol therapy in pregnancy: maternal and fetal outcome. *American Journal of Obstetrics and Gynecology*, **135**, 485–489

Rakoczi, I, Tallian, F, Bagdany, S and Gati, I (1979) Platelet life-span in normal pregnancy and pre-eclampsia as determined by a non-radioisotope technique. *Thrombosis Research*, **15**, 553–556

Ramanathan, J, Sibai, BM, Mabie, WC *et al.* (1988a) The use of labetalol for attenuation of the hypertensive response to endotracheal intubation in pre-eclampsia. *American Journal of Obstetrics and Gynecology*, **159**, 650–654

Ramanathan, J, Sibai, BM, Pillai, R and Angel, JJ (1988b) Neuromuscular transmission studies on pre-eclamptic women receiving magnesium sulfate. *American Journal of Obstetrics and Gynecology*, **158**, 40–46

Redd, J, Mosey, LM and Langford, HG (1968) Effect of posture upon sodium excretion in pre-eclampsia. *American Journal of Obstetrics and Gynecology*, **100**, 343–347

Redman, CWG (1982) A controlled trial of the treatment of hypertension in pregnancy: labetalol compared with methyldopa. In *The Investigation of Labetalol in the Management of Hypertension in Pregnancy* (edited by A Riley and EM Symonds) pp. 101–110. Amsterdam: Excerpta Medica

Redman, CWG (1986) Immunology of the placenta. *Clinics in Obstetrics and Gynecology*, **13**, 496–499

Redman, CWG (1987) The definition of pre-eclampsia. In *Hypertension in Pregnancy* (edited by F Sharp and EM Symonds) pp. 3–11. New York: Perinatology Press

Redman, CWG (1988) Eclampsia still kills. *British Medical Journal*, **296**, 1209–1210

Redman, CWG (1989) Hypertension in pregnancy. In *Medical Disorders in Obstetric Practice* (edited by M de Swiet) pp. 249–305. Oxford: Blackwell Scientific Publications

Redman, CWG and Jeffries, M (1988) Revised definition of pre-eclampsia. *Lancet*, **i**, 809–812

Redman, CWG, Beilin, LJ and Bonnar, J (1976a) Variability of blood pressure in normal and abnormal pregnancy. In *Hypertension in Pregnancy* (edited by MD Lindheimer, AI Katz and FP Zuspan) pp. 53–60. New York: John Wiley

Redman, CWG, Beilin, LJ and Bonnar, J (1976b) Renal function in pre-eclampsia. *Journal of Clinical Pathology*, **10 (suppl Royal College of Pathologists)**, 91–94

Redman, CWG, Beilin, LJ and Bonnar, J (1977) Treatment of hypertension in pregnancy with methyl-dopa: blood pressure control and side effects. *British Journal of Obstetrics and Gynaecology*, **84**, 419–426

Redman, CWG, Bonnar, J and Beilin, LJ (1978) Early platelet consumption in pre-eclampsia. *British Medical Journal*, **1**, 467–469

Redman, CWG, Beilin, LJ, Bonnar, J and Ounsted, MK (1976a) Plasma urate measurements in predicting fetal death in hypertensive pregnancy. *Lancet*, **i**, 1370–1373

Redman, CWG, Beilin, LJ, Bonnar, J and Ounsted, MK (1976b) Fetal outcome in trial of anti-hypertensive treatment in pregnancy. *Lancet*, **ii**, 753–756

Redman, CWG, Allington, MJ, Bolton, FG and Stirrat, GM (1977a) Plasma-thromboglobulin in pre-eclampsia. *Lancet*, **ii**, 248

Redman, CWG, Denson, KWE, Beilin, LJ *et al.* (1977b) Factor VIII consumption in pre-eclampsia. *Lancet*, **ii**, 1249–1252

Redman, CWG, Bodmer, JG, Bodmer, WF *et al.* (1978) HLA antigens in severe pre-eclampsia. *Lancet*, **ii**, 397–399

Remuzzi, G, Misiani, R, Muratore, D *et al.* (1979) Prostacyclin and human foetal circulation. *Prostaglandins*, **18**, 341–348

Remuzzi, G, Marchesi, D, Muratore, D *et al.* (1980) Reduced umbilical and placental vascular prostacyclin in severe pre-eclampsia. *Prostaglandins*, **20**, 105–110

Reynolds, B, Butters, L, Evans, J *et al.* (1984) First year of life after the use of atenolol in pregnancy associated hypertension. *Archives of Disease in Childhood*, **59**, 1061–1063

Richards, A, Graham, D and Bullock, R (1988) Clinicopathological study of neurological complications due to hypertensive disorders of pregnancy. *Journal of Neurology, Neurosurgery and Psychiatry*, **51**, 416–421

Ritter, JM, Farquar, C, Rodin, A and Thom, MH (1987) Low dose aspirin treatment in late pregnancy differentially inhibits cyclo-oxygenase in maternal platelets. *Prostaglandins*, **34**, 717–722

Robertson, EG (1971) The natural history of oedema during pregnancy. *Journal of Obstetrics and Gynaecology of the British Commonwealth*, **78**, 520–529

Robertson, WB and Khong, TY (1987) Pathology of the uteroplacental bed. In *Hypertension in Pregnancy* (edited by F Sharp and EM Symonds) pp. 101–113. New York: Perinatology Press

Robson, JS (1976) Proteinuria and the renal lesion of pre-eclampsia and abruptio placenta. In *Hypertension in Pregnancy* (edited by MD Lindheimer, AI Katz and FP Zuspan) pp. 61–73. New York: Wiley

Rodgers, GM, Taylor, RN and Roberts, JM (1988) Pre-eclampsia is associated with a serum factor cytotoxic to human endothelial cells. *American Journal of Obstetrics and Gynecology*, **159**, 908–914

Romero, R, Vizoso, J, Emamian, M *et al.* (1988) Clinical significance of liver dysfunction in pregnancy-induced hypertension. *American Journal of Perinatology*, **5**, 146–151

Rowlatt, RJ (1978) Effect of maternal diazepam on the newborn. *British Medical Journal*, **1**, 985

Rubin, PC (1987) Beta blockers in pregnancy. *British Journal of Obstetrics and Gynaecology*, **94**, 292–294

Rubin, PC, Butters, L and McCabe, R (1988) Nifedipine and platelets in pre-eclampsia. *American Journal of Hypertension*, **1**, 175–177

Rubin, PC, Butters, L, Clark, DM et al. (1983) Placebo controlled trial of atenolol in treatment of pregnancy associated hypertension. *Lancet*, **i**, 431–434

Rubin, PC, Butters, L, Clark, D et al. (1984) Obstetric aspects of the use in pregnancy-associated hypertension of the β-adrenoceptor antagonist atenolol. *American Journal of Obstetrics and Gynecology*, **150**, 389–392

Ryan, G, Lange, FR and Naugler, MA (1989) Clinical experience with phenytoin prophylaxis in severe pre-eclampsia. *American Journal of Obstetrics and Gynecology*, **161**, 1297–1304

Sacks, T, Moldow, CF, Craddock, PR et al. (1978) Oxygen radicals mediate endothelial cell damage by complement-stimulated granulocytes. An in vitro model of immune damage. *Journal of Clinical Investigation*, **61**, 1161–1167

Saleh, A, Bottoms, S, Norman, G et al. (1988) Haemostasis in hypertensive disorders of pregnancy. *Obstetrics and Gynecology*, **71**, 719–722

Sawyer, MM, Lipschitz, J, Anderson, GD et al. (1981) Diurnal and short term variation of blood pressure: comparison of pre-eclamptic, chronic hypertensive and normotensive patients. *Obstetrics and Gynecology*, **58**, 291–296

Schenker, JG and Chowers, I (1971) Phaeochromocytoma and pregnancy. Review of 89 cases. *Obstetrical and Gynecological Survey*, **26**, 739

Schenker, JG and Granat, M (1982) Phaeochromocytoma and pregnancy on updated appraisal. *Australian and New Zealand Journal of Obstetrics and Gynaecology*, **22**, 1–10

Scher, J, Hailey, DM and Beard, RW (1972) The effects of diazepam on the fetus. *Journal of Obstetrics and Gynaecology of the British Commonwealth*, **79**, 635–638

Schiff, E, Peleg, E, Goldenberg, M et al. (1989) The use of aspirin to prevent pregnancy-induced hypertension and lower the ratio of thromboxane A_2 to prostaglandin in relatively high risk pregnancies. *New England Journal of Medicine*, **321**, 351–356

Schmorl, G (1893) *Pathologische-Anatomische Untersuchingen uber Puerperaleklampsie*. Leipzig: FCW Vogel

Scott, JS (1952) Pregnancy toxaemia associated with hydrops fetalis, hydatidiform mole and hydramnios. *Journal of Obstetrics and Gynaecology of the British Commonwealth*, **65**, 689

Seligman, SA (1971) Diurnal blood pressure variation in pregnancy. *Journal of Obstetrics and Gynaecology of the British Commonwealth*, **78**, 417–422

Senior, JB, Fahim, I, Sullivan, FM and Robson, JM (1963) Possible role of 5 hydroxytryptamine in toxaemia of pregnancy. *Lancet*, **ii**, 553–554

Sexton, LI, Hertig, AT, Reid, DE et al. (1950) Premature separation of the normally implanted placenta. *American Journal of Obstetrics and Gynecology*, **59**, 13–24

Seymour, AE, Petrucco, OM, Clarkson, AR et al. (1976) Morphological and immunological evidence of coagulopathy in renal complications of pregnancy. In *Hypertension in Pregnancy* (edited by MD Lindheimer, AI Katz and F Zuspan) pp. 139–153. New York: Wiley

Shanklin, DR and Sibai, BM (1989) Ultrastructural aspects of pre-eclampsia. *American Journal of Obstetrics and Gynecology*, **161**, 735–741

Sheehan, HL and Lynch, JB (1973) *Pathology of Toxaemia of Pregnancy*. London: Churchill Livingstone

Sheppard, BL and Bonnar, J (1976) The ultrastructure of the arterial supply of the human placenta in pregnancy complicated by intrauterine growth retardation. *British Journal of Obstetrics and Gynaecology*, **83**, 948–959

Sheppard, BL and Bonnar, J (1981) An ultrastructural study of uteroplacental spiral arteries in hypertensive and normotensive pregnancy and fetal growth retardation. *British Journal of Obstetrics and Gynaecology*, **88**, 695–705

Sibai, BM, El-Nazer, A and Gonzalez-Ruiz, A (1986) Severe pre-eclampsia-eclampsia in young primigravid women: subsequent pregnancy outcome and remote prognosis. *American Journal of Obstetrics and Gynecology*, **155**, 1011–1016

Sibai, BM, Grossman, RA and Grossman, HG (1984) Effect of diuretics on plasma volume in pregnancies with long term hypertension. *American Journal of Obstetrics and Gynecology*, **150**, 831–835

Sibai, BM, Schneider, JM and Morrison, JC (1980) The late postpartum eclampsia controversy. *Obstetrics and Gynecology*, **55**, 1

Sibai, BM, McCubbin, JH, Anderson, GD *et al.* (1981) Eclampsia I: observations from 67 recent cases. *Obstetrics and Gynecology*, **58**, 609–613

Sibai, BM, Spinnato, JA, Watson, DL *et al.* (1984) Effect of magnesium sulphate on electroencephalographic findings in pre-eclampsia and eclampsia. *Obstetrics and Gynecology*, **64**, 261–266

Sibai, BM, Gonzalez, AR, Mabie, WC and Moretti, M (1987) A comparison of labetalol plus hospitalisation alone in the management of pre-eclampsia remote from term. *Obstetrics and Gynecology*, **70**, 323–327

Sibai, BM, Mirro, R, Chesney, CM and Leffler, C (1989) Low dose aspirin in pregnancy. *Obstetrics and Gynecology*, **74**, 551–557

Sims, EAH and Krantz, KE (1985) Serial study of renal function during pregnancy and the puerperium in normal women. *Journal of Clinical Investigation*, **37**, 1764

Sinzinger, H, Virgolini, I and Peskar, BA (1989) Response of thromboxane B_2, malondialdehyde and platelet sensitivity to 3 weeks low dose aspirin in health volunteers. *Thrombosis Research*, **53**, 261–269

Skinner, SL, Lumbers, ER and Symonds, EM (1972) Analysis of changes in the renin–angiotensin system during pregnancy. *Clinical Science*, **42**, 479

Slater, RM, Wilcox, FL, Smith, WD *et al.* (1987) Phenytoin infusion in severe pre-eclampsia. *Lancet*, **i**, 1417–1421

Socol, ML, Weiner, CP, Louis, G *et al.* (1985) Platelet activation in pre-eclampsia. *American Journal of Obstetrics and Gynecology*, **151**, 494–497

Spargo, B, McCartney, CP and Winemiller, R (1959) Glomerular capillary endotheliosis in toxemia of pregnancy. *Archives of Pathology*, **68**, 593–599

Spencer, JAD, Smith, MJ, Cederholm-Williams, SA and Wilkinson, AR (1983) Influence of pre-eclampsia on concentrations of haemostatic factors in mothers and infants. *Archives of Disease in Childhood*, **58**, 739–741

Speroff, L, Haning, RV and Levin, RM (1977) The effect of angiotensin II and indomethacin on uterine artery blood flow in pregnant monkeys. *Obstetrics and Gynecology*, **50**, 611

Spitz, B, Magness, RR, Cox, SM *et al.* (1988) Low dose aspirin 1. Effect on angiotensin II pressor responses and blood prostaglandin concentration in pregnant women sensitive to angiotensin II. *American Journal of Obstetrics and Gynecology*, **159**, 1035–1043

Stirrat, GM (1987) The immunology of hypertension in pregnancy. In *Hypertension in Pregnancy* (edited by F Sharp and EM Symonds) pp. 249–259. New York: Perinatology Press

Stuart, MJ, Clark, DA, Sunderji, SG *et al.* (1981) Decreased prostacyclin production: a characteristic of chronic placental insufficiency syndromes. *Lancet*, **i**, 1126–1128

Stuart, MJ, Gross, SJ, Elrad, H and Groeber, JE (1982) Effects of acetylsalicylic acid ingestion on maternal and neonatal hemostasis. *New England Journal of Medicine*, **307**, 909–912

Studd, JWW, Blainey, JD and Bailey, DE (1970) Serum protein changes in pre-eclampsia-eclampsia syndrome. *Journal of Obstetrics and Gynaecology of the British Commonwealth*, **77**, 796–801

Sumioki, H, Shimokowa, H, Miyamoto, D *et al.* (1989) Circadian variations of plasma atrial naturiuretic peptide in four types of hypertensive disorder during pregnancy. *British Journal of Obstetrics and Gynaecology*, **96**, 922–927

Symonds, EM and Broughton Pipkin, F (1978) Pregnancy hypertension, parity and the renin–angiotensin system. *American Journal of Obstetrics and Gynecology*, **132**, 473

Symonds, EM, Broughton Pipkin, F and Craven, DJ (1975) Changes in the renin–angiotensin system in primigravidae with hypertensive disease of pregnancy. *British Journal of Obstetrics and Gynaecology*, **82**, 643

Symonds, EM, Stanley, MA and Skinner, SL (1968) Production of renin by in vitro cultures of human chorion and uterine muscle. *Nature*, **217**, 1152

Talledo, OE, Chesley, LC and Zuspan, FP (1968) Renin angiotensin system in normal and toxaemic pregnancies III. Differential sensitivity to angiotensin II and norepinephrine in toxaemia of pregnancy. *American Journal of Obstetrics and Gynecology*, **100**, 218–221

Tateson, JE, Moncada, S and Vane, JR (1977) Effects of prostacyclin (PGX) on cyclic AMP concentrations in human platelets. *Prostaglandins*, **13**, 389–399

Taylor, D (1988) The epidemiology of hypertension during pregnancy. In *Hypertension in Pregnancy* (edited by P Rubin) pp. 223–240. Amsterdam: Elsevier

Templeton, A and Campbell, D (1977) A retrospective study of eclampsia in the Grampian Region. *Health Bulletin*, **37**, 55–59

Tervila, L, Groecke, C and Timonen, S (1973) Estimation of gestosis of pregnancy (EPH-gestosis). *Acta Obstetrica and Gynecologica Scandinavica*, **52**, 235

Theisen, R, Jackson, R, Morrissey, J *et al*. (1961) Serum enzymes in normal and toxemic pregnancies. *Obstetrics and Gynecology*, **17**, 183

Thomson, AM, Hytten, RE and Billewicz, WZ (1967) The epidemiology of oedema during pregnancy. *Journal of Obstetrics and Gynaecology of the British Commonwealth*, **74**, 1–10

Thomson, D, Paterson, WG, Smart, GE *et al*. (1972) The renal lesions of toxaemia and abrupto placentae studied by light and electron microscopy. *Journal of Obstetrics and Gynaecology of the British Commonwealth*, **79**, 311–312

Thornton, CA and Bonnar, J (1977) Factor VIII-related antigen and Factor VIII coagulant activity in normal and pre-eclamptic pregnancy. *British Journal of Obstetrics and Gynaecology*, **84**, 919–923

Toivanen, J, Ylikorkala, O and Viinikka, L (1984) One milligramme of acetylsalicylic acid daily inhibits platelet thromboxane A_2 production. *Thrombosis Research*, **35**, 681–687

Tribe, CR, Smart, GE, Davies, DR and Mackenzie, JC (1979) A renal biopsy study in toxaemia of pregnancy using light microscopy linked with immunofluorescence and immuno-electron microscopy. *Journal of Clinical Pathology*, **32**, 681–692

Trudinger, BJ (1976) Platelets and intra-uterine growth retardation in pre-eclampsia. *British Journal of Obstetrics and Gynaecology*, **83**, 284–286

Trudinger, BJ, Cook, CM, Thompson, RS, Giles, WB and Connelly, A (1988) Low-dose aspirin therapy improves fetal weight in umbilical placental insufficiency. *American Journal of Obstetrics and Gynecology*, **159**, 681–685

Tulenko, T, Schneider, J, Floro, C and Sicilla, M (1987) The in vitro effect on arterial wall function of serum from patients with pregnancy induced hypertension. *American Journal of Obstetrics and Gynecology*, **156**, 817–823

Tunstall, ME (1969) The effect of propranolol on the onset of breathing at birth. *British Journal of Anaesthesia*, **41**, 792

Tuvemo, T (1980) Role of prostaglandins, prostacyclin and thromboxanes in the control of the umbilical-placental circulation. *Seminars in Perinatology*, **4**, 91–95

Ueland, K, Novy, MJ, Peterson, EN and Metcalfe, J (1969) Maternal cardiovascular dynamics. IV The influence of gestational age on the maternal cardiovascular response to posture and exercise. *American Journal of Obstetrics and Gynecology*, **104**, 856–864

Villar, MA and Sibai, BM (1988) Eclampsia. *Obstetric and Gynecology Clinics of North America*, **15**, 355–377

Vosburgh, GJ (1976) Blood pressure, edema and proteinuria in pregnancy. Edema relationships. *Progress in Clinical and Biological Research*, **7**, 155–168

Waisman, GD, Mayorga, LM, Camera, MI *et al*. (1988) Magnesium plus nifedipine: potentiation of hypotensive effect in pre-eclampsia. *American Journal of Obstetrics and Gynecology*, **159**, 308–309

Walker, JJ (1987) The case for early recognition and intervention in pregnancy induced hypertension. In *Hypertension in Pregnancy* (edited by F Sharp and EM Symonds) pp. 289–304. New York: Perinatology Press

Walker, JJ, Greer, IA and Calder, AA (1983) Treatment of acute pregnancy related hypertension: labetalol and hydralazine compared. *Postgraduate Medical Journal*, **59 (suppl 3)**, 168–170

Wallenburg, HCS (1988) Hemodynamics in hypertensive pregnancy. In *Hypertension in Pregnancy* (edited by P Rubin) pp. 66–101. New York: Elsevier

Wallenburg, HCS and Hutchinson, DL (1979) A radioangiographic study of the effects of catecholamines on uteroplacental blood flow in the rhesus monkey. *Journal of Medical Primatology*, **8**, 57–65

Wallenburg, HCS and Rotmans, N (1982) Enhanced reactivity of the platelet thromboxane pathway in normotensive and hypertensive pregnancies with insufficient fetal growth. *American Journal of Obstetrics and Gynecology*, **144**, 523–528

Wallenburg, HCS and Rotmans, U (1987) Prevention of recurrent idiopathic fetal growth retardation by low-dose aspirin and dipyridamole. *American Journal of Obstetrics and Gynecology*, **157**, 1230–1235

Wallenburg, HCS, Dekker, GA, Makovitz, JW and Rotmans, P (1986) Low dose aspirin prevents pregnancy induced hypertension and pre-eclampsia in angiotensin-sensitive primigravidae. *Lancet*, **i**, 1–3

Walsh, SW (1985) Pre-eclampsia: an imbalance in placental prostacyclin and thromboxane production. *American Journal of Obstetrics and Gynecology*, **152**, 335–340

Walsh, SW, Behr, MJ and Allen, NH (1985) Placental prostacyclin production in normal and toxemic pregnancies. *American Journal of Obstetrics and Gynecology*, **151**, 110–115

Walters, BNJ and Redman, CWG (1984) Treatment of severe pregnancy-associated hypertension with the calcium antagonist nifedipine. *British Journal of Obstetrics and Gynaecology*, **91**, 330–336

Warren, AY, Craven, DJ and Symonds, EM (1982) Production of active and inactive renin by cultured explants from the human female genital tract. *British Journal of Obstetrics and Gynaecology*, **89**, 628

Warso, MA and Lands, WEM (1983) Lipid peroxidation in relation to prostacyclin and thromboxane physiology and pathophysiology. *British Medical Bulletin*, **39**, 277–280

Watson, DL, Sibai, BM, Shaver, DC *et al.* (1983) Late postpartum eclampsia: an update. *Southern Medical Journal*, **76**, 1487–1489

Weiner, CP and Brandt, J (1982) Plasma antithrombin III activity: an aid in the diagnosis of pre-eclampsia-eclampsia. *American Journal of Obstetrics and Gynecology*, **142**, 275–281

Weiner, CP, Kwaan, HC, Xu, C *et al.* (1985) Antithrombin III activity in women with hypertension during pregnancy. *Obstetrics and Gynecology*, **65**, 301–306

Weinstein, L (1982) Syndrome of hemolysis, elevated liver enzymes and low platelet count: a severe consequence of hypertension in pregnancy. *American Journal of Obstetrics and Gynecology*, **142**, 159–167

Weinstein, L (1985) Pre-eclampsia/eclampsia with hemolysis elevated liver enzymes and thrombocytopenia. *Obstetrics and Gynecology*, **66**, 657–660

Weir, RJ, Brown, JJ, Fraser, R *et al.* (1975) Relationship between plasma renin, renin substrate, angiotensin II, aldosterone and electrolytes in normal pregnancy. *Journal of Clinical Endocrinology and Metabolism*, **40**, 108

Weir, RJ, Fraser, R, Lever, AF *et al.* (1973) Plasma renin, renin substrate, angiotensin II and aldosterone in hypertensive disease of pregnancy. *Lancet*, **i**, 291

Weksler, BB and Jaffe, EA (1986) Prostacyclin and the endothelium. In *Vascular Endothelium in Hemostasis and Thrombosis* (edited by MA Gimbrone) pp. 40–56. Edinburgh: Churchill Livingstone

Whigham, KAE, Howie, PW, Drummond, AH and Prentice, CRM (1978) Abnormal platelet function in pre-eclampsia. *British Journal of Obstetrics and Gynaecology*, **85**, 28–32

Wichman, K, Ryulden, G and Karlberg, BE (1984) A placebo controlled trial of metoprolol in the treatment of hypertension in pregnancy. *Scandinavian Journal of Clinical and Laboratory Investigation*, (suppl) **169**, 90

Wightman, H, Hibbard, BM and Rosen, NM (1978) Perinatal mortality and morbidity associated with eclampsia. *British Medical Journal*, **2**, 235

Winter, ME and Tozer, TN (1986) Phenytoin. In Applied *Pharmacokinetics – Principles of Therapeutic Drug Monitoring* (edited by WE Evans, JJ Schentag and WJ Jusko) pp. 493–539. San Francisco: Applied Therapeutics

de Wolf, F, Brosens, I and Renaer, M (1980) Fetal growth retardation and the maternal arterial supply of the human placenta in the absence of sustained hypertension. *British Journal of Obstetrics and Gynaecology*, **87**, 678–685

de Wolf, F, Robertson, WB and Brosens, I (1975) The ultrastructure of acute atherosis in hypertensive pregnancy. *American Journal of Obstetrics and Gynecology*, **123**, 164–174

Zeek, PM and Assali, NS (1950) Vascular changes with eclamptogenic toxemia of pregnancy. *American Journal of Obstetrics and Gynecology*, **20**, 1099–1109

Chapter 3

Thrombo-embolism

Elizabeth A Letsky

Introduction

The profound changes in blood volume (Hytten, 1985) and haemostatic mechanisms (Stirling *et al.*, 1984), together with suppression of fibrinolysis (Ballegeer *et al.*, 1987) during normal pregnancy, help to combat the hazard of haemorrhage at delivery but convert pregnancy into a hypercoagulable state. Venous thrombo-embolism is one of the most serious complications that can arise in the healthy pregnant woman and the diagnosis and management present special problems. Obstetric deaths from all causes have decreased markedly over the past 30 years but pulmonary embolism has remained the first or second most important cause of maternal mortality in England and Wales (Department of Health, 1989).

Most patients with pulmonary embolism die rapidly before diagnosis can be made and treatment instituted. Often the deep vein thrombosis develops without symptoms or overt clinical signs. Until significant advances are made in early detection of venous thrombosis and prevention of thrombo-embolism, the maternal deaths from this cause are unlikely to be reduced. The absolute numbers over the past triennia have remained remarkably steady in the published *Confidential Enquiries into Maternal Deaths in England and Wales*. Similarly in Sweden maternal mortality rates from haemorrhage, pre-eclampsia and sepsis have fallen over the years but deaths from pulmonary embolism have remained stable (Hogberg, 1986).

Although pulmonary embolism is the most serious immediate result of venous thrombosis, many women who do not suffer this complication are left with chronic venous insufficiency leading to pain, leg oedema and skin changes with ulceration (Bergqvist *et al.*, 1990).

A reduction of morbidity and mortality resulting from venous thrombosis can be achieved only by recognition of predisposing factors and selective use of prophylaxis in high-risk patients. This chapter attempts to deal with these controversial issues.

Incidence and significance

Accurate figures for maternal deaths in England and Wales associated with pulmonary embolism are available over the past 30 years because of the detailed reports of *Confidential Enquiries into Maternal Deaths in England and Wales* (Department of Health, 1989). We can be confident of these data because deaths from pulmonary embolism are relatively easy to diagnose. Pulmonary embolus was also the second cause of maternal death in Massachusets, USA, between 1982 and 1985 (Sachs *et al.*, 1987) giving a mortality rate of 1.2 per 100 000.

From the Department of Health (DHS) triennial reports it is clear that overall mortalities have fallen over the past few decades, mainly because of a dramatic reduction in postpartum fatalities. However, the proportion of deaths occurring in the antenatal period has shown a sharp increase more recently.

Thrombo-embolism was previously regarded as a complication of the puerperium. Only four of the 138 women in the 1952–1954 period died during pregnancy but, since 1961, 25 per cent of the deaths at least have occurred in the antenatal period and have been distributed throughout the 40 weeks of pregnancy. The *Report of Confidential Enquiries* of 1989 described 25 deaths occurring in the triennium 1982–1984, of which one-third occurred after abortion or antenatally. However, the most recent Report (Department of Health, 1991), concerning the triennium 1985–1987 and including those deaths occurring in Scotland and Northern Ireland, demonstrated not only that pulmonary embolism was the most frequent cause of maternal mortality but that more than half, 17 of the 29 deaths, occurred during the antenatal period.

After delivery, the most dangerous period for fatal pulmonary embolism is the first week, then the second week, after which the risk decreases. A significant proportion of deaths (up to 19 per cent) occur within the first 24 hours following both vaginal delivery and caesarean section. This has important implications in terms of prophylaxis of thrombo-embolism in high-risk cases.

It is more difficult to obtain accurate figures for the incidence of non-fatal deep vein thrombosis (DVT) and, to a lesser extent, pulmonary embolism (PE). These conditions are not easy to diagnose objectively or with precision and there are particular difficulties during pregnancy (see below). Pregnancy appears to increase the risk of thrombo-embolism sixfold (Royal College of General Practitioners, 1967). In earlier published reports the incidence of thrombo-embolic complications varied between two and five per 1000 deliveries (Aaro and Juergens, 1971, 1974; Coon, 1977). An incidence of DVT of 0.19 per cent in 32 337 pregnancies at the Mayo Clinic has been reported (Aaro and Juergens, 1971). At Queen Charlotte's Maternity Hospital, there were 20 cases of DVT and 10 cases of PE associated with 35 000 deliveries in the decade 1970 to 1980, an overall incidence of 0.09 per cent. Confirmation of these diagnoses was obtained by venogram or scan in the majority of cases (de Swiet *et al.*, 1981).

There are few studies using objective methods, because of the problems of using radiographic or radio-isotope techniques during pregnancy (Ginsberg *et al.*, 1989a). In one early study, Friend and Kakkar (1970) used ^{125}I-labelled fibrinogen in the puerperium. Their results suggested an incidence of DVT of 2.6 per cent following vaginal delivery. Later studies using the less accurate but safer methods of plethysmography and thermography (Sandler and Martin, 1985) suggested incidences of 0.07 per cent during pregnancy and 1.8 per cent following caesarean section (Bergqvist, Bergqvist and Hallbrook, 1979, 1983).

We are faced therefore with the problem of managing a condition which occurs rarely during pregnancy, which is difficult to identify but which is a major cause of maternal mortality.

Epidemiological observations (Treffers *et al.*, 1983) show that the incidence of postpartum thrombo-embolism has fallen but not that of antenatal complications. This could be attributable to a number of factors: the trend towards younger mothers and smaller families; the virtual disappearance of the elderly grand multipara and traumatic operative delivery; early ambulation and better diagnosis and treatment.

On the other hand, the increase in proportion of antenatal complications could be due to increased rates of admission to hospital and the use of bed rest in the management of hypertension and antepartum haemorrhage (see below).

Risk factors

Haemostatic factors

The procoagulant factors
Increases in concentrations of factor XII, high-molecular-weight kininogen and prekallikrein have been reported (Hellgren and Blomback, 1981; Sayama *et al.*, 1981; Adam *et al.*, 1985). More important than these documented increases are the significant increases in factors VIII, VII and X and the very marked increase in fibrinogen. Both von Willebrand factor and factor VIII coagulant activity (the components of the factor VIII complex) increase progressively throughout pregnancy. The coagulation activity of factor VIII at term is approximately double that found in the non-pregnant state. Some workers have found a parallel increase in von Willebrand factor and factor VIII bioactivity (Scholtes, Gerretsen and Haak, 1983) but the majority have reported an increase in the von Willebrand factor:factor VIIIC ratio in the order of 2:1 (Hellgren and Blomback, 1981; Inglis *et al.*, 1982; Stirling *et al.*, 1984). Factor VIII is a key procoagulant factor of the intrinsic system. The increase in concentration of factor VII, the main component of the extrinsic coagulation system, may be as much as tenfold (Beller and Ebert, 1982; Stirling *et al.*, 1984). There is also an increase in factor X, one of the most important linking factors between the intrinsic and extrinsic coagulation systems. The most dramatic increase, however, occurs in the concentration of fibrinogen, which rises from a non-pregnant level of 2.5–4.0 g/l to 6.0 g/l during late pregnancy and labour. If the increase in plasma volume is taken into consideration, the amount of circulating fibrinogen during late pregnancy is at least double that present in the non-pregnant state (Hellgren and Blomback, 1981; Stirling *et al.*, 1984).

Naturally occurring anticoagulants
The three clinically important factors are antithrombin III, protein C and its co-factor protein S. Antithrombin III is the essential heparin co-factor and exerts its main influence against factors Xa and thrombin (Abildgaard, 1979). Antithrombin III activity, although thought in earlier studies to decrease in pregnancy, has now been shown to remain relatively unchanged (Weiner and Brandt, 1980; Hellgren and Blomback, 1981; Stirling *et al.*, 1984). Protein C and protein S balance the activity of the procoagulant factors V and VIII (Clouse and Comp, 1986). Protein C levels appear to remain constant or to increase slightly (Mannucci *et al.*, 1984; Gonzales, Alberca and Vincente, 1985; Malm, Laurell and Dahlback, 1988). When total protein S is measured antigenically, protein S activity is found to fall during normal pregnancy (Comp *et al.*, 1986a,b; Warwick *et al.*, 1989). The result of these physiological changes is to alter the usual balance between the procoagulants and anticoagulants in favour of the factors promoting blood clotting.

Fibrinolysis
Fibrinolytic activity appears to be reduced during healthy pregnancy, but rapidly returns to normal after delivery. This is thought to be due to the effect of placentally

derived plasminogen activator inhibitor type II (PAI-2) which is present in abundance during pregnancy (Nilsson *et al.*, 1986; Booth *et al.*, 1988). In addition, the activity of the fibrinolytic system in response to stimulation has been found to be significantly reduced in pregnancy (Ballegeer *et al.*, 1987) and this physiological impairment of fibrinolysis could contribute to the increased thrombotic risk in pregnancy.

Postpartum changes in coagulation and fibrinolysis
The dramatic changes in haemostasis revert to normal after the uterus has emptied. The most rapid effect is in fibrinolysis, which returns to non-pregnant activity within hours of separation of the placenta, following the loss of placentally derived PAI-2 (Wiman *et al.*, 1984). Immediately after delivery, there is evidence of coagulation activation and platelet consumption followed a few days later by an increase in platelet count, fibrinogen and factor VIIIC. All the components of the haemostatic system appear to return to normal within 4 weeks of delivery.

It is most likely, therefore, that the pathogenesis of venous thrombosis in pregnancy results from a combination of the increased tendency to venous stasis in the lower limbs, together with a disturbance in the balance of coagulation factors and impaired fibrinolysis which favours thrombus formation.

Other pregnancy-related risk factors

Operative delivery
There is no doubt, on analysis of the *Reports of Confidential Enquiries*, that the risk of fatal pulmonary embolism following caesarean section is on average at least ten times greater than that following vaginal delivery. It is probable that other forms of complicated instrumental delivery also increase the risk of thrombo-embolism (Aaro and Juergens, 1974). The overall incidence of thrombo-embolism following caesarean section is about 20 times greater than that following spontaneous vaginal delivery (Treffers *et al.*, 1983).

Age and parity
The risk of thrombo-embolism is greater with increasing age and parity, which operate independently of each other. Advancing age is the more potent risk factor, with a marked increase after the age of 35 years.

Obesity
This is an important risk factor in women weighing >76 kg. Analysis of the *Reports of Confidential Enquiries* reveals that approximately one in five women with fatal pulmonary embolism fell into this category.

Restricted activity
Conditions that may complicate pregnancy, such as hypertension, diabetes, placenta praevia, multiple pregnancy and heart disease, often warrant admission to hospital with restricted activity and prolonged periods of bed rest. Women with pregnancies complicated in this manner are at increased risk of thrombo-embolism.

Suppression of lactation with oestrogen
Stilboestrol treatment to suppress lactation was first shown by Daniel and colleagues

in 1967 (Daniel, Campbell and Turnbull, 1967) to increase tenfold the risk of non-fatal thrombo-embolism in women of low parity aged 25 years and more and the finding was supported by Jeffcoate and colleagues (Jeffcoate *et al.*, 1968). If drug treatment is required to suppress lactation, bromocriptine should be used rather than oestrogens.

Additional non-pregnancy-related risk factors

Previous thrombo-embolism
In a retrospective analysis, Badaracco and Vessey (1974) estimated that there was about a 12 per cent risk of developing PE or DVT in pregnancy if a woman had a history of thrombo-embolism. The risk was not affected by the circumstances of the previous event, e.g. whether associated with pregnancy or with oral contraception.

Lupus anticoagulant
The presence of lupus anticoagulant indicates a risk for both venous and arterial thrombo-embolism and the thrombi may occur in atypical sites such as the arm, portal vessels and cerebral vasculature. These women need special management during pregnancy (see below).

Paroxysmal nocturnal haemoglobinuria (PNH)
There is an increased risk of thrombo-embolism in this rare condition which occasionally complicates pregnancy (Hurd, Miodovnik and Stys, 1982) (see below). Thrombosis accounts for approximately 50 per cent of deaths in reported autopsies. The major morbidity also relates to venous thrombosis, which has been reported in peripheral as well as in mesenteric, hepatic, portal and cerebral veins.

The hypercoagulable state has been attributed to the triggering effect of intravascular haemolysis and increased activity of coagulation factors but the most relevant explanation for the enhanced thrombotic tendency is that the PNH platelets can bind much greater amounts of complement than normal platelets. Activation of the complement pathway triggers PNH platelets to undergo the release reaction and aggregate, thus initiating thrombosis (Vermylen *et al.*, 1986). The fertility rate in this uncommon condition is thought to be low and experience of pregnancies complicated by PNH is limited.

Hereditary risk factors

ABO blood group
To have an ABO blood group other than O is a risk factor for thrombo-embolism in pregnancy, as in the non-pregnant state (Jick *et al.*, 1969). Analysis of *Reports of Confidential Enquiries* shows a lower than expected incidence of blood group O in women with fatal thrombo-embolism. Only 1 of 17 patients (6 per cent) with DVT in pregnancy belonged to blood group O in a Scandinavian study (Bergqvist, Bergqvist and Hallbrook, 1983). The expected prevalence of group O in Northern Europe is approximately 45 per cent.

Homocystinuria
Patients with homocystinuria are at increased risk from both arterial and venous

thrombo-embolism (Mudd *et al.*, 1985). The risk has been demonstrated in pregnancy (Constantine and Green, 1987) but the mechanism of increased risk is unknown (Davies, 1985). In those patients in whom the metabolic defect responds to pyridoxine therapy, the risk of thrombo-embolism may be decreased by using this treatment (Constantine and Green, 1987).

Hereditary coagulopathies

Antithrombin III (ATIII), protein C and protein S deficiencies and dysfibrinogenaemia may all be associated with a hypercoagulable state (thrombophilia). ATIII deficiency is rare. Not one case was found in >500 patients screened for ATIII deficiency following severe thrombosis (Bergqvist and Hedner, 1983). However, familial ATIII deficiency often presents for the first time in pregnancy where the risk of thrombo-embolism is about 70 per cent if no prophylaxis is used (Hellgren *et al.*, 1983).

The frequency of protein C and protein S deficiencies among women with thrombo-embolism in pregnancy is as yet unknown but it is likely to be greater than that of ATIII deficiency. Protein C deficiency is present in 8 per cent of patients with a first episode of thrombo-embolism before the age of 40 years and 7 per cent of patients with recurrent episodes (Horellou *et al.*, 1984).

Protein S deficiency has been described in families with recurrent thrombo-embolism (Comp and Esmon, 1984). At Queen Charlotte's and Chelsea Hospital we are beginning to find women with protein C and protein S deficiencies who present with thrombo-embolism in pregnancy or who have a personal or family history of thrombo-embolism. Before the recent introduction of laboratory screening procedures, these women would have gone unidentified.

Women with a past history of thrombo-embolism or a family history should be screened for thrombophilia, preferably before embarking upon pregnancy, as they may need special management. It is also very important to complete screening tests once pregnancy is successfully negotiated in a woman who presents with a first episode of thrombo-embolism in the index pregnancy. Screening presents special difficulties during pregnancy because of the physiological alterations in haemostatic factors in healthy pregnancy.

Diagnosis of thrombo-embolism

Clinical features of PE and DVT are well known, although notoriously unreliable. It is particularly important to establish an objective diagnosis in pregnancy because long-term anticoagulant therapy is not without risk to both mother and fetus (see below). In addition, any thrombo-embolism in a young woman of childbearing years, whether pregnant or not, will cause concern regarding prophylaxis in future pregnancies.

Venous thrombosis

In pregnancy, DVT is much more common in the left femoral vein and tributaries than in the right. The ratio is approximately 8:1 (Bergqvist, Bergqvist and Hallbrook, 1983; Bergqvist and Hedner, 1983). It very difficult to make a diagnosis on clinical signs alone. For example, physiological swelling of the lower extremities in pregnancy is usually slowly progressive, painless and symmetrical but may occasionally cause rapid and unilateral increase without any underlying thrombosis. It has been estimated that if venography is not used for the diagnosis of DVT, two patients are treated unnecessarily for each one treated correctly (Ramsay, 1983). Approximately 50 per cent of patients who have an acutely tender swollen calf do not have a DVT (Simpson et al., 1980; Sandler et al., 1984) and some form of investigation must therefore be performed in order to support a clinical diagnosis.

Impedance plethysmography (IPG)
This method is based on the principle that blood volume changes in the calf preceded by inflation of a pneumatic thigh cuff result in changes in electrical activity that can be detected by locally placed electrodes. These electrical changes are reduced in patients with thrombosis of the popliteal or more proximal veins. This test is 95 per cent sensitive and specific for proximal DVT in non-pregnant patients (Wheeler and Anderson, 1985) but it is very insensitive for isolated calf DVT. In addition, there are two main disadvantages to the use of IPG in clinical practice: (1) it must be repeated serially in patients with an initial normal result; (2) false-positive results may occur with conditions that interfere with arterial inflow and venous emptying.

Serial IPG testing has not been evaluated in a large number of pregnant patients. The specificity and positive predictive value of the test is questionable in the third trimester because false positive results may be obtained with the uterus pressing on the iliofemoral veins (Clarke-Pearson and Jelovsek, 1981).

Doppler ultrasound
The Doppler ultrasound detector emits an ultrasound beam which is reflected from red cells at a frequency that is proportional to the velocity of blood flow. The examination starts at the common femoral vein and moves distally to the femoral, popliteal and posterior tibial veins. A number of Doppler abnormalities occur in the presence of DVT, the most common of which are loss of plasticity during the respiratory cycle and decreased or absent augmentation during compression manoeuvres (Polak and O'Leary, 1988).

In expert hands the test has a sensitivity of 87 per cent and a specificity of 95 per cent (Sandler et al., 1984) for proximal DVT; it is less sensitive for isolated calf DVT. Like IPG, Doppler ultrasound should be repeated serially in those patients with an initial normal result. In addition, false-positive results may be obtained during the third trimester of pregnancy, due to compression of the iliofemoral veins by the enlarged uterus.

Real-time ultrasonography
This method, well known in the field of cardiac imaging in cardiovascular diseases, has more recently been used in the diagnosis of DVT in lower limbs (Vogel et al., 1987). Real-time ultrasound visualizes the common femoral vein, femoral vein and popliteal vein. Although visualization of intraluminal clots can be difficult because of the difference in echogenicity depending on the age of the thrombus, when the technique is combined with external compression the identification of thrombosis is more reliable and reproducible. The accuracy of compression ultrasonography (CU) has been compared to that of contrast venography. It has the same potential drawbacks as IPG and Doppler ultrasound. In addition, it is not possible to detect isolated iliac thrombosis. This method, however, has been employed successfully in the diagnosis of DVT in pregnancy (Greer et al., 1990). It has the advantage of being non-invasive and quick and uses standard equipment that is available in most

obstetric units. The use of the equipment is easy and safe and it can be used repeatedly to monitor progress. Venography (see below) is not made redundant by this technique but a firm diagnosis of DVT using CU can allow the use of anti-coagulant therapy without recourse to venography and its potential hazards (Ginsberg *et al.*, 1989). Venography may be required to demonstrate pelvic vein thrombosis (inaccessible to this technique) or to confirm or refute the occasional equivocal result. It has been suggested (Greer *et al.*, 1990) that real-time ultrasound should be used as the investigation of choice for the primary diagnosis of DVT in antenatal patients, with venography being reserved for the further investigation of equivocal results.

Isotope methods
^{125}I-fibrinogen screening is a non-invasive imaging technique based on the incorporation of radiolabelled fibrinogen into an actively forming thrombus. ^{125}I-fibrinogen leg-screening is contraindicated in pregnancy. In the antenatal period, the isotope is trapped by the fetal thyroid and may cause hypothyroidism (Excess and Graeme, 1974) or subsequent carcinoma. It is also secreted in high concentration in the breast milk and the same risks apply to the breast-fed infant.

Contrast venography
This is the traditional reference method or 'gold standard' for the diagnosis of DVT. Radio-opaque contrast material is injected into a dorsal vein in the foot in order to visualize the entire deep venous system of the leg. It is reliable provided that it is properly performed and interpreted (Redman, 1988). The diagnostic indicators are (1) the presence of a constant intraluminal filling defect seen in two or more views; (2) an abrupt cut off in a deep vein above the knee. At present, none of the diagnostic techniques available outside specialist vascular laboratories approaches the precision of venography (Sandler *et al.*, 1984). However venography is an invasive technique with a number of disadvantages. Fetal irradiation is obviously of concern but with adequate shielding of the uterus, the direct radiation dose is very small and less than in pelvimetry (Laros and Alger, 1979). Pain may be caused by venography but this can be lessened by the use of non-ionic contrast agents (Bettman *et al.*, 1987). Post-venographic DVT may occur in a small number (<5 per cent) of patients (Albrechtsson and Olsson, 1979). The use of less-irritant water-soluble non-ionic contrast media makes it much less likely that venography itself will promote thrombo-embolism (Thomas *et al.*, 1984). In most centres the procedure is covered with intravenous heparin until the diagnosis is confirmed or refuted.

^{99}Tc^m red-cell venography
For this test, 2 ml of the patient's red blood cells are labelled *in vitro* with 20 mCi of ^{99}Tc^m pertechnetate. The labelled red cells are then reinjected in order to visualize the venous system. A recent prospective study showed that ^{99}Tc^m red blood cell venography had high sensitivity but lower specificity for the diagnosis of DVT (Leclerc *et al.*, 1988). Thus a normal ^{99}Tc^m venogram may be taken to rule out this diagnosis but an abnormal result should not be assumed to establish the diagnosis. As a result of this test, 300–400 mrad are delivered to the gonads depending on whether the bladder is full or empty. This corresponds to approximately half the dose delivered by pelvimetry and therefore ^{99}Tc^m venography should probably not be used in pregnancy (Leclerc and Roy, 1991).

Pulmonary embolism

The clinical manifestations of pulmonary embolism (PE) depend on the size, number and location of the emboli and are varied. Patients with massive PE, attributable either to multiple small emboli obstructing >50 per cent of the pulmonary vasculature or to large emboli in the main pulmonary outflow tract, collapse with hypotension, chest pain, breathlessness and cyanosis. On occasion they may present with abdominal pain only, perhaps due to diaphragmatic irritation (Hussein and Critchley, 1986). On further examination they may be found to have a third heart sound and a parasternal heave. Elevation of the jugular venous pressure helps to distinguish PE from most of the other causes of collapse in pregnant women where the diagnosis is not obvious, such as concealed antepartum haemorrhage, or rupture or inversion of the uterus. Amniotic fluid embolism, myocardial infarction and Gram-negative septicaemia all have to be considered and are dealt with elsewhere in this book. The diagnosis of major PE is rarely in doubt. Massive PE, however, is often preceded by smaller emboli and a high index of suspicion is essential if these are to be identified. Warning signs and symptoms are often ignored because they are associated with other non-thrombotic disorders. Conversely, in one prospective study, less than half of the patients with clinically suspected PE had this condition confirmed by pulmonary angiography (Hull *et al.*, 1985). The signs and symptoms that may be confusing include unexplained pyrexia, syncope, cough, chest pain and breathlessness. Pleuritic pain and rub should not be considered to be caused by underlying infection unless the patient has a high temperature and is producing purulent sputum. The patient may have to be treated with both anticoagulants and antibiotics until the diagnosis becomes clear.

Chest radiograph, electrocardiogram and blood gases
Chest radiography is often the initial diagnostic test in patients with suspected PE. It is useful to exclude other conditions which may simulate PE, such as pneumothorax or rib fracture, but it is frequently normal in patients with confirmed PE or may show non-specific abnormalities such as atelectasis or pleural effusion. The electrocardiogram may also be normal or may show features associated with healthy pregnancy, such as a deep S wave in lead I and Q wave and inverted T wave in lead III. Measurement of blood gases can be helpful but both false-positive and false-negative results can be obtained (Robin, 1977). Arterial samples should be taken with the patient sitting and not supine. Under these conditions, with a $P_{A_{O_2}}$ <70 mmHg and $P_{A_{CO_2}}$ normal or reduced, it is likely that the patient's symptoms are due to pulmonary embolus, provided that there is no other cause of reduced cardiac output or evidence of widespread pulmonary disease.

Lung scans
As it is so important to establish a diagnosis of thrombo-embolism in pregnancy, lung scans should be carried out in all cases where the diagnosis is in doubt.

Perfusion scans
Perfusion lung scans will detect areas of decreased blood flow and are performed by injecting the soft γ-emitting isotope $^{99}Tc^m$ coupled to microaggregates of human albumin; these lodge in the pulmonary capillaries. The distribution of radioactivity is measured by scanning the patient's chest with a gamma camera. A normal result

excludes PE; an abnormal result cannot confirm the diagnosis, because other pulmonary disorders can cause impaired blood flow, although in the presence of a normal chest radiograph a large perfusion defect is likely to be due to PE. The radiation to the fetus is minimal, $\approx$59 mrem ($\approx$0.59 Sv) or one-tenth of the maximum gestational exposure recommended to radiation workers in the USA (Marcus *et al.*, 1985; Ponto, 1986). The quantities of $^{99}Tc^m$ secreted in the breast milk are negligible (Tribukait and Swedjemark, 1978).

Ventilation scan
If both the perfusion scan and chest radiograph are abnormal, a ventilation scan may be helpful in determining high probability for PE. The isotopes used are ^{133}Xe or $^{81}Kr^m$ with short half-lives and the radiation is similar to that with perfusion scans. A reduction in perfusion with maintenance of ventilation indicates PE. If both ventilation and perfusion are reduced, the condition is likely to be infective in the presence of acute radiographic changes.

Pulmonary angiography
This is considered to be the most accurate method for the diagnosis of PE (Sostman *et al.*, 1986). Its safety has been greatly improved in recent years by using selective arterial catheterization and by use of magnification techniques. Pulmonary angiography can be performed during pregnancy if the abdomen of the patient has been shielded with a lead-lined apron, but in the opinion of many, a lead-lined diaphragm is necessary for this procedure to be safe in pregnancy! In the few patients in whom lung scans for PE do not show high probability, pulmonary angiography may be helpful (Leclerc and Roy, 1991).

Management of thrombo-embolism in pregnancy

Massive PE usually presents with collapse due to a catastrophic reduction in cardiac output. The standard cardiac arrest procedure should be instituted, and if it is thought likely that the arrest is due to pulmonary embolism, heparin 20 000 units should be given intravenously and prolonged cardiac massage instituted, as both measures may help to break up and reverse the effects of the original clot, thus permitting an increase in pulmonary blood flow (Hume, Sevitt and Thomas, 1970; Heimbecker, Keon and Richards, 1973).

Following emergency resuscitation for pulmonary embolus the treatment of both DVT and PE falls into two phases: the initial acute phase lasts for up to a week and the chronic phase for up to three months, the aim being to prevent further thrombo-embolism. Management of the acute phase may involve surgery, thrombolytic therapy and heparin; chronic phase treatment involves the anticoagulants heparin and warfarin. Nearly 30 years ago, maternal mortality associated with PE and DVT was reduced from 13 to 1 per cent in an uncontrolled study (Villasanta, 1965). The only controlled study in the literature of anticoagulation versus placebo had to be abandoned because of the very high death rate in the placebo group (Borrit and Jordan, 1960). It is now generally accepted that anticoagulant treatment should be instituted promptly in PE. A search of the literature showed a mortality of <1 per cent (one in 113 patients) in anticoagulated patients with PE in pregnancy (Mosely and Kerstein, 1980).

Acute-phase treatment

Surgery
Embolectomy should be considered in the occasional patient who does not die from massive PE, but who remains shocked, with a systolic blood pressure <90 mmHg; Pa_{O_2} <60mmHg and a urine output <20 ml/h (Sasahara and Barsamian, 1973). This will usually be preceded by pulmonary angiography (see above), not only to confirm the diagnosis but also to localize the embolus. The results are excellent in those who survive until surgery can be performed. The place of surgery in massive iliofemoral thrombosis is less clear. It has been suggested that this might reduce the incidence of post-phlebitic leg symptoms (Mayor, 1969) but this has not been substantiated in follow-up studies (Lansing and Davies, 1968). There may be a place for thrombectomy (Silver and Sabiston, 1975; Mogensen *et al.*, 1989) where limb swelling is so great as to cause venous gangrene, but the need for open ligation or plication in cases of recurrent pulmonary embolism (Donaldson, Wirthlin and Donaldson, 1980) has been made largely obsolete by the availability of filters or caval 'umbrellas' which are placed within the inferior vena cava (IVC) distal to the renal veins with the help of a guide wire inserted through the common jugular or common femoral vein (Mansour, Chang and Sindelar, 1985; Jones, Barnes and Greenfield, 1986; Rose *et al.*, 1987).

Thrombolytic therapy
Thrombolytic therapy has been advocated in pregnancy complicated by iliofemoral venous thrombosis or by major PE followed by shock or pulmonary hypotension (Ludwig, 1973). This suggestion was supported by the treatment of 24 patients, mainly in the third trimester, without apparent adverse effects. There is evidence that patients who have thrombolytic therapy for DVT are much less likely to develop post-phlebitic leg symptoms (Elliot *et al.*, 1979). It has been suggested (Browse, 1977) that the risk of massive PE is minimized following treatment with streptokinase in patients with extensive iliofemoral thrombosis where the proximal end is floating free, but this has not been proven.

After PE it has been shown that the pulmonary capillary volume and pulmonary diffusing capacity are normal in patients treated with thrombolytic therapy, whereas they usually remain abnormal on follow-up one year later, in patients treated with heparin and warfarin, even if they are asymptomatic (Sharma, Burlesco and Sasahara, 1980).

Streptokinase does not cross the placenta and so should not harm the fetus directly (Pfeiffer, 1970a; Ludwig, 1973) but there is concern about the effects of maternal fibrinolysis (Meissner *et al.*, 1987) on the placental bed. In addition, severe uterine bleeding would be expected if thrombolytic drugs were used postpartum; nevertheless, there have been anecdotal reports of successful treatment over the years (Pfeiffer, 1970b; Hall, Young and Sutton, 1972; Delclos and Devila, 1986).

Without objective evidence of its benefits and risks, thrombolytic therapy cannot be recommended in pregnancy, except perhaps in exceptional circumstances (Flute, 1976) such as in the case of a shocked patient with massive PE where surgery is contraindicated or unavailable.

Anticoagulants
Both oral anticoagulants and heparin are avoided during pregnancy whenever possible because of their particular hazards to both mother and fetus (see below).

Nevertheless, there are times when they have to be used, particularly if the diagnosis of venous thrombo-embolism is made during the antenatal period. In the acute phase the major problem is how to prevent thrombus extension, embolism or recurrent thrombosis without causing bleeding in either the infant or the mother. Heparin is the anticoagulant therapy of choice in the acute phase.

Heparin

The majority of cases of venous thrombo-embolism are treated initially with heparin. Heparin is a strongly electronegative glycosaminoglycan with a molecular weight of between 10 000 and 30 000 Da. It exerts its anticoagulant effect by increasing dramatically the rate at which the naturally occurring plasma serum protein inhibitor antithrombin III neutralizes several important activated clotting factors, in particular factor Xa and thrombin.

Heparin has particular advantages in pregnancy. Because it is strongly polar and non-lipid soluble, it does not cross the placenta (Flessa et al., 1965; Hirsh, Cade and O'Sullivan, 1970). Its effect in vivo can be easily and rapidly reversed by intravenous administration of protamine sulphate, which immediately neutralizes the effect of heparin so that emergency surgery can be carried out and bleeding due to overdosage dealt with promptly. In addition, its short circulating half-life (≈60 min) means that withholding therapy alone will rapidly restore coagulation and haemostasis to normal. However, this short half-life, together with the fact that heparin must be administered parenterally, is the basis for its main disadvantage even in the acute phase. The object of heparin therapy in the initial phase is to prevent further, possibly fatal, episodes. To treat an established thrombus, large doses are given intravenously, preferably by continuous infusion starting with 40 000 i.u. daily.

Although up to 40 000 units per day have been given subcutaneously (Bonnar, 1976) this is not usually practicable because of bruising or irregular absorption. Given in large therapeutic doses, heparin has a powerful antithrombin effect. It is absorbed on to the clot and prevents further conversion of fibrinogen to fibrin by thrombin. The amount of heparin required to achieve therapeutic levels varies directly with the size of the thrombus. Larger doses are required for PE or massive iliofemoral thromboses than for a small DVT in the calf.

The aim is to achieve a blood concentration of heparin of 0.5–1.0 i.u./ml. Laboratory control of heparin therapy in the pregnant patient is difficult because of the blood clotting changes which alter the sensitivity to heparin of the commonly used tests employed to monitor its anticoagulant effect and to adjust the dose.

Methods based on prolongation of various tests in vitro of coagulation cascade efficiency are not very satisfactory. It has been suggested that prolongation of the activated partial thromboplastin time (APTT) to 1.5–2.5 times the mean of the normal control plasma indicates effective safe anticoagulation. However, each individual metabolizes heparin in a different manner and the control plasma should be taken from the patient concerned, ideally before the heparin infusion is started. It has also been suggested that prolongation of the thrombin time to 2–3 times the normal control value indicates a satisfactory level of heparin in the circulation. The same drawback exists regarding the control plasma as in the APTT. In addition, the thrombin time is extremely sensitive to therapeutic levels of heparin and cannot be used to monitor safe levels in practice.

Heparin can be assayed in the plasma using an extension of the thrombin clotting time test, the protamine sulphate neutralization test. Varying concentrations of protamine sulphate are added to the patient's plasma before the addition of thrombin. When all of the heparin in the plasma has been neutralized, the thrombin clotting time will become normal. The amount of heparin in the sample can be calculated from the amount of protamine sulphate needed to neutralize its effect on the thrombin clotting time (Dacie et al., 1984). At Queen Charlotte's Hospital we have found this test for monitoring heparin levels in pregnancy by far the most helpful. It seems to bear a clear relationship to the clinical situation and aids the obstetrician to achieve satisfactory control, rather than confusing the issue. However, most coagulation laboratories in District General Hospitals are automated and do not offer the protamine sulphate neutralization test to monitor therapeutic heparin. The prolongation of the APTT will have to be relied upon to achieve control in the few pregnant among the many non-pregnant individuals which the laboratory has to investigate. If the factor Xa assay (see below) is available for monitoring prophylactic small-dose heparin, then this method may be a more satisfactory way to monitor therapeutic levels of heparin in pregnancy than prolongation of the APTT. The results are often ignored if outside the therapeutic range of 1.5–2.5 times the control partial thromboplastin time (Fennerty et al., 1985). Clinicians should be aware that such assays have significant variability between occasions even in patients on continuous intravenous infusions of heparin. The variation may be diurnal in nature with higher values at night (Decousus et al., 1985).

The only side effect of therapeutic heparin administration in the acute phase of thrombo-embolism is bleeding, but the preservative chlorbutal may cause hypotension (Bowler et al., 1986).

Because of the high risk of haematoma formation in patients who are fully anticoagulated, other parenteral therapy such as antibiotics should be given intravenously rather than intramuscularly.

If it is necessary to reverse heparin therapy, cessation of infusion will be enough in most patients because of the short half-life. In more urgent situations, protamine sulphate 1 mg for every 100 units of administered heparin may be given. With a constant infusion, twice the quantity of protamine should be given to neutralize the hourly dose (de Swiet, 1989). No more than 50 mg of protamine should be given in a 10 min period because protamine itself in excess can be a powerful anticoagulant and cause bleeding (Laros and Alger, 1979).

Acute phase high-dose therapeutic heparin is administered continuously intravenously for an arbitrary period of 3–7 days, depending on the severity of the initial episode and whether there is any evidence of recurrence.

Chronic-phase treatment

After the acute phase, the therapeutic options include two main classes of anticoagulant drugs. The first class comprises the orally administered coumarin derivatives and indanediones, which act by interfering with the synthesis in the liver of the vitamin-K-dependent pro-coagulants, factors II, VII, IX and X. Warfarin, a coumarin derivative has emerged over the last decade or so as the oral anticoagulant used almost exclusively. Indanediones, particularly phenindione, have unacceptable side effects. The second class comprises heparin and heparinoids, which have to be given parenterally. Before the introduction of self-administered subcutaneous injections for small-dose prophylaxis, heparin was used only over the short-term therapeutic period (see above and below).

Warfarin
The single advantage of warfarin is that it can be taken by mouth, but it has many disadvantages during pregnancy. It crosses the placenta and has adverse effects on the fetus throughout the antenatal period (see below), including teratogenicity in the first trimester and an increasing haemorrhagic tendency up until term, maximal during labour and delivery. A woman who is adequately anticoagulated on warfarin can bleed disastrously if an obstetric complication such as premature placental separation occurs, or if urgent caesarean section or instrumental delivery has to be performed. Warfarin has a prolonged effect and the action cannot be reversed rapidly, although administration of vitamin K will achieve reversal within 24 h. However, if warfarinization is required after the emergency is over, re-stabilization after the administration of vitamin K is very difficult; in addition, vitamin K adminis- tration may result in rebound hypercoagulability. The only rapid method of revers- ing the effect of warfarin is by the infusion of fresh frozen plasma to restore the depleted haemostatic factors. Another disadvantage is that, because of the elevated coagulation factors and increased blood volume in normal pregnancy, the require- ments during pregnancy are changing constantly and much more frequent monitor- ing and control of dosage is necessary than in the non-pregnant state. Drugs that interact with warfarin make its control more difficult and may increase the risk of bleeding in the mother and fetus. In particular, antibiotics used in the treatment of urinary tract infection, a relatively common complication, will alter the requirements of warfarin dramatically. Dangerously low levels of haemostatic factors or inad- equate anticoagulation may result if the laboratory control tests are not performed appropriately and the dose altered as necessary (Hirsh, 1986).

Laboratory control of warfarin
The purpose of laboratory control in the chronic phase of treatment is to achieve and maintain a level of hypocoagulability that is effective in preventing thrombosis but is not sufficient to make the risk of spontaneous haemorrhage appreciable. It is not realistic (or, in fact, possible) to induce a derangement of normal haemostatic mechanisms without accepting some risk of bleeding (Dacie *et al.*, 1984).

Prothrombin time
The one-stage prothrombin time of Quick is the most popular test in the United Kingdom for the control of warfarin therapy. This test is basically an examination of the integrity of the extrinsic coagulation pathway but as such is also a crude assay of the vitamin-K-dependent pro-coagulant factors II, VII and X (with the exception of factor IX). The most important variable is the thromboplastin used in the test. Thromboplastins have been used from animal sources (in particular from the rabbit) and, in the past, from human brain but this is now precluded because of the danger of transmission of viral infections. There are a number of commercial rabbit-brain thromboplastins available. These various thromboplastins give different prolonga- tions of prothrombin time with the same test plasma and it is not possible to define the therapeutic range unless the thromboplastin used is also specified. It is possible to use a reference thromboplastin to assess the sensitivity of the thromboplastin used in individual laboratories. These reference thromboplastins have all been calibrated in terms of a primary WHO human brain thromboplastin; the relative potency of each is defined by an interaction of sensitivity index (ISI). In the anticoagulant clinic the measured prothrombin time is converted to a prothrombin ratio by comparing it to the mean of a number of normal plasma prothrombin times. If the sensitivity index of

the thromboplastin used in the laboratory is known, each patient's ratio can be converted into an international normalized ratio (INR). The optimal therapeutic ratio for the INR is in general within the range of 2.0–4.0 (Poller, 1986). This is valid for all thromboplastins that have been standardized against the international reference thromboplastins supplied by WHO (Dacie *et al.*, 1984).

The thrombotest of Owren measures overall clotting activity and the result is influenced by deficiencies of all of the vitamin K dependent factors (Dacie *et al.*, 1984). The thrombotest is a satisfactory alternative to the prothrombin time for anticoagulant clinics. It can be performed on capillary blood or on uncentrifuged venous whole blood, which facilitates a speedy result while the patient is waiting. The commercial thrombotest reagent is available worldwide, so that the thrombotest, like the INR, has international appreciation. However, oral anticoagulant control for women in pregnancy is usually managed by employing the prothrombin time ratio. The laboratory control of oral anticoagulants depends very much on quality assessment and standardization of thromboplastins to an international reference thromboplastin.

A survey conducted some ten years ago (Poller and Taberner, 1982) before these stringent measures were taken, showed that in order to achieve a laboratory pro-thrombin ratio of between 2.0 and 4.0 there were wide differences in the dosage of warfarin given from centre to centre. In particular much larger daily doses of warfarin were being administered to women in the United States and Canada to achieve this laboratory ratio than in the United Kingdom. This has important implications regarding the reported incidence of adverse effects due to warfarin (see below).

Effects of warfarin on the fetus
It is established that there is a definite but variable incidence of teratogenesis associated with the use of warfarin in the first trimester of pregnancy (Kerber, Warr and Richardson, 1968; Becker, Genieser and Feingold, 1975; Pettifor and Benson, 1975; Abbott, Sibert and Weaver, 1977; Smith and Cameron, 1979; Ginsberg *et al.*, 1989b). Chondrodysplasia punctata, a syndrome characterized by abnormal cartilage and bone formation, is the most common syndrome (Shaul, Emery and Hall, 1975), although warfarin is not the only cause of this (Sheffield *et al.*, 1976; Curry *et al.*, 1984). Asplenic syndrome has also been reported after fetal exposure to warfarin (Cox, Martin and Hall, 1977). It has also been recognized for many years that the use of warfarin during late pregnancy (after 36 weeks' gestation) is associated with serious retroplacental and fetal bleeding, an important hazard to the fetus being intracerebral haemorrhage (Villasanta, 1965). These hazards can be explained by warfarin crossing the placenta together with the fact that the fetus has low levels of the clotting factors synthesized in the liver because of functional immaturity (Andrew *et al.*, 1987, 1988). For these reasons Hirsh and colleagues (Hirsh, Cade and O'Sullivan, 1970) recommended that, after an initial period of heparinization in the acute attack, prophylactic heparin should continue to be used in the first trimester followed by warfarin between 13 and 36 weeks, reverting to small-dose prophylactic heparin (see below) for the last weeks of pregnancy. These recommendations have been widely followed (Henderson, Lund and Creasman, 1972; Szekely, Turner and Snaith, 1973; Anonymous, 1975; Pridmore, Murray and McAllen, 1975; de Swiet, Letsky and Mellows, 1977; de Swiet, Bulpitt and Lewis, 1980; de Swiet *et al.*, 1981). However, as early as 1975 an editorial in the *British Medical Journal* questioned the use of oral anticoagulants even after the first trimester because of the risk

of fetal malformation. Sherman and Hall (1976) described a case of microcephaly in the newborn infant of a patient who had taken warfarin for the last 6 months of pregnancy only, and this stimulated further correspondence (Carson and Reid, 1976; Hall, 1976) culminating in a report (Holzgreve, Carey and Hall, 1976) in which a further five cases of microcephaly occurring in California were cited. They reported their own case of warfarin CNS damage and reviewed the, largely American, literature on the hazards of warfarin. The incidence of complications in the fetus was enormously high: nearly 28 per cent of those exposed were either abnormal at birth or died *in utero*. It has been suggested (Shaul and Hall, 1977) that the optic atrophy, microcephaly and mental retardation described had been caused by repeated small intracerebral haemorrhages induced by maternal warfarin therapy. Holzgreve and colleagues (Holzgreve, Carey and Hall, 1976) also made the point that there should be long-term follow up of the fetus exposed to warfarin as their reported case was apparently normal at birth but was shown subsequently to have a CNS developmental abnormality. At Queen Charlotte's Hospital we have conducted such a follow-up of 22 children for a mean of 4 years (22–67 months), who were exposed to warfarin *in utero*, two in the first trimester and 20 where the mother had taken warfarin after 14 weeks' gestation. The children were drawn from a total of 45 women who took warfarin in pregnancy between 1974 and 1978. On examination, all of the offspring were within the normal developmental parameters. Although the fetal wastage was high (8.7 per cent), our results suggested that the risk of permanent damage if the fetus survived was low (Chong, Harvey and de Swiet, 1984). An earlier study (Chen *et al.*, 1982) reported the outcome of 42 pregnancies where all of the mothers had taken warfarin in the mid-trimester; in 22 of them, warfarin had been taken in the first trimester also. Although the spontaneous abortion rate was high, there were no cases of chondrodysplasia punctata or microcephaly. The only prospective study (Iturbe-Alessio *et al.*, 1986), of 72 pregnancies exposed to warfarin in 67 women with artificial heart valves, yielded a staggering incidence of warfarin embryopathy of 28.6 per cent, but no cases of CNS malformation were reported in this series from Mexico. This series demonstrated clearly that the risk of embryopathy due to warfarin exposure was confined to the period between the sixth and 12th weeks of pregnancy. In contrast, a report in 1988 from Pavankumar and colleagues in New Delhi gave details of 10 years' experience of pregnancy in patients with cardiac valve replacements, 37 of whom had 47 pregnancies. They were managed before and throughout the antenatal period on a strictly monitored coumarin regimen through to the last week of pregnancy, when they were switched to heparin (5000 i.u. 6-hourly until delivery. Although fetal wastage was high (8.5 per cent), none of the neonates had any congenital abnormalities and they were developmentally normal on discharge, although there was no long-term follow-up.

Why are there such gross discrepancies between reports from various centres of the hazards of warfarin effects on the fetus? One simple explanation is that it may be a dosage phenomenon. The very high incidence of both chondrodysplasia punctata and mid-trimester CNS developmental effects comes mainly from North America, where it has been shown (Poller and Taberner, 1982) that at the time of treatment to achieve satisfactory laboratory control, much higher mean daily doses were being given than in the UK. This was thought to be due in part to the different laboratory reagents and the failure to submit the insensitive thromboplastins used to international standardization. Indeed, the CNS abnormalities seem to occur in those women on higher doses of warfarin (de Swiet, 1989). Certainly, in the UK it is very difficult to find a clinically obvious case of chondrodysplasia punctata and many women over the past years with cardiac abnormalities have taken warfarin through out the first trimester. I have yet to see, or hear of, a case locally of microcephaly or associated CNS abnormalities attributable to exposure to warfarin during the mid-trimester. This must be encouraging for physicians who have to manage women with artificial heart valves during pregnancy in the UK, because small dose heparin is not a safe alternative to warfarin for prevention of thrombo-embolism in these cases (see below). The risk of bleeding in both mother and fetus on warfarin therapy after 36 weeks of pregnancy is so high that this should be changed to heparin until delivery is safely negotiated. Some time in the first week postpartum, warfarin can be in-troduced or reintroduced if the mother so desires, and continued for a minimum of 6 weeks in the puerperium.

Patients may continue to breast-feed (Brambel and Hunter, 1950; McKenna, Cale and Vasan, 1983) on warfarin as there is no detectable secretion of warfarin in breast milk (Orme *et al.*, 1977). Infants who are breast-fed while their mothers are taking warfarin are not at any increased risk of abnormal bleeding. This is not so for phenindione, where maternal therapy has caused severe haemorrhage in a breast-fed infant (Eckstein and Jack, 1970).

Heparin
Heparin would appear to be the drug of choice, at least during the antenatal period, as it does not cross the placenta. Its main disadvantage is that it has to be given parenterally. Bonnar (1976) pioneered the use of self-administered subcutaneous heparin for the treatment and prophylaxis of thrombo-embolism in pregnancy. Its efficiency depends on the fact that, in doses too small to have a direct effect on thrombin in the circulation, heparin inhibits the activation of factor X to factor Xa, an action almost identical with, and potentiated by, the naturally occurring anti-coagulant ATIII. Small dose prophylactic subcutaneous heparin, when given to cover surgery, does not require monitoring in the presence of normal hepatic and renal function. A standard dose used is 5000 i.u. 8-hourly. During pregnancy, however, therapy continues for a much longer time and requirements are greater, particularly in the weeks approaching term (Whitfield, Lele and Levy, 1983). The half-life of heparin injected subcutaneously is $\approx$18 h in comparison to intravenous heparin which has a half-life of 1.5 h. The small doses of heparin used in chronic-phase therapy do not quantitatively lower the concentrations of coagulation factors in the plasma and, therefore, the effect cannot be measured by using crude tests of coagulation bioactivity such as the APTT or prothrombin time. The introduction of a more specific assay method based on the ability of heparin to accelerate the neutral-ization of factor Xa (Denson and Bonnar, 1973) has allowed these low levels of heparin in the plasma to be measured. There are now a number of commercial kits available using chromogenic substrates and most district general hospitals can offer this investigation if required. Because of the variations in renal function that may occur, it has been suggested that frequent monitoring should be undertaken so that dangerous or inadequate anticoagulation can be avoided (Bonnar, 1981). Experi-ence suggests that a plasma heparin level of 0.02–0.2 i.u./ml provides adequate prophylaxis against thrombo-embolism without the hazard of bleeding. Where subcutaneous heparin prophylaxis is used without facilities for monitoring levels, a dose of 7500 i.u. twice daily has been suggested (Bonnar, 1981). At Queen Char-lotte's Hospital we use 10 000 i.u. 12-hourly throughout the antenatal period, only altering the dose by reducing it if levels >0.2 i.u./ml are found. We take samples for heparin assay at each antenatal clinic visit. A rapid method to check that there is not

over-anticoagulation is to perform coagulation screening tests, which should be within the normal range.

A recent report from Sweden (Dahlman, Hellgren and Blomback, 1989) shows how successfully prophylactic heparin can be controlled in pregnancy, using these methods. Although patients often show initial reluctance, the majority can be taught to give themselves subcutaneous heparin and therefore can be discharged home after acute phase treatment. If ampoules of appropriate dose with needles attached are not available, the women have to be taught to draw up the appropriate dose into a tuberculin syringe. They should be given concentrated heparin 50 000 u/ml (0.2 ml of this concentration is equivalent to 10 000 i.u.). We have not found any difference in bruising between sodium and calcium heparins. Possible injection sites are the thighs or abdominal wall (Walker *et al.*, 1987).

Because of the high incidence of thrombo-embolism in the days following labour and delivery and the increased risk following operative delivery, subcutaneous heparin is continued throughout labour and delivery, whether it be normal vaginal, instrumental or by caesarean section. The heparin assay is checked in the week preceding delivery. A small controlled trial of prophylactic subcutaneous heparin therapy (Howell *et al.*, 1983) showed no excess of antenatal or postnatal bleeding associated with small dose heparin.

The question of small-dose heparin prophylaxis and epidural anaesthesia remains controversial. Since I first wrote about the subject (Letsky and de Swiet, 1984; Letsky, 1985), largely guided by the published experience of Crawford (1978), my views have completely changed. Provided that the heparin assay is within the prophylactic range (i.e. < 0.2 i.u./ml) or that there is no prolongation of coagulation screening tests (APTT, prothrombin time and particularly the thrombin time, which is peculiarly sensitive to therapeutic levels of heparin), in my opinion it is quite safe to administer epidural analgesia during heparin prophylaxis. Given in appropriate small dosage, heparin does not interfere with the activation of haemostatic mechanisms at the site of injury nor does it interfere with platelet function, which is important for achieving a haemostatic seal at the site of a needle-stick injury. The debate is well set out in a recent report (Thorburn and Letsky, 1990).

Postpartum, the dose of heparin is empirically reduced to 7500 units b.d. because of the reduction in circulating blood volume and the fact that clotting factors return to normal levels during the puerperium. The decision to switch to warfarin after one week, when the risk of secondary postpartum haemorrhage is much less, is largely a question of patient convenience. Neither anticoagulant should prevent the mother breast-feeding. Heparin has the disadvantage of daily injections, but does not require laboratory control, whereas warfarin, although taken by mouth, needs repeated prothrombin time estimations to control the dosage and the mother has to make quite frequent hospital visits in order that blood can be taken for laboratory testing.

Complications of long-term heparin therapy
Heparin would appear to be the anticoagulant of choice in pregnancy, because it does not cross the placenta and should therefore have no adverse effect on the fetus and, administered prophylactically, it creates no haemorrhagic hazard in the mother.

However, a retrospective review of the literature by Hall and colleagues in 1980 suggested that there was an adverse fetal outcome in an amazingly high proportion (30 per cent) of cases, even if heparin was used exclusively. On appraisal it was clear that in a substantial proportion of cases where heparin was being used the women had severe pre-eclampsia, glomerulonephritis or recurrent abortions. If these women were removed from the analysis, together with those fetuses who had been delivered prematurely but who were subsequently normal, the fetal outcome in women treated with heparin alone was very favourable, differing little from the general fetal loss rate in the population at large (Ginsberg and Hirsh, 1989; Ginsberg *et al.*, 1989b). The most obvious maternal complication is bruising at the injection site. This can be reduced by good injection technique using small volumes of concentrated heparin, but not entirely eliminated.

Thrombocytopenia is a well-recognized complication of heparin therapy, with a reported incidence of 1–30 per cent (Bell, 1976; Malcolm, Wigmore and Steinbrecher, 1979; King and Kelton, 1984). The pathophysiology is not well understood and remains controversial. A prospective study (Chong, Pitney and Castaldi, 1982) demonstrated that patients could be divided into two groups on clinical grounds. One group had mild symptomless thrombocytopenia of early onset, the platelet count being $>65 \times 10^9/l$. The mechanism of the development of this type of thrombocytopenia appeared to be attributable to a direct effect of heparin on the platelet. The second group had severe thrombocytopenia with delayed onset and a high incidence of thromboembolic complications with some fatalities. In all of these patients with severe thrombocytopenia of delayed onset, a heparin-dependent IgG antibody was found in the serum; this activated the platelet prostaglandin pathway releasing thromboxane, a powerful aggregating agent.

Different approaches are needed in the management of these two distinct types of heparin-induced thrombocytopenia. Patients with mild, early onset thrombocytopenia need no active treatment but those with severe thrombocytopenia ($<50 \times 10^9/l$) of delayed onset should be started on oral anticoagulants with or without antiplatelet drugs and the heparin should be stopped immediately.

There continue to be sporadic reports of heparin-associated thrombocytopenia (Cines *et al.*, 1980; Hatjis, 1984) and its pathogenesis (Wolf and Wick, 1986; Cines, Tomaski and Tannenbaum, 1987) but, in our own experience and that of others in the UK, thrombocytopenia does not appear to be a significant problem. It is thought that the lack of this complication in the UK may be due to the source of heparin that is generally used.

The most important hazard of heparin therapy to emerge over the years is that of a form of bone demineralization known as osteopenia (Jaffe and Willis, 1965; Thompson, 1973; Avioli, 1975; Squires and Pinch, 1979; Matzsch *et al.*, 1986). The cause of this osteopenia is unknown, although it has been attributed to a deficiency of 1,25-dihydrotachysterol (Aarskog, Aksnes and Lehmann, 1980; Aarskog *et al.*, 1984). One of our patients treated antenatally with heparin long term presented with severe backache that became much worse postpartum. Radiography in the puerperium revealed three collapsed vertebrae (Wise and Hall, 1980). Heparin-induced osteopenia had been reported to occur only if patients had received $>15\,000\,i.u./day$ for >6 months (Griffith *et al.*, 1965) but, more recently bone demineralization following administration of $10\,000\,i.u./day$ in pregnancy for 19 weeks has been reported (Griffiths and Liu, 1984).

A retrospective follow-up study of 20 women treated during and after pregnancy with subcutaneous heparin suggested that even those patients who are asymptomatic may have some degree of bone demineralization, as assessed by computerized tomography of the small bones of the hand (de Swiet *et al.*, 1983). The data suggested that therapy with $20\,000\,i.u./day$ for >20 weeks was associated with bone demineralization and that it is not an idiosyncratic response but may occur in all patients if treated long enough. This is particularly worrying as bone demineralization, like osteoporosis, does not appear to be reversible and because women treated with heparin for long periods in pregnancy will suffer further demineralization and increased risk of fractures following the menopause.

A very recent report questions our findings (Dahlman, Lindvall and Hellgren, 1990). The spine and hip radiographs of 70 women were examined. They had received therapeutic or prophylactic heparin for variable periods during pregnancy. There were 12 (17 per cent) with obvious osteopenia, including two with multiple fractures of the spine. Re-examination 6–12 months postpartum showed that changes were reversible in most cases. The changes did not appear to be related either to the duration of therapy or to the daily dosage in this study. These findings are surprising, in view of the recognition and incidence of osteopenia in the older literature.

Heparin remains the drug of choice for long-term treatment of thrombo-embolism during pregnancy, but whether or not prophylaxis should be instituted in women entering pregnancy with a history of previous thrombo-embolism or with other high-risk factors is a matter for debate, given the high rate of maternal bone demineralization.

Prophylaxis of thrombo-embolism

There are two groups of patients in whom prophylaxis might be considered: (1) those who are at high risk because of age, parity, obesity or operative delivery (Department of Health, 1989); (2) those who have had thrombo-embolism in the past (Badaracco and Vessey, 1974).

With regard to the first group, it is generally believed (but not proven) that the risk of thrombo-embolism is greatest in the postnatal period, so that prophylaxis need be used only to cover labour and the puerperium. It would seem reasonable to use some form of prophylaxis for all patients >30 years of age having a caesarean section, and also in women >35 years of age, even if they have a normal vaginal delivery. Although in the past we used intravenous dextran to cover labour and caesarean section in order that an epidural anaesthetic could be administered, we now administer intrapartum prophylactic subcutaneous heparin whether an epidural analgesic is being used or not, and do not believe that prophylactic heparin is a contraindication (see above) to epidural anaesthesia. In fact, dextran affects platelet function by reducing adhesiveness and aggregation and this may be more likely than prophylactic heparin to increase the hazard of bleeding in the epidural space. It has been suggested that the bleeding problems using dextran 40 can approach the frequency of those encountered with oral anticoagulants (Harris et al., 1972); nevertheless, Bonnar (1981) suggested that dextran 70 can be used in patients having epidural anaesthesia. Although there has been no systemic evaluation of efficacy and risks of dextran in pregnancy, Bergqvist, Bergqvist and Hallbrook (1979) found no cases of deep venous thrombosis in 19 patients given dextran 70 during caesarean section, whereas there were three venous thromboses out of 150 patients undergoing caesarean section who did not receive dextran.

However, there are several other drawbacks to dextran. It interferes with blood compatibility testing and therefore blood must be taken for cross-matching before the infusion is started, in case transfusion should be required. Dextran should be avoided in any obstetric patient with cardiac or renal impairment or with a history of allergic reactions, as it can cause anaphylaxis. The incidence of this possible but rare complication is said to vary between 1:400 (Paull, 1987) and 1:1400 (Ring and Messmer, 1977). A survey involving >200 clinics in Sweden showed that ≈12 per cent of physicians do not use dextran 70 for prophylaxis because of the risk of serious anaphylactic reactions (Bergqvist, 1980).

The second group of patients who may require prophylaxis are those who enter pregnancy with a history of previous thrombo-embolism. These are considered to be at risk throughout pregnancy, but the need for prophylactic anticoagulation during the total antenatal period as well as intrapartum and postpartum – once widely accepted – is now challenged.

The practice was largely based on retrospective surveys that found previous thrombo-embolism to be a powerful risk factor for thrombo-embolism in pregnancy. Badaracco and Vessey (1974) in a retrospective study estimated that the risk of recurrent DVT or PE during pregnancy was 12 per cent if there was a history of previous thrombo-embolism. This study was, however, subject to diagnostic bias. Without objective confirmation by plethysmography, Doppler examination or venography, non-specific symptoms such as ankle swelling, minor calf pain or tenderness, which are frequent complaints in pregnancy, can be misinterpreted, especially when there is a high level of suspicion because of previous thrombo-embolism. It would appear that the risk of recurrent antenatal thrombo-embolism has been over-stated in the past and the risk appears to be of the order of ≤2 per cent (de Swiet, 1989). A more recent and relevant indication of the incidence of recurrence comes from two prospective studies at Queen Charlotte's Maternity Hospital. In the first (Howell et al., 1983), 40 patients with a documented history of venous thrombosis were randomly allocated to receive 10 000 i.u. heparin subcutaneously twice daily, or no heparin during pregnancy, although all patients were given subcutaneous heparin 8000 i.u. twice daily for 6 weeks from the first postnatal day. One patient in the control group developed a DVT for which she was treated promptly. It was in this small controlled trial that one patient treated with heparin developed severe debilitating osteopenia.

This was followed by the second study of Lao and colleagues (Lao et al., 1985) in which 26 patients with a history of venous thrombosis were managed without anticoagulants in the antenatal period. They received dextran 70 during delivery, followed after delivery by subcutaneous heparin or subcutaneous heparin and warfarin. Among the total of ≈40 patients who did not receive antenatal prophylaxis, only one patient suffered a recurrent DVT during pregnancy. There were no postpartum thrombo-embolic events and no fatalities.

It becomes difficult to argue for routine antenatal prophylaxis in women with a history of simple thrombo-embolism and no extra risk factors, given the risks of warfarin administration and the substantial risk of bone demineralization when heparin is given long term. We have now managed >80 pregnancies in patients with a history of thrombo-embolism, withholding anticoagulants in the antenatal period. In recent years intrapartum dextran has been replaced by intrapartum subcutaneous heparin. There have been no further recognized recurrences of DVT or PE in either the pregnancy or the puerperium.

Our present approach is to counsel patients with a history of thrombo-embolism about the relative risks of prophylactic therapy and recurrence of thrombo-embolism in the antenatal period. All women should have been screened after the initial episode to exclude extra risk factors such as protein C, protein S, antithrombin III deficiencies and dysfibrinogenaemia, all of which may require long-term prophylaxis outside pregnancy. The lupus anticoagulant and anti-cardiolipin syndrome should also be excluded as all of these conditions require special management in pregnancy (see below).

Antenatal subcutaneous heparin is recommended only in those patients who are at particular risk, having had more than one episode in the past, or who have inherited abnormalities of the haemostatic mechanisms leading to thrombophilia. Subcutaneous heparin is also used antenatally in those patients who are particularly concerned about recurrence in the antenatal period. This is an uneasy compromise but only a large study with multicentre co-operation would answer the question of relative risks and benefits of antenatal prophylaxis of thrombo-embolism because the numbers at risk in any one centre are too small.

Experience at Queen Charlotte's Hospital has shown that a single episode of thrombo-embolism does not pose a sufficient hazard in most women to contraindicate future pregnancies, although common sense suggests a minimum interval of 6–12 months between the event and embarking on a subsequent pregnancy, if only to avoid conception on warfarin therapy.

Obviously, if there were a safe and convenient way of administering long-term anticoagulant prophylaxis there would be no question of withholding it in the antenatal period. A recently introduced new form of heparin for clinical usage – fractionated or low-molecular-weight heparin – may be what we are looking for.

Low-molecular-weight heparins (LMWH)

Low molecular weight heparins (LMWH) are prepared from standard unfractionated heparin (UH) by enzymatic degradation, chemical degradation or gel filtration. Some few preparations have been available for clinical use on an experimental basis for some years. Their advantages in terms of prophylaxis of venous thrombosis are their allegedly enhanced anti-thrombotic properties (anti-X^a activity) and reduced haemorrhagic hazards (anti-thrombin effect). It is well known that the anti-thrombin activity of heparin is critically dependent upon molecular size. There is an inverse relationship between the anticoagulant activity of heparins in terms of anti-X^a activity and molecular size. Although LMWH are commonly referred to in a generic sense, they are not completely interchangeable in terms of efficacy and safety. Reports of assessments *in vivo* are limited and there have been few randomized trials of the use of LMWH to date. These have been well reviewed (Levine and Hirsh, 1988). Over the few years in which there has been limited clinical investigation, certain facts have emerged. The biological half-life of anti-X^a activity of LMWH is approximately twice as long as that of UH and it is well absorbed from subcutaneous injection sites. This means that one injection daily is sufficient to achieve safe prophylaxis. The size of the molecule also influences its interaction with platelets and, if the heparin molecules are reduced to <5000–8000 Da, the possible reaction with platelets is blocked and therefore the incidence of heparin-associated thrombocytopenia is reduced. Most clinical trials have been devoted to finding a safe but effective dose, but the unexpected long biological half-life led to over-dosage in the early days and a high incidence of perioperative haemorrhage.

Another problem has been the monitoring of dosage *in vitro*. The assessment of the correct dose for LMWH has been made even more difficult by the lack of guidance by assays *in vitro*, because the LMWH have been calibrated against a standard composed of UH, a practice which has been shown to be inappropriate. However, it has become clear that factor X^a assays calibrated against a standard of the specific LMWH in clinical use does bear a relationship to the haemorrhagic hazard. In a series of trials performed by Samama and Combe-Tamzali (1989), the lowest haemorrhage hazard was seen in patients who received only 20 mg of enoxaparin daily, which corresponded to an anti-factor Xa level of 0.12 u/ml. It would appear that the haemorrhagic hazard can be controlled by factor Xa assays, *in vitro* with appropriate standardization of the assay using LMWH as the baseline. LMWH have now been licensed for clinical use in a variety of situations (Kakkar and Murray, 1985) but not for pregnancy. A few centres are using LMWH on a named patient basis to treat and prevent recurrence of thrombo-embolism in the antenatal period. The obvious practical advantage for the woman is the reduction in the number of the self-administered long-term injections. The correct dose has yet to be found for safe and effective prophylaxis in pregnancy but one daily injection will be sufficient. More importantly, perhaps, it is hoped that a reduction in the total dosage will reduce the risk of the serious complication of osteopenia.

At the time of writing there are only occasional sporadic case reports of the use of LMWH in pregnancy (Priollet *et al.*, 1986) but a few multicentre clinical trials are now under way. It is encouraging that there is no evidence to suggest that LMWH cross the placenta at any stage of pregnancy (Forestier, Daffos and Capella-Pavlovsky, 1984; Andrew *et al.*, 1985; Forestier *et al.*, 1987; Omri *et al.*, 1989).

Prevention of thrombo-embolism in pregnancy in women with cardiac problems

The one situation where coumarins should still be used in pregnancy is in the prevention of arterial thrombo-embolism in patients with prosthetic heart valves (Bjork and Henze, 1975; Ibarra-Perez *et al.*, 1976; Oakley and Doherty, 1976; Limit and Grondin, 1977; Lutz *et al.*, 1978; Larrea *et al.*, 1983; Oakley, 1983; Ben Ismail *et al.*, 1986; Lee *et al.*, 1986; Iturbe-Alessio and Salazar, 1987; Stein and Kantrowitz, 1989) or with mitral valve disease (Levine, Pauker and Salzman, 1989). There is no acceptable substitute for adequate oral anticoagulant therapy in patients with artificial heart valve prostheses. Despite improvements in valve design and materials, systemic embolism and valve thrombosis remain the major causes of late morbidity and mortality. Inadequate anticoagulation increases the risk of thrombo-embolism between twofold and sixfold (McLeod, Jennings and Townsend, 1978; Chesebro, Adams and Fuster, 1986; Edmunds, 1987). Although adding dipyridamole or aspirin to warfarin further reduces the risk of systemic embolism after valve replacement (Sullivan *et al.*, 1971; Dale *et al.*, 1977), there is good evidence that antiplatelet drugs are ineffective in this setting (Bjork and Henze, 1975; Brott *et al.*, 1981; Dale and Myhre, 1981). In one large series of 68 pregnancies (Salazar *et al.*, 1984) coumarins were replaced by antiplatelet drugs (aspirin and/or dipyridamole); this resulted in three fatal valve thromboses and a 20 per cent incidence of systemic embolism.

Success has been reported in a small number of cases using dipyridamole alone (Ahmad *et al.*, 1976; Biale *et al.*, 1980) but there is little experience of this and the use of small-dose heparin alone (Wang *et al.*, 1983) has been associated with disastrous and fatal thrombosis of the prosthesis (Bennett and Oakley, 1968). Effective anticoagulation must be continued whenever women become pregnant after valve replacement. The only exceptions are those women with biovalves (Bortolotti *et al.*, 1982), in whom anticoagulants can be stopped 3 months after surgery, except where mitral valve replacement is accompanied by atrial fibrillation or major left atrial enlargement (Chesebro, Adams and Fuster, 1986).

The extensive recent literature on this subject has revealed several facts. It would appear from a very careful study that the danger of chondrodysplasia punctata is confined to the period of gestation between 6 and 9 weeks and that this embryopathy occurs only in fetuses who are exposed to warfarin during this period of gestation (Iturbe-Alessio *et al.*, 1986). We also know that the embryopathy and the CNS malformations may well be dose related (Poller and Taberner, 1982) and that the incidence of these complications has perhaps, been overemphasized in the past (Holzgreve, Carey and Hall, 1976; Shaul and Hall, 1977; O'Neill and Blake, 1982). Our follow-up study (Chong, Harvey and de Swiet, 1984) and the report from Hong Kong (Chen *et al.*, 1982) suggest that the risks in terms of developmental abnormality to the fetus exposed to warfarin at any time in pregnancy are very small. The 10-year experience of Pavankumar and colleagues in New Delhi reported in 1988 would also support this contention. Even if the fetus is exposed to warfarin during the sixth to 12th week of gestation, the risk of chondrodysplasia punctata is very small if the dose of warfarin is not excessive (Pavankumar *et al.*, 1988) and laboratory control of the International Normalized Ratio conforms to international standards. Javares and colleagues (Javares *et al.*, 1984) note that using minimum doses of warfarin with a low prothrombin ratio may reduce the teratogenic and abortion risks. In the series of Iturbe-Alessio *et al.* (1986), two women whose therapy was changed to subcutaneous heparin in the early (7–12) weeks of pregnancy had valve thromboses; however, they had been managed on small doses of heparin (10 000 i.u. b.d.) and these have been shown to be ineffective in the prophylaxis of arterial thrombo-embolism. A more aggressive policy (Rabinovici *et al.*, 1987; Nelson *et al.*, 1984; Hull *et al.*, 1986) using continuous infusions of heparin might have prevented this disastrous complication.

There is no ideal solution to this problem but the incidence of side effects of warfarin in the UK appears to be very low. This, together with the fact that subcutaneous prophylactic heparin is ineffective in preventing thrombo-embolism in this situation, has led us to adopt a policy of continuing warfarin until the 36th week of pregnancy when the risk of fetal (and maternal) bleeding seems overwhelming (Hirsh, Cade and O'Sullivan, 1970). The patient is then admitted to hospital and given continuous intravenous heparin infusion in order to achieve a level of 0.4–0.6 u/ml, as measured by heparin assay. It is believed that the clotting system of the fetus will return to normal after warfarin has been withheld for 7–9 days. At that time the heparin therapy is reduced to give a level <0.2 u/ml and labour is induced. If the woman goes into labour while on warfarin, then fresh frozen plasma will correct her coagulopathy. Some recommend giving vitamin K to the mother to reverse the action of warfarin in the fetus but this is hazardous in terms of a rebound hypercoagulable effect in the mother and problems in re-establishing warfarin therapy after delivery. In extreme cases vitamin K has been given to the fetus *in utero* by transamniotic injection (Larsen *et al.*, 1978). After delivery the patient should continue to receive intravenous heparin for 7 days, maintaining a level of 0.4–0.6 u/ml; warfarin can be restarted thereafter.

Women with artificial heart valves in the reproductive years need intensive and explicit education about the potential hazards of warfarin for the infant and the need to report suspected pregnancy early, so that the switch to therapeutic heparin can be made in time, should they so desire. The suggestion that the teratogenic effect of Dindevan (phenindione), which has many unacceptable side effects, may be less than that of warfarin (Oakley and Hawkins, 1983), is entirely without foundation and there are no data to support this.

Special risks

The lupus anticoagulant, anticardiolipin antibodies and thrombo-embolism

The lupus anticoagulant (LA) is the most frequent of the various anticoagulants that may develop in systemic lupus erythematosus (SLE) (Boxer, Ellman and Carvalho, 1976) and is present in 5–10 per cent of all lupus patients. Because these anticoagulants were first identified in a series of patients with SLE, the label of 'lupus' anticoagulant has become permanently attached. In contrast to the haemorrhagic states associated with the specific inhibitors of individual clotting factors (e.g. factor VIII antibody), the clinical syndromes associated with LA are characterized paradoxically by thrombotic episodes (Bowie et al., 1963; Mueh, Herbst and Rapaport, 1980; Marchesi et al., 1981; Boey et al., 1983; Hughes, 1983; Elias and Eldor, 1984). The lupus anticoagulant is a non-specific inhibitor but interferes in vitro with the phospholipid-dependent steps in tests of integrity of the coagulation cascade. It inhibits the interaction between prothrombin activator and prothrombin but its precise mode of action is unknown. The diagnosis was originally based on finding a prolonged partial thromboplastin time that was not corrected by normal plasma. The increased risk of thrombosis paradoxically associated with prolonged coagulation times in vitro was first clearly identified by Bowie and colleagues in 1963 (Bowie et al., 1963). It was not until 1975, however, that Nilsson and co-workers described the more important pregnancy-associated complication, the first case of recurrent fetal loss associated with the lupus anticoagulant (Nilsson et al., 1975). In 1983, Harris and colleagues described the strong association between anticardiolipin antibody and thrombosis in patients with SLE (Harris et al., 1983). Reports of substantial numbers of women suffering from the 'antiphospholipid syndrome' have now appeared in an expanding literature. This syndrome consists of recurrent fetal losses, placental insufficiency and infarcts and thrombotic episodes associated with identification of either one or both of the two antiphospholipid antibodies, the lupus anticoagulant and anticardiolipin antibody.

The close association of lupus anticoagulant with anticardiolipin antibody (80–100 per cent) has raised the possibility that these antiphospholipid antibodies are identical (Harris et al., 1985). Against this is the fact that some sera with high anticardiolipin antibody concentrations do not interfere with coagulation tests and yet there is an increased incidence of thrombosis in individuals with anticardiolipin antibody. In addition, during treatment with corticosteroids the prolongation of coagulation in vitro may be corrected, whereas the anticardiolipin antibodies usually remain unchanged (Derksen et al., 1986).

Pathogenesis of clinical problems

In obstetric practice, individuals found on investigation to have the lupus anticoagulant may present with episodes of thrombo-embolism or recurrent fetal losses (Branch et al., 1985; Scott, Rote and Branch, 1987). Various mechanisms have been proposed to account for the tendency towards both venous and arterial thrombo-embolism (Vermylen et al., 1986) and almost every possible pathway contributing to haemostasis has been investigated. Among the most recent theories supported by laboratory investigation are that the lupus anticoagulant inhibits endothelial-cell-mediated protein C activation (Cariou *et al.*, 1986), causes platelet activation (Vermylen *et al.*, 1986) or impairs prostacyclin release by the endothelial cell (Carreras *et al.*, 1981; Vermylen *et al.*, 1986). Doubt has been cast on this last attractive theory by the fact that sera from patients with SLE and no lupus anti-coagulant also inhibit prostacyclin production by the endothelial cell (Rustin *et al.*, 1988).

The mechanism of fetal loss in women with lupus anticoagulant is also incompletely understood (Lubbe and Liggins, 1985). The most usual finding in women with late fetal losses is the presence of infarcts in the placenta. These may be detectable only at microscopic level or may be massive and obvious (De Wolf *et al.*, 1982). Many reports have now appeared describing infarction, intravillous thrombo-sis and decidual necrosis. However, in many instances of fetal death the placental lesions appear insufficient alone to account for the intrauterine loss (Lockshin *et al.*, 1985).

It is as yet not proven that either the lupus anticoagulant or anticardiolipin antibodies are responsible for the pathological processes observed *in vivo*. In preg-nancy the association between these phospholipid antibodies, thrombo-embolism and recurrent fetal loss is established but the antibodies may act merely as a marker for susceptibility to these conditions.

Laboratory identification of the lupus anticoagulant
There is confusion concerning the ideal test for identification of the lupus anti-coagulant and criteria are not firmly established. Failure to correct prolongation of a phospholipid-dependent coagulation test by addition of an equal volume of normal plasma remains the basis of the various laboratory procedures. In the early days the activated partial thromboplastin time (APTT) was the universal screening test but it has a variable sensitivity, depending on reagents and methods employed. In the experience of some (Lubbe and Butler, 1991), a significant number of individuals with the lupus anticoagulant detected by more sensitive methods have an APTT within normal limits.

The sensitivity of the APTT can be improved by a platelet neutralization pro-cedure (Triplett *et al.*, 1983), but a more widely used test in the United Kingdom is the kaolin clotting time (KCT) (Exner, Rickard and Kronenberg, 1978). In this test the amount of phospholipid is limited because platelet-poor plasma is used and no phospholipid is added. This test has been criticized as being too sensitive because it may be positive in individuals who have no clinical manifestation of the anti-phospholipid syndrome.

The dilute Russel viper venom time (RVVT) test is a relatively simple, reproduc-ible and sensitive method of detecting the lupus anticoagulant and has yielded promising results (Thiagarajan, Pengo and Shapiro, 1986; Mackie, Coloca and Machin, 1987) but the KCT remains the most popular identification test to date.

Management of pregnancies in women with lupus anticoagulant
The first reports, in women with a history of recurrent fetal loss, of successful outcomes of pregnancies in which the lupus anticoagulant had been suppressed (Lubbe *et al.*, 1983), have resulted in many centres managing pregnancies with steroids or other immune-suppressive therapies, including plasmapheresis and intravenous IgG. The original cases were also treated with aspirin in a dose of 75 mg

daily, a regimen which presumably exerts a beneficial effect by inhibiting platelet/ vessel wall interaction and helps to keep the placental vasculature patent. Inasmuch as small dose aspirin has been shown in pilot trials to improve outcome in pregnancies associated with placental insufficiency such as pre-eclampsia, pregnancy-induced hypertension and intrauterine growth retardation, most obstetricians would now manage all women with lupus anticoagulant and fetal loss with aspirin, whatever other therapy they use. Whether or not this therapy should be used in primigravidae with an identified lupus anticoagulant but no associated clinical manifestations is controversial (Stuart et al., 1982).

The management of recurrent fetal loss associated with the lupus anticoagulant is dealt with elsewhere in this book, but this chapter deals with the complicated problem of the woman with lupus anticoagulant who presents in pregnancy with thrombo-embolism or with a documented previous history of thrombo-embolism.

Thrombosis associated with the lupus anticoagulant and anticardiolipin antibodies may be extensive and may recur repeatedly (Mueh, Herbst and Rapaport, 1980; Harris et al., 1983). Sites of thrombosis may be unusual. Cerebrovascular involvement (Gastineau et al., 1985), pulmonary hypertension (Asherson et al., 1983; Lubbe and Butler, 1991) and myocardial infarction (Rallings, Exner and Abraham, 1989) have been described.

Heparin is used as described above for women with antiphospholipid antibody who have a history of, or who develop, venous thrombo-embolism during pregnancy. However, the control of heparin therapy in the presence of the lupus anticoagulant is difficult because the usual tests for monitoring the dose are prolonged. Heparin may have to be given empirically in doses usually employed to achieve a therapeutic or prophylactic effect, or serum levels may be assayed in order to regulate the dose.

The prophylaxis and treatment of women with lupus anticoagulant and arterial thrombo-embolism pose even more difficult problems. Long-term therapeutic heparin is difficult to manage on an outpatient basis and has the additional hazard of osteopenia, especially if the patient is also receiving steroids. Warfarin, as used for women in pregnancy with cardiac problems (see above), may be the best compromise.

The whole question remains controversial and the approach to treatment is largely empirical. Several aspects of all forms of therapy require formal clinical trial.

Paroxysmal nocturnal haemoglobinuria

This rare condition with an increased risk of thrombotic complications is occasionally seen in pregnancy (Hurd, Miodovnik and Stys, 1982), but experience is limited.

The main hazards appear to be spontaneous abortion, often following acute haemolytic episodes, and serious thrombotic events, mainly in the puerperium, the time of maximum risk. Hepatic vein thrombosis is the most common complication but antenatal pulmonary embolism has also been reported. Low-dose heparin has been shown to be ineffective prophylaxis in at least one case in the antenatal period (Spencer, 1980). It has been suggested, therefore, that full anticoagulation should be used to treat any thrombotic episode in the antenatal period and that full anticoagulation should be used prophylactically in the puerperium (Hurd, Miodovnik and Stys, 1982).

Management of inherited coagulopathies associated with thrombo-embolism in pregnancy

Antithrombin III (ATIII) deficiency

An inherited deficiency of ATIII is one of the conditions in which a familial tendency to thrombosis has been described (Hirsh, Piovella and Pini, 1989). Pregnancy and the puerperium are major risk periods for thrombo-embolism in familial ATIII deficiency (Winter *et al.*, 1982). Thromboembolism can occur during early and late pregnancy and during the puerperium. Thrombosis usually affects the lower limbs (Hellgren, Tengborn and Abildgaard, 1982) but 8 per cent of patients have had mesenteric vein thrombosis, a very rare event in pregnancy (Islam, 1984). The condition often presents for the first time during pregnancy or when women take the contraceptive pill. Approximately 75 per cent of the incidents occur antenatally (Brandt and Stenbjerg, 1979), in contrast to the incidence of thrombo-embolism in pregnancy in patients who do not have ATIII deficiency. Although a recent report (Rosendaal *et al.*, 1991) suggests that a general policy of prophylactic anticoagulation in hereditary ATIII deficiency cannot be recommended, it is clear that, during pregnancy and the puerperium, effective antithrombotic therapy in identified affected family members will be of immense benefit, whether they have had a previous thromboembolic episode or not. To this end, it is essential that ATIII deficient women are given a clear understanding of their condition so that pregnancy can be carefully planned. Oestrogen-containing oral contraceptives should not be taken, in view of their association with thrombosis in deficient individuals (Filip, Eckstein and Veltkamp, 1976). Prophylactic therapy with subcutaneous heparin should be started early in pregnancy, or before conception if the woman is already on warfarin (in view of the risk of teratogenesis). In any case, she should be asked to report suspected pregnancy early so that the change from warfarin to heparin can take place before the critical sixth week (see above). There is a marked fall in ATIII levels in early pregnancy, independently of the introduction of heparin (Samson *et al.*, 1984), which may account for the high incidence of early antenatal thrombo-embolic events reported in this condition.

Early reports in the literature described management of ATIII deficiency in pregnancy using heparin and warfarin with variable success (Van de Meer, Stoepman-van Dalen and Janset, 1973; Zucker, Gomperts and Marcus, 1976). Brandt and Stenfjerg (1979) reported the successful use of subcutaneous heparin prophylaxis in the antenatal period in two patients, one of whom, however, developed femoral vein thrombosis 24 h after delivery. Fresh frozen plasma was used as a source of ATIII to cover labour and delivery in some of these early-reported cases, but the volume required to raise the concentration of ATIII to the recommended 80 per cent of normal would be impossible to administer with safety. During the last decade, concentrates of antithrombin III have become available for clinical use and, in combination with heparin, have now become the therapeutic agents of choice in the management of ATIII-deficient pregnancies. The generally recommended pattern of prophylaxis and management is to use various regimens of heparin antenatally and a combination of ATIII concentrates and heparin to cover labour, delivery and the immediate postpartum period (Brandt, 1981), and then to continue with oral anticoagulants for a minimum of 6 weeks or long term if there has been a history of thrombo-embolism.

One of the earliest prospective studies (Hellgren, Tengborn and Abildgaard, 1982) reported the variably successful management of nine pregnancies in eight women who were treated with subcutaneous heparin twice daily from early pregnancy, to give a prolongation of the APTT of 5–10 s immediately before the next dose. During delivery and abortion, plasma ATIII levels were maintained at >80 per cent of the normal level by daily infusions of ATIII concentrate. Successful prophylaxis in pregnancy using similar regimens in ATIII-deficient women has been reported (Samson *et al.*, 1984; Massignon, Pegaz-Fiornet and Coeur, 1986).

Successful management has also been achieved using either heparin (Michiels *et al.*, 1984; Leclerc *et al.*, 1986) or ATIII concentrate alone (Tengborn and Bengtsson, 1986). The optimal dose of heparin for prophylaxis in pregnancy has not been established: high doses suppress ATIII levels and are more likely to be associated with osteoporosis, but low doses may be inadequate to prevent thrombosis. The initial dose is usually 10 000 i.u. b.d. to achieve the desired prolongation of the APTT (see above; Hellgren, Tengborn and Abildgaard, 1982) but larger doses may be required as pregnancy progresses, particularly in the third trimester when a shortening of the APTT usually occurs. At delivery, or if an obstetric complication occurs, the heparin dosage should be reduced to 5000 i.u. b.d. and ATIII concentrate infused to achieve a level of >80 per cent of the normal level (Winter and Douglas, 1991). A starting dose of 50–70 i.u./kg of ATIII (1 i.u. = 1 ml normal plasma) should be sufficient to achieve the required levels. The half-life is around 36 h and daily infusions are sufficient to maintain these levels. Mannucci *et al.* (1982) recommend a similar regimen. Daily infusions are required thereafter, the dose depending on the ATIII levels achieved; these should be measured twice daily.

If thrombosis occurs during pregnancy, ATIII and heparin should be given to achieve full anticoagulation for a minimum of 7 days; this can be followed by twice-daily subcutaneous heparin prophylaxis. However, if thrombosis occurs during heparin prophylaxis, it may be advisable to substitute warfarin after the 12th week of pregnancy (see above).

Heparin co-factor II deficiency

This protein is antigenically distinct from ATIII. It is a thrombosis inhibitor and its effect is accelerated in the presence of heparin. The physiological relevance of its role in haemostasis is not yet established but two kinships with deficiency associated with thrombosis have been described. In one family, two members had cerebrovascular disease and one had a DVT during pregnancy. In the second family, one of four affected members developed thrombosis (Sie *et al.*, 1985; Tran, Marbet and Duckert, 1985).

Protein C and protein S deficiencies

Protein C and its co-factor protein S are vitamin K-dependent, naturally occurring anticoagulants which exert their effects by inhibiting activity of the procoagulant factors V and VIII. The physiological importance is manifest clinically by a predisposition to thrombosis in individuals with deficiencies of these factors (Mannucci and Owen, 1987).

As with antithrombin III deficiency, the depressed activity of proteins C and S may be due to qualitative or quantitative disorders. There are a number of assay systems now available to assist in the identification of the precise nature of the abnormalities and this subject has been well reviewed (Preissner, 1990). It is clear that samples should be dealt with by specialist laboratories. Difficulties are encountered when diagnosis is attempted in individuals receiving coumarin derivatives, which lead to falls in proteins C and S as well as in the procoagulant factors II, VII, IX and X. Ratios of proteins C and S to these vitamin-K-dependent procoagulant factors have been used in some laboratories to establish the presence of deficiency, but it may be necessary to interrupt warfarin therapy in order to make the diagnosis.

Protein C deficiency

A homozygous form of the disorder has been described (Seligsohn *et al.*, 1984; Sharon, Tirindelli and Mariani, 1986), usually presenting with a severe coagulopathy in the neonate. In pregnancy the importance of this form of the condition is that it is susceptible to prenatal diagnosis by examination of fetal blood in the second trimester (Mibashan *et al.*, 1985). In this form of the disorder, parents have low levels of protein C but do not usually have a personal or family history of thrombo-embolism.

Pregnancies of women at risk of thrombo-embolism involve the autosomal dominant heterozygous form of the disorder. The majority of cases have a quantitative deficiency (type 1). A few patients have been reported who have normal immunoreactive protein but impaired functional activity and these are termed type 2. The clinical syndrome of purpura fulminans in the neonate, previously described in homozygotes for protein C deficiency (see above), may arise in the infant of a heterozygous mother who is receiving coumarin anticoagulants (Ogston, 1987).

The association of thrombo-embolism with heterozygous protein C deficiency is now well accepted following the first reports of families with protein C deficiency and thrombophilia (Griffin *et al.*, 1981; Bertina *et al.*, 1982; Horellou *et al.*, 1984, 1985). Isolated protein C deficiency was found in 8 per cent of a group of young patients with thrombo-embolic disease and 7 per cent of patients with recurrent episodes (Broekmans, Veltkamp and Bertina, 1983). The prevalence of protein C deficiency was calculated to be about 1 per 16 000 in western Holland from this and other data (Broekmans, Veltkamp and Bertina, 1983), but a more recent study in the United States gave a much higher prevalence (Miletich, Sherman and Bronze, 1987), namely 1 in 200–300. However, none of the protein C-deficient subjects identified had a history of thrombo-embolic disease, so that, although the overall incidence of protein C deficiency is higher than that of antithrombin III deficiency, the number of protein C-deficient individuals with no history of thrombosis is also higher than that in patients with ATIII deficiency, in whom this combination is most unusual (Vikydal *et al.*, 1985). In pregnancy as previously described, although free and total protein S levels decrease during the antenatal period (returning to normal in the puerperium), protein C levels tend to remain within normal limits or to rise slightly (Malm, Laurell and Dahlback, 1988; Warwick *et al.*, 1989). Pregnancy appears to be a particular risk period for the development of thrombosis in both protein C and protein S deficiencies. Pregnancy was an associated factor in seven out of 14 female cases of thrombo-embolism associated with protein C deficiency (Horellou *et al.*, 1984). A study of 31 women with protein C deficiency in whom 82 pregnancies occurred (Conrad *et al.*, 1987) showed that, of the 66 who proceeded to term, 17 were associated with thrombosis, with almost one-third of events occurring during the antenatal period.

Protein S deficiency

The association of thrombosis with familial protein S deficiency was first described 3 years after protein C deficiency (Comp *et al.*, 1984) and therefore there is less accumulated knowledge of the problems that arise. In the kinships described (Schwartz *et al.*, 1984; Broekmans *et al.*, 1985; Kamiya *et al.*, 1986) there seems to be a high association with thrombo-embolic disease in the subjects identified as deficient.

There are two recognized forms of protein S deficiency. In the plasma, protein S exists in two forms (Comp *et al.*, 1986a): ≈40 per cent exists as a free protein and the remainder is bound to C4b, a regulatory protein of the complement system. In the more commonly reported type of deficiency, levels of both free and bound protein S are ≈50 per cent of normal. In the rarer type of deficiency, the concentration of total protein S is normal or slightly reduced but the ratio of free to bound protein S is reduced. In healthy women, levels of both free and bound protein S fall during pregnancy, reaching lowest levels (≈60 per cent of non-pregnant levels) during the second trimester. The diagnosis of protein S deficiency during pregnancy is, therefore, particularly difficult.

Clinical features of protein C and protein S deficiencies
The clinical features of these deficiencies are much the same as those of ATIII deficiency. However, in both protein C and protein S deficiencies, superficial thrombophlebitis appears to be more common. In addition, coumarin-induced skin necrosis is a complication that has been described in both deficiencies during the induction period with warfarin. It is thought to be due to the more rapid fall in protein C together with factor VII compared with other vitamin K-dependent coagulation factors, leading to thrombosis of the venules of the skin and infarction.

Treatment and prophylaxis of thrombo-embolism during pregnancy with protein C and protein S deficiencies
Experience is lacking and published reports scanty in these relatively recently described familial thrombophilic conditions. The successful management has been reported of one case of protein C deficiency using heparin during the last month of pregnancy and the puerperium (Gonzales *et al.*, 1985). Another patient with protein C deficiency and a history of iliofemoral thrombosis in a previous pregnancy was managed successfully throughout the antenatal period with prophylactic heparin and in the puerperium with oral anticoagulants (Carter and Bellem, 1988).

Protein S deficiency has been managed without complication throughout pregnancy in two patients using oral anticoagulant therapy (Broekmans *et al.*, 1985; Michiels *et al.*, 1987).

The use of fresh frozen plasma as a source of protein C in deficient subjects involves the use of frequent large volumes and can cause problems from circulatory overload (Majer, Chisholm and Hickton, 1989). However, protein C concentrates are becoming more widely available and may have a place in management during pregnancy, particularly at delivery and for the management or prevention of skin necrosis during induction of warfarin therapy.

Meanwhile, with the evidence available, it would appear that heparin is the anticoagulant of choice for treatment and prophylaxis in both protein C and protein S deficiencies during the antenatal period and at delivery. During the puerperium, warfarin may be introduced but this must be performed slowly and with care under heparin cover, in order to avoid the hazard of skin necrosis.

Dysfibrinogenaemia
Many individuals who have a genetically abnormal fibrinogen molecule have now been identified, following investigation of an isolated prolonged thrombin time. The vast majority have no associated symptoms but ≈30 per cent have a bleeding tendency; slightly <10 per cent have a thrombotic tendency and the incidence of thrombosis in identified family members with the defect is low (Carrell *et al.*, 1983). The mechanisms leading to the thrombotic tendency are not well understood and various theories have been proposed.

Clinical information regarding thrombosis during pregnancy is scanty (Egeberg, 1967; Fuchs, Egbring and Havemann, 1977) and general recommendations regarding management cannot be given, except to follow basic guidelines for the other high-risk situations outlined above.

Rare coagulation factor deficiencies and thrombo-embolism in pregnancy
Paradoxically, deficiencies of procoagulants factor XII (Hageman factor) and factor VII have both been associated with the development of thrombo-embolism in affected individuals (Goodnough, Saito and Ratnoff, 1983; Shifter, Machtey and Creter, 1984). The pathogenesis in these cases is not clear and documented associations with pregnancy are scanty. There appears to be only one reported case of factor XII deficiency associated with thrombosis during pregnancy: a 30-year-old woman developed venous thrombosis in the puerperium (Baumann and Straub, 1968).

Inherited disorders of fibrinolysis
Venous thrombosis has been described in association with inherited abnormalities of the fibrinolytic system and rare cases of thrombosis in pregnancy have been reported. Postpartum thrombosis associated with familial plasminogen deficiency was reported in one case (Ten Cate, Peters and Buller, 1983).

Petaja and colleagues (Petaja *et al.*, 1989) described two families from Finland with impaired fibrinolysis and thrombophilia; one individual suffered venous thrombo-embolism during pregnancy.

Inborn errors of metabolism and thrombosis in pregnancy

Hyperlipidaemia

Autosomal dominant forms of familial hyperlipidaemia are common in the population and must therefore be relatively common in pregnant women. However, increased incidences of myocardial or cerebral infarctions associated with these abnormalities in pregnancy have not been reported (Winter and Douglas, 1991). Coronary artery disease in females occurs later than in males and premenopausal women seem rarely to be affected by coronary artery disease, even if they suffer from hyperlipidaemia.

Homocystinuria

Homocystinuria is the one inborn error of metabolism with a strong association with thrombo-embolism. It is inherited as an autosomal recessive disorder and has an incidence of approximately 1 in 200 000 livebirths. There is a deficiency of the enzyme cystathione β-synthetase and the condition is characterized by arachnodactyly, variable mental deficiency and skeletal and ocular abnormalities, together with an increased risk of thrombo-embolism. Both arterial and venous thrombo-embolism may occur and these may develop in the first few months of life; however, patients usually present between the ages of 15 and 30 years (Mudd *et al.*, 1985). Peripheral venous thrombosis occurs in half of the cases. Cerebrovascular events are relatively common. Arterial occlusion of peripheral vessels and coronary thrombosis have also been described. Deaths from vascular disease have been reported during the third and fourth decades (Scott, 1983).

Thrombosis may be precipitated by major surgery or by such investigations as angiography (Grobe and Balleisen, 1983) in these patients. There have been few reports associated with vascular occlusions during pregnancy. Iliofemoral thrombosis in the puerperium was reported in one case (Lamon *et al.*, 1981). One 20-year-old female developed major arterial occlusion late in the puerperium and this precipitated the diagnosis of previously unrecognized homocystinuria both in herself and her brother (Newman and Mitchell, 1984). Death occurred four days after caesarean section in one 28-year-old woman with homocystinuria (Constantine and Green, 1987).

The mechanism underlying the increased risk of thrombo-embolism is unknown and, because of this, it has been suggested that the risk may be reduced by pyridoxine administration in those cases in whom the metabolic defect responds to this therapy.

Postscript and conclusions

At the time of writing, the latest *Confidential Enquiries into Maternal Deaths* has just been released, reporting the triennium 1985–1987 (Department of Health, 1991). This report includes figures from Scotland and Northern Ireland, as well as the traditionally included figures from England and Wales. The commonest cause of death in the United Kingdom for this latest reported triennium 1985–1987 is pulmonary embolism: there were 29 deaths from this cause. Compared with previous reports for England and Wales, a higher proportion, more than half, occurred in the antenatal period. In many cases the diagnosis of thrombo-embolism did not appear to have been considered, particularly in early pregnancy. Investigation was inadequate in several cases. The majority of women who died had no clinical evidence of DVT, yet autopsy revealed thrombosis in pelvic and leg veins.

The potential dangers of anticoagulant therapy in producing antepartum and postpartum bleeding appear to have been exaggerated. There was also failure to investigate meticulously and appropriately women with suspicious symptoms.

'All those looking after or involved in the care of pregnant or recently pregnant women should consider pain in the leg, pain in the chest or dyspnoea in an otherwise healthy woman to be due to thrombosis or pulmonary embolism until proved otherwise and ensure that the appropriate treatment is instituted. Following this the onus is to confirm or refute the diagnosis as soon as possible' (Department of Health, 1991).

It is clear that thrombosis and its treatment in pregnancy, whatever the aetiology, carries special hazards for both the mother and the fetus. Those with known risk factors should be identified, preferably before pregnancy is embarked upon, so that appropriate action can be planned. Successful management can be achieved only by close continuing co-operation between obstetrician, paediatrician, physician and haematologist.

References

Aaro, KA and Juergens, JL (1971) Thrombophlebitis associated with pregnancy. *American Journal of Obstetrics and Gynecology*, **109**, 1128–1136

Aaro, KA and Juergens, JL (1974) Thrombophlebitis and pulmonary embolism as a complication of pregnancy. *Medical Clinics*, **58**, 829

Aarskog, D, Aksnes, L and Lehmann, V (1980) Low, 1,25-dihydroxyvitamin D in heparin-induced osteopenia. *Lancet*, **ii**, 650–651

Aarskog, D, Aksnes, L, Markestad, T et al. (1984) Heparin-induced inhibition of 1,25-dihydroxyvitamin D formation. *American Journal of Obstetrics and Gynecology*, **148**, 1141–1142

Abbott, A, Sibert, JR and Weaver, JB (1977) Chondrodysplasia punctata and maternal warfarin treatment. *British Medical Journal*, **1**, 1639–1640

Abildgaard, U (1979) A review of antithrombin III. In *The Physiological Inhibitors of Blood Coagulation and Fibrinolysis* (edited by D Collen, B Wiman and M Verstraete) pp. 19–29. Amsterdam. Elsevier/North Holland Biomedical Press

Adam, A, Albert, A, Boulanger, J et al. (1985) Influence of oral contraceptives and pregnancy on constituents of the Kallikrein–kininogen system in plasma. *Clinical Chemistry*, **31**, 1533–1536

Ahmad, R, Rajah, SM, Mearns, AJ and Deverall, PB (1976) Dipyridamole in successful management of pregnant women with prosthetic heart valve. Lancet, **ii**, 1414–1415

Albrechtsson, U and Olsson, CG (1979) Thrombosis after phlebography: a comparison of two contrast media. *Cardiovascular Radiology*, **2**, 9–18

Andrew, M, Boneu, B, Cade, J et al. (1985) Placental transport of low molecular weight heparin in the pregnant sheep. *British Journal of Haematology*, **59**, 103–108

Andrew, M, Paes, B, Milner, R et al. (1987) Development of the human coagulation system in the full term infant. *Blood*, **70**, 165–172

Andrew, M, Paes, B, Milner, R et al. (1988) Development of the human coagulation system in the healthy premature infant. *Blood*, **72**, 1651–1657

Anonymous (1975) Venous thrombo-embolism and anticoagulants in pregnancy. *British Medical Journal*, **2**, 421–422

Asherson, RA, Mackworth-Young, CG, Boey, ML et al. (1983) Pulmonary hypertension in systemic lupus erythematosus. *British Medical Journal*, **287**, 1024–1025

Avioli, LV (1975) Heparin-induced osteopenia: an appraisal. *Advances in Experimental Medicine and Biology*, **52**, 375–387

Badaracco, MA and Vessey, M (1974) Recurrence of venous thrombo-embolism disease and use of oral contraceptives. *British Medical Journal*, **1**, 215–217

Ballegeer, V, Mombarts, P, Declerk, PJ et al. (1987) Fibrinolytic response to venous occlusion and fibrin fragment D-dimer levels in normal and complicated pregnancy. *Thrombosis and Haemostasis*, **58**, 1030–1032

Barritt, DW and Jordan, SC (1960) Anticoagulant drugs in the treatment of pulmonary embolism: a controlled trial. *Lancet*, **i**, 1309–1312

Baumann, R and Straub, PW (1968) Congenital deficiency of Hageman factor (clotting factor XII). *Helvetica Medica Acta*, **34**, 313–326

Becker, MH, Genieser, NB and Feingold, M (1975) Chondrodysplasia punctata: is maternal warfarin therapy a factor? *American Journal of Diseases of Children*, **129**, 356–359

Bell, WR (1976) Thrombocytopenia occurring during heparin therapy. *New England Journal of Medicine*, **295**, 276–277

Beller, FK and Ebert, C (1982) The coagulation and fibrinolytic enzyme systems in normal pregnancy and the puerperium. *European Journal of Obstetrics, Gynecology and Reproductive Biology*, **13**, 177–197

Ben Ismail, M, Abid, F, Trabelsi, S et al. (1986) Cardiac valve prostheses, anticoagulation and pregnancy. *British Heart Journal*, **55**, 101–105

Bennett, GG and Oakley, CM (1968) Pregnancy in a patient with a mitral valve prosthesis. *Lancet*, **i**, 616–619

Bergqvist, D (1980) Prevention of post-operative thrombosis in Sweden. Results of a survey. *World Journal of Surgery*, **4**, 489–495

Bergqvist, D and Hedner, U (1983) Pregnancy and venous thrombo-embolism. *Acta Obstetricia et Gynecologica Scandinavica*, **62**, 499–453

Bergqvist, A, Bergqvist, D and Hallbrook, T (1979) Acute deep vein thrombosis (DVT) after caesarean section. *Acta Obstetricia et Gynecologica Scandinavica*, **Supplement 58**, 473–476

Bergqvist, A, Bergqvist, D and Hallbrook, T (1983) Deep vein thrombosis during pregnancy. A prospective study. *Acta Obstetricia et Gynecologica Scandinavica*, **62**, 443–448

Bergqvist, A, Bergqvist, D, Lindhagen, A and Matzch, T (1990) Late symptoms after pregnancy-related deep vein thrombosis. *British Journal of Obstetrics and Gynaecology*, **97**, 338–341

Bertina, RM, Broekmans, AW, Van de Linden, IK and Mortens, K (1982) Protein C deficiency in a Dutch family with thrombotic diseases. *Thrombosis and Haemostasis*, **48**, 1–5

Bettman, MA, Robbins, A, Braun, SD *et al.* (1987) Contrast venography of the leg: diagnostic efficacy, tolerance and complication rates with ionic and nonionic contrast media. *Radiology*, **165**, 113–116

Biale, Y, Cantor, A, Lewen Thal, H and Gueron, M (1980) The course of pregnancy in patients with artificial heart valves treated with dipyridamole. *International Journal of Obstetrics and Gynaecology*, **18**, 128–132

Bjork, VO and Henze, A (1975) Management of thrombo-embolism after aortic valve replacement with the Bjork-Shiley tilting disc valve. *Scandinavian Journal of Thoracic Cardiovascular Surgery*, **9**, 183–191

Boey, ML, Colaco, CB, Gharavi, AE *et al.* (1983) Thrombosis in systemic lupus erythematosus: striking association with the presence of circulating lupus anticoagulant. *British Medical Journal*, **287**, 1021–1023

Bonnar, J (1976) Long term self-administered heparin therapy for prevention and treatment of thromboembolic complications in pregnancy. In *Heparin Chemistry and Clinical Usage* (edited by VV Kakkar and DP Thomas) pp. 247–260, London: Academic Press

Bonnar, J (1981) Venous thrombo-embolism and pregnancy. *Clinics in Obstetrics and Gynaecology*, **8**, 455–473

Booth, N, Reith, A, Bennett, B *et al.* (1988) A plasminogen activator inhibitor (PA1–2) circulates in two molecular forms during pregnancy. *Thrombosis and Haemostasis*, **59**, 77–79

Bortolotti, U, Milano, A, Mazzucco, A *et al.* (1982) Pregnancy in patients with a porcine valve bioprosthesis. *American Journal of Cardiology*, **50**, 1051–1054

Bowie, EJW, Thompson, JH, Pascuzzi, CA *et al.* (1963) Thrombosis in systemic lupus erythematosus despite circulating anticoagulant. *Journal of Laboratory Clinical Medicine*, **62**, 416–430

Bowler, GMR, Galloway, DW, Meiklejohn, BH and Macintyre, CCA (1986) Sharp fall in blood pressure after injection of heparin containing chlorbutol. *Lancet*, **i**, 848–849

Boxer, M, Ellman, L and Carvalho, A (1976) The lupus anticoagulant. *Arthritis and Rheumatism*, **19**, 1244–1248

Brambel, CE and Hunter, RE (1950) Effects of dicoumarol on the nursing infant. *American Journal of Obstetrics and Gynecology*, **59**, 1153–1159

Branch, DW, Scott, JR, Kochenour, NK *et al.* (1985) Obstetric complications associated with the lupus anticoagulant. *New England Journal of Medicine*, **313**, 1322–1326

Brandt, P (1981) Observations during the treatment of antithrombin III deficient women with heparin and antithrombin concentrate during pregnancy, parturition and abortion. *Thrombosis Research*, **22**, 15–24

Brandt, P and Stenbjerg, S (1979) Subcutaneous heparin for thrombosis in pregnant women with hereditary anti-thrombin deficiency. *Lancet*, **i**, 100–101

British Medical Journal Editorial (1975) Venous thrombo-embolism and anticoagulants in pregnancy. *British Medical Journal*, **2**, 421–422

Broekmans, AW, Veltkamp, JJ and Bertina, RM (1983) Congenital protein C deficiency and venous thrombo-embolism. *New England Journal of Medicine*, **309**, 340–344

Broekmans, AW, Bertina, RM, Reinaida-Poot, J *et al.* (1985) Hereditary protein S deficiency and venous thrombo-embolism. *Thrombosis and Haemostasis*, **53**, 273–277

Brott, WH, Zajtchuk, R, Bowen, TE *et al.* (1981) Dipyridamole–aspirin as thromboembolic prophylaxis in patients with aortic valve prosthesis. *Journal of Thoracic Cardiovascular Surgery*, **81**, 623–635

Browse, NL (1977) Personal views on published facts. What should I do about deep vein thrombosis and pulmonary embolism? *Annals of the Royal College of Surgeons of England*, **59**, 138–142

Cariou, R, Tobelem, G, Soria, C *et al.* (1986) Inhibition of protein C activation by endothelial cells in the presence of lupus anticoagulant. *New England Journal of Medicine*, **314**, 1193–1194

Carrell, N, Gabriel, DA, Blatt, PM *et al.* (1983) Hereditary dysfibrinogenemia in a patient with thrombotic disease. *Blood*, **62**, 439–447

Carreras, LO, Vermylen, J, Spitz, B and Van Assche, A (1981) Lupus anticoagulant and inhibition of prostacyclin formation in patients with repeated abortion, intrauterine growth retardation and intrauterine death. *British Journal of Obstetrics and Gynaecology*, **88**, 890–894

Carson, M and Reid, M (1976) Warfarin and fetal abnormality. *Lancet*, **i**, 1127

Carter, CJ and Bellem, PJ (1988) Management of protein C deficiency in pregnancy. *Fibrinolysis (supplement)*, **1**, 161

Chen, WWC, Chan, CS, Lee, PR *et al.* (1982) Pregnancy in patients with prosthetic heart valves: an experience with 45 pregnancies. *Quarterly Journal of Medicine*, **51**, 358–365

Chesebro, JH, Adams, PC and Fuster, V (1986) Antithrombotic therapy in patients with valvular heart disease and prosthetic heart valves. *Journal of the American College of Cardiology*, **8, Supplement B**, 41B–56B

Chong, BH, Pitney, WR and Castaldi, PA (1982) Heparin-induced thrombocytopenia: association of thrombotic complications with heparin-dependent IgG antibody that induces thromboxane synthesis and platelet aggregation. *Lancet*, **ii**, 1246–1248

Chong, MKB, Harvey, D and de Swiet, M (1984) Follow-up study of children whose mothers were treated with warfarin during pregnancy. *British Journal of Obstetrics and Gynaecology*, **91**, 1070–1073

Cines, DB, Tomaski, A and Tannenbaum, S (1987) Immune endothelial cell injury in heparin-associated thrombocytopenia. *New England Journal of Medicine*, **316**, 581–589

Cines, DB, Kaywin, P, Bina, M *et al.* (1980) Heparin-associated thrombocytopenia. *New England Journal of Medicine*, **303**, 788–795

Clarke-Pearson, DL and Jelovsek, FR (1981) Alterations of occlusive cuff impedance plethysmography results in the obstetric patient. *Surgery*, **89**, 594–598

Clouse, LH and Comp, RC (1986) The regulation of haemostasis: the protein C system. *New England Journal of Medicine*, **314**, 1298–1304

Comp, PC and Esmon, CT (1984) Recurrent venous thrombo-embolism in patients with a partial deficiency of protein S. *New England Journal of Medicine*, **311**, 1525–1528

Comp, PC, Nixon, RR, Cooper, MR and Esmon, CT (1984) Familial protein S deficiency is associated with recurrent thrombosis. *Journal of Clinical Investigation*, **74**, 2082–2088

Comp, PC, Doray, D, Patton, D and Esmon, CT (1986a) An abnormal plasma distribution of protein S occurs in functional protein S deficiency. *Blood*, **67**, 504–508

Comp, PC, Thurnau, CR, Welsh, J *et al.* (1986b) Functional and immunologic protein S levels are decreased during pregnancy. *Blood*, **68**, 881–885

Conrad, J, Horellou, MH, Van Dredn, P and Samama, M (1987) Pregnancy and congenital deficiency in antithrombin III or protein C. *Thrombosis and Haemostasis* (**Abstracts of XIth International Congress on Thrombosis and Haemostasis**) 39

Constantine, G and Green, A (1987) Untreated homocystinuria: a maternal death in a woman with four pregnancies. *British Journal of Obstetrics and Gynaecology*, **94**, 803–806

Coon, WW (1977) Epidemiology of venous thromboembolism. *Annals of Surgery*, **186**, 149–164

Cox, DR, Martin, L and Hall, BD (1977) Asplenia syndrome after fetal exposure to warfarin. *Lancet*, **ii**, 1134

Crawford, JS (1978) *Principles and Practice of Obstetric Anaesthesia*, 4th edn, pp. 182–183. Oxford: Blackwell Scientific Publications

Curry, CJR, Megenis, RE, Brown, M *et al.* (1984) Inherited chondrodysplasia punctata due to a deletion of the terminal short arm of an X chromosome. *New England Journal of Medicine*, **311**, 1010–1015

Dacie, JV, Lewis, SM, Pitney, WR and Brozovic, M (1984) Laboratory control of anticoagulant and thrombolytic therapy. In *Practical Haematology*, 6th edn, edited by JV Dacie and SM Lewis, pp. 259–270. Edinburgh: Churchill Livingstone

Dahlman, TC, Hellgren, MS and Blomback, M (1989) Thrombosis prophylaxis in pregnancy with use of subcutaneous heparin adjusted by monitoring heparin concentration in plasma. *American Journal of Obstetrics and Gynecology*, **161**, 420–425

Dahlman, T, Lindvall, N and Hellgren, M (1990) Osteopenia in pregnancy during long-term heparin treatment: a radiological study post-partum. *British Journal of Obstetrics and Gynaecology*, **97**, 221–228

Dale, J and Myhre, E (1981) Can acetylsalicylic acid alone prevent arterial thrombo-embolism? A pilot study in patients with aortic ball valve prostheses. *Acta Medica Scandinavica*, **Supplement 645**, 73–78

Dale, J, Myhre, E, Storstein, O *et al.* (1977) Prevention of arterial thrombo-embolism with acetylsalicylic acid. *American Heart Journal*, **94**, 101–111

Daniel, DJ, Campbell, H and Turnbull, AC (1967) Puerperal thrombo-embolism and suppression of lactation. *Lancet*, **ii**, 287–289

Davies, JA (1985) The pre-thrombotic state. *Clinical Science*, **69**, 641–646

Decousus, HA, Croze, M, Levi, FA *et al.* (1985) Circadian changes in anticoagulant effect of heparin infused at a constant rate. *British Medical Journal*, **290**, 341–344

Delclos, GL and Davila, F (1986) Thrombolytic therapy for pulmonary embolism in pregnancy: a case report. *American Journal of Obstetrics and Gynecology*, **155**, 375–376

Denson, KWE and Bonnar, J (1973) The measurement of heparin: a method based on the potentiation of anti-factor Xa. *Thrombosis et Diathesis Haemorrhagica*, **30**, 471

Department of Health (1989) *Report on Health and Social Subjects 34. Report on Confidential Enquiries into Maternal Deaths in England and Wales 1982–1984*. London: HMSO

Department of Health (1991) *Report on Confidential Enquiries into Maternal Deaths in the United Kingdom 1985–1987*. London: HMSO

Derksen, RHWM, Biesma, D, Bouma, BN *et al.* (1986) Discordant effects of prednisone on anti-cardiolipin antibodies and the lupus anticoagulant. *Arthritis and Rheumatism*, **29**, 1295–1296

de Swiet, M (1989) Thromboembolism. In *Medical Disorders in Obstetric Practice*, 2nd edn (edited by M de Swiet) pp. 166–197. Oxford: Blackwell Scientific Publications

de Swiet, M, Bulpitt, CJ and Lewis, PJ (1980) How obstetricians use anticoagulants in the prophylaxis of thrombo-embolism. *Journal of Obstetrics and Gynaecology*, **1**, 29–32

de Swiet, M, Letsky, E and Mellows, H (1977) Drug treatment and prophylaxis of thrombo-embolism in pregnancy. In *Therapeutic Problems in Pregnancy* (edited by PJ Lewis) pp. 81–89. Lancaster: MTP Press

de Swiet M, Fidler, J, Howell, R and Letsky, E (1981) Thromboembolism in pregnancy. In *Advanced Medicine* (edited by DP Jewell) pp. 309–317. London: Pitman Medical

de Swiet, M, Dorrington Ward, P, Fidler, J *et al.* (1983) Prolonged heparin therapy in pregnancy causes bone demineralization (heparin-induced osteopenia). *British Journal of Obstetrics and Gynaecology*, **90**, 1129–1134

De Wolf, F, Carreras, LO, Moerman, P *et al.* (1982) Decidual vasculopathy and extensive placental infarction in a patient with repeated thromboembolic accidents, recurrent fetal loss, and a lupus anticoagulant. *American Journal of Obstetrics and Gynecology*, **142**, 829–834

Donaldson, MC, Wirthlin, LS and Donaldson, GA (1980) Thirty-year experience with surgical interruption of the inferior vena cava for prevention of pulmonary embolism. *Annals of Surgery*, **191**, 367–372

Eckstein, H and Jack, B (1970) Breast feeding and anticoagulant therapy. *Lancet*, **i**, 672–673

Edmunds, LH (1987) Thrombotic and bleeding complications of prosthetic heart valves. *Annals of Thoracic Surgery*, **44**, 430–445

Egeberg, O (1967) Inherited fibrinogen abnormality causing thrombophilia. *Thrombosis and Diathesis Haemorrhagica*, **17**, 176–187

Elias, M and Eldor, A (1984) Thromboembolism in patients with the 'lupus'-type circulating anti-coagulant. *Archives of Internal Medicine*, **144**, 510–515

Elliot, MS, Immelman, EJ, Jeffery, P *et al.* (1979) A comparative trial of heparin versus streptokinase in the treatment of acute proximal venous thrombosis: an interim report of a prospective trial. *British Journal of Surgery*, **66**, 838–843

Excess, R and Graeme, B (1974) Congenital athyroidism in the newborn infant from intrauterine radioactive iodine. *Biology of the Neonate*, **24**, 289–291

Exner, T, Rickard, KA and Kronenberg, H (1978) A sensitive test demonstrating lupus anticoagulant and its behavioural patterns. *British Journal of Haematology*, **40**, 143–151

Fennerty, AG, Thomas, P, Backhouse, G, Bentley, P and Campbell, IA (1985) Audit of control of heparin treatment. *British Medical Journal*, **290**, 27–28

Filip, DJ, Eckstein, JD and Veltkamp, JJ (1976) Hereditary antithrombin III deficiency and thromboembolic disease. *American Journal of Hematology*, **2**, 343–349

Flessa, HC, Kapstrom, AB, Glueck, MJ *et al*. (1965) Placental transport of heparin. *American Journal of Obstetrics and Gynecology*, **93**, 570–573

Flute, PT (1976) Thrombolytic therapy. *British Journal of Hospital Medicine*, **16**, 135–142

Forestier, F, Daffos, F and Capella-Pavlovsky, M (1984) Low molecular weight heparin (PK 10169) does not cross the placenta during the second trimester of pregnancy. Study by direct fetal blood sampling under ultrasound. *Thrombosis Research*, **34**, 557–560

Forestier, F, Daffos, F, Rainaut, M and Toulemonde, F (1987) Low molecular weight heparin (CY216) does not cross the placenta during the third trimester of pregnancy. *Thrombosis and Haemostasis*, **57**, 234

Friend, JR and Kakkar, VV (1970) The diagnosis of deep vein thrombosis in the puerperium. *Journal of Obstetrics and Gynaecology of the British Commonwealth*, **77**, 820–825

Fuchs, G, Egbring, R and Havemann, K (1977) Fibrinogen Marburg: a new genetic variant of fibrinogen. *Blut*, **34**, 107–118

Gastineau, DA, Kazmier, FJ, Nichols, WL *et al*. (1985) Lupus anticoagulant: an analysis of the clinical and laboratory features of 219 cases. *American Journal of Hematology*, **19**, 265–275

Ginsberg, JS and Hirsh, J (1989) Anticoagulants during pregnancy. *American Review of Medicine*, **40**, 79–86

Ginsberg, JS, Hirsh, J, Rainbow, AJ and Coates, G (1989a) Risks to the fetus of radiologic procedures used in the diagnosis of maternal venous thromboembolic disease. *Thrombosis and Haemostasis*, **61**, 189–196

Ginsberg, JS, Kowalchuk, G, Hirsh, J *et al*. (1989b) Heparin therapy during pregnancy. Risks to the fetus and mother. *Archives of Internal Medicine*, **149**, 2233–2236

Gonzalez, R, Alberca, I and Vincente, V (1985) Protein C levels in late pregnancy, postpartum and in women on oral contraceptives. *Thrombosis Research*, **39**, 637–640

Gonzalez, R, Alberca, I, Sala, N and Vincente, V (1985) Protein C deficiency – response to danazol and DDAVP. *Thrombosis and Haemostasis*, **53**, 320–322

Goodnough, LT, Saito, H and Ratnoff, OD (1983) Thrombosis or myocardial infarction in congenital clotting factor abnormalities and chronic thrombocytopenias: a report of 21 patients and review of 50 previously reported cases. *Medicine*, **62**, 248–255

Greer, IA, Barry, J, Macklon, N and Allan, PL (1990) Diagnosis of deep venous thrombosis in pregnancy. A new role for diagnostic ultrasound. *British Journal of Obstetrics and Gynaecology*, **97**, 53–57

Griffin, JH, Evatt, B, Zimmerman, TS *et al*. (1981) Deficiency of protein C in congenital thrombotic disease. *Journal of Clinical Investigation*, **68**, 1370–1375

Griffith, GC, Nichols, G, Asher, JD and Hanagan, B (1965) Heparin osteoporosis. *Journal of the American Medical Association*, **193**, 91–94

Griffiths, HT and Liu, DTY (1984) Severe heparin osteoporosis in pregnancy. *Postgraduate Medical Journal*, **60**, 424–425

Grobe, H and Balleisen, L (1983) Thromboembolic vessel disease in homocystinuria. In *The Thromboembolic Disorders* (edited by J van de Loo, CRM Prentice and FK Beller), pp. 513–522. Stuttgart: Schattauer Verlag

Hall, JG (1976) Warfarin and fetal abnormality. *Lancet*, **i**, 1127

Hall, JG, Pauli, RM and Wilson, KM (1980) Maternal and fetal sequelae of anticoagulation during pregnancy. *American Journal of Medicine*, **68**, 122–140

Hall, RJC, Young, C and Sutton, CG (1972) Treatment of acute massive pulmonary embolism by streptokinase during labour and delivery. *British Medical Journal*, **4**, 647–649

Harris, EN, Boey, ML, Mackworth-Young, CG *et al*. (1983) Anticardiolipin antibodies: detection by radioimmunoassay and association with thrombosis in systemic lupus erythematosus. *Lancet*, **ii**, 1211–1214

Harris, EN, Gharavi, AE, Loizou, S *et al*. (1985) Cross reactivity of antiphospholipid antibodies. *Journal of Clinical Laboratory Immunology*, **16**, 1–6

Harris, WH, Salzman, EW, De Sanctis, RW and Coutts, RD (1972) Prevention of venous thromboembolism following total hip replacement: warfarin vs dextran 40. *Journal of American Medical Association*, **220**, 1319–1322

Hatjis, CG (1984) Heparin-induced thrombocytopenia in pregnancy. A case report. *Journal of Reproductive Medicine*, **29**, 337–338

Heimbecker, RO, Keon, WJ and Richards, KU (1973) Massive pulmonary embolism: a new look at surgical management. *Archives of Surgery*, **107**, 740–746

Hellgren, M and Blomback, M (1981) Studies on blood coagulation and fibrinolysis in pregnancy, during delivery and in the puerperium. I Normal condition. *Gynecologic and Obstetric Investigation*, **12**, 141–154

Hellgren, M, Tengborn, L and Abildgaard, U (1982) Pregnancy in women with congenital antithrombin III deficiency: experience of treatment with heparin and antithrombin. *Gynaecologic and Obstetric Investigation*, **14**, 127–141

Hellgren, M, Hagnevik, K, Robbe, JH *et al.* (1983) Severe acquired antithrombin III deficiency in relation to hepatic and renal insufficiency and intrauterine fetal death in late pregnancy. *Gynecologic and Obstetric Investigation*, **16**, 107–118

Henderson, SR, Lund, CJ and Creasman, WT (1972) Antepartum pulmonary embolism. *American Journal of Obstetrics and Gynecology*, **112**, 476–486

Hirsh, J (1986) Mechanism of action and monitoring of anticoagulants. *Seminars in Thrombosis and Hemostasis*, **12**, 1–11

Hirsh, J, Cade, JF and O'Sullivan, EF (1970) Clinical experience with anticoagulant therapy during pregnancy. *British Medical Journal*, **1**, 270–273

Hirsh, J, Piovella, F and Pini, M (1989) Congenital antithrombin III deficiency. Incidence and clinical features. *American Journal of Medicine*, **87 (supplement 3B)**, 34S–38S

Hogberg, U (1986) Maternal deaths in Sweden, 1971–1980. *Acta Obstetricia et Gynecologica Scandinavica*, **65**, 161–167

Holzgreve, W, Carey, JC and Hall, BD (1976) Warfarin-induced fetal abnormalities. *Lancet*, **ii**, 914–915

Horellou, MH, Conrad, J, Bertina, RM and Samama, M (1984) Congenital protein C deficiency and thrombotic disease in nine French families. *British Medical Journal*, **289**, 1285–1287

Horellou, MH, Conrad, J, Van Dreden, P *et al.* (1985) Congenital protein C deficiency in 19 French families. *Thrombosis and Haemostasis*, **54**, 143

Howell, R, Fidler, J, Letsky, E and de Swiet, M (1983) The risks of antenatal subcutaneous heparin prophylaxis: a controlled trial. *British Journal of Obstetrics and Gynaecology*, **90**, 1124–1128

Hughes, GRV (1983) Thrombosis, abortion, cerebral disease and the lupus anticoagulant. *British Medical Journal*, **287**, 1088–1089

Hull, RD, Carter, C, Hirsh, J *et al.* (1985) Diagnostic value of ventilation-perfusion lung scanning in patients with suspected pulmonary embolism. *Chest*, **88**, 819–828

Hull, RD, Raskob, GE, Hirsh, J *et al.* (1986) Continuous intravenous heparin compared with intermittent subcutaneous heparin in the initial treatment of proximal-vein thrombosis. *New England Journal of Medicine*, **315**, 1109–1114

Hume, M, Sevitt, S and Thomas, DP (1970) *Venous Thrombosis and Pulmonary Embolism*. Cambridge, Massachusetts: Harvard University Press

Hurd, WH, Miodovnik, M and Stys, SJ (1982) Pregnancy associated with paroxysmal nocturnal haemoglobinuria. *Obstetrics and Gynecology*, **60**, 742–746

Hussein, IY and Critchley, HOD (1986) An unusual presentation of pulmonary thrombo-embolism in late pregnancy. Case report. *British Journal of Obstetrics and Gynaecology*, **93**, 1161–1162

Hytten, F (1985) Blood volume changes in normal pregnancy. In *Haematological Disorders in Pregnancy, Clinics in Haematology, Volume 14* (edited by EA Letsky) **14**, pp. 601–612. Philadelphia: Saunders

Ibarra-Perez, C, Arevalo-Toledo, N, Alvarez-De La Cadena, O *et al.* (1976) The course of pregnancy in patients with artificial heart valves. *American Journal of Medicine*, **61**, 504–512

Inglis, TCM, Stuart, J, George, AJ *et al.* (1982) Haemostatic and rheological changes in normal pregnancy and pre-eclampsia. *British Journal of Haematology*, **56**, 461–465

Islam, T (1984) Portal vein thrombosis in pregnancy. *Journal of Obstetrics and Gynaecology*, **4**, 242

Iturbe-Alessio, I and Salazar, E (1987) Anticoagulation in pregnant women with artificial heart valves. *New England Journal of Medicine*, **316**, 1663–1664

Iturbe-Alessio, I, del Carmen Fonseca, M, Mutchinik, O *et al.* (1986) Risks of anticoagulant therapy in pregnant women with artificial heart valves. *New England Journal of Medicine*, **315**, 1390–1393

Jaffe, MD and Willis, PW (1965) Multiple fractures associated with long-term sodium heparin therapy. *Journal of the American Medical Association*, **193**, 152–154

Javares, T, Coto, EC, Maiques, V *et al.* (1984) Pregnancy after heart valve replacement. *International Journal of Cardiology*, **5**, 731–739

Jeffcoate, TNA, Miller, J, Ros, RF and Tindall, VR (1968) Puerperal thrombo-embolism in relation to the inhibition of lactation by oestrogen therapy. *British Medical Journal*, **4**, 19–25

Jick, H, Stone, KD, Westerholm, B, Inman, WHW *et al.* (1969) Venous thromboembolic disease and ABO blood type. A cooperative study. *Lancet*, **i**, 359–542

Jones, TK, Barnes, RW and Greenfield, LJ (1986) Greenfield vena caval filter. Rationale and current indications. *Annals of Thoracic Surgery*, **42 (Supplement)**, 48–55

Kakkar, VV and Murray, WJG (1985) Efficacy and safety of low-molecular weight heparin (CY216) in preventing postoperative venous thrombo-embolism: a cooperative study. *British Journal of Surgery*, **72**, 786–791

Kamiya, T, Sugihara, T, Ogata, K *et al.* (1986) Inherited deficiency of protein S in a Japanese family with recurrent thrombosis: a study of three generations. *Blood*, **67**, 406–410

Kerber, IJ, Warr, OS III and Richardson, C (1968) Pregnancy in a patient with a prosthetic mitral valve associated with a fetal anomaly attributed to warfarin sodium. *Journal of the American Medical Association*, **203**, 223–225

King, DJ and Kelton, JG (1984) Heparin-associated thrombocytopenia. *Annals of Internal Medicine*, **100**, 535–540

Lamon, JM, Lenke, RR, Levy, HL *et al.* (1981) Selected metabolic diseases. In *Genetic Diseases in Pregnancy* (edited by JD Schulmann and JL Simpson) pp. 6–8. New York: Academic Press

Lao, TT, de Swiet, M, Letsky, E and Walters, BNJ (1985) Prophylaxis of thrombo-embolism in pregnancy: an alternative. *British Journal of Obstetrics and Gynaecology*, **92**, 202–206

Lansing, AM and Davies, WM (1968) Five year follow-up of iliofemoral venous thrombectomy. *Annals of Surgery*, **168**, 620–628

Laros, RK and Alger, LS (1979) Thromboembolism and pregnancy. *Clinical Obstetrics and Gynecology*, **22**, 871–888

Larrea, JL, Nunez, L, Reque, JA *et al.* (1983) Pregnancy and mechanical valve prostheses: a high-risk situation for the mother and fetus. *Annals of Thoracic Surgery*, **36**, 459–463

Larsen, JF, Jacobsen, B, Holm, HH *et al.* (1978) Intrauterine injection of vitamin K before the delivery during anticoagulant treatment of the mother. *Acta Obstetricia et Gynecologica Scandinavica*, **57**, 227–230

Leclerc, JR and Roy, J (1991) The diagnosis of venous thrombo-embolism during pregnancy and the post-partum period. In *Haemostasis and Thrombosis in Obstetrics and Gynaecology* (edited by IA Greer, AGG Turple and CD Forbes) London: Chapman and Hall, in press

Leclerc, JR, Geerts, W, Panju, A *et al.* (1986) Management of antithrombin III deficiency during pregnancy without administration of antithrombin III. *Thrombosis Research*, **41**, 567–573

Leclerc, JR, Wolfson, C, Rosenthall, L *et al.* (1988) Tc-99m red blood cell venography in patients with clinically suspected first episode of deep vein thrombosis: a prospective study. *Journal of Nuclear Medicine*, **29**, 1498–1506

Lee, PK, Wang, RYC, Chow, JSF *et al.* (1986) Combined use of warfarin and adjusted subcutaneous heparin during pregnancy in patients with an artificial heart valve. *Journal of American College of Cardiology*, **8**, 221–224

Letsky, EA (1985) Coagulation problems during pregnancy. *Current Reviews in Obstetrics and Gynaecology, 10*. Edinburgh: Churchill Livingstone

Letsky, EA and de Swiet, M (1984) Thromboembolism in pregnancy and its management. *British Journal of Haematology*, **57**, 543–552

Levine, HJ, Pauker, SC and Salzman, EW (1989) Antithrombotic therapy in valvular heart disease. *Chest*, **95, supplement**, 98S–106S

Levine, MN and Hirsh, J (1988) Clinical use of low molecular weight heparins and heparinoids. *Seminars in Thrombosis and Hemostasis*, **14**, 116–125

Limit, R and Grondin, CM (1977) Cardiac valve prosthesis, anticoagulation and pregnancy. *Annals of Thoracic Surgery*, **23**, 337–341

Lockshin, MD, Druzin, ML, Goei, S et al. (1985) Antibodies to cardiolipin as a predictor of fetal distress or death in pregnant patients with systemic lupus erythematosus. New England Journal of Medicine, 313, 152–156

Lubbe, WF and Butler, WS (1991) Acquired defects of coagulation – the lupus anticoagulant. In Haemostasis and Thrombosis in Obstetrics and Gynaecology (edited by IA Greer, AGG Turpie and CD Forbes). London: Chapman and Hall, in press

Lubbe, WF and Liggins, GC (1985) Lupus anticoagulant and pregnancy. American Journal of Obstetrics and Gynecology, 135, 322–327

Lubbe, WF, Butler, WS, Palmer, SJ and Liggins, GC (1983) Fetal survival after prednisone suppression of maternal lupus anticoagulant. Lancet, i, 1361–1363

Ludwig, H (1973) Results of streptokinase therapy in deep venous thrombosis during pregnancy. Postgraduate Medical Journal, Supplement, 65–67

Lutz, DJ, Noller, KL, Spittell, JA et al. (1978) Pregnancy and its complications following cardiac valve prosthesis. American Journal of Obstetrics and Gynecology, 131, 460–468

McKenna, R, Cale, ER and Vasan, U (1983) Is warfarin sodium contraindicated in the lactating mother? Journal of Paediatrics, 103, 325–327

Mackie, IJ, Coloca, CB and Machin, SJ (1987) Familial lupus anticoagulants. British Journal of Haematology, 67, 359–363

McLeod, AA, Jennings, KP and Townsend, ER (1978) Near fatal puerperal thrombosis on Bjork–Shiley mitral valve prosthesis. British Heart Journal, 40, 934–937

Majer, RV, Chisholm, M, and Hickton, MC (1989) Replacement therapy for protein C deficiency using fresh frozen plasma. British Journal of Haematology, 72, 475

Malcolm, ID, Wigmore, TA and Steinbrecher, UP (1979) Heparin associated thrombocytopenia low frequency in 104 patients treated with heparin of intestinal mucosal origin. Canadian Medical Association Journal, 120, 1086–1088

Malm, J, Laurell, M and Dahlback, B (1988) Changes in the plasma levels of vitamin K-dependent proteins C and S and of C4b-binding protein during pregnancy and oral contraception. British Journal of Haematology, 68, 437–443

Mannucci, PM and Owen, WG (1987) Basic and clinical aspects of proteins C and S. In Haemostasis and Thrombosis, 2nd edn (edited by AL Bloom and DP Thomas), pp. 452–464, Edinburgh: Churchill Livingstone

Mannucci, PM, Boyer, C, Wolf, M et al. (1982) Treatment of congenital antithrombin III deficiency with concentrates. British Journal of Haematology, 50, 531–535

Mannucci, PM, Vigano, S, Bottasso, B et al. (1984) Protein C antigen during pregnancy delivery and the puerperium. Thrombosis and Haemostasis, 52, 217

Mansour, M, Chang, AE and Sindelar, WF (1985) Interruption of the inferior vena cava for the prevention of recurrent pulmonary embolism. American Journal of Surgery, 51, 375–380

Marchesi, D, Parbtani, A, Frampton, G et al. (1981) Thrombotic tendency in systemic lupus erythematosus. Lancet, i, 719

Marcus, CS, Mason, GR, Kuperus, JH and Mena, I (1985) Pulmonary imaging in pregnancy maternal risk and fetal dosimetry. Clinical Nuclear Medicine, 10, 1–4

Massignon, D, Pegaz-Fiornet, M and Coeur, P (1986) Conduite thérapeutique au cours d'une grossesse avec déficit congénitale en antithrombine III associée à une néphropathie gravidique. Journal of Gynecology, Obstetrics and Reproductive Biology, 15, 299–304

Matzsch, T, Bergqvist, D, Hedner, U et al. (1986) Heparin-induced osteoporosis in rats. Thrombosis and Haemostasis, 56, 293–294

Mayor, GE (1969) Deep vein thrombosis – surgical management. British Medical Journal, 4, 680–682

Meissner, AJ, Misiak, A, Ziemski, JM et al. (1987) Hazards of thrombolytic therapy in deep vein thrombosis. British Journal of Surgery, 74, 991–993

Mibashan, RS, Millar, DS, Rodeck, CJ et al. (1985) Prenatal diagnosis of hereditary protein C deficiency. New England Journal of Medicine, 313, 1607

Michiels, JJ, Stibbe, J, Vallenga, E and van Vliet, HHDM (1984) Prophylaxis of thrombosis in anti-thrombin III-deficient women during pregnancy and delivery. European Journal of Obstetrics and Gynecology and Reproductive Biology, 18, 149–153

Michiels, JJ, Stibbe, J, Bertina, R and Brockmans, A (1987) Effectiveness of long term oral anticoagulant therapy in preventing venous thrombosis in hereditary protein S deficiency. *British Medical Journal*, **295**, 641–643

Miletich, J, Sherman, L and Broze, G (1987) Absence of thrombosis in subjects with heterozygous protein C deficiency. *New England Journal of Medicine*, **317**, 991–996

Mogensen, K, Skibsted, L, Wadt, J and Nissen, F (1989) Thrombectomy of acute iliofemoral venous thrombosis during pregnancy. *Surgery, Gynecology and Obstetrics*, **169**, 50–54

Moseley, P and Kerstein, MD (1980) Pregnancy and thrombophlebitis. *Surgery, Gynecology and Obstetrics*, **150**, 593–597

Mudd, SH, Skorby, F, Levy, HL *et al*. (1985) The natural history of homocystinaemia due to cystathionine β-synthase deficiency. *American Journal of Human Genetics*, **37**, 1–31

Mueh, JR, Herbst, KD and Rapaport, SI (1980) Thrombosis in patients with lupus anticoagulant. *Annals of Internal Medicine*, **92**, 156–159

Nelson, DM, Stempel, LE, Fabri, PJ and Talbert, M (1984) Hickman catheter use in a pregnant patient requiring therapeutic heparin anticoagulation. *American Journal of Obstetrics and Gynecology*, **149**, 461–462

Newman, G and Mitchell, JRA (1984) Homocystinuria presenting as multiple arterial occlusions. *Quarterly Journal of Medicine*, **53**, 251–258

Nilsson, IM, Astedt, B, Hedner, U and Berezin, D (1975) Intrauterine death and circulating anticoagulant 'antithromboplastin'. *Acta Medica Scandinavica*, **197**, 153–159

Nilsson, IM, Felding, P, Lecander, I *et al*. (1986) Different type of plasminogen activator inhibitors in plasma and platelets in pregnant women. *British Journal of Haematology*, **62**, 215–220

Oakley, CM (1983) Pregnancy in patients with prosthetic heart valves. *British Heart Journal*, **286**, 1680–1682

Oakley, C and Doherty, P (1976) Pregnancy in patients after valve replacement. *British Heart Journal*, **38**, 1140–1148

Oakley, CM and Hawkins, DF (1983) Pregnancy in patients with prosthetic heart valves. *British Medical Journal*, **287**, 358

Ogston, D (1987) *Venous Thrombosis. Causation and Prediction*. Chichester: Wiley Medical

Omri, A, Dalaloye, JF, Andersen, H *et al*. (1989) Low molecular weight heparin Novo (LHN-1) does not cross the placenta during the second trimester of pregnancy. *Thrombosis and Haemostasis*, **61**, 55–56

O'Neill, H and Blake, S (1982) Problems in the management of patients with artificial valves during pregnancy. *British Journal of Obstetrics and Gynaecology*, **89**, 940–943

Orme, M L'e., Lewis, M, de Swiet, M *et al*. (1977) May mothers given warfarin breast-feed their infants? *British Medical Journal*, **1**, 1564–1565

Paull, JA (1987) Retrospective study of dextran-induced anaphylactoid reactions in 5745 patients. *Anaesthesia and Intensive Care*, **15**, 163–167

Pavankumar, P, Venugopal, P, Kaul, U *et al*. (1988) Pregnancy in patients with prosthetic cardiac valve. A 10-year experience. *Scandinavian Journal of Thoracic and Cardiovascular Surgery*, **22**, 19–22

Petaja, J, Rasi, V, Myllyla, G *et al*. (1989) Familial hypofibrinolysis and venous thrombosis. *British Journal of Haematology*, **71**, 393–398

Pettifor, JM and Benson, R (1975) Congenital malformations associated with the administration of oral anticoagulants during pregnancy. *Journal of Pediatrics*, **86**, 459–462

Pfeiffer, GW (1970a) Distribution and placental transfer of [141]I streptokinase. *Australian Annals of Medicine*, **Supplement**, 17–18

Pfeiffer, GW (1970b) The use of thrombolytic therapy in obstetrics and gynaecology. *Australian Annals of Medicine*, **Supplement**, 28–31

Polak, JF and O'Leary, DH (1988) Deep venous thrombosis in pregnancy: non-invasive diagnosis. *Radiology*, **166**, 377–379

Poller, L (1986) Laboratory control of anticoagulant therapy. *Seminars in Thrombosis and Hemostasis*, **12**, 13–19

Poller, L and Taberner, DA (1982) Dosage and control of oral anticoagulants: an international collaborative survey. *British Journal of Haematology*, **51**, 479–485

Ponto, JA (1986) Fetal dosimetry from pulmonary imaging in pregnancy. Revised estimates. *Clinical Nuclear Medicine*, **11**, 108–109

Preissner, KT (1990) Biological relevance of the protein C system and laboratory diagnosis of protein C and protein S deficiencies. *Clinical Science*, **78**, 351–364

Pridmore, BR, Murray, KH and McAllen, PM (1975) The management of anticoagulant therapy during and after pregnancy. *British Journal of Obstetrics and Gynaecology*, **82**, 740–744

Priollet, P, Roncato, M, Aiach, M, Housset, E, Poissonnier, MH and Chavinie, J (1986) Low-molecular-weight heparin in venous thrombosis during pregnancy. *British Journal of Haematology*, **63**, 605–606

Rabinovici, J, Mani, A, Barkai, G *et al.* (1987) Long-term ambulatory anticoagulation by constant subcutaneous heparin infusion in pregnancy. *British Journal of Obstetrics and Gynaecology*, **94**, 89–91

Rallings, P, Exner, T and Abraham, R (1989) Coronary artery vasculitis and myocardial infarction associated with antiphospholipid antibodies in the pregnant woman. *Australian and New Zealand Journal of Medicine*, **19**, 347–350

Ramsay, LE (1983) Impact of venography on the diagnosis and management of deep vein thrombosis. *British Medical Journal*, **286**, 698–699

Redman, HC (1988) Deep venous thrombosis: is contrast venography still the diagnostic 'gold standard'? *Radiology*, **168**, 277–278

Ring, J and Messmer, K (1977) Incidence and severity of anaphylactoid reactions to colloid volume substitutes. *Lancet*, **i**, 466–469

Robin, ED (1977) Overdiagnosis and overtreatment of pulmonary embolism: the emperor may have no clothes. *Annals of Internal Medicine*, **87**, 775–781

Rose, BA, Simon, DC, Hess, ML *et al.* (1987) Percutaneous transfemoral placement of Kimray–Greenfield vena cava filter. *Radiology*, **165**, 373–376

Rosendaal, FR, Heijboer, H, Briet, E *et al.* (1991) Mortality in hereditary antithrombin III deficiency – 1830 to 1989. *Lancet*, **i**, 260–262

Royal College of General Practitioners (1967) Oral contraception and thromboembolic disease. *Journal of the Royal College of General Practitioners*, **13**, 267–279

Rustin, MHA, Bull, HA, Machin, SJ *et al.* (1988) Effects of the lupus anticoagulant in patients with systemic lupus erythematosus on endothelial cell prostacyclin release and procoagulant activity. *Journal of Investigative Dermatology*, **90**, 744–748

Sachs, BP, Brown, DAJ, Driscoll, SG *et al.* (1987) Maternal mortality in Massachusetts. Trends and prevention. *New England Journal of Medicine*, **316**, 667–672

Salazar, E, Zajarias, A, Gutierrez, N *et al.* (1984) The problem of cardiac valve prostheses, anticoagulants and pregnancy. *Circulation*, **Supplement I**, I169–I177

Samama, M and Combe-Tamzali, S (1989) Prevention of thromboembolic disease in general surgery with enoxaparin in new approaches to management of venous thrombo-embolism. *British Journal of Clinical Practice*, 43, **Symposium Supplement 65**, 9–17

Samson, D, Stirling, Y, Woolf, L *et al.* (1984) Management of planned pregnancy in a patient with congenital antithrombin III deficiency. *British Journal of Haematology*, **56**, 243–249

Sandler, DA and Martin, JF (1985) Liquid crystal thermography as a screening test for deep-vein thrombosis. *Lancet*, **i**, 665–668

Sandler, DA, Martin, JF, Duncan, JS *et al.* (1984) Diagnosis of deep-vein thrombosis: comparison of clinical evaluation, ultrasound, plethysmography and venoscan with X-ray venogram. *Lancet*, **ii**, 716–719

Sasahara, AA and Barsamian, E (1973) Another look at pulmonary embolectomy. *Annals of Thoracic Surgery*, **16**, 317–320

Sayama, S, Kashiwagi, H, Owaga, T *et al.* (1981) Circulating levels of prekallikrein and kallikrein in pregnancy and labor. *Biological Research in Pregnancy*, **2**, 90–94

Scholtes, MCW, Gerretsen, G and Haak, HL (1983) The factor VIII ratio in normal and pathological pregnancies. *European Journal of Obstetrics, Gynecology and Reproductive Biology*, **16**, 89–95

Schwartz, HP, Fischer, M, Hopmeir, P *et al.* (1984) Plasma protein S deficiency in familial thrombotic disease. *Blood*, **64**, 1297–1300

Scott, CR (1983) Disorders of amino acid metabolism. In *Principles and Practice of Medical Genetics, Volume 2* (edited by AEH Emery and DL Rimoin), pp. 1241–1266, Edinburgh: Churchill Livingstone

Scott, JR, Rote, NS and Branch, DW (1987) Immunologic aspects of recurrent abortion and fetal death. *Obstetrics and Gynecology*, **70**, 645–656

Seligsohn, U, Berger, A, Abend, M *et al.* (1984) Homozygous protein C deficiency manifested by massive venous thrombosis in the newborn. *New England Journal of Medicine*, **310**, 559–562

Sharma, GVRK, Burlesco, VA and Sasahara, AA (1980) Effect of thrombolytic therapy on pulmonary-capillary blood volume in patients with pulmonary embolism. *New England Journal of Medicine*, **303**, 842–845

Sharon, C, Tirindelli, A and Mariani, G (1986) Homozygous protein C deficiency with moderately severe clinical symptoms. *Thrombosis Research*, **41**, 483–488

Shaul, WL and Hall, JG (1977) Multiple congenital anomalies associated with oral anticoagulants. *American Journal of Obstetrics and Gynecology*, **127**, 191–198

Shaul, WL, Emery, H and Hall, JG (1975) Chondrodysplasia punctata and maternal warfarin use during pregnancy. *American Journal of Diseases in Children*, **129**, 360–362

Sheffield, LJ, Danks, DM, Mayne, KV and Hutchinson, LA (1976) Chondrodysplasia punctata – 23 cases of a mild and relatively common variety. *Journal of Pediatrics*, **89**, 916–923

Sherman, S and Hall, BD (1976) Warfarin and fetal abnormality. *Lancet*, **i**, 692

Shifter, T, Machtey, I and Creter, D (1984) Thromboembolism in congenital factor VII deficiency. *Acta Haematologica*, **71**, 60–62

Sie, P, Dupouy, D, Pichon, J and Boneu, B (1985) Constitutional heparin co-factor II deficiency associated with recurrent thrombosis. *Lancet*, **ii**, 414–416

Silver, D and Sabiston, DC (1975) The role of vena caval interruption in the management of pulmonary embolism. *Surgery*, **77**, 3–10

Simpson, FG, Robinson, PJ, Bark, M and Losowsky, MS (1980) Prospective study of thrombophlebitis and pseudo thrombophlebitis. *Lancet*, **i**, 331–333

Smith, MF and Cameron, MD (1979) Warfarin as teratogen. *Lancet*, **i**, 727

Sostman, HD, Rapdport, S, Goffschalk, A *et al.* (1986) Progress in clinical radiology. *Investigative Radiology*, **21**, 443–454

Spencer, JAD (1980) Paroxysmal nocturnal haemoglobinuria in pregnancy. *British Journal of Obstetrics and Gynaecology*, **87**, 246–248

Squires, JW and Pinch, LW (1979) Heparin-induced spinal fractures. *Journal of the American Medical Association*, **241**, 2417–2418

Stein, PD and Kantrowitz, A (1989) Antithrombotic therapy in mechanical and biological prosthetic heart valves and saphenous vein bypass grafts. *Chest*, **95 Supplement**, 107S–117S

Stirling, Y, Woolf, L, North, WRS *et al.* (1984) Haemostasis in normal pregnancy. *Thrombosis and Haemostasis*, **52**, 176–182

Stuart, MJ, Gross, SJ, Elrad, H and Graeber, JE (1982) Effects of acetylsalicylic acid ingestion on maternal and neonatal hemostasis. *New England Journal of Medicine*, **307**, 909–912

Sullivan, JM, Harken, DE and Gorlin, R (1971) Pharmacologic control of thromboembolic complications of cardiac-valve replacement. *New England Journal of Medicine*, **284**, 1391–1394

Szekely, P, Turner, R, and Snaith, L (1973) Pregnancy and the changing pattern of rheumatic heart disease. *British Heart Journal*, **35**, 1293–1303

Ten Cate, JW, Peters, M and Buller, H (1983) Isolated plasminogen deficiency in a patient with recurrent thrombotic complications. *Thrombosis and Haemostasis*, **50**, 59

Tengborn, L and Bengtsson, T (1986) Antithrombin III thromboprophylaxis during pregnancy in a patient with congenital antithrombin III deficiency. *Acta Obstetricia et Gynecologica Scandinavica*, **65**, 375–376

Thiagarajan, P, Pengo, V and Shapiro, S (1986) The use of the dilute Russel Viper Venom Time for the diagnosis of lupus anticoagulants. *Blood*, **68**, 869–874

Thomas, ML, Keeling, FP, Piaggio, RB and Treweeke, PS (1984) Contrast agent induced thrombophlebitis following leg phlebography: iopamidol versus meglumine iothalamate. *British Journal of Radiology*, **57**, 205–207

Thompson, RC (1973) Heparin osteoporosis. *Journal of Bone and Joint Surgery*, **55A**, 606–612

Thorburn, J and Letsky, E (1990) Epidural anaesthesia is contraindicated in mothers on low-dose heparin. In *Controversies in Obstetric Anaesthesia* (edited by B Morgan) pp. 49–61. London: Edward Arnold

Tran, TT, Marbet, GA and Duckert, F (1985) Association of hereditary heparin co-factor II deficiency with thrombosis. *Lancet*, **ii**, 413–414

Treffers, PE, Huidekoper, BL, Weenik, GH and Kloosterman, GJ (1983) Epidemiological observations of thromboembolic disease during pregnancy and in the puerperium in 56,022 women. *International Journal of Gynaecology and Obstetrics*, **21**, 327–331

Tribukait, B and Swedjemark, GA (1978) Secretion of Tc^{99m} in breast milk after intravenous injection of marked macroaggregated albumin. *Acta Radiologica: Oncology*, **17**, 379–382

Triplett, DA, Brandt, JJ, Kaczor, D *et al*. (1983) Laboratory diagnosis of lupus inhibitors: a comparison of the Tissue Thromboplastin Inhibition Procedures with a new platelet neutralization procedure. *American Journal of Clinical Pathology*, **79**, 678–682

Van de Meer, J, Stoepman-van Dalen, EA and Janset, JMS (1973) Antithrombin III deficiency in a Dutch family. *Journal of Clinical Pathology*, **26**, 532–538

Vermylen, J, Blockmans, D, Spitz, B and Deckmyn, H (1986) Thrombosis and immune disorders. In *Clinics in Haematology* (edited by N Chesterman), pp. 393–412. Eastbourne: Saunders

Vikydal, R, Korninger, C, Kyrle, PA *et al*. (1985) The prevalence of hereditary antithrombin III deficiency in patients with a history of venous thrombo-embolism. *Thrombosis and Haemostasis*, **54**, 744–745

Villasanta, U (1965) Thromboembolic disease in pregnancy. *American Journal of Obstetrics and Gynecology*, **93**, 142–160

Vogel, P, Laing, FC, Jeffrey, RB *et al*. (1987) Deep venous thrombosis of the lower extremity: US evaluation. *Radiology*, **163**, 747–751

Walker, MG, Shaw, JW, Thomson, GJL *et al*. (1987) Subcutaneous calcium heparin versus intravenous sodium heparin in treatment of established acute deep vein thrombosis of the legs: a multicentre prospective randomized trial. *British Medical Journal*, **294**, 1189–1192

Wang, RYC, Lee, PK, Chow, JSF and Chen, WWC (1983) Efficacy of low-dose, subcutaneously administered heparin in treatment of pregnant women with artificial heart valves. *Medical Journal of Australia*, **2**, 126–128

Warwick, R, Hutton, RA, Goff, L *et al*. (1989) Changes in protein C and free protein S during pregnancy and following hysterectomy. *Journal of the Royal Society of Medicine*, **82**, 591–594

Weiner, CP and Brandt, J (1980) Plasma antithrombin III activity in normal pregnancy. *Obstetrics and Gynecology*, **56**, 601–603

Wheeler, HR and Anderson, FA Jr (1985) Can non-invasive tests be used as the basis for treatment of deep vein thrombosis? In *Non-Invasive Diagnostic Techniques in Vascular Disease* (edited by FF Bernstein) pp. 805–818. St. Louis: CV Mosby

Whitfield, LR, Lele, AS and Levy, G (1983) Effect of pregnancy on the relationship between concentration and anticoagulant action of heparin. *Clinical Pharmacology and Therapeutics*, **34**, 23–28

Wiman, B, Csemiczky, G, Marsk, L *et al*. (1984) The fast inhibitor of tissue plasminogen activator in plasma during pregnancy. *Thrombosis and Haemostasis*, **52**, 124–126

Winter, JH and Douglas, AS (1991) Congenital thrombotic problems in obstetrics and gynaecology. In *Haemostasis and Thrombosis in Obstetrics and Gynaecology* (edited by IA Greer, AGG Turpie and CD Forbes). London: Chapman and Hall, in press

Winter, JH, Fenech, A, Ridley, W *et al*. (1982) Familial antithrombin III deficiency. *Quarterly Journal of Medicine*, **51**, 373–395

Wise, PH and Hall, AJ (1980) Heparin-induced osteopenia in pregnancy. *British Medical Journal*, **2**, 110–112

Wolf, H and Wick, G (1986) Antibodies interacting with, and corresponding binding site for heparin on human thrombocytes. *Lancet*, **ii**, 222–223

Zucker, ML, Gomperts, ED and Marcus, RG (1976) Prophylactic and therapeutic use of anticoagulants in inherited antithrombin III deficiency. *South African Medical Journal*, **50**, 1743–1748

Chapter 4

Heart disease
Michael de Swiet

PART 1. GENERAL CONSIDERATIONS

Physiology

The most obvious haemodynamic change in pregnancy is a rise in cardiac output of approximately 40 per cent, i.e. from about 3.5 l/min to 6.0 l/min when the patient is at rest. Such data derived from the cardiac catheter laboratory must be viewed with objectivity, and too much reliability must not be placed on individual measurements. There is considerable variation between individuals, and the experimental conditions under which investigations have been made are not always relevant to the situations of clinical importance, such as labour or other forms of exercise. The time of this rise in cardiac output is also open to discussion. However, those investigators that have measured cardiac output early in pregnancy find that it is already markedly elevated in the first trimester.

What is disputed is whether the cardiac output falls at the end of pregnancy and, if so, by how much. It was originally thought that falls in cardiac output demonstrated in late pregnancy were spurious and associated with measurements made in the supine position (Lees *et al.*, 1967). However the fall in cardiac output associated with lying in the supine position may be no more than 3% (Newman, Derrington and Sore, 1983). Furthermore, Ueland *et al.* (1969) and Pyörälä (1966) were aware of these possibilities, and both measured cardiac output in the lateral position, showing falls in cardiac output of 4–20 per cent of the non-pregnant level in the last 10 weeks of pregnancy.

More recently, non-invasive studies, using electrical impedance cardiography (Davies *et al.*, 1986) and Doppler estimation of aortic velocity (James *et al.*, 1985), have again suggested that cardiac output falls to non-pregnant levels at term. Both these techniques are subject to criticism, the former because of changes that may occur in pregnancy in the pulmonary blood vessels (de Swiet and Talbert, 1986), which lead to underestimation of cardiac output (Milsom *et al.*, 1983), and the latter because the aorta dilates in pregnancy (Hart *et al.*, 1986).

However, the most recent Doppler studies that have also measured the cross-sectional area through which the blood is flowing [usually at the pulmonary, aortic or mitral valves (Robson *et al.*, 1987a, b)] have shown a high cardiac output at the onset of labour (7 l/min mean), rising further within labour and falling markedly with the first 2 weeks of delivery (Robson *et al.*, 1987a). Echocardiographic studies measuring volume changes in the heart during the cardiac cycle have also shown a 30 per cent increase in cardiac output in the third trimester, declining rapidly after delivery (Mashini *et al.*, 1987). At 24 weeks after delivery the cardiac output has fallen further to 5 l/min (Robson *et al.*, 1987b), which is approximately normal for a non-pregnant woman. Current data, therefore, do not favour any great decrease in cardiac output at the end of pregnancy.

Cardiac output (assessed by the Doppler technique) is not affected by breast feeding (Robson *et al.*, 1989). Clinicians should not be concerned, therefore, that breast-feeding will 'put an extra strain on the heart' and breast-feeding should be encouraged in patients with heart disease. The increase in cardiac output in pregnancy is caused partly by an increase in heart rate (Clapp, 1985) and partly by an increase in stroke volume.

There is no change in pulmonary capillary pressure in pregnancy (Mashini *et al.*, 1987), although it rises in labour (see below). The increase in cardiac output is, therefore, unlikely to be caused by increased filling of the heart (increased preload) in association with the increased circulating blood volume. Rather, as blood pressure does not rise in pregnancy and usually falls, the increase in cardiac output is related to a marked fall in peripheral vascular resistance (decreased afterload). Indeed, it is likely that the fall in peripheral resistance is one (if not the major) factor that causes the rise in cardiac output (Phippard *et al.*, 1986; Schrier, 1988).

Only part of the change in peripheral vascular resistance can be accounted for by blood flow through the low resistance shunt of the pregnant uterus, as cardiac output is elevated during the first trimester, at a time when there is very little change in uterine blood flow. Oestrogen (Slater *et al.*, 1986), progesterone, and prostaglandins, including prostacyclin, are other probable mediators of the alterations in haemodynamics caused by pregnancy. More recently, a very potent vasodilator – calcitonin gene-related peptide – has been described, which also increases in concentration in pregnancy and which may contribute to the increase in cardiac output (Stevenson *et al.*, 1986). (For further reviews of these changes, see de Swiet, 1980, 1988; Schrier, 1988).

In contrast to the considerable volume of studies of the haemodynamics of pregnancy in normal individuals, there has been little information concerning patients with heart disease. Ueland and his colleagues showed that patients with asymptomatic mitral valve disease are unable to increase their cardiac outputs on exercise in pregnancy to the same level as normal patients at rest (Ueland, Novy and Metcalfe, 1972).

More recently, the application of Swan–Ganz catheterization to obstetric patients (Clark *et al.*, 1985a) has begun to yield further information. This technique involves the placing of a catheter, usually via the jugular or subclavian vein, without radiographic screening, in the pulmonary artery and wedged pulmonary artery positions, the latter for the indirect measurement of left atrial pressure. Injection of cold saline in the right atrium and subsequent measurement of temperature in the pulmonary artery allows measurement of cardiac output by the dilution technique. This technique should be performed only by those skilled in its use because there are many complications such as pneumothorax. Using this technique, Clark *et al.* (1985b) demonstrated a sharp (10 mmHg) rise in left atrial pressure in patients with mitral stenosis immediately after delivery. Similar data have been published in a patient in labour following myocardial infarction in pregnancy (Hankins *et al.*, 1985). Even Braxton Hicks' contractions cause elevation in left atrial pressure (Jakobi *et al.*, 1989), presumably due to blood expelled by the contracting uterus.

The Starling relation in pregnancy

The nett capillary filtration (F) of fluid (outwards from the capillary values positive) can be written:

$$F = L_p.A \, ((P_c - P_i) - r \, (COP_p - COP_i))$$

where L_p = membrane hydraulic conductivity per unit area
A = exchanging surface area
P_c = capillary hydrostatic pressure
P_i = interstitial hydrostatic pressure
COP_p = colloid osmotic pressure of plasma
COP_i = colloid osmotic pressure of interstitial fluid
r = capillary reflection coefficient for plasma proteins

(Oian et al., 1985; MacLennan, 1986).

Oian et al. (1985) measured P_i, COP_p and COP_i in the subcutaneous tissue of the thorax and the ankle of patients in the first and third trimesters. They found that although COP_p fell between the first and third trimesters from 23 to 21 mmHg (3.1–2.8 kPa) the other variables, P_i and COP_i, changed in direction to offset this effect. Oedema formation in the systemic circulation must, therefore, relate to an increase either in membrane hydraulic conductivity or in the capillary pressure. As membrane hydraulic conductivity does not change (Spetz, 1965), an increase in capillary pressure is more likely to be the cause (Oian et al., 1985).

The analysis by Oian et al. (1985) discussed above applies only to oedema in the systemic circulation. The tendency of pregnant women to form pulmonary oedema has also been described by MacLennan (1986), using the Starling formula. Unfortunately, even fewer of the variables can be measured in the pulmonary circuit but a rise in pulmonary wedge pressure (pulmonary capillary pressure), which is equivalent to capillary hydrostatic pressure, has been documented in labour in patients with mitral stenosis (Clark et al., 1985b); this, coupled with the fall in osmotic pressure of pregnancy, could account for the high risk of pulmonary oedema at this time. Furthermore, Gonik and colleagues (Gonik and Cotton, 1982; Gonik et al., 1985; Cotton et al., 1986) have demonstrated falls in colloid osmotic pressure from about 22 mmHg at the onset of labour to a nadir with a mean of about 16 mmHg, 6 h after delivery. These falls occur in women delivered vaginally or abdominally, under epidural or general anaesthesia, but seem particularly marked in those women given excessive quantities of crystalloid intravenously at delivery. This fall in colloid osmotic pressure, if it does not also occur in pulmonary interstitial fluid plus the rise in pulmonary capillary pressure, should give pulmonary oedema more often than occurs clinically. Typically, non-cardiogenic pulmonary oedema occurs at colloid osmotic pressures of 13–16 mmHg (Stein et al., 1975; Rackow, Fein and Lippo, 1977). It is, therefore, surprising that the modern management of labour with liberal use of crystalloid does not cause symptoms more frequently than it does. However, those patients with pre-eclampsia who develop pulmonary oedema have usually been given large quantities of crystalloid (Sibai et al., 1987), which is certainly in keeping with the above analysis.

Maternal mortality

Although sporadic fatalities will be seen in all forms of heart disease in pregnancy, maternal mortality is most likely in those conditions where pulmonary blood flow cannot be increased (Jewett, 1979). This occurs because of obstruction, either within the pulmonary blood vessels or at the mitral valve. The situation is documented clearly in Eisenmenger's syndrome, where up to now there has been no effective treatment and where the maternal mortality is between 30 per cent and 50 per cent (Morgan Jones and Howitt, 1965; Neilson, Galea and Blunt, 1970; Pitts, Crosby and Basta, 1977; Gleicher et al., 1978). Elevations in pulmonary vascular resistance are also found in pregnancy in cor pulmonale (Rush, Verjans and Spracklen, 1979), patients with single ventricle (Stiller et al., 1984), pulmonary veno-occlusive disease (Tsou et al., 1984) and in primary pulmonary hypertension. In the last condition the maternal mortality is about 50 per cent (McCaffrey and Dunn, 1964; Morgan Jones and Howitt, 1965; Sinnenberg, 1980; Abboud et al., 1983).

In contrast, in Fallot's tetralogy where the pulmonary vascular resistance is normal, the reported maternal mortality varies between 4 per cent and 20 per cent (Mendelson, 1960; Jacoby, 1964; Morgan Jones and Howitt, 1965). Furthermore, the figure of 20 per cent is based on only one maternal death in five pregnancies in the study of Jacoby.

The Connecticut series (Whittemore, Hobbins and Engle, 1982) of patients with congenital heart disease shows how good the results can be with obsessional care, as in 482 pregnancies from 233 women, including eight mothers with Eisenmenger's syndrome, there were no maternal deaths.

In rheumatic heart disease the maternal mortality can also now be very low. Szekely, Turner and Snaith (1973) reported 26 mortalities in 2856 pregnancies (about 1 per cent) complicated by rheumatic heart disease between 1942 and 1969. Half of the deaths were due to pulmonary oedema, which became much less common once mitral valvotomy was freely available. These authors reported no maternal deaths in about 1000 pregnancies occurring after 1960. Rush, Verjans and Spracklen (1979) also reported a maternal mortality of 0.7 per cent in 450 mothers with rheumatic heart disease in South Africa.

Pregnancy does not affect the long-term survival of a woman with rheumatic heart disease, provided that she survives pregnancy itself (Chesley, 1980).

Fetal outcome

The fetal outcome in rheumatic heart disease in pregnancy is usually good, and little different from that in patients who do not have heart disease (Rush, Verjans and Spracklen, 1979; Sugrue, Blake and MacDonald, 1981; McNab and Macafee, 1985). However, the babies are likely to be lighter by about 200 g on average (Ho, Chen and Wong, 1980).

In patients with congenital heart disease there is no excess fetal mortality except in the group with cyanotic congenital heart disease, whether associated with pulmonary hypertension or not: here the babies are generally growth retarded (Schaefer et al., 1968; Batson, 1974; Whittemore, Hobbins and Engle, 1982), and the fetal loss, including abortion, may be as high as 45 per cent (Copeland et al., 1963; Batson, 1974; Gleicher et al., 1979; Whittemore, Hobbins and Engle, 1982). Even in the tetralogy of Fallot, which does not have a particularly high maternal mortality, the fetal loss rate may be as high as 57 per cent (Copeland et al., 1963) and the majority of the babies are growth retarded (Jacoby, 1964). This is hardly surprising in view of the mechanisms of placental exchange, which cannot compensate for maternal systemic hypoxaemia. It is likely that the fetus dies because of inadequate oxygen supply or because of prematurity. In contrast, the fetal results following total correction of Fallot's tetralogy are excellent (Singh, Bolton and Oakley, 1982).

Women or men who themselves have congenital heart disease are naturally concerned that their children may be similarly afflicted. Earlier studies suggested that for most forms of congenital heart disease the risk to the fetus was 2–4 per cent if either parent was affected (Nora and Nora, 1978), which is at least double the risk in the normal population. However, in mothers (not fathers) with atrioventricular defects (ostium primum atrial septal defect, common atrioventricular canal, single atrium) the risk of congenital heart disease in the infant is much greater (8–14 per cent); the defect is usually concordant, i.e. of the same nature as in the mother (Emmanuel et al., 1983). Conversely, it may be possible to quote a lower risk if the mother herself was exposed to an adverse environmental agent (e.g. rubella or lithium therapy in her own fetal life, that will not be operating in the index pregnancy (Burn, 1987). It is, therefore, difficult to counsel women about the precise risk of congenital heart disease in their infant; perhaps 5–10 per cent would be a fair estimate (Burn, 1987). The majority of these lesions would be amendable to surgery.

Clinical management

Patients should be seen in a combined clinic attended by an obstetrician and a cardiologist and the nature and severity of the heart lesion assessed.

Because of the mortality statistics indicated above, Eisenmenger's syndrome, primary pulmonary hypertension and pulmonary veno-occlusive disease are absolute indications for termination of pregnancy. Termination may also be indicated very occasionally in patients with such severe pulmonary disease that they have pulmonary hypertension. In all other cases, the decision whether the pregnancy should continue depends on an individual assessment of the risk of pregnancy compared with the patient's desire to have children. (See below for termination of pregnancy because of fetal heart disease.)

In general, the indications for surgery in pregnancy are similar to those in the non-pregnant state: failure of medical treatment with either intractable heart failure or intolerable symptoms. However, because of the bad reputation of severe mitral stenosis in pregnancy, mitral valvotomy is performed relatively freely in patients with suitable heart valves, whereas open-heart surgery is done with reluctance because of anxiety about the fetus. Nevertheless, mitral valvotomy has become a rare procedure in the UK: none have been performed in patients referred to Queen Charlotte's Maternity Hospital in the last 10 years, and Sugrue, Blake and Mac-Donald (1981) reported only three cases from Dublin in 387 pregnancies complicated by rheumatic heart disease. As very few cardiac surgeons now perform closed mitral valvotomies, preferring the improved control offered by open heart surgery, this trend seems likely to continue.

A review of open heart surgery during pregnancy by Zitnik et al. (1969) indicated that, although maternal results were reasonable (5 per cent mortality in a group of 22 women with severely affected hearts), the fetal results were not, with a perinatal mortality of 33 per cent, possibly due to inadequate perfusion of the placenta during cardiopulmonary bypass (Farmakides et al., 1987), or to artificially induced hypothermia. These earlier reports were all of surgery performed early in pregnancy with a high abortion rate. More recently, Eilen et al. (1981) have reviewed the literature and found no fetal losses in patients operated on after the first trimester.

Becker (1983) found only one maternal and 20 per cent fetal loss in 68 patients operated on at all stages of pregnancy. Nevertheless, the indication for open-heart surgery in pregnancy is usually life-threatening pulmonary oedema that cannot be managed medically.

Antenatal care

After the initial assessment of the patient, the remainder of medical management during pregnancy is associated with avoiding, if possible, those factors which increase the risk of heart failure, and treating failure vigorously if it occurs.

Obstetric management before labour includes early ultrasound examination of the conceptus to confirm gestational age and, in women with congenital heart disease (see above), second-trimester examination of the fetal heart by ultrasound to exclude congenital malformations. In experienced hands this technique will diagnose or exclude all major congenital malformations by 18 weeks' gestation (Allan et al., 1986) allowing termination in selected cases or reassurance of the mother in the majority.

Those women who do not have haemodynamically significant heart disease require no special obstetric antenatal management. However, if there is haemodynamically significant heart disease and particularly if maternal arterial P_{O_2} is reduced, as in cyanotic congenital heart disease, the fetus should be monitored for growth retardation and intrauterine asphyxia. This would currently entail assessment of fetal growth and amniotic fluid volume clinically and by ultrasound, measurements of abnormalities in fetal heart rate by ultrasound (cardiotocography), measurement of fetal and maternal placental blood flow indices by Doppler ultrasound and, possibly, fetal blood sampling for direct assessment of fetal hypoxia.

Treatment of heart failure and dysrhythmias

The principles of treatment of heart failure in pregnancy are the same as those in the non-pregnant state.

Digoxin

Dosage requirements for digoxin are believed to be the same in pregnancy as in the non-pregnant state (Conradsson and Werkö, 1974). Both digoxin (Rogers et al., 1972) and digitoxin (Okita, Plotz and Davis, 1956) cross the placenta, and produce drug levels in the fetus similar to those seen in the mother (Rogers et al., 1972; Saarikosi, 1976) (although not necessarily in the hydropic fetus where placental exchange may be compromised (Younis and Granat, 1987)). Digoxin enters the umbilical circulation within 5 min of intravenous administration to the mother (Saarikosi, 1976). In general, there is no evidence that therapeutic maternal drug levels of digoxin affect the neonatal electrocardiogram (Mendelson, 1960; Rogers et al., 1972) or cause any harm to the fetus. Indeed, maternal digoxin therapy is the treatment of choice for the fetus presenting with tachyarrhythmia in utero (Maxwell et al., 1988). Although therapeutic maternal drug levels do not harm the fetus, toxic levels do, as was shown in one case of maternal digitoxin poisoning where electrocardiographic changes of digitalis toxicity were demonstrated in the neonate which died aged 3 days (Sherman and Locke, 1960). The recent demonstration of the production of digoxin-like immunoreactive substance by the fetus questions the validity of some of the above statements (Weiner et al., 1987).

Digoxin is secreted in breast milk, but as the total daily excretion in the mother with therapeutic blood levels would not exceed 2 µg (Levy, Grait and Laufer, 1977) this is unlikely to cause any harm to the neonate, unless it has any other predisposing causes of digitalis toxicity, such as hypokalaemia.

Diuretic therapy
Frusemide is the most commonly used and rapidly acting loop diuretic for the treatment of pulmonary oedema. Ethacrynic acid has also been used successfully in the management of pulmonary oedema associated with mitral stenosis in labour (Young and Haft, 1970). In congestive cardiac failure, where speed of action is not as important, oral thiazides are usually used in the first instance, although the extra potency of the loop diuretics may be necessary in a minority of cases. Andersen (1970) showed that the use of thiazide in late pregnancy was not associated with any significant salt or water depletion in the neonate.

There are no risks to the use of diuretics in the treatment of heart failure that are specific to pregnancy, but, as in the non-pregnant state, hypokalaemia is an important complication in a patient who may also be taking digoxin.

Treatment of pulmonary oedema should also include opiates such as morphine. If the patient does not respond to these measures, vasodilating drugs should be used to unload the left ventricle. These include nitrates (causes venous dilatation and reduces preload), angiotensin-converting enzyme inhibitors such as captopril or enalapril and hydralazine (cause arteriolar dilatation and reduce afterload). In this desperate situation the risks, to the fetus, of captopril and nitrates are not as important as the maternal risk. Life-threatening pulmonary oedema that does not respond to drug therapy may be helped by mechanical ventilation. If this is successful, and in other cases that do not respond to medical treatment, cardiac surgery should be considered, if the patient has a potentially operable lesion.

Dysrhythmias
Most dysrhythmias that require treatment are due to ischaemic heart disease, which usually presents in women after their childbearing years and is rare in pregnancy (Ginz, 1970; Husaini, 1971); There is, therefore, limited experience in the treatment of dysrhythmias during pregnancy. Nevertheless, the problem does exist, particularly in patients who have non-ischaemic abnormalities of cardiac-conducting tissue, such as are believed to occur in the Wolff–Parkinson–White and Lown–Ganong–Levine sydnromes.

The antidysrhythmic drugs that have been used most frequently in pregnancy are digoxin (discussed above), quinidine and β-adrenergic blocking agents, in particular propranolol, atenolol and oxprenolol. The indications for the use of these drugs are unaltered by pregnancy. Other β-blocking drugs such as pindolol (Storstein, 1972) have been used occasionally.

Although there are isolated case reports of intrauterine growth retardation, acute fetal distress in labour and hypoglycaemia in the neonate, in patients taking β-adrenergic blocking agents (Gladstone, Hordof and Gersony, 1975; Cotrill, McAllister and Pentecost, 1977; Habib and McArthy, 1977), these have not been confirmed in clinical trials of oxprenolol (Gallery *et al.*, 1979; Fidler *et al.*, 1983), atenolol (Rubin *et al.*, 1983) or labetalol (Plovin *et al.*, 1988) when used for hypertension in the latter half of pregnancy. A recent study of atenolol in the treatment of hypertension throughout pregnancy has demonstrated an increased risk of intrauterine growth retardation with this drug (Butters, Kennedy and Rubin, 1990). It would seem reasonable, therefore, to use propranolol, oxprenolol or atenolol in the acute treatment of supraventricular and ventricular tachycardia in pregnancy and oxprenolol with caution for long-term treatment (see also Chapter 2).

Quinidine is used to maintain or induce sinus rhythm in patients either after DC conversion or when taking digoxin. It is well tolerated in pregnancy (Ueland *et al.*, 1981) and has only minimal oxytocic effect (Mendelson, 1956). The only adverse reports concern the inhibitory effect of quinidine on pseudo-cholinesterase activity which is already lowered in normal pregnancy (Kambam, Franks and Smith, 1987). Pseudo-cholinesterase is necessary to allow reversal of succinycholine; caution is necessary, therefore, if patients taking quinidine in pregnancy have a general anaesthetic. There may also be enhanced toxicity of ester-type local anaesthetics (e.g. chloroprocaine) used in epidural anaesthesia.

Although there is little documentary evidence of the safety of verapamil in pregnancy, it has been widely used. There is much less experience of other antidysrhythmic drugs such as bretylium tosylate, disopyramide or amiodarone; however, a case report has suggested that mexiletine is safe in pregnancy for the treatment of ventricular dysrhythmias and has shown that mexiletine levels in cord blood are similar to those in maternal plasma (Timmis, Jackson and Holt, 1980). Mexiletine is secreted in fairly high proportion in breast milk (concentration 4.5 times that in maternal plasma) (Lownes and Ives, 1987), so caution is necessary concerning breast feeding. The use of disopyramide has been associated with hypertonic uterine activity on one occasion (Leonard, Braun and Levy, 1978) but not in others (Finlay and Edmunds, 1979); disopyramide should be used in pregnancy with caution, therefore. The long-term risks of phenytoin are well known; however, this drug is likely to be used only in the acute treatment of dysrhythmias, particularly those induced by digitalis intoxication. Szekely and Snaith (1974) have also used procainamide successfully to abolish atrial fibrillation in pregnancy.

The use of amiodarone has been reviewed in 18 pregnancies (Barrett and Pen, 1986) and a total of about 30 cases are known to the manufacturers. There is no evidence of teratogenicity in the relatively few pregnancies reported. Amiodarone contains large quantities of iodine, is known to affect the maternal thyroid and might affect the fetal thyroid producing hypo- or hyperthyroidism. Although neonatal hypothyroidism has been noted in one poorly documented case (Haffaje, 1983), other abnormalities have been mild and transient (Penn *et al.*, 1985). In addition, neonatal bradycardia and prolongation of the infants' QT intervals have also been found (McKenna *et al.*, 1983; Penn *et al.*, 1985). These abnormalities have also been transient and do not seem to have caused any harm. Amiodarone is a potentially dangerous drug but, on the basis of these reports, it would seem reasonable to use amiodarone to treat arrhythmias resistant to all other therapy in late pregnancy. Patients should not breast feed when they are taking amiodarone.

The difficulty arises in considering long-term prophylactic treatment with antidysrhythmic drugs that have not been extensively used in pregnancy. Here each case must be considered on its own merits, paying particular attention to the frequency and severity of the attacks of the dysrhythmia. A single short episode of supraventricular tachycardia associated with no other symptoms does not require prophylactic treatment. Frequent attacks of ventricular tachycardia associated with syncope would require prophylaxis – whatever the outcome in the fetus.

DC conversion for tachyarrhythmias is safe in pregnancy and does not harm the fetus (Finlay and Edmunds, 1979).

Cardiopulmonary resuscitation

In patients with cardiac arrest, external cardiac massage is usually performed with the patient lying supine on a hard surface. However, in late pregnancy, lying supine will cause obstruction of the vena cava and seriously reduce venous return in this critical situation. The patient should therefore be turned to the left before starting cardiac massage, but if she fails to recover after 5 min, caesarean section should be performed as part of the resuscitation procedure (Hoffenberg *et al.*, 1987; Oates, Williams and Rees, 1988). Not only will this reduce caval compression and improve maternal prognosis but also there is the chance of delivery of a live and healthy baby; 70 per cent of fetuses delivered within 5 min of maternal death survive (Katz, Dotters and Droegemueller, 1986) and healthy survivors have been reported delivered up to 15 min after maternal cardiac arrest.

Anticoagulant therapy

This is a major problem in the management of patients with heart disease in pregnancy. Anticoagulant therapy may be necessary in patients with congenital heart disease who have pulmonary hypertension due to pulmonary vascular disease, those with atrial fibrillation and those who have artificial heart valve replacement. The risk of a woman having an embolic episode if she has an aritificial valve and does not take anticoagulants is about 1 per 100 months of exposure (Limet and Crondin, 1977).

For conditions such as pulmonary embolus, subcutaneous heparin is safer than warfarin: there appears to be less maternal bleeding and no fetal risk of congenital abnormalities, such as chondrodysplasia punctata or optic atrophy. However, where there is a risk of systemic thromboembolism, as in heart disease, subcutaneous heparin treatment does not seem to be adequate (Vitalli *et al.*, 1986); there are also reports of Starr Edward aortic and Björk–Shiley mitral prosthetic valves that thrombosed during pregnancy when the mothers were either managed with subcutaneous heparin (Bennett and Oakley, 1968; McLeod, Jennings and Townsend, 1978) or were not given anticoagulant therapy (Chen *et al.*, 1982). Such disasters have been treated with emergency cardiopulmonary bypass and caesarean section (assuming fetal maturity) followed by prosthetic valve replacement (Antunes, Myer and Santos, 1984).

Ahmad *et al.* (1976) and Biale *et al.* (1980) have reported one and four cases respectively, where patients with artificial heart valves have been treated with dipyridamole alone during pregnancy. There were no incidents of thromboembolism, but as the data of Limet and Crondin (1977) suggest that risk is only one in ten pregnancies if no anticoagulants are used, larger series are necessary to establish the effectiveness of this form of treatment. There is no ideal solution to this problem. Even though the risk of fetal malformations such as optic atrophy may persist after 16 weeks' gestation (Shaul and Hall, 1977), I believe that warfarin should be used until about 37 weeks' gestation because subcutaneous heparin does not give adequate protection. Furthermore, even subcutaneous heparin therapy has the risk of bone demineralization and the fetal risks of warfarin have probably been overestimated. In Javares' series of 42 pregnancies in patients receiving warfarin throughout pregnancy until 34–36 weeks, for artificial heart valves, there was the expected abortion rate (29 per cent); however, there were only two other fetal losses (one stillbirth and one preterm), one case of cerebral haemorrhage, one case of nasal hypoplasia and three growth-retarded fetuses (Javares *et al.*, 1984). Similar data have been described elsewhere (Ibarra-Perez *et al.*, 1976; Lutz *et al.*, 1978; Ben Ismail *et al.*, 1986). The data of Javares *et al.* and Lee *et al.* (1986) suggest that patients with mitral valve replacement, where cardiac function remains more impaired than in aortic valve replacement, may be particularly at risk from abortion. Furthermore, use of the minimum dose of warfarin, maintaining a prothrombin ratio of 1.5:2 rather than 2:2.5, may decrease the teratogenic and abortion risks of warfarin (Javares *et al.*, 1984). The deleterious effect of heart disease and anticoagulants was clearly shown by Sanchez-Cascos (1987) in a large series of 1002 pregnancies in Spain. The overall fetal mortality (abortions, stillbirths, malformations) was 18 per cent before surgery, 28 per cent after the first valvotomy, 33 per cent after implanting biological valves and 41 per cent after implanting artificial valves and with long-term anticoagulation.

It is also possible that the teratogenic effect of dindevan may be less than that of warfarin (Oakley and Hawkins, 1983) but there are not the data to prove this and, as there is more experience in general with warfarin, I would suggest that this drug should be used in preference. At 37 weeks, when the risk of fetal bleeding associated with labour seems to be too great, the patient should be admitted to hospital and given continuous intravenous heparin to achieve a heparin level, as assayed by protamine sulphate neutralization, of 0.4–0.6 units/ml (Dacie, 1975). Heparin does not cross the placenta (Flessa *et al.*, 1965) and therefore will not cause bleeding in the fetus. It is believed that the clotting system of the fetus will return to normal after warfarin has been withheld for one week. At that time, maternal heparin therapy should be reduced to give a heparin level of <0.4 units/ml or a normal thrombin time, and labour should be induced. If the patient inadvertently goes into labour taking warfarin, she should be given vitamin K to reverse the action of warfarin in the fetus and started on heparin therapy as above. In extreme cases, vitamin K has been given intramuscularly to the fetus *in utero* by transamniotic injection (Larsen *et al.*, 1978).

After delivery, because of the risk of maternal postpartum haemorrhage, the patient should continue to receive heparin for 7 days; then warfarin may be restarted. This is not a contraindication to breast feeding, because insignificant quantities of warfarin are secreted in breast milk (Orme *et al.*, 1977). However, dindevan is excreted in breast milk (Eckstein and Jack, 1970) and patients taking dindevan should not breast-feed.

An alternative approach to anticoagulation in the early part of pregnancy was that of Iturbe-Alessio *et al.* (1986) in Mexico. They discontinued warfarin in 35 women as soon as they reported in pregnancy and substituted subcutaneous heparin (5000 units twice daily) until the end of the 12th week. At this stage warfarin was started, to be replaced by heparin at the end of pregnancy. The results were compared with those in 37 women who continued warfarin throughout the early part of pregnancy. In the control group there was an extraordinarily high rate of embryopathy (30 per cent), mostly diagnosed on the basis of minor abnormalities of the face; there were no cases of embryopathy and only two abortions in 23 women who discontinued warfarin before 7 weeks; there were two cases of embryopathy in eight continuing pregnancies where warfarin was discontinued between 7 and 12 weeks. The price to pay for this form of treatment was two massive valve thromboses in the heparin-treated group. Although the diagnosis of warfarin embryopathy must be questioned because of its very high incidence in the control group, it does appear that it may be prevented by stopping warfarin between 7 and 12 weeks. Ten thousand units of heparin per day is a very low dose in pregnancy and a more aggressive policy, possibly with continuous intravenous infusion (Nelson *et al.*, 1984) or subcutaneous heparin therapy adjusted to achieve a partial thromboplastin time of 1.5 times control (Lee *et al.*, 1986) might have reduced the incidence of embolism. However, this form of management has not yet been fully evaluated.

Anticoagulation is, therefore, the major problem in patients with artificial heart valves. Those patients who have successful isolated aortic or mitral valve replacement usually have near-normal cardiac function and do not incur haemodynamic problems in pregnancy (Oakley, 1983). Even those patients with multiple valve replacements usually have sufficient cardiac reserve for a successful pregnancy (Andrinopoulos and Arias, 1980). Although it is clear that the long-term outlook is not as good for patients with tissue heart valves (Kirklin, 1981), mainly because of calcification in porcine xenografts when implanted in young people (Sanders *et al.*, 1980), there is no doubt that these are superior in pregnancy. In addition, if the valve does require replacement, second porcine valves are not rejected sooner and possibly last longer than the first (Magilligan *et al.*, 1983).

Labour

Patients with significant heart disease require care concerning fluid balance in labour. Many women in labour are given copious quantities of intravenous crystalloid fluids. If they have normal hearts, they can cope with the resultant increase in circulating blood volume and decrease in colloid osmotic pressure (Gonik *et al.*, 1985); patients with heart disease cannot, and may easily develop pulmonary oedema.

Some centres are gaining increasing experience in the use of elective central catheterization (Swan–Ganz technique) to measure right atrial pressure, wedge pressure (indirect left atrial pressure) and cardiac output in labour in patients with heart disease. There is no doubt that this technique allows a much more rational use of fluid therapy, diuretics and inotropic agents. Preliminary results would also suggest that measurement of central venous pressure alone is so misleading as an index of left ventricular filling pressure that it should not be used for this purpose (although it is still invaluable in patients with bleeding problems). However, the technique of Swan–Ganz catheterization is quite difficult and it has a significant morbidity; it should, therefore, be used only in centres where there is sufficient experience.

In the majority of patients with heart disease, analgesia is best given by epidural anaesthesia which not only decreases cardiac output and heart rate because it is an effective analgesic, but also decreases cardiac output by causing peripheral vasodilatation and decreasing venous return. However, the use of epidural anaesthesia is questioned in Eisenmenger's syndrome and contraindicated in hypertrophic cardiomyopathy (see below). Most obstetric emergencies arising in labour, including the need for caesarean section, can be managed using epidural anaesthesia. However, if epidural anaesthesia is not available, or if elective caesarean section is advised, general anaesthesia probably causes less haemodynamic derangement than does epidural anaesthesia. However, there are few adequate comparisons of these forms of anaesthesia in comparable patients, and more depends on the skill and preference of the anaesthetist.

The *Confidential Enquiries into Maternal Death in England and Wales* show that there were ten maternal deaths from endocarditis between 1970 and 1975 (Department of Health and Social Security, 1982). In the majority of the 124 cases that have been reported in obstetric and gynaecological practice, the organism was a streptococcus (Seaworth and Durack, 1986). However, the case for antibiotic pro-phylaxis in labour has not been proven. There are several large series of patients with heart disease in pregnancy, where no antibiotics have been given and where no endocarditis has been observed (Smith *et al.*, 1976; Fleming, 1977; Sugrue, Blake and MacDonald, 1982). It is difficult to document bacteraemia in labour (Burwell and Metcalfe, 1958; Redleaf and Farell, 1959). Several authors have argued persuas-ively against antibiotic prophylaxis (Fleming, 1977; Sugrue *et al.*, 1980). A recent British working party recommended antibiotic prophylaxis in labour only in women with artificial heart valves, who are a particularly high-risk group if they do contract endocarditis (Working Party, 1982).

Nevertheless, from the data of the Confidential Maternal Mortality series, it would seem that women are at increased risk from endocarditis in pregnancy. What is not clear from these data is whether endocarditis was contracted during labour, and was potentially preventable by antibiotics, or whether it arose at some other time. The one case that is described in detail in the 1973–1975 report concerns a woman who did appear to develop endocarditis during a normal delivery, and other similar non-fatal cases have been reported (de Swiet, de Louvois and Hurley, 1975), even in a patient with normal heart valves (Hughes, McFadyen and Raftery, 1988). Until more details are available, I will continue to advise antibiotic prophylaxis in all patients with structural heart disease, except mitral valve prolapse without regurgitation where there appears to be no risk of endocarditis (Hickey, Macmahon and Wilcken, 1985). The antibiotics that we use are intramuscular ampicillin (500 mg) and intramuscular gentamicin (80 mg), three injections given every 8 h at the onset or induction of labour (Durack, 1975). The patient who is pencillin sensitive receives one in-travenous injection of vancomycin (1 g) (Garrod and Waterworth, 1962; Durack, 1975) or two intravenous injections of vancomycin (500 mg) 12-hourly. Vancomycin should be given over 60 min (Simmons *et al.*, 1986) because of the risk of idiosyn-cratic hypotensive reactions (Hill, 1985). An alternative compromise is to use prophylactic antibiotics only in those cases at high risk, i.e. those with previous endocarditis, valve replacement, instrumental delivery or delivery following pro-longed rupture of membranes.

PART 2. SPECIFIC CONDITIONS OCCURRING DURING PREGNANCY

Acquired heart disease

Chronic rheumatic heart disease

As already indicated, this form of heart disease has been commenest in pregnancy in the UK and still is in many parts of the world. By far the most important lesion is mitral stenosis, which may be the only lesion or the dominant abnormality among several others. Women with mitral stenosis are particularly likely to develop pulmo-nary oedema in pregnancy because of the increase in cardiac output, the increase in heart rate preventing ventricular filling and the increase in pulmonary blood volume (Burwell and Metcalfe, 1958). Mitral stenosis is the lesion that is most likely to require treatment for pulmonary oedema, or heart failure (see above), and also to require surgery during pregnancy. The haemodynamic changes associated with labour in patients with mitral stenosis have been documented by Swan–Ganz catheterization. Patients entering labour with a wedge pressure (indirect left atrial pressure) <14 mmHg are unlikely to develop pulmonary oedema (Clark *et al.*, 1985b). Mitral regurgitation puts a volume load on the left atrium and left ventricle, but it does not cause pulmonary hypertension until late in the condition, and heart failure is rare in pregnancy; it usually occurs in older women.

Rheumatic aortic valve disease is much less common in women than in men, and much less common than mitral valve disease in pregnancy. Severe aortic regurgitation causes pulmonary oedema; aortic stenosis may be associated with chest pain, syncope and sudden death; although both conditions are usually not severe enough to be a problem in pregnancy, critical aortic stenosis may cause maternal death.

Disease of the tricuspid valve hardly ever occurs in isolation. In addition, tricuspid valve disease rarely requires specific treatment: the patient improves when the rheumatic disease of the other valves is treated, either medically or surgically. Although there are case reports of successful pregnancy following triple valve replacement (aortic, mitral and tricuspid), it is unusual for such surgery to be necessary in patients within the reproductive age group (Nagorney and Field, 1981).

Myocardial infarction

Myocardial infarction is rare in pregnancy and in young women in general. Only 1 per cent of admissions for myocardial infarction occur in women younger than 45 years (Peterson, Thomson and Chinn, 1972). Cortis *et al.* (1979) cite only 76 cases of myocardial infarction in pregnancy in the literature since 1922; most of these cases were in women aged 30–40 years. However, the increasing incidence of myocardial infarction in women and the increasing age at which women become pregnant may result in an increased incidence of myocardial infarction in pregnancy. Patients with diabetes and vascular disease are also particularly at risk (Reece *et al.*, 1986).

The precise mechanism of myocardial infarction in many patients is open to speculation. Women have a particularly high incidence of coronary spasm, and atypical mechanisms seem to be common in pregnancy. Beary, Summer and Buckley (1979) suggest that the group of patients with myocardial infarction occurring in the puerperium are those that are most likely to have spasm or coronary artery thrombosis unassociated with atherosclerotic narrowing, as documented by Ciraulo and Markovitz (1979). The syndrome of myocardial infarction with normal coronary arteries occurring in young women is well documented. In the non-pregnant state the prognosis is good if they survive the initial episode (Fox, 1983). Other possible causes of myocardial infarction in pregnancy are primary dissection of the coronary arteries (Bulkley and Roberts, 1973) and anomalous origin of the coronary arteries (Klein *et al.*, 1984).

Left ventricular aneurysm formation may complicate myocardial infarction but is not an absolute contraindication to further pregnancies (Roberts *et al.*, 1983). Successful pregnancy is also possible following severe myocardial infarction, which may include cardiac arrest (Stokes, Evans and Stone, 1984); termination of pregnancy is, therefore, not mandatory under these circumstances.

It is difficult to be dogmatic about management, as there is little experience and the pathology may be diverse. It would be sensible to treat the initial episode in a coronary care unit, with conventional opiate analgesics and medication for complications such as dysrhythmias. Because of the possibility of coronary spasm, nitroglycerine or other vasodilators should be used early in patients with continuing pain.

Early treatment with low-dose aspirin and streptokinase each reduce mortality by about 15 per cent in non-pregnant patients (ISIS, 1988). The use of low-dose aspirin is probably justified in pregnancy; the use of streptokinase is not, because of the bleeding risk and the irritant effect of fibrin degradation products (FDPs) on the uterus (Amias, 1977). Once the patient has been delivered (again in an intensive care environment), coronary arteriography should be performed to delineate the pathology which may be atypical. The angiographic demonstration of coronary embolus would be an indication for anticoagulant therapy but, otherwise, the benefits of anticoagulation in myocardial infarction unassociated with pregnancy do not seem great enough to justify the considerable extra risks imposed on the pregnancy. Patients should be allowed a spontaneous vaginal delivery, preferably with epidural anaesthesia, unless there are good obstetric reasons for interfering. However, as in other cases of heart disease, the second stage should be limited by forceps delivery. Syntocinon infusion should be used rather than ergometrine in the third stage, as ergometrine is more likely to cause coronary artery spasm. There is no evidence that pregnancy predisposes to myocardial infarction; unless it is thought that the patient has had a coronary embolus, pregnancy should not be discouraged in patients who have had myocardial infarction in the past.

Cardiomyopathy

Hypertrophic obstructive cardiomyopathy (HOCM)

Extensive experience of the management of this condition in pregnancy has been reported by Oakley and colleagues from the Hammersmith Hospital (Oakley et al., 1979). These authors originally advocated β-adrenergic blockade in all cases to reduce the risk of syncope caused by obstruction of the left ventricular outflow tract (Turner, Oakley and Dixon, 1968); this is now reserved for symptomatic patients only. Patients should not be allowed to become hypovolaemic, as this, too, increases the risk of obstruction of the left ventricular outflow tract. They should not lie supine, because of the risk of caval obstruction and subsequent decrease in venous return. Particular care should be taken to give adequate fluid replacement if there is antepartum haemorrhage and also to avoid postpartum haemorrhage. During labour, patients with hypertrophic obstructive cardiomyopathy should be given epidural anaesthesia with great caution, as this causes relative hypovolaemia by increasing venous capacitance in the lower limbs.

Peripartum cardiomyopathy

The incidence of peripartum cardiomyopathy in the United Kingdom is about 1 in 5000 or less. If the condition does arise in the puerperium, which is usually the case, the patient is almost invariably breast feeding (Stuart, 1968). There is no predisposing cause for the heart failure and the heart is grossly dilated. The patients are usually, although not inevitably (O'Connell et al., 1986), multiparous, Black, relatively elderly and of poor social class; pregnancy has often been complicated by hypertension. Pulmonary, peripheral and particularly cerebral embolization is a major cause of morbidity and mortality, which is 25–50 per cent (Homans, 1985). The majority of deaths occur around the time of presentation but some women have protracted illnesses and die up to 8 years later; however, if the patients recover fully from the initial episode, the long-term prognosis is good. The condition is likely to recur in future pregnancies (Demarkis *et al.*, 1971), which are, therefore, contraindicated in view of the overall bad prognosis.

The pathogenesis of this condition is unknown (Homans, 1985); some authors have denied, however, that peripartum cardiomyopathy is a specific entity (Brown *et al.*, 1967) and have considered the condition to be another form of congestive cardiomyopathy caused by hypertension (Benchimol, Carneiro and Schlesinger, 1959). Rand, Jenkins and Scott (1975), on the basis of antibodies to heart muscle present in cord blood and serum from the mother in a case of pregnancy cardiomyopathy, postulate an immunological cause, possibly autoimmunity attributable to cross-reaction between antibodies to uterine actinomysin and cardiac tissue (Knobel, Melamud and Kishon, 1984). Alternatively, the combination of multiparity and low social class has suggested that the condition is due to an undefined nutritional defect; nevertheless, well-nourished patients may develop peripartum cardiomyopathy (O'Connell *et al.*, 1986). Melvin *et al.* (1982) described three cases of peripartum cardiomyopathy due to myocarditis, confirmed by endomyocardial biopsy at cardiac catheterization, and these authors propose that infection may be an important cause. Sanderson, Olsen and Gate (1986) performed a similar study, showing myocarditis in 5 of 11 women with peripartum cardiomyopathy. Cunningham *et al.* (1986) reviewed 28 cases of obscure cardiomyopathy occurring in 106 000 pregnancies in Texas: in only seven cases was the condition really idiopathic, emphasizing the rarity of the condition, but these patients fared very badly; four were dead within 8 years.

The distinction of peripartum cardiomyopathy from other forms of cardiomyopathy depends on the history and associated clinical features; the diagnosis is based on the exclusion of other known causes of cardiomyopathy. Apart from conventional antifailure treatment, these patients should also receive anticoagulant therapy until the heart size has returned to normal, and until they have no further dysrhythmias. The place of immunosuppressive therapy with either prednisone or azathioprine is not clear. This has been used successfully in cases associated with acute myocarditis demonstrated by endomyocardial biopsy (Melvin *et al.*, 1982) but such treatment cannot be routinely recommended (Homans, 1985).

Those few patients who present before delivery should be electively delivered because, in the long term, the demand on their hearts will decrease after pregnancy. If the cervix is in a favourable condition, vaginal delivery should be chosen; if not, the patient should be delivered by caesarean section. Skilled epidural anaesthesia is preferred for both routes of delivery. There is no evidence that breast feeding influences the course of peripartum cardiomyopathy.

Because of the bad prognosis of peripartum cardiomyopathy, the patients' young age and their social responsibilities having just been delivered, they should receive early consideration and high priority for cardiac transplantation. The indication for this is intractable pump failure despite optimal medical therapy.

Davidson and Parry (1978) have described a specific form of peripartum cardiac failure occurring in the Hausa tribe in Northern Nigeria. The peak incidence is 4 weeks postpartum. During this period, for up to 40 days after delivery, the Hausa woman spends 18 h/day lying on a mud bed, heated so that the ambient temperature reaches 40°C. She also increases her sodium intake to 450 mmol/day by eating kanwa salt from Lake Chad. The condition has a much better prognosis than other forms of peripartum cardiomyopathy and is likely to be an extreme example of volume overload.

Pericardial disease

This is a rare complication of pregnancy but should be considered because of its specific haemodynamic problems (Blake *et al.*, 1984). Acute pericarditis is normally not of any haemodynamic consequence and is of importance only because it must be considered in patients presenting with chest pain and because of the necessity to diagnose the underlying cause. However, patients with significant pericardial effusion or, more commonly, with calcific pericarditis, suffer because they cannot increase ventricular filling above the limit restricted by the pericardium: they can, therefore, increase cardiac output only by increasing heart rate, and they are dependent on maintaining both venous filling and heart rate in pregnancy.

Patients usually present with oedema, hepatomegaly, ascites and raised jugular venous pressure. Symptoms and signs of pulmonary oedema are a late finding. The diagnosis is often suggested by seeing calcification in the pericardium on radiography and is confirmed by echocardiography.

Patients should be treated with diuretics only if they develop pulmonary oedema or if peripheral oedema is a major problem; digoxin is indicated only for atrial tachyarrhythmias; β-adrenergic blocking agents should not be used. Patients should not become hypovolaemic; the condition improves when circulating blood volume decreases after delivery. Definitive treatment is pericardiectomy, which can usually be deferred until after delivery (Sachs *et al.*, 1986).

Congenital heart disease

Eisenmenger's syndrome and other causes of pulmonary vascular disease

Eisenmenger's syndrome has a very high maternal mortality. Only recently has there been any form of surgical treatment and this, heart and lung transplantation, must be considered to be experimental (Reitz *et al.*, 1982).

Most maternal mortalities in patients with Eisenmenger's syndrome occur in the puerperium. Although deaths are occasionally sudden, due to thromboembolism, this is not usually so: more frequently, these patients die because of a slowly falling systemic $P_{A_{O_2}}$ with associated decrease in cardiac output.

What can be offered to the pregnant patient with Eisenmenger's syndrome? Unfortunately, abortion would appear to be the answer. The maternal mortality associated with abortion is only 7 per cent, in comparison to 30 per cent for continuing pregnancy (Gleicher *et al.*, 1979). Nevertheless, note that, in normal patients second-trimester termination with prostaglandin E_2 is associated with an increase of cardiac output, measured by Doppler, averaging 64 per cent: in this procedure some patients have cardiac outputs as high as 21 l/min (Willis *et al.*, 1987). Surgical dilatation and evacuation is preferable, therefore, in these and all other cases where termination is performed because of maternal heart disease.

If the patient nevertheless decides to continue with pregnancy, prophylactic anticoagulation, probably with subcutaneous heparin, should be offered, because of the risk of thromboembolism, both systemic and pulmonary. Labour should not be induced unless there are good obstetric reasons.

There is controversy concerning the place of epidural anaesthesia for the management of labour. Although epidural anaesthesia could shunt blood away from the lungs by decreasing the systemic vascular resistance, this does not occur – at least it did not in the one case studied by Midwall *et al.* (1978). On balance, a carefully administered elective epidural anaesthetic at the beginning of labour is probably preferable to emergency epidural or general anaesthesia, if it is suddenly decided that instrumental delivery is necessary (Crawford, Mills and Pentecost 1971; Gleicher et al., 1979).

If the patient does become hypotensive, with increasing cyanosis and decreasing cardiac output, it has been shown that high inspired oxygen concentrations can decrease pulmonary vascular resistance, increasing pulmonary blood flow, and can increase peripheral oxygen saturation (Midwall et al., 1978). In addition, α-sympathomimetic agents, such as phenylephrine, methoxamine and noradrenaline, will increase systemic resistance and also shunt blood to the lungs (Devitt and Noble, 1980). However, drugs such as tolazoline, phentolamine, nitroprusside and isoprenaline, which have been used to decrease pulmonary vascular resistance in other clinical situations, probably should not be given, because they will also decrease the systemic vascular resistance (Devitt and Noble, 1980). If systemic resistance decreases more than pulmonary resistance, pulmonary blood flow will decrease rather than increase. The same problem occurs with dopamine and β-sympathomimetic drugs, which have been given to increase cardiac output: they, too, will decrease systemic resistance and, if systemic resistance decreases more than cardiac output increases, pulmonary blood flow will fall. In summary, the management of the deteriorating patient with Eisenmenger's syndrome depends on giving oxygen and α-sympathomimetic amines.

In Eisenmenger's syndrome, pulmonary hypertension is due to increased pulmonary vascular resistance. However, pulmonary hypertension may also occur with a high blood flow and normal pulmonary resistance. Under these circumstances, the maternal outcome is much better, because the high pulmonary blood flow allows adequate oxygenation. The importance of pulmonary vascular resistance rather than pulmonary hypertension has been emphasized by Johnston and de Bono (1989), who describe successful pregnancy in a patient with single ventricle and pulmonary hypertension but relatively normal pulmonary vascular resistance. In this rather well-documented condition (Leibrand, Muench and Gander, 1982; Stiller et al., 1984; Baumann et al., 1987), the maternal outcome depends on the pulmonary vascular resistance and the fetal outcome on the degree of maternal hypoxaemia.

Cor pulmonale, pulmonary veno-occlusive disease, primary pulmonary hypertension

In cor pulmonale, pulmonary veno-occlusive disease and primary pulmonary hypertension, where there is pulmonary hypertension and vascular disease in small blood vessels, the maternal mortality is still high. The problem in these conditions still appears to be one of maintaining adequate pulmonary blood flow for adequate oxygenation. Even though blood cannot be shunted directly from the pulmonary to the systemic circuit, as in Eisenmenger's syndrome, excessive vasodilatation in the systemic circulation during epidural anaesthesia could still decrease preload to the right ventricle and therefore further decrease pulmonary blood flow. Unfortunately, as in Eisenmenger's syndrome, selective pulmonary vasodilators are not available; the options include nitroprusside (Nelson et al., 1983), oxygen and prostacyclin. In addition, manoeuvres that suddenly increase venous return (ergometrine injection, movement from supine to left lateral position) should be avoided, as should those which increase vagal tone (e.g. catheterization). Several patients with primary pulmonary hypertension have died in association with bradycardia and atrioventricular block, which suggest vagally mediated mechanisms. These patients should be delivered in an intensive care environment, with elective insertion of a Swan–Ganz catheter (notwithstanding the risk in patients with pulmonary hypertension) and facilities for pacing (Nelson *et al.*, 1983).

Coarctation of the aorta

In both coarctation of the aorta and Marfan's syndrome (see below) the maternal risk is of dissection of the aorta, associated with the hyperdynamic circulation of pregnancy, and possibly with an increased risk of medial degeneration due to the hormonal environment of pregnancy (Konishi *et al.*, 1980). Patients with coarctation also have the specific risk of cerebral haemorrhage due to ruptured berry aneurysm. The maternal mortality in coarctation has been stated to be as high as 17 per cent (Mendelson, 1940). However, Mendelson's series dates from 1858 to 1939, and there have only been 14 maternal deaths reported in the whole literature, none of which occurred in the 83 patients studied since 1960 (Deal and Wooley, 1973). The risk of dissection has, therefore, probably been exaggerated and good obstetric care and effective antihypertensive therapy would decrease the risk still further. It is probable that we no longer see the patients similar to those of Mendelson's series, as most patients with severe coarctation are operated on in infancy. Only those patients who already have evidence of dissection should have the coarctation repaired in pregnancy. Any upper limb hypertension should be treated aggressively with antihypertensive drugs (Benny, Prasao and MacVicar, 1980). If there is gross widening of the ascending aorta, suggesting intrinsic disease of the aorta, the patient should be delivered by elective caesarean section to reduce the risk of dissection associated with labour.

Marfan's syndrome

Some authors consider the risk of dissection to be so high in Marfan's syndrome that they advise avoidance of pregnancy, or termination, if there is any degree of aortic dilatation (Pyeritz and McKuisick, 1979). This seems an extreme attitude, which Pyeritz has modified to suggest that dilatation of the aorta to >40 mm (as determined echocardiographically) should be the limit at which pregnancy is contraindicated (Pyeritz, 1981). In a series of pregnancies in 26 women with Marfan's syndrome, there was only one fatality and that patient died from endocarditis.

As in coarctation of the aorta, any associated hypertension should be treated aggressively with β-blockade to decrease the haemodynamic load on the ascending aorta. β-Blocking drugs (propranolol) should also be used, even in the absence of hypertension, if there is any dilatation of the aorta. Delivery should be by caesarean section if there is evidence of aortic disease.

Congenital heart block

Congenital heart block is usually no problem in pregnancy. Although part of the normal response to pregnancy includes an increase in heart rate to increase the cardiac output, this is not obligatory. There are many records of successful pregnancy in patients with heart block, both paced (Ginns and Holinrake, 1970) and not paced (Szekely and Snaith, 1974). Presumably, patients are able to increase stroke volume sufficiently to cope with the increased demands of pregnancy. A few patients are unable to increase cardiac output sufficiently at the end of pregnancy or during labour (Bowman and Millar-Craig, 1980); patients with heart block who are not paced, or those where there is any question of pacemaker failure, should be managed, therefore, in obstetric units where there is access to pacing facilities.

References

Abboud, TK, Raya, J, Noueihed, R and Daniel, J (1983) Intrathecal morphine for relief of labour pain in a parturient with severe pulmonary hypertension. *Anaesthesiology*, **59**, 477–479

Ahmad, R, Rajah, SM, Mearns, AJ and Deverall, PB (1976)Dipyridamole in successful management of pregnant women with prosthetic heart valve. *Lancet*, **ii**, 1414–1415

Allan, LD, Crawford, DC, Chita, SK *et al.* (1986) Familial recurrences of congenital heart disease in the prospective series of mothers referred for fetal echocardiography. *American Journal of Cardiology*, **58**, 334–337

Amias, AG (1977) Streptokinase, cerebral vascular disease – and triplets. *British Medical Journal*, **1**, 1414–1415

Andersen, JB (1970) The effect of diuretics in late pregnancy on the new born infant. *Acta Paediatrica Scandinavica*, **59**, 659–663

Andrinopoulos, GC and Arias, F (1980) Triple heart valve prosthesis and pregnancy. *Obstetrics and Gynaecology*, **55**, 762–764

Antunes, MJ, Myer, IG and Santos, LP (1984) Thrombosis of mitral valve replacement: management by simultaneous Caesarean section and mitral valve replacement. Case report. *British Journal of Obstetrics and Gynaecology*, **91**, 716–718

Barrett, PA and Penn, IM (1986) Amiodarone in pregnancy. *Clinical Progress in Electrophysiology and Pacing*, **4**, 158–159

Batson, GA (1974) Cyanotic congenital heart disease and pregnancy. *British Journal of Obstetrics and Gynaecology*, **81**, 549–553

Baumann, H, Schneider, H, Drack, G *et al.* (1987) Pregnancy and delivery by Caesarean section in a patient with transposition of the great arteries and single ventricle. Case report. *British Journal of Obstetrics and Gynaecology*, **94**, 704–708

Beary, JF, Sumner, WR, and Bulkley, BH (1979) Postpartum acute myocardial infarction: a rare occurrence of uncertain etiology. *American Journal of Cardiology*, **43**, 158–160

Becker, RM (1983) Intracardiac surgery in pregnant women. *Annals of Thoracic Surgery*, **36**, 453–458

Benchimol, AB, Carneiro, RD and Schlesinger, P (1959) Post-partum heart disease. *British Heart Journal*, **21**, 89–100

Ben Ismail, M, Abid, F, Travelsi, S *et al.* (1986) Cardiac valve prosthesis, anticoagulation and pregnancy. *British Heart Journal*, **55**, 101–105

Bennett, GG and Oakley, CM (1968) Pregnancy in a patient with a mitral valve prosthesis. *Lancet*, **i**, 616–619

Benny, PS, Prasao, J, and MacVicar, J (1980) Pregnancy and coarctation of the aorta. Case report. *British Journal of Obstetrics and Gynaecology*, **87**, 1159–1161

Biale, Y, Lewenthal, H, Gueron, M and Ben-Adereth, W (1977) Caesarean section in patients with mitral valve prosthesis. *Lancet*, **i**, 907

Blake, S, Bonar, F, MacDonald, D *et al.* (1984) Pregnancy with constrictive pericarditis. *British Journal of Obstetrics and Gynaecology*, **91**, 404–406

Bowman, PR and Millar-Craig, MW (1980) Congenital heart block and pregnancy: a further case report. *Journal of Obstetrics and Gynaecology*, **1**, 98–99

Brown, AK, Doukas, N, Riding, WD and Wyn Jones, E (1967) Cardiomyopathy and pregnancy. *British Heart Journal*, **29**, 387–393

Bulkley, BH and Roberts, WC (1973) Dissecting aneurysm (haematoma) limited to coronary artery. *American Journal of Medicine*, **55**, 747–756

Burn, J (1987) The next lady has a heart defect. *British Journal of Obstetrics and Gynaecology*, **94**, 97–99

Burwell, CS and Metcalfe, J (1958) In *Heart Disease and Pregnancy; Physiology and Management*, p 125. Boston Massachusetts: Little Brown

Butters, L, Kennedy, S and Rubin PC (1990) Atenolol in essential hypertension during pregnancy. *British Medical Journal*, **301**, 587–589

Chen, WWC, Chan, CS, Lee, PR *et al.* (1982) Pregnancy in patients with prosthetic heart valves: an experience with 45 pregnancies. *Quarterly Journal of Medicine*, **51**, 358–365

Chesley, LC (1980) Severe rheumatic cardiac disease and pregnancy: the ultimate prognosis. *American Journal of Obstetrics and Gynecology*, **136**, 552–558

Ciraulo, DA and Markovitz, A (1979) Myocardial infarction in pregnancy associated with a coronary artery thrombosis. *Archives of Internal Medicine*, **139**, 1046–1047

Clapp, JF III (1985) Maternal heart rate in pregnancy. *American Journal of Obstetrics and Gynecology*, **152**, 659–660

Clark, SL, Hortenstein, JM, Phelan, JP *et al.* (1985a) Experience with the pulmonary artery catheter in obstetrics and gynecology. *American Journal of Obstetrics and Gynecology*, **152**, 374–378

Clark, SL, Phelan, JP, Greenspoon, J *et al.* (1985b) Labor and delivery in the presence of mitral stenosis: central hemodynamic observations. *American Journal of Obstetrics and Gynecology*, **152**, 984–988

Conradsson, TB and Werkö, L (1974) Management of heart disease in pregnancy. *Progress in Cardiovascular Disease*, **16**, 407–419

Copeland, WE, Wooley, CF, Ryan, JM *et al.* (1963) Pregnancy and congenital heart disease. *American Journal of Obstetrics and Gynecology*, **86**, 107–110

Cortis, BS, Freese, E, Luisada, AA *et al.* (1979) Precordial pain and myocardial infarction in pregnancy. *Giornale Italiano Cardiologica*, **9**, 532–534

Cotrill, CM, McAllister, RG and Pentecost, BL (1977) Propranolol therapy during pregnancy, labor and delivery: evidence for transplacental drug transfer and impaired neonatal drug disposition. *Journal of Pediatrics*, **91**, 812–814

Cotton, DB, Longmire, S, Jones, MM *et al.* (1986) Cardiovascular alterations in severe pregnancy-induced hypertension: effects of intravenous nitroglycerine coupled with blood volume expansion. *American Journal of Obstetrics and Gynecology*, **145**, 1053–1059

Crawford, JS, Mills, WG and Pentecost, BL (1971) A pregnant patient with Eisenmenger's syndrome. *British Journal of Anaesthesia*, **43**, 1091–1094

Cunningham, FG, Pritchard, JA, Hankins, GDV *et al.* (1986) Peripartum heart failure: idiopathic cardiomyopathy compounding cardiovascular events. *Obstetrics and Gynecology*, **67**, 157–168

Dacie, J (1975) *Practical Haematology*, pp. 413–414. Edinburgh: Churchill Livingstone

Davidson, NMcD and Parry, EHO (1978) Peri-partum cardiac failure. *Quarterly Journal of Medicine*, **47**, 431–461

Davies, P, Francis, RI, Docker, MF *et al.* (1986) Analysis of impedance cardiography longitudinally applied in pregnancy. *British Journal of Obstetrics and Gynaecology*, **93**, 717–720

Deal, K and Wooley, CF (1973) Coarctation of the aorta and pregnancy. *Annals of Internal Medicine*, **78**, 706–710

Demarkis, JG, Rahimtoola, SH, Sutton, GC *et al.* (1971) Natural course of peri-partum cardiomyopathy. *Circulation*, **44**, 1053–1061

Department of Health and Social Security (1982) *Report on Confidential Enquiries into Maternal Deaths in England and Wales 1976–1978*. London: HMSO

de Swiet, M (1980) The cardiovascular system. In *Clinical Physiology in Obstetrics* (edited by F Hytten and GVP Chamberlain) pp. 3–35. Oxford: Blackwell Scientific Publications

de Swiet, M (1988) The physiology of normal pregnancy. In *The Handbook of Hypertension Volume 12: Hypertension in Pregnancy* (edited by PC Rubin), pp. 1–9. Amsterdam: Elsevier Science Publishers BV

de Swiet, M and Talbert, DG (1986) The measurement of cardiac output by electrical impedance plethysmography in pregnancy. Are the assumptions valid? *British Journal of Obstetrics and Gynaecology*, **93**, 721–726

de Swiet, M, de Louvois, J and Hurley, R (1975) Failure of cephalosporins to prevent bacterial endocarditis during labour. *Lancet*, **ii**, 186

Devitt, JH and Noble, WH (1980) Eisenmemger's syndrome and pregnancy. *New England Journal of Medicine*, **302**, 751

Durack, DT (1975) Current practice in prevention of bacterial endocarditis. *British Heart Journal*, **37**, 478–481

Eckstein, H and Jack, B (1970) Breast feeding and anticoagulant therapy. *Lancet*, **i**, 672–673

Eilen, B, Kaiser, IH, Becker, RM and Cohen, MN (1981) Aortic valve replacement in the third trimester of pregnancy: case report and review of the literature. *Obstetrics and Gynecology*, **57**, 119–121

Emmanuel, R, Somerville, J, Inns, A and Withers, R (1983) Evidence of congenital heart disease in the offspring of parents with atrioventricular defects. *British Heart Journal*, **49**, 144–147

Farmakides, G, Schulman, H, Mohtashemi, M *et al.* (1987) Uterine–umbilical velocimetry in open heart surgery. *American Journal of Obstetrics and Gynecology*, **156**, 1221–1222

Fidler, J, Smith, V, Fayers, P and de Swiet, M (1983) Randomised controlled comparative study of methyldopa and oxprenolol for the treatment of hypertension in pregnancy. *British Medical Journal*, **286**, 1927–1930

Finlay, AY and Edmunds, V (1979) DC cardioversion in pregnancy. *British Journal of Clinical Practice*, **33**, 88–94

Fleming, HA (1977) Antibiotic prophylaxis against infective endocarditis after delivery. *Lancet*, **i**, 144–145

Flessa, HJ, Kapstrom, AB, Glueck, HI and Will, JJ (1965) Placental transport of heparin. *American Journal of Obstetrics and Gynecology*, **93**, 570–573

Fox, KM (1983) Myocardial infarction and the normal coronary arteriogram. *British Medical Journal*, **287**, 446–447

Gallery, EDM, Saunders, DM, Hunyor, SN and Györy, AL (1979) Randomised comparison of methyldopa and oxprenolol for treatment of hypertension in pregnancy. *British Medical Journal*, **1**, 1591–1594

Garrod, LP and Waterworth, PM (1962) The risks of dental extraction during penicillin treatment. *British Heart Journal*, **24**, 39–46

Ginns, HM and Holinrake, K (1970) Complete heart block in pregnancy treated with an internal cardiac pacemaker. *Journal of Obstetrics and Gynaecology of the British Commonwealth*, **77**, 710

Ginz, B (1970) Myocardial infarction in pregnancy. *Journal of Obstetrics and Gynaecology of the British Commonwealth*, **77**, 610

Gladstone, GR, Hordof, A and Gersony, WM (1975) Propranolol administration during pregnancy: effects on the fetus. *Journal of Pediatrics*, **86**, 962–964

Gleicher, N, Midwall, J, Hockberger, D and Jaffin, H (1979) Eisenmenger's syndrome and pregnancy. *Obstetrical and Gynecological Survey*, **34**, 721–741

Gonik, B and Cotton, DB (1982) Peripartum colloid osmotic pressure changes: influence of intravenous hydration. *American Journal of Obstetrics and Gynecology*, **150**, 99–100

Gonik, B, Cotton, D, Spillman, T, Abouleish, E and Zavisca, F (1985) Peripartum colloid osmotic pressure changes: effects of controlled fluid management. *American Journal of Obstetrics and Gynecology*, **151**, 812–815

Habib, A and McArthy, JS (1977) Effects on the neonate of propranolol administered during pregnancy. *Journal of Pediatrics*, **91**, 808–811

Haffaje, E (1983) In discussion – amiodarone pharmacokinetics. *American Heart Journal*, **106**, 847

Hart, MV, Morton, MJ, Hosenpud, JD and Metcalfe, J (1986) Aortic function during normal pregnancy. *American Journal of Obstetrics and Gynecology*, **154**, 887–891

Hankins, GDV, Wendel, GD, Leveno, KJ and Stoneham, J (1985) Myocardial infarction during pregnancy: a review. *Obstetrics and Gynecology*, **65**, 139–147

Hickey, AJ, Macmahon, SW and Wilcken, DEL (1985) Mitral valve prolapse and bacterial endocarditis: when is antibiotic prophylaxis necessary? *American Heart Journal*, **109**, 431–435

Hill, LM (1985) Fetal distress secondary to vancomycin-induced maternal hypotension. *American Journal of Obstetrics and Gynecology*, **153**, 74–75

Ho, PC, Chen, TY and Wong, V (1980) The effect of maternal cardiac disease and digoxin administration on labour, fetal weight and maturity at birth. *Australia and New Zealand Journal of Obstetrics and Gynecology*, **20**, 24–27

Hoffenberg, R, Evans, TR, Adgey, J *et al.* (1987) Resuscitation from cardiopulmonary arrest: training and organisation. *Journal of the Royal College of Physicians of London*, **21**, 175–181

Homans, DC (1985) Peripartum cardiomyopathy. *New England Journal of Medicine*, **312**, 1432–1437

Hughes, LO, McFadyen, IR and Raftery, EB (1988) Acute bacterial endocarditis in a normal aortic valve following vaginal delivery. *International Journal of Cardiology*, **18**, 261–262

Husaini, MH (1971) Myocardial infarction during pregnancy: report of two cases and review of the literature. *Postgraduate Medical Journal*, **47**, 660

Ibarra-Perez, C, Arevalo-Toledo, N, Alvarez-De Lacadena, O and Noriega-Guerra, L (1976) The course of pregnancy in patients with artificial heart valves. *American Journal of Medicine*, **61**, 504–512

ISIS (1988) Randomised trial of intravenous streptokinase, oral aspirin, both or neither among 17,187 cases of suspected acute myocardial infarction: ISIS 2. *Lancet*, **ii**, 349–360

Iturbe-Alessio, I, Fonseca, M, Mutchinik, O *et al.* (1986) Risks of anticoagulant therapy in pregnant women with artificial heart valves. *New England Journal of Medicine*, **315**, 1390–1393

Jakobi, P, Adler, Z, Zimmer, EZ and Milo, S (1989) Effect of uterine contractions on left atrial pressure in a pregnant woman with mitral stenosis. *British Medical Journal*, **298**, 27

Jacoby, WJ (1964) Pregnancy with tetralogy and pentalogy of Fallot. *American Journal of Cardiology*, **14**, 866–873

James, CF, Banner, T, Levelle, P and Caton, D (1985) Noninvasive determination of cardiac output throughout pregnancy. *Anaesthesiology*, **63**, 434

Javares, T, Coto, EC, Maiques, V *et al.* (1984) Pregnancy after heart valve replacement. *International Journal of Cardiology*, **5**, 731–739

Jewett, JF (1979) Pulmonary hypertension and pre-eclampsia. *New England Journal of Medicine*, **301**, 1063–1064

Johnston, TA and de Bono, D (1989) Single ventricle and pulmonary hypertension – a successful pregnancy. *British Journal of Obstetrics and Gynaecology*, **96**, 731–734

Kambam, JR, Franks, JJ and Smith, BE (1987) Inhibitory effect of quinidine on plasma pseudocholinesterase activity in pregnant women. *American Journal of Obstetrics and Gynecology*, **157**, 897–899

Katz, VL, Dotters, D and Droegemueller, W (1986) Perimortem Cesarean delivery. *Obstetrics and Gynecology*, **68**, 571–576

Kirklin, JW (1981) The replacement of cardiac valves. *New England Journal of Medicine*, **304**, 291–292

Klein, VR, Repke, JT, Marquette, GP and Niebyl, JR (1984) The Bland–White–Garland syndrome in pregnancy. *American Journal of Obstetrics and Gynecology*, **150**, 106–107

Knobel, B, Melamud,E and Kishon, T (1984) Peripartum cardiomyopathy. *Israel Journal of Medical Science*, **20**, 1061–1063

Konishi, Y, Tatsuta, N, Kumada, K *et al.* (1980) Dissecting aneurysm during pregnancy and the puerperium. *Japanese Circulation Journal*, **44**, 726–732

Larsen, JF, Jacobsen, B, Holm, HH *et al.* (1978) Intrauterine injection of vitamin K before the delivery during anticoagulant treatment of the mother. *Acta Obstetrica Gynecologica Scandinavica*, **57**, 227–230

Lee, P, Wang, R, Chow, J, Cheung, K, Wong, VCW and Chan, T (1986) Combined use of warfarin and injected subcutaneous heparin during pregnancy in patients with an artificial heart valve. *Journal of the American College of Cardiology*, **8**, 221–224

Lees, MM, Scott, DB, Kerr, MG and Taylor, SH (1967) The circulatory effects of recumbent postural change in late pregnancy. *Clinical Science*, **32**, 453–463

Leibrand, G, Muench, U and Gander, M (1982) Two successful pregnancies in a patient with a single ventricle and transposition of the great arteries. *International Journal of Cardiology*, **1**, 257–262

Leonard, RF, Braun, TE and Levy, AM (1978) Initiation of uterine contractions by disopyramide during pregnancy. *New England Journal of Medicine*, **299**, 84

Levy, M, Grait, L and Laufer, N (1977) Excretion of drugs in human milk. *New England Journal of Medicine*, **297**, 789

Limet, R and Crondin, CM (1977) Cardiac valve prosthesis, anticoagulation and pregnancy. *Annals of Thoracic Surgery*, **23**, 337–431

Lownes, HE and Ives, TJ (1987) Mexiletine use in pregnancy and lactation. *American Journal of Obstetrics and Gynecology*, **157**, 446–447

Lutz, DJ, Noller, KL, Spittell, JA *et al.* (1978) Pregnancy and its complications following cardiac valve prosthesis. *American Journal of Obstetrics and Gynecology*, **131**, 460–468

McCaffrey, RM and Dunn, LJ (1964) Primary pulmonary hypertension and pregnancy. *Obstetric and Gynecological Survey*, **19**, 567–591

McKenna, WJ, Harris, L, Rowland, E *et al.* (1983) Amiodarone therapy during pregnancy. *American Journal of Cardiology*, **51**, 1231–1233

MacLennan, FM (1986) Maternal mortality from Mendelson's syndrome: an explanation. *Lancet*, **i**, 587–589

McLeod, AA, Jennings, KP and Townsend, ER (1978) Near fatal puerperal thrombosis on Björk–Shiley mitral valve prosthesis. *British Heart Journal*, **40**, 934–937

MacNab, G and MacAfee, CAJ (1985) A changing pattern of heart disease associated with pregnancy. *Journal of Obstetrics and Gynaecology*, **5**, 139–142

Magilligan, DJ, Lewis, JW, Heinzerling, RM and Smith, D (1983) Fate of a second porcine bioprosthetic valve. *Journal of Thoracic Cardiovascular Surgery*, **95**, 362–370

Mashini, IS, Albazzaz, SJ, Fadel, HE *et al.* (1987) Serial noninvasive evaluation of cardiovascular hemodynamics during pregnancy. *American Journal of Obstetrics and Gynecology*, **156**, 1208–1213

Maxwell, DJ, Crawford, DC, Curry, PVM *et al.* (1988) Obstetric importance, diagnosis and management of fetal tachycardias. *British Medical Journal*, **297**, 107–110

Melvin, KR, Richardson, PJ, Olsen, EGJ *et al.* (1982) Peripartum cardiomyopathy due to myocarditis. *New England Journal of Medicine*, **307**, 731–734

Mendelson, CL (1940) Pregnancy and coarctation of the aorta. *American Journal of Obstetrics and Gynecology*, **39**, 1014–1021

Mendelson, CL (1956) Disorders of the heart beat during pregnancy. *American Journal of Obstetrics and Gynecology*, **72**, 1268

Mendelson, CL (1960) *Cardiac Disease in Pregnancy*. Philadelphia: Davis

Midwall, J, Jaffin, H, Herman, MV and Kuper Smith, J (1978) Shunt flow and pulmonary hemodynamics during labor and delivery in the Eisenmenger syndrome. *American Journal of Cardiology*, **42**, 299–303

Milsom, I, Forssman, L, Sivertsson, R and Dottori, O (1983) Measurement of cardiac stroke volume by impedance cardiography in the last trimester of pregnancy. *Acta Obstetrica Gynecologica Scandinavica*, **62**, 473–479

Morgan Jones, A and Howitt, G (1965) Eisenmenger syndrome in pregnancy. *British Medical Journal*, **1**, 1627–1631

Nagorney, DM and Field, CS (1981) Successful pregnancy 10 years after triple cardiac valve replacement. *Obstetrics and Gynecology*, **57**, 386–388

Neilson, G, Galea, EG and Blunt, A (1970) Congenital heart disease and pregnancy. *Medical Journal of Australia*, **1**, 1086–1088

Nelson, DM, Main, E, Crafford, W and Ahumada, GG (1983) Peripartum heart failure due to primary pulmonary hypertension. *Obstetrics and Gynecology*, **62**, 58S–63S

Nelson, DM, Stempel, LE, Fabri, PJ and Talbert, M (1984) Hickman catheter use in a pregnant patient requiring therapeutic heparin anticoagulation. *American Journal of Obstetrics and Gynecology*, **149**, 461–462

Newman, B, Derrington, C and Sore, C (1983) Cardiac output and the recumbent position in late pregnancy. *Anaesthesia*, **38**, 332–335

Nora, JJ and Nora, AH (1978) The evolution of specific genetic and environmental counselling in congenital heart diseases. *Circulation*, **57**, 205–213

Oakley, CM (1983) Pregnancy in patients with prosthetic heart valves. *British Medical Journal*, **286**, 1680–1682

Oakley, CM and Hawkins, DF (1983) Pregnancy in patients with prosthetic heart valves. *British Medical Journal*, **287**, 358

Oakley, GDG, McGarry, K, Limb, DG and Oakley, CM (1979) Management of pregnancy in patients with hypertrophic cardiomyopathy. *British Medical Journal*, **1**, 1749–1750

Oates, S, Williams, GL and Rees, GAD (1988) Cardiopulmonary resuscitation in late pregnancy. *British Medical Journal*, **297**, 404–405

O'Connell, JB, Costanzo-Nordin, MR, Subramanian, R *et al.* (1986) Peripartum cardiomyopathy: clinical, hemodynamic, histologic and prognostic characteristics. *Journal of the American College of Cardiology*, **8**, 52–56

Oian, P, Malthau, JM, Noddeland, H and Fadnes, HO (1985) Oedema-preventing mechanisms in subcutaneous tissue of normal pregnant women. *British Journal of Obstetrics and Gynaecology*, **92**, 113–119

Okita, GT, Plotz, EJ and Davis, ME (1956) Placental transfer of radioactive digitoxin in pregnant woman and its fetal distribution. *Circulation Research*, **4**, 376–380

Orme, ML'E, Lewis, PJ, de Swiet, M *et al.* (1977) May mothers given warfarin breast-feed their infants? *British Medical Journal*, **1**, 1564–1565

Penn, IM, Barrett, PA, Pannikote, V *et al.* (1985) Amiodarone in pregnancy. *American Journal of Cardiology*, **56**, 196–197

Peterson, DR, Thomson, DJ and Chinn, N (1972) Ischaemic heart disease prognosis. A community-made assessment (1966–1969). *Journal of the American Medical Association*, **219**, 1423–1427

Phippard, AF, Horvath, JS, Glynn, EM *et al.* (1986) Circulatory adaptation to pregnancy – serial studies of haemodynamics, blood volume, renin and aldosterone in the baboon (*Papio hamadryas*). *Journal of Hypertension*, **4**, 773–779

Pitts, JA, Crosby, WM and Basta, LC (1977) Eisenmenger's syndrome in pregnancy. *American Heart Journal*, **93**, 321–326

Plovin, P, Breart, G, Maillard, F *et al.* The Labetalol Methyldopa Study Group (1988) Comparison of antihypertensive efficacy and safety of labetalol and methyldopa in the treatment of hypertension in pregnancy: a randomized controlled trial. *British Journal of Obstetrics and Gynaecology*, **95**, 868–876

Pyeritz, RE (1981) Maternal and fetal complications of pregnancy in the Marfan syndrome. *American Journal of Medicine*, **71**, 784–790

Pyeritz, RE and McKuisick, VA (1979) The Marfan syndrome: diagnosis and management. *New England Journal of Medicine*, **300**, 772–777

Pyörälä, T (1966) Cardiovascular response to the upright position during pregnancy. *Acta Obstetrica et Gynecologica Scandinavica*, **45**, Suppl. 5, 1–116

Rackow, EC, Fein, AI and Lippo, J (1977) Colloid osmotic pressure as a prognostic indicator of pulmonary edema and mortality in the critically ill. *Chest*, **72**, 709–713

Rand, RJ, Jenkins, DM and Scott, DG (1975) Maternal cardiomyopathy of pregnancy causing stillbirth. *British Journal of Obstetrics and Gynaecology*, **82**, 172–175

Redleaf, PD and Farell, EJ (1959) Bacteremia during parturition – prevention of subacute bacterial endocarditis. *Journal of the American Medical Association*, **169**, 1284–1285

Reece, EA, Egan, JFX, Coustan, DR *et al.* (1986) Coronary artery disease in diabetic pregnancy. *American Journal of Obstetrics and Gynecology*, **154**, 150–151

Reitz, BA, Wallwork, JL, Hunt, SA *et al.* (1982) Heart-lung transplantation. Successful therapy with pulmonary vascular disease. *New England Journal of Medicine*, **306**, 557–564

Roberts, ADG, Low, RAL, Rae, AP and Hillis, WS (1983) Left ventricular aneurysm complicating myocardial infarction occurring during pregnancy. Case report. *British Journal of Obstetrics and Gynaecology*, **90**, 969–970

Robson, SC, Dunlop W, Boys, RJ and Hunter, S (1989) Haemodynamic effects of breast feeding. *British Journal of Obstetrics and Gynaecology*, **96**, 1106–1107

Robson, SC, Dunlop, W, Boys, RJ and Hunter, S (1987a) Cardiac output during labour. *British Medical Journal*, **295**, 1169–1172

Robson, SC, Hunter, S, Moore, M and Dunlop, W (1987b) Haemodynamic changes during the puerperium; a Doppler and M-mode echocardiographic study. *British Journal of Obstetrics and Gynaecology*, **94**, 1028–1039

Rogers, ME, Willerson, JT, Goldblatt, A and Smith, TW (1972) Serum digoxin concentrations in the human fetus, neonate and infant. *New England Journal of Medicine*, **287**, 1010–1013

Rubin, PC, Butters, L, Clark, DM *et al.* (1983) Placebo-controlled trial of atenolol in the treatment of pregnancy-associated hypertension. *Lancet*, **i**, 431–434

Rush, RW, Verjans, M and Spracklen, FHN (1979) Incidence of heart disease in pregnancy. A study done at Peninsular Maternity Services Hospital. *South African Medical Journal*, **55**, 808–810

Saarikoski, S (1976) Placental transfer and fetal uptake of ^{3}H-digoxin in humans. *British Journal of Obstetrics and Gynaecology*, **83**, 879–884

Sachs, BP, Lorell, BH, Mehrez, M and Damien, M (1986) Constrictive pericarditis and pregnancy. *American Journal of Obstetrics and Gynecology*, **154**, 156–157

Sanchez-Cascos, A (1987) Offspring from women with rheumatic valve disease. *European Heart Journal*, **8**, 245–246

Sanders, SP, Levy, RJ, Freed, MD *et al.* (1980) Use of Hancock Porcine Xenografts in children and adolescents. *American Journal of Cardiology*, **46**, 429–438

Sanderson, JE, Olsen, EGJ and Gate, D (1986) Peripartum heart disease: an endomyocardial biopsy study. *British Heart Journal*, **56**, 285–291

Schaefer, G, Arditi, LI Solomon, HA and Ringland, JE (1968) Congenital heart disease and pregnancy. *Clinical Obstetrics and Gynecology*, **11**, 1048–1063

Schrier, RW (1988) Pathogenesis of sodium and water retention in high-output and low-output cardiac failure, nephrotic syndrome, cirrhosis and pregnancy. (Second of two parts). *New England Journal of Medicine*, **319**, 1127–1134

Seaworth, BJ and Durack, DT (1986) Infective endocarditis in obstetric and gynecologic practice. *American Journal of Obstetrics and Gynecology*, **154**, 180–188

Shaul, WL and Hall, JG (1977) Multiple congenital anomalies associated with anticoagulants. *American Journal of Obstetrics and Gynecology*, **127**, 191–198

Sherman, JL and Locke, RV (1960) Transplacental neonatal digitalis intoxication. *American Journal of Cardiology*, **6**, 834

Sibai, BM, Mabie, BC, Harvey, CJ and Gonzalez, AR (1987) Pulmonary edema in severe pre-eclampsia–eclampsia: analysis of thirty-seven sensitive cases. *American Journal of Obstetrics and Gynecology*, **156**, 1174–1179

Simmons, NA, Cawson, RA, Clarke, CA *et al.* (1986) Prophylaxis of infective endocarditis. *Lancet*, **i**, 1267

Singh, H, Bolton, PJ and Oakley, CM (1982) Pregnancy after surgical correction of tetralogy of Fallot. *British Medical Journal*, **285**, 168–170

Sinnenberg, RJ (1980) Pulmonary hypertension in pregnancy. *Southern Medical Journal*, **73**, 1529–1531

Slater, AJ, Gude, N, Clarke, IJ and Walters, WAW (1986) Haemodynamic changes in left ventricular performance during high-dose oestrogen administration in transsexuals. *British Journal of Obstetrics and Gynaecology*, **93**, 532–538

Smith, RH, Radford, DJ, Clark, RA and Julian, DG (1976) Infective endocarditis: a survey of cases in the South-East region of Scotland 1969–1972. *Thorax*, **31**, 373–379

Spetz, S (1965) Capillary filtration during normal pregnancy. *Acta Obstetrica Gynecologica Scandinavica*, **44**, 227–242

Stein, L, Beraud, JJ, Morisette, M *et al.* (1975) Pulmonary edema during volume infusion. *Circulation*, **52**, 483–489

Stevenson, JC, MacDonald, DWR, Warren, RC *et al.* (1986) Increased concentration of circulating calcitonin related peptide during normal human pregnancy. *British Medical Journal*, **294**, 1329–1330

Stiller, RJ, Vintzkeos, AM, Nochimson, DJ *et al.* (1984) Single ventricle in pregnancy: case report and review of the literature. *Obstetrics and Gynecology*, **(Supplement)** 19S–20S

Stokes, IM, Evans, J and Stone, M (1984) Myocardial infarction and cardiac output in the second trimester followed by assisted vaginal delivery under epidural anaesthesia at 38 weeks gestation. Case report. *British Journal of Obstetrics and Gynaecology*, **91**, 197–198

Storstein, L (1972) LB-46, a new β-adrenergic receptor blocking agent in cardiac arrhythmias. *Acta medica scandinavica*, **191**, 423–428

Stuart, KL (1968) Cardiomyopathy of pregnancy and the puerperium. *Quarterly Journal of Medicine*, **37**, 463–478

Sugrue, D, Blake, S and MacDonald, D (1981) Pregnancy complicated by maternal heart disease at the National Maternity Hospital, Dublin, Ireland, 1969 to 1978. *American Journal of Obstetrics and Gynecology*, **139**, 1–6

Sugrue, DD, Blake, S and MacDonald, D (1982) Infective endocarditis during pregnancy. *Journal of Obstetrics and Gynecology*, **2**, 210–214

Sugrue, D, Blake, S, Troy, P and MacDonald, D (1980) Antibiotic prophylaxis against infective endocarditis after normal delivery – is it necessary? *British Heart Journal*, **44**, 499–502

Szekely, P and Snaith, L (1974) *Heart Disease and Pregnancy*. Edinburgh: Churchill Livingstone

Szekely, P, Turner, R and Snaith, L (1973) Pregnancy and the changing pattern of rheumatic heart disease. *British Heart Journal*, **35**, 1293–1303

Timmis, AD, Jackson, G and Holt, OW (1980) Mexiletine for control of ventricular dysrhythmias in pregnancy. *Lancet*, **ii**, 647–648

Tsou, E, Waldhorn, RE, Kerwin, DM *et al.* (1984) Pulmonary venoocclusive disease in pregnancy. *Obstetrics and Gynecology*, **64**, 281–284

Turner, GM, Oakley, CM and Dixon, HG (1968) Management of pregnancy complicated by hypertrophic obstructive cardiomyopathy. *British Medical Journal*, **4**, 281–284

Ueland, K, Novy, MJ and Metcalfe, S (1972) Hemodynamic responses of patients with heart disease to pregnancy and exercise. *American Journal of Obstetrics and Gynecology*, **113**, 47–59

Ueland, K, McAnulty, JH, Ueland, FR and Metcalfe, J (1981) Special considerations in the use of cardiovascular drugs. *Clinical Obstetrics and Gynecology*, **24**, 809–823

Ueland, K, Novy, MJ, Peterson, EN and Metcalfe, J (1969) Maternal cardiovascular dynamics IV. The influence of gestational age on the maternal cardiovascular response to posture and exercise. *American Journal of Obstetrics and Gynecology*, **104**, 856–864

Vitalli, E Donatelli, F, Quaini, E *et al.* (1986) Pregnancy in patients with mechanical prosthetic heart valves. Our experience regarding 98 pregnancies in 57 patients. *Journal of Cardiovascular Surgery*, **27**, 221–227

Weiner, CP, Landas, S and Persoon, TJ (1987) Digoxin-like immunoreactive substance in fetuses with and without cardiac pathology. *American Journal of Obstetrics and Gynecology*, **157**, 368–371

Whittemore, R, Hobbins, JC and Engle, MA (1982) Pregnancy and its outcome in women with and without surgical treatment of congenital heart disease. *American Journal of Cardiology*, **50**, 641–651

Willis, DC, Caton, D, Levelle, JP and Banner, T (1987) Cardiac output response to prostaglandin E$_2$-induced abortion in the second trimester. *American Journal of Obstetrics and Gynecology*, **156**, 170–173

Working Party (1982) The antibiotic prophylaxis of infective endocarditis. *Lancet*, **ii**, 1326

Young, BK and Haft, JI (1970) Treatment of pulmonary edema with ethacrynic acid during labour. *American Journal of Obstetrics and Gynecology*, **107**, 330–331

Younis, JS and Granat, M (1987) Insufficient transplacental digoxin transfer in severe hydrops fetalis. *American Journal of Obstetrics and Gynecology*, **157**, 1268–1269

Zitnik, RS, Brandenburg, RO, Sheldon, R and Wallace, RB (1969) Pregnancy and open heart surgery. *Circulation*, **39 (Suppl)**, 257

Chapter 5

Renal disorders

JM Davison

Introduction

A *Lancet* editorial in 1975 stated that 'children of women with renal disease used to be born dangerously, or not at all – not at all, if their doctors had their way'. That quotation, reflecting the pessimism surrounding women with renal disorders for the preceding 30 years also signalled the change to a more optimistic view. The old attitudes had led to many unnecessary therapeutic abortions and sterilizations, without women even questioning this advice. Present attitudes are that most women who have minimal renal dysfunction can go ahead with pregnancy in the knowledge that the chances of a successful outcome, although reduced, are still over 90 per cent and that there is usually no adverse effect on the natural history of their disease.

Despite the new approach during the last 15 years, there are still dilemmas, discussed in another *Lancet* editorial (1989a), which reminds the clinician that counselling a patient is still not straightforward and that '. . . the thoughtful doctor . . . should still admit his difficulties, more so nowadays because . . . the thoughtful woman demands straight answers to apparently straight questions'. With this in mind, this chapter focuses on prevailing controversies and attempts to provide some straight answers for the management of renal disorders in pregnancy.

CHANGES IN THE RENAL TRACT IN NORMAL PREGNANCY

Pregnancy is associated with major anatomical and functional changes in the renal tract. Many of the changes are of such an unusual nature and magnitude that, on the one hand, the unwary obstetrician may fail to realize their importance when interpreting data from pregnant women with renal disorders and, on the other hand, may diagnose a renal problem where only the extremes of adaptation are displayed (Dunlop and Davison, 1987).

Anatomical changes

Kidney volume, weight and size increase in pregnancy, renal length increasing by 1 cm when measured radiographically (Rasmussen and Nielsen, 1988). More striking changes, however, occur in the collecting system, where calyces, renal pelves and ureters all dilate markedly. Dilatation observed as early as the first trimester is more marked on the right, affects 90 per cent of women at term and may persist 3–4 months after delivery. The aetiology of these changes has been ascribed to both humoral (e.g. progesterone, oestrogens, prostaglandins) and mechanical (the enlarged uterus) factors. Ultrasonic evidence indicating that dilatation occurs before the uterus has enlarged sufficiently to become an obstructive factor favours the former view, but the bulk of the evidence supports the mechanical hypothesis. For instance, increased ureteral pressure, provoked by having third-trimester women stand or lie supine, is present above the pelvic brim and then decreases when the obstructive effect of the enlarged uterus is removed by assumption of a lateral decubitus or knee–chest position. Other studies have reported that ureteral dilatation terminates at the level of the pelvic brim, suggesting that obstruction there is due to the uterus pressing on the ureter when it crosses the iliac artery, the so-called 'illiacii sign' being a pyelographic filling defect (Dure-Smith, 1970). These anatomical changes have several clinical implications:

1. Acceptable norms of kidney size should be increased by 1 cm if estimated during pregnancy or in the immediate puerperium. Reductions in renal length noted several months postpartum need not be attributed to pathological decrements in renal parenchymal mass.
2. There may be substantial errors in the collection of timed urine volumes. This is because large quantities of urine may remain in the dilated collecting system and this may result in large timing errors, as well as collection errors, especially in hydropenic patients.
3. Urinary obstruction or stasis may explain why pregnant women with asymptomatic bacteriuria are more prone to develop pyelonephritis. There may also be a higher frequency of vesico-ureteral reflux, which further disposes the pregnant women to symptomatic infection.
4. Frank urinary tract obstruction may be difficult to diagnose during pregnancy. There is an 'overdistension syndrome' in late pregnancy characterized by abdominal pain, demonstration of marked hydronephrosis and variable increases in serum creatinine levels (Meyers, Lee and Munschauser, 1985).

Functional changes

Renal haemodynamics

Both glomerular filtration rate (GFR) and effective renal plasma flow (ERPF) increase to values 50–80 per cent above those measured in non-pregnant women. Twenty-four-hour creatinine clearance rises immediately after the first missed menstrual period, becomes significantly elevated by gestational week 4 and peaks at 40–50 per cent above preconception values by 9–10 weeks. This increment is sustained until late pregnancy, when a 15–20 per cent decrease occurs and sometimes non-pregnant levels are reached by term. Increases in GFR of a similar magnitude have been confirmed during short-term inulin infusion studies. ERPF increases by 60–80 per cent in pregnancy and, although decreasing approximately 25 per cent near term, it is still considerably above non-pregnant values.

Reasons why renal haemodynamics increase during pregnancy are obscure. It is of interest that the stimulus appears to be maternal in origin and micropuncture studies in the rat demonstrate that gestational vasodilatation involves equal reductions in the tone of the pre- and postglomerular arterioles, so that intraglomerular blood pressure is maintained constant. If the latter is true in humans, this would suggest that 9 months of hyperfiltration will have few, if any, adverse effects on the kidney.

The increments in renal haemodynamics have clinical implications:

1. Levels of creatinine and urea decrease from a mean of 62 μmol/l and 4.5 mmol/l to 44 μmol/l and 3.2 mmol/l, respectively, while values of 80 μmol/l and 5.0 mmol/l suggest underlying renal disease and prompt further evaluation.
2. Increases in GFR and ERPF may also explain, in part, why urinary excretion of several solutes, including glucose, amino acids, water-soluble vitamins and protein, increase during pregnancy. The upper limit defining normal proteinuria should be doubled in pregnancy, with 300 mg/24 h not considered abnormal.
3. Women with underlying renal lesions may experience marked increments in protein excretion during pregnancy, which should not be misconstrued as exacerbation of disease.

Tubular function

There may be decrements in the tubular reabsorption of glucose which, when combined with the marked increase in this solute's filtered load, explain why many women with normal carbohydrate metabolism have measurable glycosuria during pregnancy (Davison and Dunlop, 1984). The same may be true for the renal handling of several amino acids, as substantial amnioaciduria also characterizes normal pregnancy. Plasma urate levels decrease in pregnancy and levels exceeding 300 μmol/l are abnormal. This decrement reflects not only decreases in the fractional reabsorption of urate, but also increases in GFR (Dunlop and Davison, 1977).

The relevance of these tubular changes is as follows:

1. Glycosuria, when present, is intermittent and bears no consistent relationship to plasma glucose levels; thus, urine glucose measurements are unreliable for managing diabetic women (a practice rarely employed any more in non-pregnant populations with easy access to glucometers).
2. Increased excretion of glucose and amino acids may partially explain why pregnant women with asymptomatic bacteriuria often develop symptomatic disease.
3. An increase in plasma urate may be an early sign of pre-eclampsia.

Acid–base regulation

Renal bicarbonate reclamation and hydrogen ion secretion appear to be intact during normal gestation. However, a mild alkalaemia is present, blood hydrogen levels decreasing by 2–4 nmol/l and arterial (or arterialized capillary) blood pH increasing to 7.42–7.44 units (Lim, Katz and Lindheimer, 1976). The changes occur early in pregnancy and are sustained until term. The alkalaemia is respiratory in origin, for pregnant women normally hyperventilate and arterial P_{CO_2} decreases from a mean of 36 torr, before conception, to 31 torr during pregnancy. In addition, plasma bicarbonate decreases by approximately 4 mEq/l and values of 18–22 mEq/l are normal.

Alterations in acid–base metabolism have several consequences:

1. Because P_{CO_2} is already reduced, the pregnant woman will be at a disadvantage in defending pH in the face of acute metabolic acidosis.
2. A pregnant woman may be hypercapnoeic with a P_{CO_2} considered normal in the non-pregnant state: for example, a pregnant asthmatic whose P_{CO_2} is 40 torr already has CO_2 retention.

Osmoregulation

Plasma osmolality (P_{osmol}) decreases early in pregnancy and by gestational week 10 reaches a nadir 8–10 mosmol/kg below non-pregnant values, which is maintained through term. Most of the change is due to a decline in plasma sodium and its attendant anions and only about 1.5 mosmol/kg of this decrement represents decreased urea levels. These changes in tonicity are attributable to decrements in the osmotic thresholds for thirst and for vasopressin (AVP) release, both of which also decrease by 8–10 mosmol/kg in pregnancy; pregnant women therefore concentrate and dilute their urines around a P_{osmol} that is 10 mosmol/kg below that present before conception (reviewed in Lindheimer, Barron and Davison, 1989).

Other osmoregulatory changes include a substantial rise in the metabolic clearance rate (MCR) of AVP, which increases fourfold between gestational week 10 and mid-pregnancy. The rise appears to parallel the appearance, and marked increase in circulating levels, of the placental enzyme vasopressinase (also called oxytocinase), which is a cystine aminopeptidase capable of inactivating large quantities of AVP *in vitro*. The MCR of 1-deamino-8-D-AVP(dDAVP), an analogue resistant to degradation by vasopressinase, is hardly altered in gestation, suggesting that the aminopeptidase enzymes are also active *in vivo* (Lindheimer, Barron and Davision, 1989).

The osmoregulatory changes of pregnancy have clinical relevance. First, the necessity of maintaining a decreased P_{osmol} must be taken into account when managing women with known central diabetes insipidus (DI). If AVP (pitressin) is used, a substantial increment in dose schedule may be required. However, most patients are now managed with dDAVP and little change in therapy is required. Second, a syndrome labelled transient DI of pregnancy can appear during the second half of pregnancy, remitting post partum (Krege, Katz and Bouts, 1989). Some women with this complication appear to have had subclinical lesions of central DI, brought to the fore by the increased MCR of AVP late in pregnancy. Even more intriguing are patients in whom transient DI seems to reflect massive destruction of AVP *in vivo* due, perhaps, to extremely high levels of, or to exaggerated effects of, vasopressinase. These are women whose disorder, characterized by marked polyuria and polydipsia and the presence of dilute urine, is resistant to pharmacological quantities of AVP. The patients, however, can be managed, and concentrate urine appropriately when treated with dDAVP, which, as noted, is resistant to degradation by vasopressinase.

Volume regulation

There are changes in both volume homoeostasis and the regulation of blood pressure in normal pregnancy (Gallery and Brown, 1987). Most healthy women gain approximately 12.5 kg during first pregnancies and 1 kg less during subsequent gestations. Generations of clinicians have considered these averages as upper limits of permissible weight gain, ignoring the fact that there is a plus and a minus to deviations about a mean. As a result many pregnant women have been unnecessarily admonished for excessive weight gain and their salt intake and/or calories restricted.

Most of the weight increase is in fluid, total body water increasing by 6–8 litres, 4–6 of which are extracellular. Plasma volume increases by 40–50 per cent during pregnancy, the largest rate of increment occurring during the second trimester, whereas increments in the interstitial space are greatest in the third trimester. There is also a gradual cumulative retention of approximately 900 mmol of sodium, distributed between the products of conception and the maternal extracellular space.

Table 5.1.   Changes in the renal tract in normal pregnancy

Change	Manifestation	Clinical implications
Increased renal size	Renal length 1 cm greater on intravenous urography (IVU)	Postpartum decreases in size should not be mistaken for parenchymal loss
Dilatation of pelves, calyces and ureters	Resembles hydronephrosis on IVU (more marked on right)	Not obstructive uropathy (see Tables 5.2 and 5.3) Retained urine causes collection errors Delay intravenous urography until 12–16 weeks. Upper urinary tract infections are more virulent
Increased renal haemodynamics	ERPF and GFR increase by 50–80%	Plasma creatinine (P_{cr}) and urea decrease in normal pregnancy; P_{cr} >80 μmol/l is suspect. There is increased excretion of glucose, aminoacids and protein
Changes in acid–base metabolism	Renal bicarbonate threshold decreases	Plasma bicarbonate is 4–5 mM/l lower
Renal water handling	Osmoregulation altered	Plasma osmolality decreases by 10 mosm/kg and sodium by 5 mmol/l

These increases in maternal intravascular and interstitial compartments produce a physiologic hypervolaemia, yet the volume receptors sense these changes as normal and, when sodium restriction or diuretic therapy limits this physiological expansion, maternal responses resemble those in salt-depleted non-pregnant subjects. This is one reason why sodium restriction has little or no place in modern antenatal care and women should be advised to salt their food to taste. In fact, some researchers believe that a liberal sodium intake is beneficial during pregnancy.

The influence of humoral changes during normal pregnancy, including activation of the renin–angiotensin system and increases in the circulating levels of several mineralocorticoids, on renal sodium handling and volume regulation, is incompletely understood. The increment in GFR means that >10 000 additional mmol of sodium must be reabsorbed by the renal tubules each day, a quantity considerably greater than the expected salt-retaining effects of high circulating levels of oestrogens, aldosterone and deoxycorticosterone.

Finally, the practical consequences of volume changes are that (1) increments in intravascular volume and a concomitant physiological haemodilution are positive signs when managing renal disease in pregnancy and (2) the physiological volume changes of pregnancy must also be taken into account when managing women undergoing dialysis after acute renal failure, or for end-stage renal disease.

Table 5.1 summarizes the major anatomical and functional alterations discussed in this section, once again underscoring the need to be familiar with the normal adaptations in pregnancy, before disease can be defined.

DETECTION OF RENAL DISEASE IN PREGNANCY

Examination of the urine

Healthy non-pregnant women excrete considerably less than 100 mg of protein in the urine each day but, owing to the relative imprecision and variability of testing methods used by hospital laboratories, proteinuria is not considered abnormal until it exceeds 150 mg/day. There is increased protein excretion during pregnancy and amounts of up to 300 mg/day (some accept 500 mg/day) may still be normal (Davison, 1985). Furthermore, approximately 5 per cent of healthy adolescents and young adults have postural proteinuria, which may become apparent or first be detected in pregnancy. Postural proteinuria may also appear or increase near term when women tend to assume a more lordotic posture, which aggravates the condition.

There are only sporadic reports concerning the excretion of small-molecular-weight proteins or enzymuria in normal and abnormal pregnancies and, therefore, these tests have little current value in gestation. It is also not clear whether urinary albumin excretion increases in normal pregnancy, a research area of interest because the detection of microalbuminuria is one of the earliest signs of renal dysfunction in diseases such as diabetes and may have predictive value for the occurrence of pre-eclampsia (Rodriguez et al., 1988).

There have been few attempts to quantitate urinary sediment in pregnancy. The excretion of red blood cells may increase, but it is not clear whether leucocyturia also occurs. Spontaneous gross or microscopic haematuria can be attributable to a variety of causes (Danielli et al., 1987): rupture of small veins about the dilated renal pelvis may cause bleeding; urinary infection associated with congenital urinary tract anomalies can be difficult to eradicate and may predispose to haematuria. Very occasionally, haematuria may be secondary to acute glomerulonephritis, primary or metastatic neoplasm, haemangioma, calculus or fungal disease (Klein, 1983); a bleeding ureteral stump after a nephrectomy (for either benign or malignant disease), should not be forgotten. Endometriosis, inflammatory bowel lesions, leucoplakia, amyloidosis and granulomas may involve the urinary tract and produce haematuria.

Investigation, which includes ultrasound and radiological and endoscopic assessments, can usually be deferred until after delivery. In the absence of any demonstrable cause, haematuria can be classified as idiopathic and recurrences are unlikely in either the current or a subsequent pregnancy.

Renal function tests

Clearance of endogenous creatinine, which is the primary way of assessing GFR in non-pregnant subjects, is useful for evaluating renal function in pregnant women. The lower limit of normal for creatinine clearances measured during pregnancy should be 30 per cent above that for non-pregnant women, which in most hospitals averages 110–115 ml/min. One should be aware, however, that urinary creatinine results from tubular secretion, as well as from glomerular filtration. When renal dysfunction is moderate (plasma creatinine of 125–250 µmol/l) or severe, a substantial proportion of the clearance may be due to secretion, resulting in considerable overestimation of the GFR.

Acid excretion and urinary concentration and dilution are similar in pregnant and non-pregnant women: thus, tests such as ammonium chloride loading (rarely indicated in pregnancy) give values similar to those in non-pregnant women. Supine posture can interfere with tests of maximal urinary dilution, while lateral recumbency interferes with urinary concentration and it is perhaps best to perform these studies with the patient seated quietly in a comfortable chair.

URINARY TRACT INFECTIONS: DIAGNOSIS AND TERMINOLOGY

The analysis of urine specimens during pregnancy can be hampered by contamination at the time of collection with bacteria from urethra, vagina and/or perineum. This problem can be overcome by obtaining a fresh midstream urine (MSU) collected by a clean-catch technique or by suprapubic aspiration of bladder urine, this latter procedure being unacceptable to some patients and clinicians. *True bacteriuria* is then traditionally defined as the presence of >100 000 bacteria of the same species per millilitre of urine in two consecutive MSU samples, or in a single suprapubic aspiration. Some recent evidence, however, indicates that lower colony counts may represent active infection (Stamm, Counts and Running, 1982). Various presumptive tests based on changes in chemical indicators are not reliable enough for clinical practice.

Asymptomatic or *covert bacteriuria* designates true bacteriuria in the absence of symptoms or signs of acute urinary tract infection (UTI). Where there is *symptomatic UTI*, two clinical syndromes are recognized: *lower UTI* or *cystitis* and *upper UTI* or *acute pyelonephritis*. It must be remembered, however, that pregnant women often complain of, or will admit to, frequency of micturition, dysuria, urgency or nocturia, singly or in combination and that such symptoms are not in themselves diagnostic of UTI (*Lancet* editorial, 1985).

It is probable that bacteria originate from the large bowel and colonize the urinary tract transperineally. By far the commonest infecting organism is *Escherichia coli*, which is responsible for 75–90 per cent of bacteriuria during pregnancy. The pathogenic virulence of this organism, which is not the most plentiful in faeces, appears to derive from a number of factors including resistance to vaginal acidity, rapid division in urine, possession of adhesions (characterized as fimbriae) allowing adherence to uro-epithelial cells and production of chemicals which decrease ureteric peristalsis and inhibit phagocytosis (McFadyean, 1986; Cunningham, 1987). Other organisms frequently responsible for UTI include species of *Klebsiella*, *Proteus*, coagulase-negative *Staphylococcus* and *Pseudomonas*.

The stasis associated with ureteropelvic dilatation and/or partial ureteric obstruction increases the nutrient content of the urine, and although potential pathogens are present in most women, only a small minority develop bacteriuria. Susceptible women may differ immunologically from those who resist infection: they are less likely to express antibody to the O antigen of *E. coli* on the vaginal epithelium and may display less effective leucocyte activity against the organism.

Asymptomatic bacteriuria

Localization of infection

Asymptomatic or covert bacteriuria is a heterogeneous entity. Several methods have been used to try to differentiate between upper and lower urinary tract bacteriuria, e.g. renal biopsy, ureteral catheterization, bladder washout tests, urinary concentration tests and serum antibody tests. The first two methods are too invasive for clinical practice and the remainder are insufficiently precise to localize infection confidently. The determination of antibody-coated bacteria in the urine as a predictor of the presence and site of a UTI, also remains controversial.

Significance and importance of diagnosis

The reservoir of young women with covert bacteriuria acquired during childhood is about 5 per cent, but only 1.2 per cent are infected at any one time. The incidence increases after puberty and is approximately equal in both the pregnant and non-pregnant populations (2–10 per cent). During pregnancy, 40 per cent of the infected group, if left untreated, develop acute symptoms, accounting for 60–70 per cent of all cases of symptomatic UTI. Of those with initial negative cultures, 1.5 per cent develop acute infections accounting for the remaining 30–40 per cent of all cases of acute UTI.

Thus not all untreated bacteriuric women will develop symptoms of acute UTI during pregnancy, and those who are found to have sterile urine when screened at antenatal booking can contribute substantially to the pool of symptomatic women. A view has emerged that screening programmes are not cost-effective (Lawson and Miller, 1973; Campbell-Brown et al., 1987). Furthermore, it has been shown that as a predictor of symptomatic urinary infection, the presence of bacteriuria has a specificity of 89 per cent but a sensitivity of only 33 per cent and a false-positive rate of almost 90 per cent (Chng and Hall, 1982); this population, however, was screened by means of a single urine test only and an unusually high prevalence (11.8 per cent) of bacteriuria was detected. It has been suggested that women with a history of previous UTI as well as current bacteriuria are ten times more likely to develop symptoms during pregnancy than women without either feature.

Asymptomatic bacteriuria has been alleged to be associated with several complications of pregnancy such as low birthweight, fetal loss, pre-eclampsia and maternal anaemia. Several of these apparent correlations may have resulted from inaccuracies in matching cases and controls and none appears to be supported by more recent studies (Davison, Sprott and Selkon, 1984).

Management in pregnancy

Choice of drug
The sensitivity of the isolated organism(s) is important and short-acting sulphonamides or nitrofurantoin derivatives are usually the initial therapy (Cunningham, 1987). Other antibiotics are reserved for the treatment of failures and for symptomatic infection. Ampicillin and the cephalosporins can safely be used throughout pregnancy. Tetracyclines are contraindicated because of the staining of the teeth of infants by binding with orthophosphates as well as the rare maternal complication of acute fatty liver of pregnancy (AFLP). If sulphonamides are still being prescribed in late pregnancy, they should be withheld during the last 2–3 weeks because they compete with bilirubin for albumin-binding sites, increasing the risk of fetal hyperbilirubinaemia and kernicterus. Nitrofurantoin used during the last few weeks may precipitate haemolysis due to erythrocyte phosphate dehydrogenase deficiency in the newborn.

Treatment regimen
There are differing opinions on optimal duration of therapy. Continuous antibiotic therapy was once recommended from the time of diagnosis until after delivery, based

on belief that relapse rate can be high because of problems of renal parenchymal involvement. As at least 60 per cent of patients only have bladder involvement, however, short-term therapy (2 weeks) is satisfactory. If follow-up is meticulous, there is no advantage to long-term antibiotics and the possible hazards of such therapy to the fetus are avoided (Cunningham, Lucas and Hankins, 1987). Many new antibiotics have been administered to pregnant women but the clinician should preferably limit himself to those with a proven record during pregnancy. Follow-up urine culture should be obtained 1 week after therapy is stopped and then at 4-weekly intervals throughout pregnancy.

Relapses and reinfection
Relapse is the recurrence of bacteriuria caused by the same organism, usually within 6 weeks of the initial infection. Reinfection is the recurrence of bacteriuria involving a different strain of bacteria, after successful eradication of the initial infection. Most patients with a reinfection pattern have infections limited to the bladder, usually occurring at least 6 weeks after therapy.

Approximately 25 per cent of patients will have a recurrence during pregnancy and a second course of treatment should be given, based on a repeat culture with sensitivity testing. As *E. coli* causes the majority of initial infections as well as recurrences, it is sometimes desirable to employ an *E. coli* serotyping system to distinguish different strains precisely. In the group of patients who relapse or who are resistant to the first course of therapy, only about 40 per cent will have the asymptomatic bacteriuria cleared with subsequent therapy.

Long-term management

Importance of follow-up
With increasing interval between treatment of bacteriuria in pregnancy and post-delivery review, the influence of the bacteriuria becomes less noticeable. Ten or more years after an initial episode of bacteriuria in pregnancy, the prevalence of bacteriuria (29 per cent) in women not treated during pregnancy is virtually the same as in those women who were treated (25 per cent). Women who were never bacteriuric during pregnancy have subsequent rates of bacteriuria of around 5 per cent. Thus a single course of treatment during the index pregnancy does not appear to protect against persistent or recurrent bacteriuria years later (*Lancet* editorial, 1985).

There are few prospective studies, but available evidence does not suggest that persistent asymptomatic bacteriuria in women with normal urinary tracts causes long-term renal damage or that treatment reduces the incidence of chronic renal disease (McFadyean *et al.*, 1973; Cunningham, 1987).

FURTHER INVESTIGATION AND POSTPARTUM EVALUATION
It is known that 20 per cent of all patients with asymptomatic bacteriuria have radiological abnormalities and the percentage is increased among patients with acute infections and/or infections that are difficult to eradicate during pregnancy (Gower *et al.*, 1968). This may indicate a predisposition to infection, it may result from infection or it may be unrelated to infection (Gower *et al.*, 1968; Briedahl *et al.*, 1972). An intravenous urogram should be performed on one occasion, no earlier than 4 months post-delivery, to document a non-obstructed urinary tract in women

who have had asymptomatic bacteriuria during pregnancy with the following additional criteria: (1) difficulty in eradicating the bacteriuria; (2) episode(s) of acute symptomatic UTI; (3) history of acute symptomatic UTI before pregnancy, and (4) persistent and/or recurrent asymptomatic bacteriuria or acute UTI. This will ensure detection of about 90 per cent of women with major urinary tract abnormalities.

Acute cystitis

This occurs in about 1 per cent of pregnant women of whom 60 per cent have had negative initial screening. The symptoms are often difficult to distinguish from those attributable to pregnancy itself. Features indicating a true infection include haematuria, dysuria and suprapubic discomfort, as well as a positive urine culture. The bacteriology is the same as in women with asymptomatic bacteriuria and similar treatment is recommended, with the aims of abolishing symptoms and preventing occurrence of acute pyelonephritis. It is too early to gauge the success of single-dose therapy for pregnant women with cystitis.

Acute pyelonephritis

Significance and importance of diagnosis

The differential diagnosis includes other urinary tract pathology, other causes of pyrexia such as respiratory tract infection, viraemia or toxoplasmosis (appropriate serological screening should be performed) and other causes of acute abdominal pain such as acute appendicitis, biliary colic, gastro-enteritis, uterine fibroid degeneration or abruptio placentae (Baker, Madeley and Symonds, 1989).

Acute appendicitis can be a difficult diagnosis to make, especially in the third trimester. Usually, at the onset of appendicitis, the pain is referred to the centre of the abdomen, vomiting is not a marked feature, pyrexia is not great and rigors do not occur.

Pneumonia on the affected side should present no difficulties if attention is paid to the type of respiration, the respiratory rate and the physical signs in the chest. It should be noted, however, that so-called adult respiratory distress syndrome (ARDS), with accompanying liver and haematopoietic dysfunction, can be a significant complication of pyelonephritis (Cunningham, Lucas and Hankins, 1987; Pruett and Faro, 1987).

Acute hydro-ureter and hydronephrosis
With the so-called 'overdistension syndrome' (Meyers, Lee and Munschauser, 1985) obstruction may occur at varying levels at or above the pelvic brim (Tables 5.2 and 5.3). Some women have only transient mild loin pain whereas others have recurrent episodes of severe loin pain or lower abdominal pain radiating to the groin. The variation in symptoms with changes in posture and position are hallmarks of this condition. Urinalysis contains few or no red cells and repeat MSU specimens are sterile. Diagnosis can be confirmed using ultrasound sonar scanning or limited excretory urography. Positioning of the patient in lateral recumbency or the knee–chest position often gives relief but if this fails ureteral catheterization or nephrostomy may be necessary. Corrective surgery is best delayed until the postpartum period.

Table 5.2.   Clinical implications of pregnancy-induced urinary tract dilatation

Clinical entity	Clinical features
Overdistension syndrome	Flank pain, renal colic
Pyelonephritis	Flank pain, fever, bacteriuria
Rupture of the urinary tract (see Table 5.3)	
Retroperitoneal	
Parenchymal	Flank pain
	Mass: abscess, haematoma
	Anaemia/hypotension due to blood loss
	Haematuria
Collecting system	Flank pain
	Mass: perinephric or subcapsular urinoma
	Haematuria (microscopic)
Intraperitoneal	
Parenchymal	Peritonitis
Collecting system	Flank pain
	Anaemia/hypotension due to blood loss
	Haematuria

Non-traumatic rupture of the urinary tract
The intrusion of unremitting pain and haematuria upon the course of pyelonephritis or the 'overdistension syndrome' suggests rupture of the urinary tract (Tables 5.2 and 5.3). Furthermore, this complication can masquerade as other obstetrical and surgical abdominal catastrophes, including acute appendicitis, pelvic abscess, cholecystitis, urolithiasis or abruptio placentae. Prompt recognition may prevent a small tear and urine leak, treatable by postural or tube drainage, from extending and/or expanding. Rupture of the renal parenchyma, with haemorrhagic shock, formation of a flank mass or dissection of the urinary tract contents intraperitoneally compels prompt surgical intervention, usually with nephrectomy (Meyers, Lee and Munschauser, 1985).

Management of acute pyelonephritis in pregnancy

A midstream urine sample should be sent for culture and sensitivity tests immediately. Treatment should be aggressive, undertaken in a hospital setting and backed up by good nursing care.

Fluid balance
If the patient is dehydrated through vomiting and sweating, she will require intravenous fluid therapy. Regular assessment of renal function and plasma urea and

Table 5.3.   Rupture of the urinary tract

Pregnancy-related	
Traumatic	
Non-traumatic	
Parenchymal	Tumour, especially haematoma
	Abscess
	Vascularities: polyarteritis nodosa
	Cystic disease
	Congenital: tuberous sclerosis
Non-parenchymal	Obstruction due to urolithiasis, infection, reflux or stricture

electrolytes should be undertaken. Infectious episodes have little effect on renal haemodynamics in non-pregnant patients but such attacks during pregnancy cause transient but marked decrements in creatinine clearance (Whalley, Cunningham and Martin, 1975).

Choice of drug

Treatment should aim at administering the most effective drug to eradicate a particular infection without exposing the fetus to an unnecessarily harmful agent. Antibiotics producing high blood levels and resulting in high renal parenchymal concentrations are favoured. Two antibiotics that give appropriate blood levels are ampicillin and the cephalosporins; *E. coli*, the most common organism isolated in urinary infections, is usually sensitive to these antibiotics. Until the patient is afebrile, it is preferable to give intravenous antibiotics, to be continued orally thereafter.

Time course of treatment

The duration of therapy should be 2 weeks for lower tract UTI and a minimum of 3 weeks for acute pyelonephritis. Antibiotic sensitivity should be reviewed within 48 h. In patients showing clinical deterioration or whose urine cultures reveal bacterial resistance to the selected antibiotic, a repeat urine culture is necessary and alternative antibiotic therapy should be considered. In severely ill patients, blood specimens should be taken for culture. After the completion of treatment, urine for culture should be taken at every antenatal visit for the rest of the pregnancy.

Gram-negative sepsis

This can occur with acute pyelonephritis but the situation is commonly associated with instrumentation of an infected urinary tract. An aminoglycoside antibiotic is best because it is effective against nearly all of the Gram-negative urinary bacteria. Enterococci less commonly cause bacteraemia but, because of possible resistance to aminoglycosides, ampicillin can be used combined with an aminoglycoside until culture results are available.

CHRONIC RENAL DISEASE

The consensus is that, if non-pregnant renal function is only mildly compromised, proteinuria is minimal and hypertension is absent or minimal, then there is usually a successful obstetrical outcome and no adverse effect on remote renal prognosis, except in a few specific disease entities (see later) (*Lancet* editorials, 1975, 1989a; Lindheimer and Katz, 1987; Packham *et al.*, 1989).

Chronic renal dysfunction and its clinical implications

A woman may lose approximately 50 per cent of renal function and yet maintain a plasma creatinine level of $<125 \, \mu mol/l$. If there is more severe renal dysfunction, however, further small decreases in glomerular filtration rate (GFR) cause plasma creatinine to increase markedly (Levey, Perrone and Madias, 1988). Nevertheless, a woman who has lost 75 per cent of her nephrons may have lost only 50 per cent of function and may have a deceptively normal plasma creatinine due to hyperfiltration in the remaining nephrons. With renal disease, most women will remain symptom free until GFR declines to <25 per cent of normal, and many plasma constituents are frequently normal until a late stage of the disease. Decreases in renal function are accompanied by reduced fertility and decreased ability to sustain a viable pregnancy (Abe *et al.*, 1985; Kincaid-Smith and Fairley, 1987; Lindheimer and Katz, 1987). Normal pregnancy is rare when non-pregnant levels of plasma creatinine and urea exceed 275 µmol/l and 10 mmol/l, respectively, a degree of functional impairment that may not cause symptoms or disrupt homoeostasis in a non-pregnant woman but that invariably jeopardizes pregnancy.

The question for a woman with renal disease must be: 'Is pregnancy advisable?' If it is, then the sooner she starts to have her family the better, because in many cases renal function will continue to decline with time. The question for a woman with suspected or known renal disease, not counselled before pregnancy and presenting as a *fait accompli*, must be: 'Should pregnancy continue?'

Chronic renal dysfunction and its impact on pregnancy

Both obstetrical and remote renal prognoses depend on the degree of renal dysfunction and the impact of pregnancy is best considered by categories of pre-pregnancy renal impairment (Tables 5.4 and 5.5).

Table 5.4.   **Pre-pregnancy renal status**

Status	Plasma creatinine (µmol/l)
Mild	<125
Moderate	125–250
Severe	>250

Preserved/mildly impaired renal function

When pre-pregnancy plasma creatinine is 125 µmol/l there is usually a good obstetric outcome and no adverse long-term renal effect (Jungers, Huiller and Forget, 1987; Lindheimer and Katz, 1987). This statement should, however, be tempered somewhat in lupus nephropathy, membranoproliferative glomerulonephritis, focal glomerulosclerosis and perhaps IgA nephropathy and reflux nephropathy, all of which can be adversely influenced by intercurrent pregnancy.

Most women will have GFR increments during pregnancy but less than in normal pregnancy. Increased proteinuria occurs in 50 per cent of pregnancies (although rarely in women with chronic pyelonephritis) and occasionally is massive (often exceeding 3 g in 24 h), leading to nephrotic oedema.

Table 5.5.   **Pregnancy prospects for women with chronic renal disease**

Renal status	Problems in pregnancy (%)	Successful obstetric outcome (%)	Problems in long term (%)
Mild	27	95 (85)	<5 (9)
Moderate	49	90 (59)	25 (71)
Severe	84	48 (8)	53 (92)

Estimates based on 1586 women/2244 pregnancies (1973–1991) which attained at least 28 weeks' gestation. Figures in parentheses refer to prospects when complications developed before 28 weeks' gestation. Collagen diseases are not included (JM Davison, unpublished)

Moderate renal insufficiency

When pre-pregnancy plasma creatinine is 125–250 μmol/l, prognosis is more guarded (Hou, Grossman and Madias, 1985; Hou, 1987). The major worries are serious renal deterioration (particularly early in pregnancy), uncontrolled hypertension, variable obstetric outcome and accelerated postpartum decline in renal function (Surian *et al.*, 1984; Jungers *et al.*, 1986).

Severe renal insufficiency

When plasma creatinine >250 μmol/l, most women have amenorrhoea and/or are anovulatory (Lim, 1987). The likelihood of conception, let alone having a normal pregnancy and outcome is low but not, as some have been misled to believe, impossible (Hou, 1987). The chance of a successful obstetrical outcome is less than the risk of severe maternal complications and perhaps such women should not therefore be taking additional health risks. The aim should be to preserve what little renal function remains and/or to achieve renal rehabilitation via a dialysis and transplant programme, after which the question of pregnancy can be reconsidered, if appropriate (Davison, Katz and Lindheimer, 1986).

Antenatal problems and their management

Antenatal visits should be at 2-week intervals until 32 weeks' gestation, after which assessment should be weekly. Routine serial antenatal observations should be supplemented by (1) assessment of renal function by 24-h creatinine clearance and protein excretion, (2) careful monitoring of blood pressure for early detection of hypertension and then assessment of its severity, (3) early detection of pre-eclampsia, (4) assessment of fetal size, development and well-being.

Renal function

If renal function deteriorates significantly at any stage of pregnancy, reversible causes, such as urinary tract infection, subtle dehydration or electrolyte imbalance (occasionally precipitated by inadvertent diuretic therapy) should be sought. Near term, as in normal pregnancy, a 15–20 per cent decrement in function, which affects blood creatinine minimally, is nothing to worry about. Failure to detect a reversible cause of a significant decrement is a reason for ending the pregnancy by elective delivery. When proteinuria occurs and persists, but blood pressure is normal and renal function preserved, pregnancy can be allowed to continue.

Blood pressure

Most of the specific risks of hypertension in pregnancy appear to be mediated through superimposed pre-eclampsia in women with pre-existing renal disease. This is because the diagnosis cannot be made with certainty on clinical grounds alone, as hypertension and proteinuria may be manifestations of the underlying renal disease. Treatment of mild hypertension (diastolic blood pressure <95 mmHg in the second trimester or <100 mmHg in the third trimester) is not necessary during normal pregnancy, but many experts would treat women with underlying renal disease more aggressively, believing that this preserves renal function.

Monitoring the fetus and timing of delivery

Regular assessment of fetal well-being is mandatory because renal disease can be associated with intrauterine growth retardation and, when complications do arise, the judicious moment for intervention can be best assessed by changes in the fetal status. Current technology should minimize intrauterine fetal death as well as neonatal morbidity and mortality. Regardless of gestational age, most babies weighing 1500 g or more survive better in a special care nursery than in a hostile intrauterine environment. Planned preterm delivery may also be necessary if renal function deteriorates substantially, if uncontrollable hypertension supervenes or if eclampsia occurs.

Role of renal biopsy in pregnancy

Experience of renal biopsy during pregnancy is slight, mainly because clinical circumstances rarely justify the risks: biopsy is therefore usually deferred until after delivery. Reports of excessive bleeding and other complications in pregnant women have led some to consider pregnancy as a relative contraindication to renal biopsy (Schewitz, Friedman and Pollak, 1965), although others have not observed any increased morbidity (Lindheimer, Spargo and Katz, 1975; Lindheimer *et al.*, 1981). When renal biopsy is undertaken in the immediate post-delivery phase with well-controlled blood pressure and normal coagulation indices, the morbidity is no different to that reported in non-pregnant patients.

The latest account of renal biopsy in pregnancy, involving 111 women, all preterm, confirms and extends the impression that the risks of the procedure resemble those in the non-pregnant population (Packham and Fairley, 1987). The incidence of transient haematuria was 0.9 per cent (considerably less than the 3–5 per cent for non-pregnant patients), a statistic that no doubt reflects the experience and technical skills of the unit and careful pre-biopsy evaluation of the women. However, these results should not be used to encourage inexperienced clinicians to undertake biopsy in pregnancy.

It is important to have specific indications for renal biopsy in pregnancy. Packham and Fairley (1987) suggest that closed (percutaneous) needle biopsy should be undertaken more often, because they believe that certain glomerular disorders are adversely influenced by pregnancy and that specific therapy, such as anti-platelet agents, might be beneficial. The consensus, however, goes against such broad indications and defends the traditional position that renal biopsy should be performed infrequently during pregnancy.

The few widely agreed indications for antenatal biopsy are as follows:

1. Sudden deterioration of renal function before 30–32 weeks' gestation, with no obvious cause. Certain forms of rapidly progressive glomerulonephritis may respond to aggressive treatment with steroid 'pulses', chemotherapy and perhaps plasma exchange, when diagnosed early.
2. Symptomatic nephrotic syndrome before 30–32 weeks' gestation. Although some might consider a therapeutic trial of steroids in such cases, it is best to determine beforehand whether the lesion is likely to respond to steroids, because pregnancy is itself a hypercoagulable state prone to deterioration by such treatment. On the other hand, proteinuria alone with well-preserved renal function in non-pre-eclamptic pregnant women without gross oedema and/or

hypoalbuminaemia, suggests the need for close monitoring with biopsy deferred until the puerperium.
3. Presentation characterized by 'active urinary sediment', proteinuria and border-line renal function in a woman who has not been evaluated in the past. This is a controversial area and it could be argued that diagnosis of a collagen disorder such as scleroderma or periarteritis would be grounds for terminating the pregnancy, or that classifying the type of lesion in a woman with lupus would determine the type of therapy.

Problems associated with specific renal diseases

These are summarized in Table 5.6

Table 5.6.   Pregnancy and specific renal diseases

Renal disease	Effects
Chronic glomerulonephritis	Usually no adverse effect in the absence of hypertension. One view is that glomerulonephritis is adversely affected by the coagulation changes of pregnancy. Urinary tract infections may occur more frequently
Pyelonephritis	Bacteriuria can lead to exacerbation
Reflux nephropathy	Risks of sudden escalating hypertension and worsening of renal function
Urolithiasis	Infections can be more frequent, but ureteral dilatation and stasis do not seem to affect the natural history
Polycystic renal disease	Functional impairment and hypertension usually minimal in childbearing years
Diabetic nephropathy	No adverse effect on the renal lesion, but there is increased frequency of infection, oedema, and/or pre-eclampsia
Permanent urinary diversion	May be associated with other malformations of the genital tract. Urinary tract infection common during pregnancy. Renal function may undergo reversible decrease. No significant obstructive problem but caesarean section often needed for abnormal presentation
After nephrectomy, solitary and pelvic kidney	May be associated with other malformations of urogenital tract. Pregnancy well tolerated. Dystocia rarely occurs with a pelvic kidney
Periarteritis nodosa	Fetal prognosis is dismal. Maternal death often occurs
Scleroderma (SS)	If onset during pregnancy then can be rapid overall deterioration. Reactivation of quiescent scleroderma may occur *post partum*
Wegener's granulomatosis	Paucity of information. Avoid cytotoxics in early pregnancy. Proteinuria ($\pm$ hypertension) common from early in pregnancy

Acute glomerulonephritis and chronic glomerular disease

The acute disease is a rare complication of pregnancy but it can be mistaken for pre-eclampsia. With chronic glomerular disease, one view warns of aggravation because of the hypercoagulable state accompanying pregnancy, with women more prone to superimposed pre-eclampsia or hypertensive crisis earlier in pregnancy (Packham *et al.*, 1989). The consensus, however, is that renal function decreases only in patients with diffuse glomerulonephritis, where hypertension is invariably both more common and severe; none the less, most pregnancies are successful (Lindheimer and Katz, 1987).

The course of pregnancy in women with IgA nephropathy is controversial. Some emphasize the substantial and occasionally irreversible deterioration in renal function (Kincaid-Smith and Fairley, 1987; Packham and Fairley, 1987; Packham *et al.*, 1989), whereas others argue that pregnancy outcome and long-term renal prognosis are excellent when hypertension is absent before pregnancy and GFR is preserved (Abe *et al.*, 1985; Barcelo *et al.*, 1986; Jungers, Huiller and Forget, 1987).

Hereditary nephritis is an uncommon disorder that may first become manifest or may be exacerbated during pregnancy; however, most pregnancies succeed. There is a variant of hereditary nephritis involving disordered platelet morphology and function where pregnancy, although usually successful, can be complicated by bleeding problems.

Pyelonephritis (tubulo-interstitial disease)

Acute pyelonephritis has been dealt with earlier. GFR may be reduced during an acute episode in pregnancy, in contradistinction to the usual lack of change in non-pregnant patients. Also specific to pregnancy is a form of adult respiratory distress syndrome (ARDS), as well as haematopoietic and liver dysfunction (Cunningham, Lucas and Hankins, 1987; Pruett and Faro, 1987).

In patients with chronic pyelonephritis, the prognosis in pregnancy is similar to that for patients with glomerular disease, with a better outcome in women with adequate renal function and normal blood pressure. The number of symptomatic infections increases in pregnancy but, overall, the antenatal course is more benign than in women with glomerular disease.

Reflux nephropathy

This term is used to describe renal morphological and functional changes that relate to past (and usually present) vesico-ureteric reflux, often complicated by recurrent infection. It is frequently associated with hypertension and moderate or severe renal dysfunction, features which, as discussed earlier, adversely affect the outcome of pregnancy (Jungers, Huiller and Forget, 1987). Specific obstetric worries in these patients include severe fetal intrauterine growth retardation and the risk of sudden rapid deterioration in blood pressure and renal function with accelerated progression to renal failure (Becker *et al.*, 1986).

Urolithiasis

The prevalence of urolithiasis in pregnancy is 0.03–0.35 per cent (Maikrantz *et al.*, 1987). Renal and ureteric calculi are one of the most common causes of non-uterine abdominal pain severe enough to need hospital admission during pregnancy. Management should be conservative initially, with adequate hydration, appropriate antibiotic therapy and pain relief with systemic analgesics. The use of continuous segmental (T11–L2) epidural block has been advocated and may even favourably influence spontaneous passage of the stone(s). With good pain relief, the woman micturates without difficulty, moves without assistance and is less at risk from thromboembolic problems than if drowsy, nauseated and bedridden with pain.

When there are complications that might need surgical intervention, ultrasound examination can be helpful and pregnancy should not be a deterrent to intravenous urography (IVU). There are, however, specific clinical criteria for undertaking an IVU: (1) microscopic haematuria, (2) recurrent urinary tract symptoms and (3) sterile urine culture when pyelonephritis is suspected. The presence of two of these features indicates a diagnosis of calculi in 60 per cent of women (Miller and Kakkis, 1982).

Alternative management involves the cystoscopic placement with local anaesthesia of an internal ureteral tube, or stent, between bladder and kidney (Loughlin and Bailey, 1986). The stent retains its position because of a pigtail or J-like curve at each end (double-J) and it can be changed every 8 weeks (to prevent encrustation). Early empirical use for presumed stone obstruction in patients with flank pain is recommended, especially when hydration, analgesia and antibiotics do not resolve pain and/or fever. When the pregnancy is over, standard management is resumed.

In patients with cystinuria, assiduous maintenance of high fluid intake is the mainstay of management. Although D-pencillinamine appears to be relatively safe it should be used only for severe cases, where urinary cystine excretion is known to be significantly increased (Gregory and Mansell, 1983).

Polycystic renal disease

This autosomal dominant disease may remain undiagnosed during pregnancy. Careful questioning for a history of familiar problems and the use of ultrasound could, however, lead to earlier detection. Patients do well when functional impairment is minimal and hypertension absent, as is often the case in childbearing years. There is, however, an increased incidence of hypertension late in pregnancy and a higher perinatal mortality compared with the pregnancies of sisters unaffected by the disease. If one or other parent has polycystic renal disease, they may seek genetic counselling, as there will be a 50 per cent chance of transmitting the disease to their offspring. On the one hand DNA probe techniques allow antenatal diagnosis from chorionic villus sampling, so that women can undergo selective termination of pregnancy (Reeders et al., 1986) and on the other hand, it has been argued that routine genetic screening is unnecessary (Watson, MacNichol and Wright, 1990).

Diabetic nephropathy

Women who have been diabetic since childhood may already have renal microangiopathic changes (Hayslett and Reece, 1987). Even so, most patients with diabetic nephropathy demonstrate the normal gestational increment in GFR and pregnancy does not appear to accelerate renal deterioration (Reece et al., 1988). There is an increased prevalence of covert bacteriuria (and possibly susceptibility to urinary tract infection), peripheral oedema and pre-eclampsia (Cousins, 1987). Whether or not hypertension should be treated more aggressively, especially before conception, is still a matter of debate.

Systemic lupus erythematosus (SLE)

This relatively common disease has a predilection for women of childbearing age and is thus of importance in nephrological obstetrics. Coincidence with pregnancy poses complex clinical problems owing to the profound disturbance of the immunological system, the multiple organ involvement and the complicated immunology of pregnancy itself (Mor-Josef *et al.*, 1984; *Lancet* Editorial, 1989b; Out, Derksen and Christiaeus, 1989).

Effect of pregnancy on SLE

As far as the disease process itself is concerned, transient improvements, no change and a tendency to relapse have all been reported during pregnancy (Out, Derksen and Christiaeus, 1989). As is the case with most illnesses that run a fluctuating course, it is difficult to document any special effect of pregnancy on SLE. The general consensus is that pregnancy does not affect the long-term prognosis of SLE, but pregnancy itself may be associated with more exacerbations, particularly in the puerperium. As women are usually observed more closely during pregnancy, this is not surprising. In addition, women with SLE are normally advised against conceiving during an active phase of the disease and therefore conceive when they are well. If the effect of pregnancy is judged by comparing the state in pregnancy with that before pregnancy, their condition can only stay unchanged, if they were well before pregnancy, or deteriorate; this is a further source of bias. Where comparisons with the pre-pregnancy period have been made, however, the exacerbation rate was three times greater in the first half of pregnancy, twice as great in the second half, and at least six times greater in the puerperium (Garsenstein, Pollak and Kark, 1962) – the time when the majority of maternal deaths occur (Kochenour *et al.*, 1987).

Decisions regarding the status of the disease and the importance to the woman and her partner of having a baby, should be made on an individual basis. The majority of pregnancies succeed, especially when the maternal disease has been in clinical remission for 6 months before conception, even if there were severe pathological changes in the original renal biopsy and heavy proteinuria in the early stage of the disease (Jungers, Dougados and Pellissies, 1982). Women should be discouraged from becoming pregnant until disease control is established or offered therapeutic abortion if they become pregnant during active disease. Continued signs of disease activity and/or increasing renal dysfunction certainly reduce the likelihood of an uncomplicated pregnancy.

Antiphospholipid and anticardiolipin antibodies

SLE sera may contain a bewildering array of autoantibodies against nucleic acids, nucleoproteins, cell surface antigens and phospholipids. The levels of all antibodies may be elevated quite disproportionately to the clinical severity of the SLE and some women with a bad obstetric history as well as high antibody titres display hardly any clinical evidence of SLE.

Antiphospholipid antibodies (APA or aPL-Ab) are directed against negatively charged phospholipids and exert a complicated effect on the coagulation system, which has led to the rather enigmatic definition of a lupus anticoagulant that is found in 5–10 per cent of patients with SLE (Schleider *et al.*, 1986; Lockshin and Druzin, 1985). *In vitro* there is prolongation of the kaolin-cephalin and the activated partial thromboplastin clotting times, even when the plasma is mixed with an equal quantity of normal plasma (Scott, 1984). Paradoxically, the lupus anticoagulant is associated with increased risk of thromboembolism, both arterial and venous, and excessive bleeding is very rare.

Anticardiolipin antibodies, which may belong to both IgG and IgM subtypes, are active against certain phospholipid components of cell walls. They are responsible for the 'false positive Wasserman reaction' [Venereal Disease Research Laboratories (VDRL) serological test] that can occur in SLE.

The fetus of a woman who has lupus anticoagulant or anticardiolipin antibodies is at risk in all three trimesters of pregnancy. It is, therefore, no surprise that in women with a bad obstetric history both antibodies are often present in high titre. If not, the level of anticardiolipin antibodies, particularly the IgG subtype, is usually considered to be a better predictor of fetal outcome, probably because it is subject to less variability (Harris et al., 1986; Lockwood et al., 1986).

The mortality risk if the mother has lupus anticoagulant has been put at 85–92 per cent (Branch et al., 1985; Lubbe and Liggins, 1985). However, when data have been culled from the literature, the women identified have often had the lupus anticoagulant measured because of a bad obstetric history. In a group of women attending a rheumatology clinic for SLE who have the lupus anticoagulant (or anticardiolipin antibodies), the risk to the fetus may be much less, although one retrospective study of anticardiolipin antibodies in women with SLE does not support this concept (Lockshin et al., 1985). It should be borne in mind that in the general obstetric population the incidence of lupus anticoagulant is very low, probably <1 per cent, but in women presenting with unexplained recurrent abortion the incidence of subclinical autoimmune disease ranges from 1 to 29 per cent and autoantibodies may be important.

The mechanism(s) by which these antibodies might affect the fetus is unknown. The antibodies can bind to cell surface phospholipids of a variety of cell types, including platelets, vascular endothelial cells and possibly trophoblastic cells. Furthermore, there may be an overlap with lymphocytotoxic antibodies (cLCTA) also found in SLE (McIntyre et al., 1984). The possible mechanisms of action in recurrent fetal death might include platelet damage with increased adhesiveness, interference with the phospholipid part of the prothrombin activator complex and inhibition of prostacyclin (PGI_2) production by vascular tissues leading to decidual vasculopathy and placental infarction (Branch et al., 1985).

Anti-Ro antibodies

This IgG autoantibody to soluble ribonucleoprotein is found in about 24 per cent of SLE patients (Scott, 1984). Sixty per cent of all mothers who deliver a baby with congenital heart block have anti-Ro (as well as anti-La) antibodies and anti-Ro autoantibodies are almost always present in women with SLE whose neonates have heart block (Maddison et al., 1983). After transplacental passage, the IgG is deposited in the fetal heart, initiating immune inflammatory responses leading to fibrosis and calcification of the atrioventricular node and bundle of His (Esscher and Scott, 1979), endocardial fibroelastosis, cardiomyopathy and, occasionally, multiple structural abnormalities (Taylor et al., 1986). The critical damage presumably occurs during cardiac organogenesis at 6 weeks of pregnancy. As the mother's heart is usually unaffected, this suggests that the fetal heart is more vulnerable to antibody-mediated damage because it may possess phase-specific antigens; alternatively, blocking (maternal) antibodies may be lacking, as IgA and IgM are not transferred to the fetus. There is a report of maternal SLE becoming apparent, clinically and serologically, many years after the birth of a baby with heart block (Kasinath and Katz, 1983).

Abortion
Although the incidence of abortion in women with SLE may be as high as 40 per cent, the risk is not clearly related to the severity of the condition nor is it shared by other connective tissue diseases (Fraga *et al.*, 1974). Furthermore, abortion often occurs later than the normal 10–14 weeks' gestation and, indeed, may occur at any gestation up to 28 weeks. In these women there can be a high titre of lymphocytotoxic antibodies, the absorption of which on to trophoblast could initiate a number of abortion mechanisms (Baesnihan *et al.*, 1977); for example, necrotizing decidual vascular lesions with immunoglobulin deposition have been described (Abramowsky *et al.*, 1980).

Hypertension and renal failure
In SLE, renal involvement is an unfavourable prognosticator. Normal renal function and normotension are associated with a successful obstetrical outcome in 88 per cent of cases (Hayslett and Lynn, 1980). Neither proteinuria nor the development of the nephrotic syndrome influence fetal prognosis but when renal function is impaired (plasma creatinine >130 μmol/l), there is a 50 per cent fetal loss (Fine, Barnett and Danovitch, 1981).

The differentiation of pre-eclampsia from a renal 'flare' of SLE is difficult but important with respect to treatment. About 30 per cent of SLE patients with a history of renal involvement develop hypertension and worsening proteinuria in pregnancy (Gimovsky, Montoro and Paul, 1984) and 50–80 per cent of all pregnant SLE patients with pre-eclamptic features have a history of nephritis (Zulman *et al.*, 1980; Lockshin, Reuitz and Druzin, 1984). Irreversible loss of renal function occurs, especially in the latter group of women (Zulman *et al.*, 1980). Serological findings do not distinguish a 'flare' but the occurrence of an active urine sediment and extrarenal exacerbation(s) strongly support the diagnosis of active nephritis.

Lupus nephropathy may sometimes become manifest for the first time during pregnancy and, when accompanied by hypertension and renal dysfunction, may again be mistaken for pre-eclampsia. Such patients are at high risk of fetal loss and in some instances a fulminant illness leads to maternal death. Some patients have a definite tendency to relapse, occasionally severely, in the puerperium and it is therefore usually considered prudent to prescribe or increase steroid therapy at this time (Leikin, Arof and Pearlman, 1986), even although a carefully performed case-controlled study does not seem to confirm this advice (Lockshin, Reuitz and Druzin, 1984). Very occasionally, a particularly severe postpartum syndrome may develop, consisting of pleural haemorrhages, effusion(s) and infiltration with fever, ECG abnormalities and even cardiomyopathy typified by extensive IgG, IgM, IgA and C3 deposition in the myocardium (Kochenour *et al.*, 1987).

Heart block and other cardiac defects in the newborn
About one in three mothers (38 per cent) who deliver babies with congenital heart block have, or will have, a connective tissue disease (Esscher and Scott, 1979) and most frequently that disease is SLE. Fetal outcome cannot be correlated with fetal (or maternal) antibody levels, apart from the relationship between congenital heart block and anti-Ro. The anti-Ro antibody involvement may explain why the fetal

prognosis is not invariably good even in the absence of recognized well-established markers for fetal death such as anticardiolipin antibodies (Singsen *et al.*, 1985). The baby with heart block usually survives and often does not require pacing. In a few cases with congenital heart block (and without anticardiolipin antibodies), however, the fetus dies *in utero* or in labour (Watson, Lane and Barnett, 1984).

Neonatal lupus syndrome
It is generally thought that neonatal lupus syndrome is associated with the presence of anti-Ro antibodies in the maternal blood and up to 5 per cent of these babies develop problems. The cardiac abnormalities are emphasized but there can be haemolytic anaemia, leucopenia, thrombocytopenia and discoid skin lesions on the face or scalp, all of which are usually transient (Nathan and Snapper, 1958; Vonderheid *et al.*, 1976). Occasionally a neonate develops SLE in the absence of any involvement in the mother. Cord and neonatal blood samples may show positive lupus-related antibodies and in particular a positive ANF and raised DNA-binding may persist for a week or two after delivery.

Monitoring SLE in pregnancy
Even though the nephrological involvement and the need for serial surveillance may seem the most significant features in a patient, it is prudent to screen for lupus anticoagulant in all women with SLE by some phospholipid-dependent coagulation test such as the activated partial thromboplastin time (APTT) and for anticardiolipin antibody by an enzyme-linked immunosorbent assay (ELISA) or a radioimmunoassay (RIA). The problem of which antibody is the best predictor of fetal loss is compounded by considerable methodological variation in assay procedures (Out, Derksen and Christiaeus, 1989). As the ESR is elevated in normal pregnancy, reduction of C_3 complement can be used as an objective index of disease activity (Zurier *et al.*, 1978).

The higher the titre of anticardiolipin antibodies, the greater the risk to the fetus, with the IgG subtype probably a better predictor of fetal outcome. Anti-Ro and the fetal cardiac implications may explain why fetal prognosis is not always good even in the absence of anticardiolipin antibodies. Even if the fetus does not die it can be jeopardized *in utero*, as judged by abnormal fetal heart rate traces (Lockshin *et al.*, 1985; Davison and Radford, 1989).

Treatment regimens in pregnancy
The drugs most frequently used for the treatment of SLE are simple analgesics such as paracetamol and non-steroidal anti-inflammatory drugs including aspirin. In more severe cases antimalarial drugs, corticosteroids, other immunosuppressives and cytotoxic agents are used. It was originally hoped that the use of corticosteroids would decrease the high abortion rate associated with SLE but in general this has not been the case (Fraga *et al.*, 1974). Recent reports, however, suggest that aggressive treatment with aspirin 75–300 mg/day and prednisone in doses increasing to 60 mg/day can suppress lupus anticoagulant and anticardiolipin antibodies and consequently improve outcome (Lubbe *et al.*, 1984; Branch *et al.*, 1985). This dose of prednisone often makes the woman cushingoid and can induce diabetes, which will require further treatment. The pregnancies are still usually complicated by hypertension or growth retardation and require very careful monitoring.

A standard approach nowadays is to reserve steroid therapy for patients who have antibodies and a bad obstetric history. Patients who have antibodies but a good obstetric history or no obstetric history (primigravidae) can be treated with aspirin 75 mg/day only, unless it is judged that they also require steroids for fetal reasons. In patients where steroid and aspirin therapy has been unsuccessful, a variety of additional therapies have been tried including azathioprine, heparin and plasma exchange, but their place is even less clear than the place of aspirin and steroid therapy (Lubbe *et al.*, 1984; Chan, Marris and Hughes, 1986; Gregorini, Setti and Remuzzi, 1986). Non-steroid anti-inflammatory agents are best avoided in normal therapeutic doses during the last trimester and if a patient requires extra therapy for this relatively short time, corticosteroids should be used.

Patients who also have a past history of thromboembolism, arterial or venous, should be treated with subcutaneous heparin throughout pregnancy in addition to any aspirin and prednisone therapy that might be considered necessary. Although heparin may exacerbate the bone loss associated with steroid therapy, it is necessary in view of the potential dire consequences, particularly of cerebral arterial thrombosis (Farquharson, Compston and Bloom, 1984).

The removal of anticardiolipin antibodies and lupus anticoagulant is not a guarantee of success nor is failure to remove the antibodies a guarantee of fetal demise (Reece *et al.*, 1984; Kilpatrick, 1986). Prospective attempts to reduce the effects of anti-Ro antibody in the fetus (and possibly the mother) have involved plasma exchange supplemented with high dose steroids (1 mg/kg/day), antiplatelet drugs as well as thromboxane-suppressing drugs (Barclay *et al.*, 1987). Success is very rare, however, and anti-Ro antibody is not necessarily completely removed from the maternal serum and is invariably detected in cord blood (Venning *et al.*, 1988).

Monitoring the fetus and timing of delivery
The timing of delivery depends on the severity of the clinical condition, which antibodies are present and the degree of renal involvement and/or hypertension. If there are no complications, the patient should be delivered at term. Increasing degrees of renal failure or hypertension will necessitate early delivery, either for these reasons alone or because of evidence of fetal compromise, as judged by poor growth, cardiotocography or Doppler ultrasound measurement of fetal and maternal placental blood flow.

Congenital heart block can be diagnosed before delivery from routine auscultation of the fetal heart and subsequent cardiotocography when bradycardia is discovered. A detailed ultrasound examination of the fetal heart should reveal atrioventricular dissociation confirming complete heart block and any structural heart disease, present in 15–20 per cent of cases (Stephenson, Clelland and Hallidive-Smith, 1981; Davison and Radford, 1989). If the fetus has complete heart block, it is difficult to monitor its general condition *in utero*, both antenatally and in labour, as accurate assessment usually depends on measurement of fetal heart rate and its variability. It is possible, however, to measure the atrial rate and its variability by detailed ultrasound. Measurement of umbilical blood flow by Doppler ultrasound and antenatal fetal blood sampling (cordocentesis or percutaneous umbilical blood sampling (PUBS)) for the measurement of fetal blood gases may be of value in this situation (Soothill *et al.*, 1986; Kleinmen, Copel and Hobbins, 1987). Labour can be monitored by repeated fetal scalp blood sampling but many such fetuses are understandably delivered by elective caesarean section. In patients taking long-term steroids, parenteral cover should be given for delivery.

Periarteritis nodosa

Obstetric outcome in women with renal involvement attributable to periarteritis nodosa is very poor, largely because of the associated hypertension, frequently of a malignant nature. Very few successful pregnancies have been reported and usually fetal prognosis is dismal. Many pregnancies end in maternal death, which may reflect the nature of the disease itself. Early therapeutic termination has less maternal risk.

Permanent urinary diversion

Although permanent urinary diversion is still used in the management of patients with congenital lower urinary tract defects, its use has declined for neurogenic bladders because of the introduction of self-catheterization. The most common complication of pregnancy is urinary tract infection and the use of prophylactic antibiotic therapy throughout pregnancy may reduce its incidence. Decline in renal function may occur, invariably related to infection or intermittent obstruction. With an ileal conduit, elevation and compression by the expanding uterus can cause outflow obstruction, whereas with a utero–sigmoid anastomosis, actual ureteric obstruction may occur (Barrett and Peters, 1983). After delivery the changes usually reverse.

Premature labour occurs in 20 per cent, possibly related to urinary tract infection. The mode of delivery depends on obstetrical considerations. Abnormal presentation, related to genital abnormalities, accounts for a caesarean section rate of 25 per cent. Vaginal delivery is safe but as continence with a urethro–sigmoid anastomosis depends on an intact anal sphincter, this must be protected with a mediolateral episiotomy.

Solitary kidney

Ablation of renal mass results in hypertrophy of the remnant kidney together with compensatory renal vasodilatation and hence increases plasma flow rate and filtration in surviving nephrons (Finkelstein and Hayslett, 1979). It has been suggested, largely on the basis of animal studies, that in the long term this compensatory renal vasodilation provides a damaging stimulus to the remaining nephrons (Brenner, 1985). The extent of compensatory vasodilatation in the remnant kidney is proportional to the amount of renal mass removed (Finkelstein and Hayslett, 1979) and available evidence in 'single-kidney man' suggests that the hyperfiltration secondary to removal of 50 per cent of renal mass (i.e. one kidney) has little long-term impact on the remaining kidney (Fotino, 1989).

It is important to know the indication for, and the time since, the nephrectomy (Klein, 1983). In patients with an infectious and/or structural renal problem, sequential pre-pregnancy investigation is needed for detection of any persistent infection. Despite the renal hypertrophy and compensatory hyperfiltration following uninephrectomy, women with single kidneys (removed owing to renal trauma) exhibit a further gestational increase in GFR (Davison, 1978). It makes no difference whether the right or left kidney remains, as long as it is located in the normal anatomical position. If function is normal and stable, women with single kidneys seem to tolerate pregnancy well.

If infection occurs in a solitary kidney during pregnancy and does not quickly respond to antibiotics, termination of pregnancy may have to be considered for the preservation of renal function. Ectopic kidneys (usually pelvic) are more vulnerable to infection and are associated with decreased fetal salvage, probably because of associated malformations of the genital tract. Follow-up of a group of women kidney donors who subsequently underwent 1–3 pregnancies, has indicated that the intermittent periods of gestational hyperfiltration have no long-term damaging effects on the remaining kidney (Buszta *et al.*, 1985).

Scleroderma or systemic sclerosis

Scleroderma is a term that includes a heterogeneous group of systemic conditions causing hardening of the skin. Systemic sclerosis implies involvement both of skin and of other sites, particularly certain internal organs: renal involvement occurs in at least 60 per cent of patients, usually within 3–4 years of diagnosis. The presentation may be the sudden onset of malignant hypertension, rapidly progressive renal failure or slowly worsening proteinuria or azotaemia.

The combination with pregnancy is rare, as systemic sclerosis occurs most often in the fourth and fifth decades and younger patients with systemic sclerosis are usually infertile. Where systemic sclerosis has its onset in pregnancy, there is a greater tendency for deterioration. There are also instances when pregnancy has been uneventful and successful but marked reactivation occurred unexpectedly post-delivery (Smith, 1982). Most maternal deaths involve rapidly progressive scleroderma with severe pulmonary complications, infections, hypertension or renal failure.

The extent of systemic involvement is probably more important than the duration of the disease and limited mild disease carries a better prognosis. The sclerotic process usually spares the abdominal wall skin and the expanding girth can be accommodated. There is one report of hydronephrosis, however, presumed to be secondary to a thickened abdominal wall and therefore decreased abdominal wall skin compliance, in a twin pregnancy complicated by polyhydramnios (Moore, Saffron and Barof, 1985).

Wegener's granulomatosis

Wegener's granulomatosis is a rare disease of unknown cause, consisting of necrotizing granulomata with vasculitis of the respiratory tract, systemic vasculitis and focal necrotizing glomerulitis, as well as an elevated serum anti-neutrophil cytoplasmic antibody titre (ANCA). Without treatment 90 per cent of patients die within 2 years of onset. The use of cytotoxic drugs with or without immunosuppression has greatly improved remission rates. A successful outcome, when complicating pregnancy, has been reported on three occasions. In one case labour was induced at 28 weeks' gestation because of severe hypertension (Talbot, Main and Levinson, 1984) but in the other two the pregnancy was allowed to go to term (Cooper, Stafford and Warwick, 1970; Murty, Davison and Cameron, 1990). Proteinuria, without hypertension or severe renal dysfunction, was a feature of these two pregnancies. In one case a tracheostomy, although predisposing to respiratory tract infection, did not otherwise complicate the course of pregnancy and labour, and even allowed the production of sufficient intra-abdominal pressure to achieve a normal vaginal delivery (Murty, Davison and Cameron, 1990). Millford and Belini (1986) reported a maternal death from intracerebral haemorrhage in the second trimester, preceded by escalating hypertension.

Although experience is very limited, the consensus is that if conception occurs while the woman is receiving cytotoxic therapy, particularly cyclophosphamide, therapeutic abortion should be considered. Routine immunosuppression, however, is not a problem and can be continued throughout the pregnancy.

CLINICAL CONTROVERSIES ASSOCIATED WITH RENAL DISEASE

Long-term effects of pregnancy

Pregnancy does not cause any deterioration or otherwise affect the rate of progression of the disease beyond what might be expected in the non-pregnant state, provided that pre-pregnancy kidney dysfunction was minimal and hypertension absent during pregnancy. An important factor in long-term prognosis could be the sclerotic effect that hyperfiltration might already have had in the residual (intact) glomeruli of the kidneys of these women. The situation may be worse in a single diseased kidney where, frequently, more sclerosis has occurred within the fewer (intact) glomeruli. Theoretically, further progressive loss of renal function could ensue in pregnancy. Although animal work (Baylis, 1987; Baylis and Reckelhoff, 1991) and the limited evidence in women with renal disease argue against hyperfiltration-induced damage in pregnancy (Davison, 1989), there can be little doubt that in some women with moderate dysfunction there can be unpredicted, accelerated and irreversible renal decline in pregnancy or immediately afterwards.

Nephrotic syndrome in pregnancy

This term is still commonly used but it is non-specific. In fact the most common cause of nephrotic syndrome in late pregnancy is pre-eclampsia and fetal prognosis declines with increasing proteinuria (Fisher *et al.*, 1981). Other causes include proliferative or membranoproliferative glomerulonephritis, lipid nephrosis, lupus nephropathy, hereditary nephritis, diabetic nephropathy, renal vein thrombosis and amyloidosis. Some of these conditions do not respond to steroids and may even be seriously aggravated by their use, emphasizing the importance of a biopsy diagnosis before initiating steroid therapy.

If renal function is adequate and hypertension is absent, there should be few complications during pregnancy. Several of the physiological changes occurring during pregnancy may, however, simulate exacerbation or aggravation of the disease. For example, increments in renal haemodynamics as well as increases in renal vein pressure may enhance protein excretion. Serum albumin usually decreases by 5–10 g/l during normal pregnancy, and further decreases attributable to nephrotic syndrome may enhance the tendency towards fluid retention. Because of decreased intravascular volume, diuretic therapy probably compromises uteroplacental perfusion or aggravates the increased tendency to thrombotic episodes.

PREGNANCY IN HAEMODIALYSIS PATIENTS

Although libido is reduced and there is relative infertility, women on haemodialysis can conceive; they must therefore use contraception if they wish to avoid pregnancy.

Conception is not common (an incidence of 1 in 200 patients has been quoted), but its true frequency is unknown because most pregnancies in these women probably end in early spontaneous abortion (Hou, 1987). There is also a high therapeutic abortion rate in these women, suggesting that those who become pregnant do so inadvertently, probably because they are unaware that pregnancy is possible.

Despite the fact that viable infants are occasionally delivered, most authorities do not advise attempts at pregnancy or its continuation if it occurs inadvertently. Women on haemodialysis are at risk of volume overloading and severe exacerbations of their hypertension or superimposed pre-eclampsia. Clinicians are reluctant to publish unsuccessful cases as well as those that end in disaster, so that the true incidence of successful pregnancies is probably less than suggested in the few selective reports (Brem *et al.*, 1988; Gaucherand *et al.*, 1988). There is high fetal wastage at all stages of pregnancy and even when therapeutic terminations are excluded, the live birth outcome is at best 19 per cent (Davison, 1990).

Antenatal problems and their management

Women frequently present for care well advanced in pregnancy because the diagnosis was not suspected. Irregular menstruation is common and missed periods are usually ignored (Lim, 1987). Urine pregnancy tests are unreliable (even if urine is available). Ultrasonic evaluation is needed to confirm and to date the pregnancy.

For a successful outcome, scrupulous attention must be paid to dialysis strategy, problems of anaemia, fluid balance, blood pressure control and provision of good nutrition (Yasin and Bey Doun, 1988).

Dialysis strategy

Some patients show a gestational increment in their regular GFR but this is academic because all will require a 50 per cent increase in hours and frequency of dialysis. The planning of dialysis strategy has several aims:

1. To maintain plasma urea <20 mmol/l (some would argue <15 mmol/l), for intrauterine death is more likely if values exceed this critical mark. Success has occasionally been achieved despite levels of 25 mmol/l for several weeks.
2. To avoid hypotension during dialysis, which could be damaging to the fetus. In late pregnancy the enlarging uterus or the supine posture may aggravate this problem by decreasing venous return.
3. To avoid rapid fluctuations in intravascular volume, by limiting inter-dialysis weight gain to about 1 kg until late pregnancy.
4. To ensure rigid control of blood pressure.
5. To observe carefully for preterm labour, as dialysis and uterine contractions are associated.
6. To watch plasma calcium closely to avoid hypercalcaemia.

Anaemia

Dialysis patients are invariably anaemic and this is further aggravated in pregnancy. Unnecessary blood sampling should be avoided in the face of anaemia and lack of venepuncture sites. Blood transfusion is needed in 35 per cent of cases, especially before delivery. Caution is necessary because transfusion may exacerbate hypertension and impair the ability to control circulatory overload, even with extra dialysis. Fluctuations in blood volume can be minimized if packed red cells are transfused during dialysis.

Hypertension

A normotensive state before pregnancy is reassuring. As a generalization, blood pressure tends to be labile and hypertension is common, although control may be possible by careful dialysis. Some patients have abnormal lipid profiles and possibly accelerated atherogenesis, so that it is difficult to predict the cardiovascular capacity to tolerate pregnancy. Women with diabetic nephropathy as their original renal pathology are those in whom cardiovascular problems are most evident.

Nutrition

Despite more frequent dialysis, an uncontrolled dietary intake should be discouraged. A daily oral intake of 70 g protein, 1500 mg calcium, 50 mmol potassium and 80 mmol sodium is advised, with supplements of dialysable vitamins. Vitamin D supplements can be difficult to judge in patients who have had parathyroidectomy.

Monitoring the fetus and timing of delivery

The guidelines discussed for chronic renal disease apply here. Preterm labour is generally the rule and it may begin during haemodialysis. Caesarean section should be necessary only for purely obstetrical reasons. It has been argued, however, that elective caesarean section in all cases would minimize potential problems during labour.

Pregnancy in chronic ambulatory peritoneal dialysis (CAPD) patients

A few successful pregnancies have been reported (Kioko et al., 1983; Hou, 1987). Although anticoagulation and some of the fluid balance and volume problems of haemodialysis are avoided, the other major problems persist: hypertension, anaemia, placental abruption, sudden intrauterine death and premature labour. Furthermore, it should be remembered that peritonitis can be a severe complication of CAPD and accounts for the majority of therapeutic failures. This, superimposed on a pregnancy, can present a confusing diagnostic picture as well as a whole series of management dilemmas.

PREGNANCY IN RENAL ALLOGRAFT RECIPIENTS

Once they have received a renal transplant, most women have a rapid return of renal, endocrine and sexual functions and 1 woman in 50 of childbearing age with a functioning graft becomes pregnant. Of the conceptions, 40 per cent do not go beyond the first trimester because of spontaneous or therapeutic abortion. However, over 90 per cent of pregnancies that do continue past early pregnancy end successfully (Davison, 1990).

Transplants have been performed with the surgeons unaware that the recipient was in early pregnancy. Obstetric success in such cases does not diminish the

Table 5.7. Pregnancy prospects for renal allograft recipients

Problems in pregnancy (%)	Successful obstetrical outcome (%)	Problems in long term (%)
50	93 (73)	10 (29)

Estimates based on 1164 women in 1408 pregnancies which attained at least 28 weeks' gestation (1961–1990). Figures in parentheses refer to prospects when complications developed before 28 weeks' gestation. (From Davison, 1990)

importance of contraceptive (and other) counselling for all women in renal failure before surgery.

Ectopic pregnancy occurs in about 0.5 per cent of all of these conceptions. The diagnosis can be difficult because irregular bleeding and amenorrhoea accompany deteriorating renal function or even an intrauterine pregnancy. These patients may be at higher risk because of pelvic adhesions due to previous urological surgery, peritoneal dialysis, pelvic inflammatory disease or the use of intrauterine contraceptive devices. The main clinical problem is that symptoms secondary to genuine pelvic pathology are erroneously attributed to the graft.

Pre-pregnancy counselling

A woman must be counselled from the time she is taken on to a programme for treatment of her renal failure when the potential for optimal rehabilitation needs to be fully discussed (Davison and Lindheimer, 1989). Couples who want a child need to know all the implications, including the harsh realities of maternal survival prospects (Table 5.7). A post-transplant wait of 18 months to 2 years is advised so that the woman will have recovered from the surgery and any sequelae, graft function will have stabilized and immunosuppression will be at maintenance levels. Furthermore, if function is well maintained at 2 years, there is a high probability of allograft survival at 5 years.

A suitable set of guidelines is given here, but the criteria are only relative:

1. Good general health for about 2 years after transplantation.
2. Stature compatible with good obstetric outcome.
3. Minimal proteinuria.
4. No hypertension.
5. No evidence of graft rejection.
6. No pelvicalyceal distension on a recent intravenous urogram.
7. Stable renal function with plasma creatinine of $\leq 180\,\mu\text{mol/l}$ (preferably $< 130\,\mu\text{mol/l}$)
8. Drug therapy reduced to maintenance levels: prednisone, $\leq 15\,\text{mg/day}$ and azathioprine $\leq 2\,\text{mg/kg/body weight/day}$ has been quoted anecdotally. Limited experience has precluded recommending a safe dose of cyclosporin A but anecdotally $5\,\text{mg/kg/day}$ is quoted, or even a change to routine immunosuppression before, or in early, pregnancy.

Antenatal problems and their management

Any strategy must incorporate serial assessment of renal function, early diagnosis and treatment of rejection, control of blood pressure, early diagnosis or prevention of anaemia, treatment of any infection and meticulous assessment of fetal well-being (Hadi, 1986; Hou, 1989). Liver function tests, plasma proteins, calcium and phosphate should be checked at 6-weekly intervals (Davison, 1987). Screening for cytomegalovirus and herpes hominis virus should be undertaken during each trimester.

Allograft function

The sustained increase in GFR characteristic of early pregnancy in normal women is evident in renal transplant recipients, even though the transplant is ectopic, denervated, often derived from a male donor, potentially damaged by previous ischaemia and immunologically different from both the recipient and her fetus. The more rapidly the graft functions after transplant and the better the pre-pregnancy GFR, then the greater the increment in renal function during pregnancy.

Transient GFR reduction can occur during the third trimester without leading to permanent impairment. In 15 per cent of women, however, significant renal impairment does develop during pregnancy and may persist following delivery. As a gradual decline in function is common in non-pregnant patients, it is difficult to delineate the specific role of pregnancy, especially as sub-clinical chronic rejection with declining renal function may occur as a late result of acute rejection or when immunosuppression has not been adequate.

Proteinuria occurs near term in 40 per cent of women but disappears post partum and in the absence of hypertension is not significant. Whether or not cyclosporin A is more nephrotoxic in pregnancy compared with the non-pregnant state is not known (Bennett, Elzinga and Kelley, 1988); consequently, advice to switch to standard immunosuppressive regimens is based purely on clinical anecdote and evaluations are urgently needed in pregnancy.

Allograft rejection

In pregnancy the incidence of serious rejection is 9 per cent. Although this is no greater than that seen in non-pregnant individuals, it is unexpected because the privileged immunological status of pregnancy might have been expected to benefit the allograft. Rejection often occurs in the puerperium and this may be due to a return to a normal immune status (despite immunosuppression) or possibly may be a rebound effect from the altered gestational immunoresponsiveness.

Chronic rejection may be a problem in all recipients, having a progressive subclinical course, but the influence of a pregnancy is unknown and there are no predictive factors. There may be a non-immune contribution to chronic graft failure due to the damaging effect of hyperfiltration through remnant nephrons, perhaps even exacerbated during pregnancy (Feehally, Bennett and Harris, 1986). From the clinical viewpoint the following points are important: (1) rejection is difficult to diagnose; (2) if any of the clinical hallmarks are present (fever, oliguria, deteriorating renal function, renal enlargement and tenderness) then rejection should be considered; (3) although ultrasound may be helpful, without renal biopsy rejection cannot be distinguished from acute pyelonephritis, recurrent glomerulopathy, possibly severe pre-eclampsia and even cyclosporin A nephrotoxicity; (4) renal biopsy is indicated before embarking upon anti-rejection therapy.

Immunosuppressive therapy

This is usually maintained at pre-pregnancy levels, but adjustments may be needed if maternal leucocyte or platelet counts decrease. When white blood cell count is maintained within physiological limits for pregnancy, the neonate usually is born with a normal blood count (Davison, Dellagrammatikas and Parkin, 1985). Azathioprine-induced liver toxicity has been noted occasionally during pregnancy and the condition responds to dose reduction.

There is a paucity of good data on pregnancies in patients taking cyclosporin A (Flechner et al., 1985; Pickerell, Sawers and Michael, 1988; Derfler et al., 1989). Numerous adverse effects are attributed to this drug in non-pregnant transplant recipients including renal toxicity, hepatic dysfunction, tremor, convulsions, diabetogenic effects, haemolytic uraemic syndrome and neoplasia.

Hypertension and pre-eclampsia

Hypertension in the third trimester, its relationship to renal deterioration, chronic underlying pathology and pre-eclampsia is a diagnostic problem. On clinical grounds, pre-eclampsia is diagnosed in about 30 per cent of pregnancies.

Infections

Throughout pregnancy, patients should be carefully monitored for all types of infection, bacterial and viral. Prophylactic antibiotics must be given before any surgical procedure, however trivial.

Diabetes mellitus

The results of renal transplantation have been progressively improving in women whose renal failure was caused by diabetes mellitus. Pregnancies are now being reported and there is no doubt that problems occur with at least twice the frequency seen in non-diabetic, pregnant renal allograft recipients (Vimicor et al., 1984) possibly because of the generalized cardiovascular pathology that can accompany diabetes (Ogburn et al., 1986).

Interestingly, a few successful pregnancies have been reported after combined kidney–pancreas transplantation (Cahne et al., 1988; Tyden et al., 1989). In one woman, however, the pancreatic graft was rejected unexpectedly shortly after delivery, having functioned normally for 3 years before pregnancy.

Monitoring of the fetus and timing of delivery

The guidelines for chronic renal disease are equally applicable here. Preterm delivery is common (45–60 per cent), not only because of intervention for obstetric reasons but also because of the common occurrence of premature labour or premature rupture of membranes.

Delivery and management in labour

Vaginal delivery should be the aim. There should be no obstructive problems or mechanical injury to the transplant. In the absence of specific obstetrical problems, the spontaneous onset of labour can be awaited.

Careful monitoring of fluid balance, cardiovascular status and temperature is mandatory. Aseptic technique is essential for every procedure. Surgical induction of labour (by amniotomy) and episiotomy warrant antibiotic cover. Pain relief can be conducted as for healthy women. Augmentation of steroids should not be neglected.

Caesarean section is necessary for obstetrical reasons only. Occasionally, transplant patients have pelvic osteodystrophy related to previous renal failure (and dialysis) or prolonged steroid therapy (particularly before puberty) and antenatal recognition is essential. If there is a question of disproportion or kidney compression, simultaneous intravenous urogram and X-ray pelvimetry may be performed at 36 weeks' gestation. Remember that when a caesarean section is performed, a lower segment approach is usually feasible but previous urological surgery may make it difficult.

PAEDIATRIC MANAGEMENT

Over 50 per cent of liveborn babies have no neonatal problems (Hadi, 1986; Davison, 1987). Preterm delivery is common (45–60 per cent) and small-for-gestational-age infants are delivered in at least 20–30 per cent of pregnancies; occasionally, the two problems coexist.

Breast-feeding

Regarding azathioprine, little is known about the quantities in breast milk. Even less is known about cyclosporin A, except that levels in breast milk are usually greater than those in a simultaneously taken blood sample (Flechner et al., 1985). Until the many uncertainties are resolved, breast feeding should not be encouraged.

Long-term assessment

Azathioprine can cause leucocyte abnormalities, which may take almost 2 years to disappear spontaneously. In tissues not yet studied, however, these anomalies may not be temporary. The sequelae could be the eventual development of malignancies in affected offspring or abnormalities in the reproductive performance of the next generation (reviewed by Davison, 1987).

MATERNAL FOLLOW-UP AFTER PREGNANCY

Ultimate transplant success is the long-term survival of the woman and the transplant. It is only 25–30 years since this procedure became widely employed in the management of end-stage renal failure and so there are few long-term data from sufficiently large series from which to draw conclusions. Furthermore, it must be remembered that today's long-term results relate to a period of renal transplantation when many aspects of management would be unacceptable by current standards. Average international figures indicate that 70–80 per cent of the recipients of kidneys from related living donors are alive 5 years after transplantation; with cadaver kidneys the figure is 40–50 per cent. Furthermore, if renal function is normal 2 years after transplantation, then survival increases to about 80 per cent, which is another good reason for women to wait for about 2 years before attempting conception.

A major concern is that she may not survive or remain well enough to rear the child she bears. Pregnancy occasionally causes unpredictable irreversible renal decline. Even though the consensus is that pregnancy has no effect on graft function or survival (Sturgiss *et al.*, 1990), 10 per cent of mothers have died within 7 years of pregnancy.

Contraception

It is unwise to offer the option of sterilization at the time of transplantation. Oral contraception can cause or aggravate hypertension or thrombo-embolism and can also produce subtle changes in the immune system, but this does not necessarily contraindicate its use. An intrauterine contraceptive device (IUCD) may aggravate menstrual problems, which in turn may obscure symptoms and signs of early preg- nancy abnormalities, such as threatened miscarriage or ectopic pregnancy. The increased risk of chronic pelvic infection in an immunosuppressed patient with an IUCD is a substantial problem, for insertion or replacement of an IUCD in healthy women is associated with bacteraemia of vaginal origin in at least 13 per cent; antibiotic cover is therefore essential at this time (Murray, Hickey and Houang, 1987). Lastly, the efficacy of the IUCD is reduced in women taking immunosuppres- sive and anti-inflammatory agents.

Gynaecological problems

There is a danger that symptoms secondary to genuine pelvic pathology may be attributed erroneously to the transplant, owing to its location near the pelvis. Allograft recipients receiving immunosuppressive therapy have a malignancy rate many times greater than normal and the female genital tract is no exception (Alloub *et al.*, 1989). This association is probably related to factors such as loss of immune surveillance, chronic immunosuppression allowing tumour proliferation and pro- longed antigenic stimulation of the reticuloendothelial system. Regular gynaecologi- cal assessment is therefore essential. Management should be along conventional lines, with the outcome unlikely to be influenced by stopping or reducing immunosuppression.

OBSTETRICAL ACUTE RENAL FAILURE

For the most part, acute renal failure (ARF) occurs in women with previously healthy kidneys but it may also complicate the course of women with pre-existing renal disease (see Table 5.8). Before anuria or oliguria is ascribed to acute renal failure, obstruction of the urinary tract must be excluded. This is particularly pertinent in obstetric practice, because it is all too easy to damage the urinary tract unwittingly when performing emergency surgery for obstetric disasters such as postpartum haemorrhage, which are themselves causes of acute renal failure.

In recent years there have been marked declines in cases of acute renal failure related to obstetrics and the current incidence is probably <0.01 per cent (Grunfeld and Pertuiset, 1987). These decreases have been attributed chiefly to declines in the number of septic abortions and improvements in perinatal care, with clinicians ready

Table 5.8.   Causes of obstetrical acute renal failure (ARF)

Volume contraction/hypotension	Abortion Hyperemesis gravidarum Antepartum haemorrhage due to placenta praevia Postpartum haemorrhage, from uterus or extensive soft tissue trauma Adrenocortical failure: usually failure to augment steroids to cover delivery
Volume contraction/hypotension and coagulopathy	Antepartum haemorrhage due to abruptio placentae Pre-eclampsia/eclampsia Amniotic fluid embolism Incompatible blood transfusion Drug reactions Acute fatty liver of pregnancy (AFLP) Haemolytic uraemic syndrome (HUS)
Volume contraction/hypotension, coagulopathy and infection	Pyelonephritis Septic abortion Chorioamnionitis Puerperal sepsis
Urinary tract obstruction	Damage to ureters during caesarean section or repair of cervical/vaginal lacerations Pelvic and/or broad ligament haematomas

to intervene quickly and aggressively in situations that could potentially lead to renal failure. Such situations include placental abruption, acute pyelonephritis, pre-eclampsia, postpartum haemorrhage and any disease that may lead to systemic infection, dehydration or hypotension (Chugh *et al.*, 1976; Pertuiset and Grunfeld, 1987). The reasons for this disposition remain unknown. Two entities associated with pregnancy – acute fatty liver and idiopathic postpartum renal failure (haemolytic uraemic syndrome) – are fortunately rare.

Diagnostic pitfalls

A carefully taken history and physical examination may reveal a background of abortion, severe hyperemesis gravidarum, haemorrhage, sensitization to drugs, incompatible blood transfusion or pre-eclampsia. Once the diagnosis of ARF has been considered to be a possibility, then exploration of its many causes must be pursued (Table 5.8). A full initial assessment is essential remembering that, ante-natally, a decision will also be needed regarding the timing and route of delivery. Laboratory values should be interpreted in terms of relation to norms for pregnancy: for example, normal values for arterial pH, sodium and bicarbonate levels are 7.44, 135 mmol/l and 20 mmol/l respectively, whereas P_{CO2} is only 28–30 torr.

It is difficult, and often impossible, to decide on the aetiology of the ARF. Total anuria or alternating periods of anuria and polyuria strongly suggests obstruction, but normal urine volumes do not exclude obstruction. Complete anuria or evidence of disseminated intravascular coagulation (DIC) is suggestive of acute cortical necrosis (ACN), but this diagnosis can be established firmly only by renal biopsy. Teamwork is the key to success with nephrologists and obstetricians working together within the proper clinical environment.

Role of dialysis in pregnancy

Both haemodialysis and peritoneal dialysis have been used in patients with obstetrical renal failure. Some authors (Miller and Tassitro, 1969) prefer the peritoneal route and comment that '... neither pelvic peritonitis nor an enlarged uterus is a contraindication to the method'. Certainly, the procedure is safe if the catheter is inserted high in the abdomen under direct vision through a small incision. As both routes are safe, the choice should be determined by the underlying clinical condition (e.g. peritoneal dialysis may be preferable in the patient with septic shock or any other hypotensive complications) or by the facilities available in a given unit. If protracted dialysis is likely in a woman with an immature fetus (<24 weeks of pregnancy), CAPD can be offered, as it keeps rapid fluid and metabolic alterations to a minimum, compared with other modes of therapy (Hou, 1987).

Urea, creatinine and many other metabolites cross the placenta, so that dialysis should be undertaken early with the aim of maintaining plasma urea at around 10 mmol/l (Yasin and Bey Doun, 1988). Thus the advantages of dialysis become even more germane during pregnancy and make the argument for 'prophylactic' dialysis more compelling.

Renal failure and septic shock

Septic abortion

This condition, especially with clostridial infection, may result in a life-threatening syndrome (Pertuiset and Grunfeld, 1987; Lindheimer et al., 1988). The onset may be sudden, a few hours to 2 days after the abortion. The disease is characterized by an abrupt rise in temperature (≥40°C), together with the presence of myalgia, vomiting and bloody diarrhoea. Muscular pains are most intense in the arms, thorax and abdomen. The clinical picture may be confused with intra-abdominal inflammatory disease, especially when a history of provoked abortion is denied or not detected. Vaginal bleeding may be absent and clostridial organisms may be difficult to culture or to detect in the smear. The situation is further confounded by the normal presence of *Clostridia* species in the female genital tract. Once signs and symptoms develop, hypotension, dyspnoea and progression to shock occur rapidly. Furthermore, the patient is often jaundiced, and may have a peculiar bronze colour caused by the association of jaundice with cutaneous vasodilation, cyanosis and pallor.

Laboratory findings include severe anaemia with markedly elevated bilirubin levels (due to haemolysis), evidence of DIC and a striking leucocytosis (>50 000 mm^3). Hypocalcaemia of sufficient severity to provoke tetany has been described, and an abdominal radiograph may demonstrate gas in the uterus or abdomen, due to gas-forming organisms or perforation.

In a small percentage of the women, death occurs in hours; most respond to antibiotic treatment and volume replacement but leave the problem of ARF to be managed. The cause of the latter is usually acute tubular necrosis (ATN) but on occasion the more ominous acute cortical necrosis (ACN) may occur. The oliguric phase in women with tubular necrosis due to septic abortion may be prolonged to 3 or more weeks, and total anuria may occur in this period. In fact, it is often just when there are worries that the patient has underlying ACN rather than ATN that the diuretic phase begins.

The initial phase of treatment requires vigorous supportive therapy and anti-biotics. The use of antitoxin, hyperbaric oxygen and exchange transfusion in the treatment of clostridial infections remains controversial. There are also major dis-agreements about the role of surgical intervention: some consider the uterus to be a huge culture medium for bacterial growth and toxin formation, resistant to treat-ment, and so recommend its rapid removal as crucial if the mother is to survive (Bartlett and Yahia, 1969); others note that modern-day antibiotic therapy suffices, and that surgery in these critically ill women may be too risky (Hawkins, Sevitt and Fairbrother, 1975).

Acute pyelonephritis

Acute pyelonephritis, the most common renal complication during pregnancy, is an extremely rare cause of ARF in non-pregnant subjects in the absence of complicating features such as obstruction, calculi, papillary necrosis and analgesic nephropathy. However, the association appears to be more frequent in pregnant women (Grunfeld and Pertuiset, 1987; Lindheimer et al., 1988). The reason is obscure. It is known that in pregnant women acute pyelonephritis is accompanied by marked decrements in GFR (Whalley, Cunningham and Martin, 1975), in contrast to the situation in non-pregnant patients. It has been suggested that the vasculature in pregnancy may be more sensitive to the vasoactive effect of bacterial endotoxins (Whalley, Cunning-ham and Martin, 1975; Pertuiset and Grunfeld, 1987).

Acute tubular necrosis (ATN)

Volume depletion is the precipitating cause of ATN. It may therefore complicate hyperemesis gravidarum or severe vomiting associated with pyelonephritis (Pertui-set and Grunfeld, 1987), the latter condition also involving increased sensitivity of the vasculature to antitoxin in pregnancy. Uterine haemorrhage is another major cause of renal failure in late pregnancy and the immediate puerperium. Antepartum bleeding may be difficult to diagnose or may be underestimated when most of the blood loss remains concealed behind the placenta and suspicion of this requires rapid ultrasonic assessment. Uterine haemorrhage most often leads to ATN but, especially when associated with abruption, ACN may ensue (see below).

Pre-eclampsia, characterized by generalized vasoconstriction, is a major cause of renal dysfunction in pregnancy. The reduction in GFR is usually mild (approxi-mately 30 per cent) (Chesley and Lindheimer, 1988). On rare occasions, however, especially when the disease is neglected and accompanied by a marked coagulo-pathy, pre-eclampsia may progress to ATN and even ACN (Lindheimer et al., 1988; Stratta, Camarese and Dogiana, 1989).

Acute cortical necrosis (ACN)

Cortical necrosis, characterized by tissue death throughout the cortex with sparing of the medullary portions of the kidney, is fortunately a rare cause of ARF, but when it occurs it is more apt to be associated with pregnancy (Grunfeld and Pertuiset, 1987). Its incidence has declined markedly in industrialized nations: for instance, statistics from the National Maternity Hospital in Dublin demonstrate a decrease from 1 in 10 000 (1961–1970) to <1 in 80 000 (1971–1980) (Madias, Donohoe and Harrington, 1988).

ACN is most common in late pregnancy, most frequently after placental abruption and less commonly following prolonged intrauterine death or with pre-eclampsia. Abruption should always be considered when ARF develops suddenly between the 26th and 30th gestational week, as 45 per cent of the patients in one series had concealed haemorrhage (Kleinknecht *et al.*, 1973).

Although ACN may involve the entire renal cortex, with resultant irreversible renal failure, it is the incomplete or 'patchy' variety that occurs more often in pregnancy. The latter condition is characterized by an initial episode of severe oliguria or even anuria, lasting longer than in uncomplicated ATN. This is followed by a variable return of function and a stable period of moderate renal insufficiency, which in some cases progresses years later to end-stage disease (Pertuiset and Grunfeld, 1987).

Why pregnant women are more prone to develop ACN than non-pregnant patients, is obscure. Many of the women are older multigravidae who may have had pre-existing nephrosclerosis, rendering their kidneys more vulnerable to such inciting factors as ischaemia or DIC.

Acute renal failure specific to pregnancy

Acute fatty liver of pregnancy (AFLP)

This disease of the third trimester or puerperium is characterized by jaundice and severe hepatic dysfunction (Pertuiset and Grunfeld, 1987; Lindheimer *et al.*, 1988). The earliest manifestations are nausea and vomiting, important clues that are frequently overlooked and considered benign because the woman is pregnant. Laboratory investigation often reveals evidence of DIC, including decrements in antithrombin III concentration (Reily, Latham and Romero, 1987). Serum urate levels may be elevated out of proportion to the degree of renal dysfunction, and hyperuricaemia may precede the clinical onset of the disease. Ultrasonography and computed tomography may also aid diagnosis (Lindheimer *et al.*, 1988).

Because this disease is uncommon, it may be misdiagnosed as septicaemia or as pre-eclampsia complicated by liver involvement – and some suggest that AFLP and pre-eclampsia frequently coexist (Grunfeld and Pertuiset, 1987; Reily, Latham and Romero, 1987). The incidence of ARF in women with AFLP, once as high as 60 per cent, is now considerably less. This may be due to earlier recognition of the disease followed by rapid intervention to end the pregnancy (Lindheimer *et al.*, 1988). The mortality rate for mother and fetus, once quoted as >70–75 per cent, probably reflected an older literature selective of patients with the poorest outcomes. Currently the prognosis is improving, with survival >80–90 per cent possibly because milder forms of the disease are being recognized (Kaplan, 1985).

The aetiology of AFLP is unknown, although in the past tetracycline toxicity was implicated in several instances. Reversible urea cycle enzyme abnormalities resembling those seen in Reye's syndrome have also been described, and it has been suggested that this condition may be an adult form of Reye's syndrome provoked by the metabolic stress of pregnancy (Weber, Snodgrass and Powell, 1979; Rolfes and Ishak, 1985). Against this, however, is the fact that women surviving AFLP have had subsequent uneventful pregnancies (Pertuiset and Grunfeld, 1987).

The characteristic hepatic lesion is deposition of fat microdroplets within the hepatocytes. Inflammation and necrosis are usually absent but there are exceptions (Reily, Latham and Romero, 1987), and some cases of AFLP may be misdiagnosed as hepatitis. Such errors can be avoided by studying freshly frozen tissue, using special fat stains. The renal lesion is mild and kidney structure may be within normal limits or abnormalities may be limited to fatty vacuolization and other non-specific changes in the tubule cells. The cause of the renal failure is obscure: it may be attributable to haemodynamic factors, as in the 'hepatorenal syndrome', or may perhaps be a consequence of the DIC.

Haemolytic uraemic syndrome (HUS)

Many other names have been applied to this syndrome, including idiopathic post-partum renal failure, irreversible postpartum renal failure and postpartum malignant sclerosis. Less than 200 cases had been reported since its delineation in 1960 until 1988 (Lindheimer *et al.*, 1988). The condition may occur between one day and several weeks after delivery. A typical patient presents with oliguria, or at times anuria, rapidly progressive azotaemia, and often with evidence of microangiopathic haemolytic anaemia or a consumption coagulopathy. Blood pressure on admission varies from only minimal elevation to presentation with severe accelerated hypertension. Some patients exhibit extrarenal manifestations involving the cardiovascular system (cardiac dilatation and congestive heart failure) and central nervous system (lethargy, convulsions) which appear disproportionate to the degree of uraemia, hypertension or volume overload present.

The aetiology of this syndrome is unknown. Suggestions include a preceding viral illness, retained placental fragments or drugs such as ergotamine compounds, oxytocin agents and oral contraceptives prescribed shortly after delivery (Pertuiset and Grunfeld, 1987). Several women have manifested hypocomplementaemia, suggesting a possible immunological cause, and deficiencies in prostaglandin production and antithrombin III levels akin to those described in non-pregnant HUS have been ascribed to the postpartum renal variant as well.

HUS has been compared in pathophysiology to thrombotic thrombocytopenic purpura, as well as to other diseases characterized by DIC, as is the case with HUS in the non-pregnant. This disease has also been compared to the generalized Shwartzman reaction, which, as previously noted, develops more readily in pregnant animals (Conger, Falk and Guggenheim, 1981). The kidney changes fall into two general categories – changes in the glomerular capillaries resembling those seen in HUS in the non-pregnant, and arteriolar lesions reminiscent of malignant nephrosclerosis or scleroderma. Some believe that glomerular lesions suggesting thrombotic microangiopathy are more apt to be noted in specimens obtained soon after the disease begins, whereas those resembling accelerated nephrosclerosis are seen in biopsy material taken later in the course. Of practical importance, an increased incidence of post-biopsy bleeding has also been reported.

Treatment is primarily aimed at controlling hypertension and general supportive measures used for all patients with ARF. In view of the possible contributing role of retained placental fragments, dilatation and curettage should be considered for women in whom the syndrome occurs close to delivery. In the past, bilateral nephrectomy was used as a life-saving measure in a few women with accelerated hypertension unresponsive to treatment. This should be unnecessary today with the potent vasodilators, angiotensin-converting enzyme inhibitors and calcium-channel-blocking agents that are available. The early use of anticoagulant therapy such as heparin and fibrinolytic agents may reverse the renal failure, but data thus far have not been convincing, and it should be kept in mind that such drugs are not harmless.

Other regimens including anti-platelet therapy (which may be of use in a possible variant of postpartum renal failure linked to circulating lupus anticoagulant), infusion of blood products, including concentrates of antithrombin III, or exchange transfusions have been advocated on the basis of their alleged success in patients with thrombotic thrombocytopenic purpura.

The prognosis of this disease is guarded. Most women have succumbed, have required chronic dialysis or have survived with severely reduced renal function; only a few have recovered. Of interest is a woman reported to have a mild form of 'postpartum haemolytic syndrome', whose disease occurred in two successive pregnancies (Gomperts *et al.*, 1978).

Miscellaneous causes

These include intra-amniotic saline administration, amniotic fluid embolism and illnesses or accidents unrelated to that pregnancy such as drug ingestion, bacterial endocarditis and incompatible blood transfusions. Sudden ARF during pregnancy has also complicated sarcoidosis (Warren, Sprague and Corwen, 1988), various nephritides and collagen disorders and it can also be due to obstructive uropathy related to the enlarged uterus with or without polyhydramnios (Eika and Skajaa, 1988). Most of the latter problems have been in women with solitary kidneys, but there have also been instances of bilateral obstruction. These cases may be managed conservatively by placement of intraureteral stents under local anaesthesia (Loughlin and Bailey, 1986; Eika and Skajaa, 1988). Finally, it should always be borne in mind that some pregnant women with mild underlying renal disease are more susceptible to develop ATN, especially when their pregnancy is complicated by superimposed pre-eclampsia or another cause of increased blood pressure.

References

Abe, S, Amagosocki, Y, Konishi, K *et al.* (1985) The influence of antecedent renal disease on pregnancy. *American Journal of Obstetrics and Gynecology*, **153**, 508–514

Abramowsky, CR, Vegas, ME, Swinehart, G *et al.* (1980) Decidual vasculopathy of the placenta in lupus erythematosus. *New England Journal of Medicine*, **303**, 668–672

Alloub, MI, Sarr, BBB, McLaren, KM *et al.* (1989) Human papilloma virus infection and cervical intraepithelial neoplasia in women with renal allografts. *British Medical Journal*, **298**, 153

Baesnihan, B, Grigor, RR, Oliver, M *et al.* (1977) Immunological mechanisms for spontaneous abortion in systemic lupus erythematosus. *Lancet*, **ii**, 1205–1207

Baker, PN, Madeley, RJ and Symonds, EM (1989) Abdominal pain of unknown aetiology. *British Journal of Obstetrics and Gynaecology*, **96**, 688–691

Barcelo, P, Lopez-Lillo, J, Cabero. L *et al.* (1986) Successful pregnancy in primary glomerular disease. *Kidney International*, **30**, 914–919

Barclay, CS, French, MAH, Ross, LD *et al.* (1987) Successful pregnancy following steroid therapy and plasma exchange in a woman with anti-Ro(SS-A) antibodies. Case report. *British Journal of Obstetrics and Gynaecology*, **94**, 369–371

Barrett, RJ and Peters, WA (1983) Pregnancy following urinary diversion. *Obstetrics and Gynecology*, **62**, 582–586

Bartlett, RH and Yahia, C (1969) Management of septic abortion with renal failure: report of 5 consecutive cases with 5 survivors. *New England Journal of Medicine*, **292**, 722–725

Baylis, C (1987) Renal disease in gravid animals. *American Journal of Kidney Disease*, **9**, 350–353

Baylis, C, Reese, R and Wilson, CB (1989) Glomerular effects of pregnancy in a model of glomerulonephritis (GN) in the rat. *American Journal of Kidney Disease*, **17**, 127–132

Baylis, C and Reckelhoff, JF (1991) Renal haemodynamics in normal and hypertensive pregnancy: lessons from micropuncture. *American Journal of Kidney Diseases*, **17**, 98–104

Becker, GJ, Ihle, BV, Fairley, KF *et al.* (1986) Effect of pregnancy on moderate renal failure in reflux nephropathy. *British Medical Journal*, **292**, 796–798

Bennett, WM, Elzinga, L and Kelley, V (1988) Pathophysiology of cyclosporine toxicity: role of eicosanoids. *Transplantation Proceedings*, **20**, 628–633

Branch, WD, Scott, JR, Kochenour, NK *et al.* (1985) Obstetric complications associated with the lupus anticoagulant. *New England Journal of Medicine*, **313**, 1322–1326

Brem, AS, Singer, D, Anderson, L *et al.* (1988) Infants of azotemic mothers: a report of 3 live births. *American Journal of Kidney Disease*, **12**, 299–303

Brenner, BM (1985) Nephron adaptation to renal injury or ablation. *American Journal of Physiology*, **249**, F324–F337

Briedahl, P, Hurst, PE, Martin, JD and Vivian, AB (1972) The post-partum investigation of pregnancy bacteriuria. *Medical Journal of Australia*, **2**, 1174–1177

Buszta, C, Steinmuller, DR, Nogick, AC *et al.* (1985) Pregnancy after donor nephrectomy. *Transplantation*, **40**, 651–655

Cahne, RY, Brons, EGM, Williams, PF, Evans, EB, Robinson, RE and Dossa, M (1988) Successful pregnancy after paratopic segmental pancreas and kidney transplantation. *British Medical Journal*, **296**, 1709

Campbell-Brown, M, McFadyean, IR, Seal, DV and Stephenson, ML (1987) Is screening for bacteriuria in pregnancy worthwhile? *British Medical Journal*, **294**, 1579–1582

Chan, JKM, Marris, EN and Hughes, GRV (1986) Successful pregnancy following suppression of cardiolipin antibodies and lupus anticoagulant and azathioprine in systemic lupus erythematosus. *Journal of Obstetrics and Gynaecology*, **7**, 16–17

Chesley, LS and Lindheimer, MD (1988) Renal hemodynamics and intravascular volume in normal and hypertensive pregnancy. In *Handbook of Hypertension: Volume 10, Hypertension in Pregnancy* (edited by PC Rubin), pp. 38–65. Amsterdam: Elsevier

Chng, PK and Hall, MH (1982) Antenatal prediction of urinary tract infection in pregnancy. *British Journal of Obstetrics and Gynaecology*, **89**, 8–11

Chugh, KS, Singhal, PC, Shamra, BK *et al.* (1976) Acute renal failure of obstetric original. *Obstetrics and Gynecology*, **48**, 642–646

Conger, JD, Falk, S and Guggenheim, SJ (1981) Glomerular dynamics and morphologic changes in the generalized Schwartzman reaction in postpartum rat. *Journal of Clinical Investigation*, **67**, 1334–1336

Cooper, K, Stafford, J and Warwick, MT (1970) Wegener's granuloma complicating pregnancy. *Journal of Obstetrics and Gynaecology of the British Commonwealth*, **77**, 1028–1030

Cousins, L (1987) Pregnancy complications among diabetic women: review 1965–1985. *Obstetrical and Gynaecological Survey*, **42**, 140–149

Cunningham, FG (1987) Urinary tract infections complicating pregnancy. *Bailliere's Clinical Obstetrics and Gynaecology*, **1**, 891–908

Cunningham, FG, Lucas, MJ and Hankins, GDV (1987) Pulmonary injury complicating antepartum pyelonephritis. *American Journal of Obstetrics and Gynaecology*, **156**, 797–807

Danielli, L, Korchazak, L, Beyar, H and Lotan, M (1987) Recurrent haematuria during multiple pregnancies. *Obstetrics and Gynecology*, **69**, 446–448

Davison, JM (1978) Changes in renal function in early pregnancy in women with one kidney. *Yale Journal of Biology and Medicine*, **51**, 347–349

Davison, JM (1985) The effect of pregnancy on kidney function in renal allograft recipients. *Kidney International*, **27**, 74–79

Davison, JM (1987) Pregnancy in renal allograft recipients: prognosis and management. *Baillière's Clinical Obstetrics and Gynaecology*, **1**, 1027–1045

Davison, JM (1989) The effect of pregnancy on long term renal function in women with chronic renal disease and single kidneys. *Clinical and Experimental Hypertension*, **B8**, 226

Davison, JM (1991) Dialysis, transplantation and pregnancy. *American Journal of Kidney Diseases*, **17**, 127–132

Davison, JM and Dunlop, W (1984) Changes in renal haemodynamics and tubular function induced by normal human pregnancy. *Seminars in Nephrology*, **4**, 198–207

Davison, JM and Lindheimer, MD (1989) Pregnancy and renal transplantation: look before you leap. *International Journal of Artificial Organs*, **12**, 144–146

Davison, JM, Dellagrammatikas, H and Parkin, JM (1985) Maternal azathioprine therapy and depressed haemopoiesis in babies of renal allograft patients. *British Journal of Obstetrics and Gynaecology*, **92**, 233–239

Davison, JM, Katz, AI and Lindheimer, MD (1986) Pregnancy in women with renal disease and renal transplants. *Proceedings EDTA and ERA*, **22**, 439A

Davison, JM, Sprott, MS and Selkon, JB (1984) The effect of covert bacteriuria in schoolgirls on renal function at 18 years and during pregnancy. *Lancet*, **ii**, 651–655

Davison, M and Radford, DJ (1989) Fetal and congenital complete heart block. *Medical Journal of Australia*, **150**, 192–196

Derfler, K, Schaller, A, Herold, CH *et al.* (1989) Successful outcome of a complicated pregnancy in a renal transplant recipient taking cyclosporine-A. *Clinical Nephrology*, **29**, 96–102

Dunlop, W and Davison, JM (1977) The effect of normal pregnancy upon the renal handling of uric acid. *British Journal of Obstetrics and Gynaecology*, **84**, 13–21

Dunlop, W and Davison, JM (1987) Renal haemodynamics and tubular function in human pregnancy. *Baillière's Clinical Obstetrics and Gynaecology*, **1**, 769–787

Dure-Smith, P (1970) Pregnancy dilatation of the urinary tract. The iliac sign and its significance. *Radiology*, **96**, 545–550

Eika, B and Skajaa, K (1988) Acute renal failure due to bilateral ureteral obstruction by the pregnant uterus. *Urology International*, **43**, 315–317

Esscher, S and Scott, JS (1979) Congenital heart block and maternal lupus erythematosus. *British Medical Journal*, **1**, 1235–1238

Farquharson, RG, Compston, A and Bloom, AL (1984) Lupus anticoagulant: a place for pregnancy treatment? *Lancet*, **ii**, 842–843

Feehally, J, Bennett, SE and Harris, PKG (1986) Is chronic renal transplant rejection a non-immunological phenomenon? *Lancet*, **2**, 486–488

Fine, LG, Barnett, EV and Danovitch, GM (1981) Systemic lupus erythematosus in pregnancy. *American Journal of Medicine*, **94**, 667–677

Finkelstein, FO and Hayslett, JP (1979) Structural and functional adaptations after reduction of population. *Yale Journal of Biology and Medicine*, **52**, 271–287

Fisher, KA, Luger, A, Spargo, BH *et al.* (1981) Hypertension in pregnancy: clinical–pathological correlation and late prognosis. *Medicine*, **60**, 267–276

Flechner, SM, Katz, AR, Van Buren, C *et al.* (1985) The presence of cyclosporine in body tissues and fluids during pregnancy. *American Journal of Kidney Diseases*, **5**, 60–63

Fotino, S (1989) The solitary kidney: a model of chronic hyperfiltration in humans. *American Journal of Kidney Diseases*, **13**, 88–98

Fraga, A, Mintz, G, Orozco, J *et al.* (1974) Sterility and fertility rates, fetal wastage and maternal morbidity in systemic lupus erythematosis. *Journal of Rheumatology*, **1**, 1293–1298

Gallery, EDM and Brown, MA (1987) Volume homeostasis in normal and hypertensive pregnancy. *Baillière's Clinical Obstetrics and Gynaecology*, **1**, 835–851

Garsenstein, M, Pollak, VE and Kark, RM (1962) Systemic lupus erythematosus and pregnancy. *New England Journal of Medicine*, **267**, 165–169

Gaucherand, P, Chalasreysse, JP, Audra, P *et al.* (1988) Pregnancy in women undergoing dialysis in chronic renal insufficiency. *Journal de Gynécologie, Obstétrique et Biologie de la Reproduction*, **17**, 889–895

Gimovsky, ML, Montoro, M and Paul, RH (1984) Pregnancy outcome in women with systemic lupus erythematosus. *Obstetrics and Gynecology*, **63**, 686–690

Gomperts, D, Sessel, L, DuPlessis, V and Hersch, C (1978) Recurrent postpartum haemolytic uraemic syndrome. *Lancet*, **i**, 48

Gower, PE, Hawell, B, Sidaway, ME and De Wardener, HE (1968) Follow-up of 164 patients with bacteriuria of pregnancy. *Lancet*, **i**, 990–1004

Gregorini, G, Setti, G and Remuzzi, G (1986) Recurrent abortion with lupus anticoagulant and pre-eclampsia: a common final pathway for two different diseases? Case report. *British Journal of Obstetrics and Gynaecology*, **93**, 194–196

Gregory, MC and Mansell, MA (1983) Pregnancy and cystinuria. *Lancet*, **ii**, 1958–1960

Grunfeld, JP and Pertuiset, N (1987) Acute renal failure in pregnancy. *American Journal of Kidney Diseases*, **9**, 359–362

Hadi, HA (1986) Pregnancy in renal transplant recipients: a review. *Obstetrical and Gynecological Survey*, **41**, 264–271

Harris, EN, Chan, J, Anderson, R *et al.* (1986) Predictive value of anticardiolipin antibody for thrombosis, fetal loss and thrombocytopenia. *Clinical Science*, **70**, 56P

Hawkins, OF, Sevitt, LH and Fairbrother, DF (1975) Management of chemical septic abortion with renal failure. Use of a conservative regimen. *New England Journal of Medicine*, **292**, 722–725

Hayslett, JP and Lynn, RI (1980) Effect of pregnancy in patients with lupus nephropathy. *Kidney International*, **18**, 207–220

Hayslett, JP and Reece, EA (1987) Managing diabetic patients with nephropathy and other vascular complications. *Baillière's Clinical Obstetrics and Gynaecology*, **1**, 939–954

Hou, S (1987) Peritoneal dialysis and haemodialysis in pregnancy. *Baillière's Clinical Obstetrics and Gynaecology*, **1**, 1009–1025

Hou, S (1989) Pregnancy in organ transplant recipients. *Medical Clinics of North America*, **73**, 667–683

Hou, SH, Grossman, SD and Madias, N (1985) Pregnancy in women with renal disease and moderate renal insufficiency. *American Journal of Medicine*, **78**, 186–194

Jungers, P, Dougados, M and Pellissies, C (1982) Lupus nephropathy and pregnancy. *Archives of Internal Medicine*, **142**, 771–776

Jungers, P, Huiller, P and Forget, D (1987) Reflux nephropathy and pregnancy. *Baillière's Clinical Obstetrics and Gynaecology*, **1**, 953–969

Jungers, P, Forget, D, Henry-Amer, M *et al.* (1986) Chronic kidney disease and pregnancy. *Advances in Nephrology*, **15**, 103–141

Kaplan, ML (1985) Acute fatty liver in pregnancy. *New England Journal of Medicine*, **313**, 367–370

Kasinath, BS and Katz, AI (1983) Delayed maternal lupus after delivery of offspring with congenital heart block. *Archives of Internal Medicine*, **142**, 1217–1218

Kilpatrick, DC (1986) Anti-phospholipid antibodies and pregnancy wastage. *Lancet*, **ii**, 185–186

Kincaid-Smith, P and Fairley, KF (1987) Renal diseases in pregnancy. Three controversial areas. Mesangial IgA nephropathy, focal glomerular sclerosis (focal and segmental hyalinosis and sclerosis), and reflux nephropathy. *American Journal of Kidney Diseases*, **9**, 328–333

Kioko, EM, Shaw, KM, Clark, AD *et al.* (1983) Successful pregnancy in a diabetic patient treated with continuous ambulatory peritoneal dialysis. *Diabetes Care*, **6**, 298–300

Klein, EA (1983) Urologic problems of pregnancy. *Obstetric and Gynecological Survey*, **39**, 605–615

Kleinknecht, D, Grunfeld, JP, Gomez, PC *et al.* (1973) Diagnostic procedures and longterm prognosis in bilateral renal necrosis. *Kidney International*, **4**, 390–400

Kleinmen, CS, Copel, JA and Hobbins, JC (1987) Combined echocardiographic and Doppler assessment of fetal congenital atrioventricular block. *British Journal of Obstetrics and Gynaecology*, **94**, 967–974

Kochenour, NK, Branch, WD, Role, NS *et al.* (1987) A new postpartum syndrome associated with antilipid antibodies. *Obstetrics and Gynecology*, **69**, 460–468

Krege, J, Katz, VL and Bouts, WA (1989) *Obstetric and Gynecological Review*, **44**, 789–795

Lancet editorial (1975) Pregnancy and renal disease. *Lancet*, **ii**, 801–802

Lancet editorial (1985) Pregnancy and renal disease. *Lancet*, **i**, 1157–1158

Lancet editorial (1989a) Pregnancy and glomerulonephritis. *Lancet*, **ii**, 253–254

Lancet editorial (1989b) Lupus nephritis and pregnancy. *Lancet*, **ii**, 82–83

Lawson, DH and Miller, AWF (1973) Screening for bacteriuria in pregnancy: a critical reappraisal. *Archives of Internal Medicine*, **132**, 925–928

Leikin, JB, Arof, HM and Pearlman, LM (1986) Acute lupus pneumonitis in the postpartum period. A case history and review of the literature. *Obstetrics and Gynecology*, **68**, 293–315

Levey, AS, Perrone, RD and Madias, NE (1988) Serum creatinine and renal function. *Annual Review of Medicine*, **39**, 465–490

Lim, VS (1987) Reproductive endocrinology in uremia. *Clinical Obstetrics and Gynaecology*, **1**, 997–1010

Lim, VS, Katz, AI and Lindheimer, MD (1976) Acid-base regulation in pregnancy. *American Journal of Physiology*, **231**, 1764–1770

Lindheimer, MD and Katz, AI (1987) Gestation in women with kidney disease: prognosis and management. *Clinical Obstetrics and Gynecology*, **1**, 921–937

Lindheimer, MD, Barron, WM and Davison, JM (1989) Osmoregulation of thirst and vasopressin release in pregnancy. *American Journal of Physiology*, **257**, F159–F169

Lindheimer, MD, Spargo, BH and Katz, AI (1975) Renal biopsy in pregnancy-induced hypertension. *Journal of Reproductive Medicine*, **15**, 189–194

Lindheimer, MD, Fisher, KA, Spargo, BH *et al.* (1981) Hypertension in pregnancy: a biopsy study with longterm follow-up. *Contributions to Nephrology*, **25**, 71–77

Lindheimer, MD, Katz, AI, Ganavel, D and Grunfeld, JP (1988) Acute renal failure in pregnancy. In *Acute Renal Failure*, 2nd edn (edited by BM Brenner and JM Lazarus) pp. 597–620. New York: Churchill Livingstone

Lockshin, MD and Druzin, NL (1985) Antiphospholipid antibodies and pregnancy. *New England Journal of Medicine*, **313**, 1351

Lockshin, MD, Reuitz, E and Druzin, NL (1984) Case control prospective study demonstrating absence of lupus exacerbation during and after pregnancy. *American Journal of Medicine*, **77**, 893–898

Lockshin, MD, Druzin, HL, Goei, S *et al.* (1985) Antibody to cardiolipin as a predictor of fetal distress or death in pregnant patients with systemic lupus erythematosus. *New England Journal of Medicine*, **313**, 152–156

Lockwood, CJ, Reece, EA, Romero, R *et al.* (1986) Antiphospholipid antibody and pregnancy wastage. *Lancet*, **ii**, 742–743

Loughlin, KR and Bailey, RB (1986) Internal ureteral stents for conservative management of ureteral calculi during pregnancy. *New England Journal of Medicine*, **315**, 1647–1649

Lubbe, WF and Liggins, GC (1985) Lupus anticoagulant and pregnancy. *American Journal of Obstetrics and Gynecology*, **153**, 322–327

Lubbe, WF, Butler, WS, Palmer, SJ *et al.* (1984) Lupus anticoagulant in pregnancy. *British Journal of Obstetrics and Gynaecology*, **91**, 357–363

MacFadyean, I (1986) Urinary tract infection in pregnancy. In *The Kidney in Pregnancy* (edited by VE Andreucci) pp. 205–229. Boston: Martinus Nijhoff

MacFadyean, IR, Eykkryn, SJ, Gardner, NHN *et al.* (1973) Bacteriuria of pregnancy. *Journal of Obstetrics and Gynaecology of the British Commonwealth*, **80**, 385–405

McIntyre, JA, Faulk, WP, Nichols-Johnson, VR *et al.* (1984) Immunologic testing and immunotherapy in recurrent spontaneous abortion. *Obstetrics and Gynecology*, **67**, 169–175

Maddison, PJ, Skinner, RP, Esscher, E *et al.* (1983) Serological studies on congenital heart block. *Annals of the Rheumatic Diseases*, **42**, 218–219

Madias, NE, Donohoe, JF and Harrington, JT (1988) Postischemic acute renal failure. In *Acute Renal Failure* (edited by BM Brenner and JM Lazarus) pp. 597–620. New York: Churchill Livingstone

Maikrantz, P, Coe, L, Parks, JH *et al.* (1987) Nephrolithiases and gestation. *Clinics in Obstetrics and Gynaecology*, **1**, 909–919

Meyers, SJ, Lee, RV and Munschauser, RW (1985) Dilatation and nontraumatic rupture of the urinary tract during pregnancy. A review. *Obstetrics and Gynecology*, **66**, 809–815

Miller, DR, Kakkis, J (1982) Prognosis, management and outcome of obstructive renal disease in pregnancy. *Journal of Reproductive Medicine*, **27**, 199–201

Miller, RB and Tassitro, CR (1969) Peritoneal dialysis. *New England Journal of Medicine*, **281**, 945–947

Millford, SL and Belini, JW (1986) Maternal death associated with Wegener's granulomatosis in pregnancy. *Journal of Laryngology and Otology*, **100**, 475–476

Moore, M, Saffron, JE and Barof, HSB (1985) Systemic sclerosis and pregnancy complicated by obstructive uropathy. *American Journal of Obstetrics and Gynecology*, **153**, 893–895

Mor-Josef, S, Navot, D, Rabinowitz, R and Schenker, JG (1984) Collagen disease in pregnancy. *Obstetrical and Gynecological Survey*, **39**, 67–83

Murray, S, Hickey, J and Houang, E (1987) Significant bacteremia associated with replacement of intrauterine contraceptive device. *American Journal of Obstetrics and Gynecology*, **156**, 698–699

Murty, GE, Davison, JM and Cameron, DS (1990) Wegener's granulomatosus complicating pregnancy: first report of a case with a tracheostomy. *Journal of Obstetrics and Gynaecology*, **10**, 399–403

Nathan, DJ and Snapper, I (1958) Simultaneous placental transfer of factors responsible for LE cell formation and thrombocytopenia. *American Journal of Medicine*, **25**, 647

Ogburn, PL, Kitzmiller, JL, Williams, PP *et al.* (1986) Pregnancy following renal transplantation in Class T diabetes mellitus. *Journal of the American Medical Association*, **255**, 911–915

Out, HJ, Derksen, RHWM and Christiaeus, GCML (1989) Systemic lupus erythematosus and pregnancy. *Obstetrical and Gynecological Survey*, **44**, 585–591

Packham, D and Fairley, KF (1987) Renal biopsy: indications and complications in pregnancy. *British Journal of Obstetrics and Gynaecology*, **94**, 935–940

Packham, DK, North, RA, Fairley, KF *et al.* (1989) Primary glomerulonephritis and pregnancy. *Quarterly Journal of Medicine*, **266**, 537–553

Pertuiset, N and Grunfeld, JP (1987) Acute renal failure in pregnancy. *Clinics in Obstetrics and Gynaecology*, **1**, 873–890

Pickerell, MD, Sawers, R and Michael, J (1988) Pregnancy after renal transplantation: severe intrauterine growth retardation. *British Medical Journal*, **296**, 825

Pruett, K and Faro, S (1987) Pyelonephritis associated with respiratory distress. *Obstetrics and Gynecology*, **69**, 444–446

Rasmussen, PE and Nielsen, FR (1988) Hydronephrosis during pregnancy: a literature survey. *European Journal of Obstetrics, Gynecology and Reproductive Biology*, **27**, 249–259

Reece, EA, Romero, R, Colyne, LP *et al.* (1984) Lupus like anticoagulant in pregnancy. *Lancet*, **i**, 344–345

Reece, EA, Constan, DR, Hayslett, JP *et al.* (1988) Diabetic nephropathy: pregnancy performance and maternal outcome. *American Journal of Obstetrics and Gynecology*, **159**, 56–66

Reeders, ST, Zerres, K, Gal, A *et al.* (1986) Prenatal diagnosis of autosomal dominant polycystic kidney disease with a DNA probe. *Lancet*, **ii**, 6–7

Reily, CA, Latham, PS and Romero, R (1987) Acute fatty liver of pregnancy. A reassessment based on observations in 9 patients. *Annals of Internal Medicine*, **106**, 703–706

Rodriguez, MH, Masak, DI, Mestman, J *et al.* (1988) Calcium/creatinine ratio and microalbuminuria in the prediction of pre-eclampsia. *American Journal of Obstetrics and Gynecology*, **159**, 1452–1455

Rolfes, DB and Ishak, KG (1985) Acute fatty liver of pregnancy: a clinicopathologic study of 35 cases. *Hepatology*, **5**, 1149–1158

Schewitz, LJ, Friedman, EA and Pollak, VE (1965) Bleeding after renal biopsy in pregnancy. *Obstetrics and Gynecology*, **26**, 295–304

Schleider, MA, Nachman, RL, Jaffe, EA and Coleman, MA (1986) Clinical study of the lupus anticoagulant. *Blood*, **48**, 499–509

Scott, JS (1984) Connective tissue disease antibodies and pregnancy. *American Journal of Reproductive Immunology*, **6**, 19–24

Singsen, BH, Akhter, JE, Weinstein, MM *et al.* (1985) Congenital complete heart block and SSA antibodies: obstetric implications. *American Journal of Obstetrics and Gynecology*, **155**, 655–659

Smith, CA (1982) Progressive systemic sclerosis and post-partum renal failure complicated by peripheral gangrene. *Journal of Rheumatology*, **9**, 455–460

Soothill, PW, Nicolaides, KH, Rodeck, CH *et al.* (1986) The effect of gestational age on blood gas and acid–base values in human pregnancy. *Fetal Therapy*, **7**, 166–173

Stamm, WE, Counts, GW and Running, KR (1982) Diagnosis of coliform infection in acutely dysuric women. *New England Journal of Medicine*, **307**, 463–465

Stephenson, O, Clelland, WP and Hallidive-Smith, K (1981) Congenital heart block and persistent ductus arteriosus associated with maternal systemic lupus erythematosus. *British Heart Journal*, **46**, 104

Stratta, P, Camarese, C and Dogiana, M (1989) Pregnancy-related acute renal failure. *Clinical Nephrology*, **32**, 14–20

Sturgiss, SN, Wilkinson, R, Taylor, RMR and Davison, JM (1990) Pregnancy, remote renal prognosis and hypertension in renal allograft recipients. *Clinical and Experimental Hypertension, Series B*, **10**, 145

Surian, M, Imbasciati, E, Bonfi, G *et al.* (1984) Glomerular disease and pregnancy. A study of 123 pregnancies in patients with primary and secondary glomerular diseases. *Nephron*, **36**, 101–105

Talbot, SF, Main, DM and Levinson, AI (1984) Wegener's granulomatosis – first report of its onset during pregnancy. *Arthritis and Rheumatism*, **27**, 109–112

Taylor, PV, Scott, JS, Gerlis, LM *et al.* (1986) Maternal antibodies against fetal cardiac antigens in congenital complete heart block. *New England Journal of Medicine*, **315**, 667–672

Tyden, G, Brattstrom, C, Bjorkman, U *et al.* (1989) Pregnancy after combined pancreas-kidney transplantation. *Diabetes*, **38 (suppl 1)**, 43–45

Venning, MC, Burn, DJ, Ward, RM *et al.* (1988) Neonatal lupus syndrome: optimism justified? *Lancet*, **i**, 640

Vimicor, F, Golichowski, A, Filo, R *et al.* (1984) Pregnancy following renal transplantation in a patient with insulin-dependent diabetes mellitus. *Diabetes Care*, **7**, 280–284

Vonderheid, EC, Koblenzer, PJ, Ming, P *et al.* (1976) Neonatal lupus erythematosus, report of 4 cases with a review of the literature. *Archives of Dermatology*, **112**, 698–705

Warren, GV, Sprague, SM and Corwen, HL (1988) Sarcoidosis presenting as acute renal failure in pregnancy. *American Journal of Kidney Disease*, **12**, 161–167

Watson, ML, MacNichol, AN and Wright, AF (1990) Adult polycystic kidney disease. *British Medical Journal*, **300**, 61–62

Watson, RM, Lane, AT and Barnett, NK (1984) Neonatal lupus erythematosus. *Medicine*, **63**, 363–364

Weber, FL, Snodgrass, PJ and Powell, DE (1979) Abnormalities of hepatic mitochondrial urea-cycle enzyme activities in acute fatty liver of pregnancy. *Journal of Laboratory and Clinical Medicine*, **94**, 27–41

Whalley, PJ, Cunningham, FG and Martin, FG (1975) Transient renal dysfunction associated with acute pyelonephritis of pregnancy. *Obstetrics and Gynecology*, **46**, 174–177

Yasin, SY and Bey Doun, SN (1988) Hemodialysis in pregnancy. *Obstetrical and Gynecological Survey*, **43**, 655–668

Zulman, JI, Talal, N, Hoffman, GS *et al.* (1980) Problems associated with the management of pregnancies in patients with systemic lupus erythematosus. *Journal of Rheumatology*, **7**, 37–49

Zurier, RB, Argyros, TG, Urman, JD *et al.* (1978) Systemic lupus erythematosus: management during pregnancy. *Obstetrics and Gynecology*, **51**, 178–180

Chapter 6

Pregnancy and the liver

James R Gray and Ian AD Bouchier

Introduction

The role of liver disease in pregnancy can be conveniently considered in four ways: First, the expected changes in the normal liver and its function in normal pregnancy; secondly, pregnancy occurring in the face of pre-existing liver disease; thirdly, liver disease developing in, but coincidental to, pregnancy; and fourthly liver diseases peculiar to pregnancy. It is no longer satisfactory to discuss only jaundice in pregnancy, as many previous reviews have done. One must consider the broader manifestations of liver disease. This chapter ends with an overall approach to the diagnosis of liver disease as suspected in the pregnant patient.

The liver in normal pregnancy

Anatomy and histology

There is no gross change in the liver during normal pregnancy. In spite of increases in plasma volume and cardiac output, there is no change in hepatic blood flow (Munnel and Taylor, 1947). There is, however, a redistribution of venous return to the heart due to compression of the inferior vena cava in late pregnancy. This leads to increased flow through the azygos and vertebral veins which will be important in later discussion of variceal bleeding in pregnancy (Kerr, Scott and Samuel, 1964).

In studies unlikely to be repeated today, Ingerslev and Teilum (1946) showed no change in liver biopsies of 17 normal pregnant women. Antia and co-workers (1958) biopsied 10 normal pregnant women and also were unable to identify any specific changes. Only using the electron microscope can proliferation of endoplasmic reticulum and, occasionally, enlarged mitochondria be seen in the liver of normal pregnant women (Perez et al., 1971).

Biochemistry

Little change in liver enzymes occurs throughout pregnancy. Serum glutamic oxaloacetic transaminase levels remain normal throughout pregnancy (Haemmerli, 1966). Alkaline phosphatase concentration may double by the third trimester but this is due to increases in both the placental and bone isoenzymes (Adeniyi and Olatunbosun, 1984). By contrast, there is no elevation in γ-glutamyl transpeptidase (GGT) activity in normal pregnancy, making this a useful test to rule out suspected biliary tract disease in pregnancy (Walker *et al.*, 1974). The only exception to this is in viral hepatitis in the first half of pregnancy, where there is a blunted rise in GGT, but the overall picture in this situation would be of hepatocellular damage rather than purely an obstructive injury (Combes *et al.*, 1977). Bilirubin levels remain normal or may even fall during pregnancy (McNair and Jaynes, 1960). Secondary to dilution caused by rising plasma volume, total protein and albumin concentrations fall by about 13 per cent, reaching a nadir at term.

Plasma cholesterol concentration rises by an average of 50 per cent, particularly in the second trimester of pregnancy. Triglyceride levels rise by a factor of 3 but both cholesterol and triglyceride levels rapidly fall to normal after delivery (Potter and Nestel, 1979). There is a rise in biliary cholesterol secretion and a fall in bile acid secretion due to a slowing of the enterohepatic circulation. This leads to conditions which favour gallstone formation, as discussed further below (Kern *et al.*, 1981; Fulton *et al.*, 1983).

Gallbladder

Arising from these biochemical changes, a great deal of interest in gallbladder function in pregnancy has developed. Ultrasonography has shown incomplete emptying of the gallbladder at a reduced rate during the second and third trimesters. This effect is not seen with oral contraceptives and is probably mediated by progesterone (Braverman, Johnson and Kern, 1980; Cohen, 1980). In spite of this increased risk for cholelithiasis, only 3.5 per cent of obstetric patients screened by ultrasonography in a large series were found to have gallstones during their pregnancies (Stauffer *et al.*, 1982).

Physical examination

There should be no change in liver or spleen size in normal pregnancy, although palpation of the liver obviously becomes more difficult as the gravid uterus rises towards the epigastrium. Two findings often associated with liver disease deserve mentioning: careful examination by Bean (1949) revealed spider angiomas in 67 per cent of White pregnant women against 12 per cent in non-pregnant controls; similarly two-thirds of pregnant patients had palmar erythema. Both of these changes settle considerably or disappear after delivery and do not suggest the presence of chronic liver disease in the context of pregnancy.

Pregnancy and previous liver disease

The whole range of chronic liver diseases must be considered here from the standpoint of the effect of a pregnancy upon these patients as well as the effect of the liver disease upon the pregnancy itself. It is generally believed that fertility is reduced in women with chronic liver disease, owing to anovulation (Cuddihy and Whelton, 1987). This is especially true in ongoing active liver disease but not so important in stable treated liver disease (Steven, Buckley and Mackay, 1979; Britton, 1982). The topic of viral hepatitis, applicable to both this and the next section, is discussed under 'Liver disease beginning in pregnancy'.

Chronic persistent hepatitis

This represents a chronic hepatitis of unknown aetiology manifest by non-specific symptoms, mild to moderate elevation of serum transaminases and characteristic liver histology. It does not require therapy and does not progress to cirrhosis. In ten pregnancies in seven women with chronic persistent hepatitis, Infeld and co-authors (Infeld, Borkowf and Varma, 1979) found no increased risk of mortality or morbidity to fetus or mother.

Chronic active hepatitis and cirrhosis

In contrast to chronic persistent hepatitis, chronic active hepatitis is more aggressive and progresses to cirrhosis if untreated. The aetiology can be viral (hepatitis B, D or non-A, non-B), Wilson's disease, drug toxicity, α_1-anti-trypsin deficiency, or idiopathic 'autoimmune'. This last cause is the commonest in women of childbearing age in the Western world whereas the sequelae of hepatitis B infection are more prevalent in Asia.

Chronic alcohol abuse is the most common cause of cirrhosis alone but affects men much more frequently than women. Excess alcohol intake will have an adverse effect on any pre-existing liver disease as well as having direct adverse effects on the pregnancy and the fetus as discussed elsewhere (Chapter 8).

Pregnancy, once achieved, is unlikely to have an adverse effect on chronic active hepatitis or cirrhosis, of whatever underlying cause. Earlier reports suggested that the increased metabolic demands of pregnancy on the liver made interruption of pregnancy advisable but this is no longer believed to be true. There may well be increased fetal loss and premature deliveries but there is no evidence of detriment to the mother with chronic pre-existing liver disease (Steven, Buckley and Mackay, 1979). In terms of fetal outcome it should also be recognized that, although rare, kernicterus can develop in an infant born of a mother with severe hyperbilirubinaemia irrespective of the cause of the underlying disorder (Waffarn et al., 1982).

Oesophageal varices

The formation of oesophageal varices is one of the most serious complications of portal hypertension. Portal hypertension occurs in the presence of chronic liver disease, such as cirrhosis, stemming from any cause, as well as in relation to extrahepatic portal vein obstruction. Haemorrhage from oesophageal varices has a mortality rate approaching 50 per cent in some series (Graham and Smith, 1981). The precise trigger for bleeding has not been elucidated but intravascular volume expansion may be important. Certainly, in pregnancy, blood volume has been shown to increase by up to 40–45 per cent (Schreyer et al., 1982). When this is combined with impaired drainage of the inferior vena cava, one will see a marked rise in flow through collateral veins including the azygos veins which are a major component of oesophageal varices (Kerr, Scott and Samuel, 1964). This should logically increase the risk of variceal bleeding. Indeed, some have demonstrated the development of transient oesophageal varices in normal pregnancy, presumably due to this increased azygos flow (Varma et al., 1977). In addition, the increased abdominal pressure during labour might increase azygos blood flow. However, in spite of this, there is no proof either of raised portal pressure or of increased risk of variceal haemorrhage in pregnancy.

Earlier reviews suggest a risk for variceal bleeding of 43 per cent in pregnant women with extrahepatic portal vein obstruction and 23 per cent with cirrhosis, with a maternal mortality rate of 18 per cent (Varma *et al.*, 1977). A more recent review described 83 pregnancies in 53 cirrhotic patients with 13 episodes of variceal haemorrhage and three maternal deaths. Moreover, 38 patients with non-cirrhotic portal hypertension carried 77 pregnancies and had only four variceal bleeds with one death (Britton, 1982). This is probably little different from what one would expect in such a high-risk population if not pregnant. The early recommendation that pregnancy be avoided and sterilization be advised for a woman with chronic liver disease is a view which, therefore, cannot now be supported.

In the non-pregnant patient with oesophageal varices that have not bled, prophylactic portosystemic shunts or injection sclerotherapy have not been of proven benefit (Burroughs, 1988; Santangclo *et al.*, 1988). However, for varices that have bled, injection sclerotherapy, followed by portacaval shunt if unsuccessful, is an effective means of controlling haemorrhage and preventing further bleeding. There are no similar data for the pregnant patient but it would seem reasonable to extrapolate the same therapeutic plan.

The recommendation for a woman with oesophageal varices that have not yet bled would be, therefore, to embark on pregnancy with the knowledge that she has a similar risk of bleeding with or without pregnancy. These bleeds should be treated with injection sclerotherapy. A woman with a previous history of bleeding oesophageal varices should undergo a complete course of sclerotherapy with the goal of complete obliteration of all varices before becoming pregnant. There are no data with which to evaluate the risk of further bleeding in this group. β-Blocking drugs have been used to prevent variceal bleeding but no data are available for their use in the pregnant woman with portal hypertension.

Wilson's disease

Wilson's disease is an autosomal recessive inheritable disorder of copper metabolism. It usually presents at a young age with haemolysis and hepatic or neurological dysfunction. In women, fertility is impaired, with almost invariable primary or secondary amenorrhoea (Kaushansky *et al.*, 1987). However, with therapy using D-penicillamine there is usually a return of normal reproductive function. Two papers have demonstrated that pregnancy is well tolerated in these patients once under treatment but that it is critical that therapy be continued throughout pregnancy. There is no risk to the fetus (Scheinberg and Sternlieb, 1975; Walshe, 1977).

Hepatic adenomas and focal nodular hyperplasia

Liver adenomas have increased in prevalence and are related to the use of oral contraceptives. They do not always require resection if they are asymptomatic and diminish in size on stopping the contraceptive preparation. However, there is a risk of regrowth and expansion of these adenomas during pregnancy. There are several reports of spontaneous rupture of these tumours in pregnancy with serious or fatal consequences (Kent *et al.*, 1975; Stock, Labudovich and Ducatman, 1985). It is, therefore advised that women with known liver adenomas should not become pregnant until the tumour has been resected or confirmed to have resolved entirely.

Focal nodular hyperplasia is another benign liver tumour which is not as clearly related to contraceptive steroid ingestion or the hormonal changes of pregnancy. Nevertheless there is at least one report of such a lesion increasing in size during pregnancy to the point that excision was required (Scott *et al.*, 1984). Ultrasonography is an easy method of monitoring the disorder through a pregnancy.

Other pre-existing liver conditions

Perhaps the most common liver disorder world wide is Gilbert's syndrome, which manifests as a fluctuating but minimal elevation of serum unconjugated bilirubin. It affects 5 per cent of the general population and is a totally benign condition. It is mentioned to serve as a reminder that no special investigations or precautions are required for these patients before or during pregnancy.

The Dubin–Johnson syndrome, an inherited cause of conjugated hyperbilirubinaemia, is also benign and requires no therapy. Pregnancy may unmask this condition and present in an otherwise well patient, as mild unconjugated hyperbilirubinaemia (Cohen, Lewis and Arias, 1972).

With increasing use of liver transplantation in the treatment of multiple liver diseases, reports have appeared of pregnancies in six women with previous hepatic transplants. A successful outcome of the pregnancy is probable, although obstetric complications have been reported. Maintenance of immunosuppression is vital and appears to have little adverse effect on the fetus (Colonna *et al.*, 1988; Newton *et al.*, 1988).

Counselling

An important point of discussion for a woman diagnosed as having chronic liver disease regards the advisability of future pregnancies. First, one would expect a reduction in fertility, particularly if the liver disease is active. Secondly, women with stable, treated, and uncomplicated chronic liver disease can expect an uneventful pregnancy but that treatments such as D-penicillinamine or steroids should be maintained through pregnancy. However, there is an added risk to the fetus with a fourfold increase in prematurity, fetal distress and stillbirth (Hardison, 1988). Babies born of mothers with hepatitis B or D will require immunoprophylaxis as discussed below. Lastly, women with liver disease complicated by oesophageal varices might bleed from these in the course of their pregnancies. Certainly, a course of injection sclerotherapy should be completed before pregnancy for those who have already suffered a variceal haemorrhage.

Liver disease beginning in pregnancy

This section considers the appearance of liver or biliary tract disease during pregnancy although not necessarily of a form unique to the pregnant state. Consideration is given to effects of the liver disease on the fetus and neonate as well as on the mother. Some of this discussion is considered under the section on 'Pregnancy and previous liver disease'.

Viral hepatitis

This represents the most frequent cause of jaundice in pregnancy, being responsible for 50 per cent of cases (Haemmerli, 1966). One must consider at least six different types of viral hepatitis including those caused by hepatitis A, B, D and three types of non-A, non-B viruses.

Hepatitis A

This infection is typically spread by faecal–oral contamination and is marked by nausea, vomiting, anorexia and a rise in serum transaminase levels. Diagnosis is confirmed by the detection of IgM antibody to hepatitis A (IgM anti-HAV). In many developing countries, almost universal childhood infection leads to lifelong immunity (Kwast and Stevens, 1987). Acute hepatitis A infection does not lead to chronic infection or cirrhosis. Apart from the rare but serious complication of fulminant hepatic failure, there does not appear to be any significant serious risk to either the mother or fetus even with third trimester infection (Tong et al., 1981). Rarely is it transmitted to the fetus, probably owing to the brief viraemic period and the lack of a chronic infectious state.

Hepatitis B

By virtue of its world-wide prevalence, transmissibility and ability to cause chronic liver disease, hepatitis B is the most important viral liver infection. It is estimated that, world wide, 200 million individuals are infected with hepatitis B. Acute infection develops from parenteral exposure to infected blood or secretions such as by blood transfusions, shared illicit needles, tattoos, sexual intercourse or, in the case of neonates, parturition. Acute infection may be self-limited or progress to a chronic carrier state. This state is indicated by the presence of a variety of viral antigens or their antibodies, hepatitis B surface antigen (HBsAg), hepatitis Be antigen (HBeAg) or hepatitis B core antibody (anti HBcAg) (Koff and Galambos, 1987). If maternal infection occurs in the first or second trimesters, it rarely is transmitted to the fetus, but with a third trimester infection the risk of transmission rises to 60 per cent (Schweitzer et al., 1973). Furthermore, in contradistinction to hepatitis A, where there is no form of chronic infection, acute hepatitis B can lead to chronic infection. In Taiwan the asymptomatic chronic carrier rate of hepatitis B affects 5–20 per cent of the general population, one of the highest in the world. If a pregnant woman is HBsAg positive, there is a 40 per cent risk of neonatal infection developing (Stevens et al., 1975). This risk of infant infection rises to 90 per cent if the mother is also HBeAg positive and, in addition, up to 90 per cent of these babies will then become chronic hepatitis B carriers (Centers for Disease Control, 1985). Having chronic hepatitis B from infancy increases the risk of developing cirrhosis and primary hepatocellular carcinoma by 200-fold (Beasley et al., 1981).

The source of this neonatal infection is controversial. Some evidence suggests it to be transplacental leakage of infected maternal blood (Lin et al., 1987). However, this antepartum transmission probably accounts for only 10 per cent of fetal infections (Wong, Lee and Ip, 1980). The majority of fetal infections arise from fetal contamination during delivery (Goudea et al., 1983). This has led to the proposal that delivery should be by caesarean section in mothers who are highly infectious as demonstrated by the presence of HBeAg (Wong, Lee and Ip, 1980; Lee et al., 1988). More recently, the introduction of hepatitis B vaccines has made this practice obsolete in many centres. If infection is not acquired at birth, further risk occurs postnatally at an annual rate of 26 per cent up to the third year of life especially, again, when the mother is HBeAg positive (Beasley et al., 1983b). Where there is no maternal hepatitis Be marker or the mother has antibody to hepatitis Be antigen, the risk of neonatal infection falls to 12 and 25 per cent, respectively and the risk of becoming a chronic carrier is also much reduced (Stevens, Buckley and Mackay, 1979; Snydman, 1985).

Older reports suggested that maternal hepatitis B infection during pregnancy increased the incidence of stillbirth and prematurity (Bornhanmanesh *et al.*, 1973). This is probably a reflection of the severity of the effect of hepatitis on the mother, as most of those reported cases suffered fulminant hepatitis. More recent work indicates no increased rates of fetal wastage, congenital malformations, or intrauterine growth retardation in pregnancies complicated by maternal acute viral hepatitis (Siegel, 1973; Hieber *et al.*, 1977; Pastorek, Miller and Summers, 1988).

With serological markers and prophylactic immunotherapy for hepatitis B infection being readily available, screening programmes for women at high risk have been advocated. The initial recommendations were to screen for HBsAg in women belonging to certain high risk groups (Table 6.1) at one prenatal visit or, failing that, at time of delivery (Centers for Disease Control, 1985). However, failure to obtain a history suggesting membership of a high risk group led to 47 per cent of HBsAg positive mothers being missed in one study (Jonas *et al*, 1987). Factors such as this, plus a cost-effectiveness analysis for the United States, has led to the recommendation that all pregnant women be screened for HBsAg (Kumar *et al.*, 1987; Arevalo and Washington, 1988).

The value of universal screening for hepatitis B rests on the availability of effective vaccines for the neonate. Prophylaxis of all infants born to HBsAg-positive mothers regardless of the mother's HBeAg or anti-HBe status is advised. Hepatitis B immunoglobulin (HBIG) 0.5 ml should be administered intramuscularly within 12 h of birth. Hepatitis B vaccine is subsequently given by three intramuscular injections of 0.5 ml each: the first dose is given concurrently with the HBIG but at a different site, with subsequent doses to follow at 1 and 6 months (Centers for Disease Control, 1985). The child's HBsAg and anti-HBs status should be checked at 12 months to evaluate the success of the therapy. A programme such as this would, at least in Asia, reduce the number of hepatitis B carriers by 20 per cent and, in turn, the morbidity and mortality of chronic liver disease (Beasley *et al.*, 1983a). Other treatment regimens are under review (Lee *et al.*, 1987).

There is no need to isolate infants born to hepatitis B positive mothers as they rarely demonstrate the antigen in the immediate neonatal period. Even though HBsAg can be found in breast milk, there is little evidence to support transmission by this route. Avoidance of breast feeding by mothers with hepatitis B is, therefore, not required (Beasley *et al.*, 1975; Snydman, 1985).

Hepatitis D
Delta hepatitis is caused by the hepatitis D agent, a virus that can affect only individuals also infected with hepatitis B. Both the acute and chronic forms of hepatitis involving this agent are more severe than hepatitis B alone. Perinatal

Table 6.1. Women who should be screened for HBsAg during pregnancy

1 Asian, Pacific Island or Eskimo descent
2 Haitian or sub-Saharan African birthplace
3 History of acute or chronic liver disease
4 Work exposure (e.g. dialysis unit, institution for mentally retarded)
5 Parenteral drug abuse
6 Multiple blood transfusions
7 Rejection as a blood donor
8 Intimate or household contact with hepatitis B patient
9 Multiple episodes of venereal disease

Adapted from Centers for Disease Control (1985)

transmission has been reported (Zanetti *et al.*, 1982). There is no specific immuno-therapy for the neonate but the same regimen as for hepatitis B should be given.

Non-A, non-B hepatitis (hepatitis C)

There are at least three agents responsible for this form of hepatitis: two bloodborne, one of which is hepatitis C (HCV), and one transmitted by the faecal-oral route. By definition these infections are not associated with the serological markers for hepatitis A or B. The importance of non-A, non-B hepatitis is that it is the cause of most cases of transfusion-related hepatitis and the aetiology of 80 per cent of cases of fulminant hepatitis (Bal *et al.*, 1987). Sources of this infection are the same as for hepatitis B, with the addition of sporadic and, in South East Asia, waterborne epidemics (Dienstag, 1983).

As with other forms of viral hepatitis, there is little evidence to suggest a direct adverse effect of non-A, non-B hepatitis on the fetus except in so far as there may be serious maternal morbidity (Khuroo *et al.*, 1981). Six of nine infants born to mothers with acute non-A, non-B hepatitis in the third trimester had elevated serum ALT levels, with two persisting beyond 8 weeks; however, there was no clinical evidence of liver disease (Tong *et al.*, 1981). From this has come the somewhat empirical recommendation that babies born of mothers with non-A, non-B hepatitis be given immune serum globulin within 24 h of birth and again 28 days later (Rustgi and Hoofnagle, 1987).

The major complications of non-A, non-B hepatitis are maternal. Fulminant hepatic failure developed in 22 per cent of pregnant women against 0 per cent of non-pregnant women and 2.8 per cent of men in one series (Khuroo *et al.*, 1981). This marked difference in susceptibility for pregnant women is particularly true in the epidemic forms of this hepatitis as found in South East Asia. There is a 10 per cent fatality rate for pregnant women compared with other groups in which it is generally self-limiting (Ramalingaswami and Purcell, 1988). Labour is often the event that precipitates liver failure.

There is no specific therapy for non-A, non-B hepatitis. As with all forms of hepatitis overly aggressive and invasive investigations are not generally needed. Unless absolutely necessary, amniocentesis should be avoided in order to prevent inadvertent parenteral contamination of the fetus. Fulminant liver failure in pregnancy is treated in the conventional fashion with ventilatory nutritional and haemodynamic support (Hoyumpa *et al.*, 1979; Dienstag, 1983).

Drugs

Just as increasing numbers of drugs are being found to cause liver disease in the non-pregnant patient, medications must be carefully ruled out as the aetiology of hepatic disease in the pregnant woman (Zimmerman and Maddrey, 1987). The trend towards minimal use of medication in pregnancy makes this task easier. Some previous cases of acute idiopathic fatty liver of pregnancy were probably due to intravenous tetracycline, which can lead to a very similar histological picture. Such intravenous therapy is rarely used now; however, erythromycin is still in common use and in all forms is potentially hepatotoxic (McCormack *et al.*, 1977).

Budd–Chiari syndrome
Hepatic venous outflow obstruction (the Budd–Chiari syndrome) is increasingly being recognized, although it remains an uncommon condition. The increased risk in

women taking oral contraceptives and in pregnancy has been well appreciated (Khuroo, 1980). There are many other aetiological factors which include paroxysmal nocturnal haemoglobinuria, use of herbal medications, inferior vena caval webs and malignant invasion of the inferior vena cava. A common feature in many cases is an increased thrombotic tendency. In six of 11 women under the age of 30 with Budd–Chiari syndrome, oral contraceptives or pregnancy were implicated (Powell-Jackson *et al.*, 1982).

Usually the onset of symptoms is acute but it may be insidious over a period of several months. Where pregnancy is involved, the onset is usually in the postpartum period. Almost all patients have ascites, hepatomegaly and upper abdominal pain. Jaundice appears rarely and late in the disease. Aminotransferase concentrations are usually less than twice normal; alkaline phosphatase may be up to five times normal. Liver biopsy was characteristic in three of 11 patients in one series, showing congestion, patchy necrosis and venular thrombosis (Mitchell *et al.*, 1982). Hepatic venography and, occasionally, ultrasound examination are the most valuable diagnostic tests: these modalities will confirm the diagnosis and rule out surgically correctable aetiologies such as inferior vena caval webs.

Treatment involves portosystemic shunting or liver transplantation in most patients. Medical management using diuretics to control the ascites may relieve symptoms in mild cases.

The prognosis in Budd–Chiari syndrome is dismal, with eight of 16 pregnant patients dead within one year in one series (Khuroo and Datta, 1980). Fortunately, liver transplantation improves the outlook. As pregnancy-related Budd–Chiari syndrome almost always develops after delivery, there is little fetal morbidity or mortality. Usually, women who survive the Budd–Chiari syndrome are advised to avoid oral contraception or further pregnancies; there is, however, one report of three uneventful subsequent pregnancies in two women with this syndrome (Vons *et al.*, 1984).

Gallbladder disease

The function of the gallbladder in pregnancy is of interest because of the long-known association between gallstones and parity. Women are known to have increased biliary cholesterol and a reduced bile salt pool, and, during pregnancy, impaired gallbladder contraction (Braverman, Johnson and Kern, 1980). Although the pathogenesis of gallstones is poorly understood, these changes are felt to be major factors. In one sonographic survey of 338 obstetric patients, 3.5 per cent were found to have cholelithiasis (Stauffer *et al.*, 1982). It must be noted, however, that many of these gallstones remain asymptomatic both during pregnancy and after, and require no therapy. Biliary colic or cholecystitis is unusual in pregnancy, with only 13 cases found in one series of 91 500 confinements (O'Neill, 1969). In many instances, symptomatic gallbladder disease can be treated conservatively. However, surgery may be required if there is no improvement with medical therapy or if complications arise. Overall fetal salvage is 75 per cent with surgical management of gallbladder disease. However, biliary tract surgery in the first trimester led to the loss of five out of seven pregnancies in one series, suggesting that delaying surgery until the latter two trimesters would be beneficial (Hiatt *et al.*, 1986).

Pancreatitis has rarely been reported to occur in pregnancy and initially was thought to be caused by the pregnancy. However, a large survey showed 18 of 20 cases of pancreatitis in pregnancy to be due to gallstones (McKay, O'Neill and Imrie,

1980). Diagnosis and treatment are the same as in the non-pregnant state. There was very little risk to mother or fetus in that series although severe pancreatitis can be a serious illness with profoundly deleterious effects on the fetus.

Liver disease of pregnancy

This section considers those conditions affecting the liver that are peculiar to pregnancy. Although uncommon, these are serious conditions, which profoundly affect the management of the index pregnancy and, potentially, future pregnancies.

Acute fatty liver of pregnancy

This is an uncommon condition that has been increasingly diagnosed during the past decade. It was first recognized in 1934 (Stander and Cadden) but fully described by Sheehan in 1940. Early estimates of incidence were less than three cases per million pregnancies (Haemmerli, 1966) with only 85 cases in the world literature by 1980. More recent surveys reflect an increased awareness of the disease and show an increased incidence to one case per 13 328 deliveries (Pockros, Peters and Reynolds, 1984).

The aetiology of this condition remains unknown. The initial implication of intravenous tetracycline therapy has not proved correct, in spite of the histological similarities of the ensuing hepatic disorders (Kunelis, Peters and Edmondson, 1965). There is no known infectious, metabolic or familial component (Kaplan, 1985; Rolfes and Ishak, 1985) and subsequent uncomplicated pregnancies have been reported (Breen *et al.*, 1972).

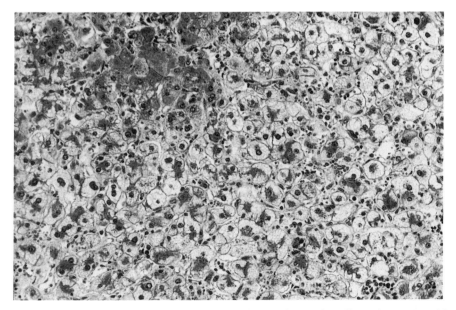

Figure 6.1. Post-mortem biopsy of liver from a fatal case of acute fatty liver of pregnancy. Note microvesicular fat droplets in the swollen hepatocytes with centrizonal hepatocyte necrosis. (H + E, × 160, courtesy Dr J Piris)

Although the clinical presentation is non-specific and similar to the more common viral hepatitis, the histological picture is characteristically different. The findings on liver biopsy are of microvesicular fat accumulation and centrizonal hepatocellular necrosis (Figure 6.1). At times the fat can be recognized only with special stains such as oil red O. Other causes of microvesicular fat disease include Reye's syndrome, valproic acid toxicity, tetracycline toxicity, and vomiting disease of Jamaica, all of which can usually be differentiated on clinical grounds.

More specifically, the findings of giant hepatic mitochondria, urea-cycle enzyme abnormalities (Weber *et al.*, 1979) and systemic carnitine deficiency (Feller *et al.*, 1983) have been demonstrated. It has been suggested that these intracellular abnormalities lead to the accumulation of toxic free fatty acids in the liver (Eisele, Barker and Smuckler, 1975; Rolfes and Ishak, 1985).

The clinical presentation of acute fatty liver of pregnancy is initially quite non-specific. There are no risk factors based on maternal age, race, or previous obstetric history. Most commonly it begins in the 35th week of gestation and never occurs before the 30th week. An increased incidence is seen in twin pregnancies and those with male offspring. There is a rapid onset, over a few days, of malaise, nausea, vomiting and non-specific upper abdominal pain. This is followed within a few more days by jaundice and the disease can progress to hepatocellular failure as manifest by coagulopathy and encephalopathy.

Physical examination is not diagnostically helpful although rapid progression to hepatic failure is quite characteristic. Seventy-eight per cent of women will have encephalopathy ranging from grade I to grade IV (Hague, Fenton and Duncan, 1983). Up to 40 per cent of patients will have evidence of pre-eclampsia with hypertension and proteinuria (Pockros, Peters and Reynolds, 1984). The time from first symptoms to death is usually 1–2 weeks but can range from 3 days to 6 weeks (Varner and Rinderknecht, 1980).

In one series, 19 of 35 women had evidence of significant upper gastrointestinal bleeding, with seven patients developing oliguric renal failure (Rolfes and Ishak, 1985).

Laboratory abnormalities are quite typical, although not diagnostic. There is a moderate thrombocytopenia $<100 \times 10^9/l$ and the presence of giant platelets, nucleated RBCs and basophilic stippling are common. Serum transaminases are minimally increased and rarely rise above 500 i.u./l except with profound hypotension. This finding is important, as severe viral hepatitis, a major differential diagnosis, often leads to serum transaminase levels >1000 i.u./l. Alkaline phosphatase levels are usually elevated. Hypoalbuminaemia and a prolonged prothrombin time are common and reflect severe hepatic synthetic dysfunction.

Disseminated intravascular coagulation has been reported (Holzbach, 1974; Liebman *et al.*, 1983). Bilirubin levels may be normal early in the disease, rarely exceed 200 µmol/l, and quickly fall after termination of the pregnancy (Burroughs *et al.*, 1982). One may see a rapid fall in transaminase and glucose levels as liver destruction progresses, precluding production of these substrates. Such findings suggest a poor prognosis.

Diagnosis of acute fatty liver of pregnancy is based on a combination of the clinical and laboratory features noted above. Liver biopsy is important for diagnosis but may not be possible with coagulation disturbances. In some centres, transjugular liver biopsies can be performed safely in the face of a coagulopathy. The biopsy findings described above are diagnostic in this clinical picture, and can be used to differentiate from such conditions as acute viral hepatitis (Figure 6.2).

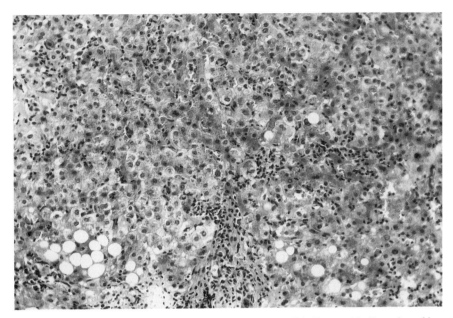

Figure 6.2. Acute viral hepatitis. Note marked inflammatory cell infiltrate with disruption of hepatic architecture and degeneration of hepatocytes. (H + E, × 160, courtesy Dr J Piris)

The differential diagnosis in the setting of rapid and profound hepatic dysfunction in the third trimester of pregnancy is between fulminant hepatitis caused by viruses or drugs including alcohol, and acute fatty liver of pregnancy. Alcoholic hepatitis is uncommon in pregnancy and historical evidence of heavy alcohol use along with typical hepatic histology would be required to make the diagnosis. Viral hepatitis can be very difficult to differentiate from acute fatty liver of pregnancy (Brown *et al.*, 1987).

Appropriate serological tests are available and are vital in the diagnosis of hepatitis A, B, C or D. Usually, serum transaminase levels are >1000 i.u./l in viral hepatitis and it is unusual to find evidence of pre-eclampsia or thrombocytopenia. Drug hepatotoxicities such as those due to paracetamol overdose, intravenous tetracycline, or valproic acid should be considered and investigated by history and serum drug levels.

Reports are now appearing, describing the use of computed tomography and ultrasound in the diagnosis of acute fatty liver of pregnancy. Both of those modalities, although not submitted to formal evaluation in this condition, are safe, rapid and effective means of detecting excess liver fat. A diffuse increased echogenicity on ultrasonography, or reduced attenuation on computed tomography, are valuable indicators of fatty infiltration, although an absence of these changes does not rule out involvement (Campillo *et al.*, 1986; McKee *et al.*, 1986).

Confirmation of the diagnosis of acute fatty liver of pregnancy is vital because therapy requires rapid termination of the pregnancy. On the other hand, in the case of fulminant hepatic failure due to viral infection, there is no benefit in rapid delivery. Most authorities advocate urgent caesarean section (Ebert *et al.*, 1984; Hou *et al.*, 1984), although others have found induced vaginal delivery satisfactory if placental function is not impaired (Davies *et al.*, 1980). This form of management has not been subjected to controlled trial. It is based rather on the prompt and striking improvement in maternal liver function after delivery and the dismal outcome without termination of the pregnancy.

Early reports described maternal and fetal mortality rates as high as 85 per cent (Varner and Rinderknecht, 1980; Scully, 1981). Stillbirth in the face of serious maternal deterioration was common even though neonatal liver function is usually normal. With earlier recognition, diagnosis and improved medical and neonatal support, the maternal and neonatal mortality rates have fallen to 8 per cent and 14 per cent respectively (Berneau et al., 1983; Rolfes and Ishak, 1985; Riely et al., 1987).

Maternal liver function returns to normal following delivery, with hepatic fat being undetectable within one month. There is no liver scarring and there are no chronic liver sequelae (Rolfes and Ishak, 1986a). Subsequent pregnancies have been reported in 13 women surviving acute fatty liver of pregnancy, including two further pregnancies in four cases. All women had normal pregnancies without recurrence of liver dysfunction (Burroughs et al., 1982). This information allows some measure of reassurance when advising on the safety of further pregnancies.

Liver disease in pre-eclampsia

Pre-eclampsia is a hypertensive disorder of pregnancy that is associated with proteinuria and oedema (see Chapter 2). It affects 5–10 per cent of all pregnancies, occurs primarily in nulliparous women, usually after the 20th week of gestation, but most commonly closer to term (Lindheimer and Katz, 1985). The major target organs are the brain, kidney and liver. This discussion focuses only on the complications of pre-eclampsia in the latter organ system.

The liver is not generally involved in pre-eclampsia until it is either severe or has progressed to frank eclampsia, at which stage liver involvement occurs in >70 per cent of cases (Haemmerli, 1966; Riely, 1986). Symptoms associated with hepatic involvement include upper abdominal pain, nausea, vomiting and jaundice in addition to the other features such as headache and oedema. Jaundice, however, occurs only in 40 per cent of patients (Rolfes and Ishak, 1986b). On examination there is generally hypertension and proteinuria but both of these classic features can be mild or absent in spite of severe pre-eclampsia.

Laboratory studies in one large survey showed a universal elevation in serum transaminases from 350 to 3720 i.u./l with most being >500 i.u./l. Bilirubin was elevated 4–16 times above normal (Rolfes and Ishak, 1986b). A well-described constellation of laboratory findings [Haemolysis, Elevated Liver enzymes, and Low Platelet count (the HELLP syndrome)] has been described in pre-eclampsia (Weinstein, 1982). Women with this syndrome differ from the usual population with pre-eclampsia in that they tend to be older, multiparous, and, importantly, often may not have hypertension, proteinuria or oedema; consequently the significance of their often non-specific complaints may be missed (Baca and Gibbons, 1988).

The aetiology of pre-eclampsia is not known. However, the histopathology of pre-eclamptic liver disease comprises combinations of periportal fibrin deposition, haemorrhage, and hepatocellular necrosis. The finding of fibrin deposits is partially responsible for one of the yet unproven theories of the pathogenesis of pre-eclampsia: this holds that there is severe vasospasm, particularly in the kidney and liver, which, in the presence of intravascular coagulation allows precipitation of fibrin and fibrinogen (Arias and Mancilla-Jimenez, 1976). Other pathogenic theories include an initial episode of liver cell necrosis or, alternatively, intrahepatic haemorrhage. Rolfes and Ishak (1986a) suggest that segmental hepatic vasospasm leads to a localized consumptive coagulopathy allowing fibrin deposition while endothelial and liver cell necrosis produce haemorrhage.

It has recently been suggested that there are clinical and histological similarities between mild cases of acute fatty liver of pregnancy and pre-eclampsia with hepatic involvement (Riely et al., 1987). This is based on reports of cases of acute fatty liver of pregnancy with hypertension, HELLP syndrome, or rupture of the liver. Furthermore, cases of pre-eclampsia with fatty liver infiltration have been reported (Berneau et al., 1983; Rolfes and Ishak, 1986a; Minuk, Liu and Kelly, 1987). However, in spite of these clinical similarities suggesting a spectrum of liver disease in pregnancy, the histological appearances remain distinctly different (Rolfes and Ishak, 1986a).

The diagnosis of liver involvement in pre-eclampsia is based on the findings of abnormal liver enzymes in the face of hypertension, proteinuria or oedema. Using autopsy samples, the majority of livers will have the histological findings discussed above. However, liver samples taken by needle biopsy will be abnormal in only 25 per cent of cases, presumably because of sampling error and less severe disease (Rolfes and Ishak, 1986a).

Specific therapy for the liver involvement is not usually required and indications for urgent delivery are dictated by the hypertensive and neurological status. Steroids are not effective in correcting the thrombocytopenia (Sibai et al., 1986). Hepatic rupture is the one situation where urgent and specific therapy is required. This typically presents with the triad of right upper quadrant pain, sudden hypotension, and pre-eclampsia. The pathogenesis of this complication has been speculated to include liver necrosis, hypervascularity and vessel rupture leading to a subcapsular haematoma or haemoperitoneum (Henny et al., 1983). In distinction to the non-pregnant state, hepatic rupture of pregnancy is rarely due to trauma. Eighty per cent of pregnant women with hepatic rupture have pre-eclampsia (British Medical Journal Editorial, 1976). After resuscitation and transfusion, emergency exploratory laparotomy is almost invariably required (Manas et al., 1985). The complication carries a maternal and fetal mortality rate of about 60 per cent (Bis and Waxman, 1976). Hepatic infarction also can develop very occasionally in pre-eclampsia. This rare but very serious outcome presumably reflects the intense hepatic vasospasm (Dammann et al., 1982).

The overall outcome at a tertiary referral centre in a recent large series of patients with liver involvement in pre-eclampsia or eclampsia demonstrated a maternal mortality rate of 2 per cent and a fetal mortality rate of 33 per cent. On follow-up, 44 patients used oral contraceptives without morbidity, and 38 patients had 49 subsequent pregnancies with only one patient having a recurrence of the syndrome (Sibai et al., 1986). There have been few reports of follow-up liver biopsies but it is believed that the liver histology returns to normal.

Intrahepatic cholestasis of pregnancy

After viral hepatitis, this condition is the second most common cause of jaundice in pregnancy, accounting for 20 per cent of cases (Haemmerli, 1966). Originally called 'recurrent jaundice of pregnancy' (even if manifesting for the first time) the present designation is 'idiopathic intrahepatic cholestasis of pregnancy'. The aetiology of this condition, as with all the liver diseases of pregnancy, is unknown.

There is a distinct regional variation in prevalence, with Chile (12–22 per cent of all pregnancies), Bolivia (9 per cent), and Sweden (2–3 per cent) reporting the highest rates (Vore, 1987). France (0.2 per cent) and Canada (0.1 per cent) report lower prevalence rates, whereas no data are available for the United Kingdom (Lunzer *et al.*, 1986). There is clearly a genetic influence, in that large kindreds have been described with cholestasis of pregnancy, but the exact mode of transmission is obscure (Reyes, 1982). This difficulty stems from variability of expression, in that one or more pregnancies may be unaffected between appearances of the syndrome. Holzbach, Sivak and Braun (1983) showed it to be transmitted as a dominant trait, but could not clarify whether it was autosomal or X-linked. Certainly, both men and women with a family history of the disease responded differently to exogenous oestrogen administration, compared with a control group (Reyes *et al.*, 1981).

Intrahepatic cholestasis occurs in a small number of women using oral contraceptives and up to one half of these women will develop the same condition subsequently during pregnancy (Vore, 1987). It is now believed that increased oestrogen levels in these susceptible women inhibit the movement of organic anions and bile acids across the hepatic canalicular membrane.

It is this reduced excretion of bilirubin and bile salts that produces the symptoms of jaundice and pruritus. Symptoms may appear at any stage of pregnancy but most commonly occur during the third trimester. Pruritus, initially nocturnal only, is generalized and distressing; it usually precedes the jaundice by 2 weeks but may remain the sole symptom (de Pagter *et al.*, 1976). The pruritus correlates with the dramatic increase in serum bile acids by up to 100 times (Laatikainen and Ikonen, 1977). In fact, serum bile acid concentrations are a sensitive means of diagnosing intrahepatic cholestasis of pregnancy (Lunzer *et al.*, 1986).

When hyperbilirubinaemia appears, it is generally mild ($<60\,\mu mol/l$) and conjugated. Urine colour may darken. In keeping with the cholestasis, the serum alkaline phosphatase level may be markedly increased. Serum transaminase levels are rarely $>250\,i.u./l$ (Krejs, 1983). Fat malabsorption, often asymptomatic, has been reported in 10 of 12 patients, with this condition beginning within 3 weeks of the first symptoms of cholestasis (Reyes *et al.*, 1987). This is presumably related to the reduction in the intestinal bile salt pool and may lead to maternal malnutrition. Specific vitamin deficiencies (in particular vitamin K) may ensue, leading to coagulation disturbances.

Physical examination in intrahepatic cholestasis is unremarkable except for mild jaundice and scratch marks. There should be no change in liver or spleen size. Other than pruritus and mild malaise, there are few symptoms, in distinction to the abdominal pain, nausea and vomiting of the other hepatic disorders of pregnancy.

Liver biopsy (which is not generally necessary) shows dilated bile canaliculi and enlarged mitochondria in an irregular and focal distribution. These changes resolve within a few months of delivery resulting in a histologically normal liver (Adlercreutz, Svanborg and Anberg, 1967).

Following delivery, the serum bilirubin, bile acid, and transaminase levels rapidly fall to normal, although the alkaline phosphatase concentration may continue to rise for up to 10 days (Haemmerli, 1966). All of these serum parameters should be normal within 2 months of delivery.

The maternal outcome for this condition is excellent with no reports of mortality. The pruritus can be treated with oral cholestyramine if troublesome (Dacus and Muram, 1987). Postpartum haemorrhage due to reduced hepatic synthesis of coagulation factors may be severe (Reid *et al.*, 1976). Careful monitoring of the prothrombin time towards term is necessary, with parenteral vitamin K replacement if abnormal. Cholestyramine will potentiate the malabsorption of vitamin K and its use makes vitamin K supplementation at the start of labour mandatory.

Unfortunately the fetal outcome is not as good, with 18 of 50 infants being premature in one series (Reid *et al.*, 1976). Up to 10 per cent of pregnancies resulted in stillbirths in another series (Reyes, 1982). Fetal distress has been correlated with the elevation in maternal serum bile acid levels (Laatikainen and Tulenheimo, 1984). However, this assay is not readily available and is therefore not a useful monitor of fetal progress in most hospitals. Short-term monitoring of fetal heart variability before term has been recommended with a view to induction of labour once fetal maturity has been established (Ammala and Kariniema, 1981).

Intrahepatic cholestasis of pregnancy may, as has been noted, recur unpredictably with subsequent pregnancies or following the use of oral oestrogens or contraceptives. Except for the need to monitor the fetus closely towards term and the nuisance of pruritus, there is no reason for a woman with such a history to avoid further pregnancies.

Hyperemesis gravidarum

Nausea and vomiting are common, particularly in early pregnancy, but rarely seriously affect the pregnancy. However, when symptoms are very severe, malnutrition, dehydration and liver dysfunction can occur. There may be mild hyperbilirubinaemia but this is rarely more than a fourfold increase. Serum transaminase levels will also be slightly elevated. These biochemical changes should resolve with control of the vomiting and improvement in hydration and nutrition. The mechanism behind the changes is not clear (Adams, Gordon and Coombes, 1968; Larrey *et al.*, 1984).

An approach to liver disease in pregnancy

From this discussion it can be seen that liver disease can present in pregnancy as non-specific complaints of malaise and nausea or as jaundice, pruritus and hepatic encephalopathy. One must carefully review the history for evidence of pre-existing liver disease or risk factors for it. Evidence of exposure to drugs, blood products or alcohol must be sought. Efforts should be made to differentiate intercurrent liver diseases complicating the pregnancy from pre-existing liver disease or from a hepatic disorder unique to pregnancy. The onset of disease in relation to the stage of pregnancy is important.

Investigations should be considered in terms of confirming the impression of liver disease, of assessing hepatic function and anticipating complications, and of determining an aetiology. Primary elevation of the transaminases or alkaline phosphatase will differentiate a hepatocellular disease from a cholestatic disorder. Viral hepatitis serology allows for easy diagnosis of hepatitis A, B, C or D infections. Abdominal ultrasound is a safe and effective means of evaluating the hepatic parenchyma for evidence of fatty infiltration, biliary obstruction, gallstones, haematomas or tumours. Liver biopsies may be safely performed only in the absence of coagulopathy and are, in fact, infrequently required; their main value is in confirming a diagnosis for which specific therapy, including early termination of the pregnancy, would be beneficial. From the maternal standpoint, early termination is helpful only for acute fatty liver of pregnancy, severe pre-eclampsia or cirrhosis with progressive liver failure. The fetal outcome, on the other hand, will be balanced between the hazards

Table 6.2.   Summary of features of liver disease and pregnancy

Feature	Acute fatty liver of pregnancy	Intrahepatic cholestasis	Viral hepatitis	Pre-eclampsia	Budd–Chiari
Onset (trimester)	3	3	1,2,3	3	Post partum
Family history	0	++	+	0	0
Abdominal pain	++	0	0	+	++
Vomiting	+++	0	0	0	0
Pruritus	0	+++	+	0	0
Bilirubin	+	+	+++	++	0
Transaminases	+	+	+++	++	+
Alkaline phosphatase	+	+++	+	0	++
Encephalopathy	+++	0	+	+	+
Special laboratory tests		Bile acids	HBsAg, HAV		
Pathology	Microvesicular fat	Centrilobular cholestasis	Necrosis	Fibrin deposition; haemorrhage	
Other				$\uparrow$BP, oedema	Ascites

of premature birth and the placental insufficiency that accompanies severe systemic liver disease and, rarely, hyperbilirubinaemia. Table 6.2 summarizes some of the features of the major hepatic conditions seen in pregnancy.

Apart from prompt delivery by caesarean section or induction, therapy of liver disease in pregnancy involves the removal of inciting agents such as drugs or alcohol, recognition and treatment of complications such as variceal haemorrhage, and, at times, specific modalities. These latter may include steroids in autoimmune hepatitis, pencillamine in Wilson's disease or surgery in persistent cholecystitis, and differ little from the management in the non-pregnant state.

Also of importance in the pregnant patient with liver disease is counselling as to the advisability of further pregnancies. Thus, in the case of intrahepatic cholestasis of pregnancy, one could anticipate pruritus but a good maternal and fetal outcome, whereas, following pre-eclamptic liver disease or the Budd–Chiari syndrome, the chance for a satisfactory outcome is very low. Finally, consideration should be given to the woman with chronic liver disease who may desire a pregnancy. She should be aware that her fertility will be reduced, especially with active liver disease, but there is little likelihood of the pregnancy adversely affecting her liver function. She will be at risk for variceal bleeding if portal hypertension is present. Maintenance therapy such as steroids or penicillamine should be continued, with only azathioprine being stopped before pregnancy.

Special consideration must be given to the neonate in the face of maternal hepatitis B or non-A, non-B and in the rare circumstances of severe and prolonged maternal hyperbilirubinaemia. Appropriate vaccinations are vital and have been reviewed above.

In summary, it is apparent that liver disease in pregnancy can no longer simply be thought of as 'jaundice in pregnancy'. An awareness of the varied presentations of hepatic disorders will provide more rapid diagnosis. Specific therapy is available for both mother and infant in many instances. Certainly, there are important differences in maternal and fetal outcomes, as well as in the implications for future pregnancies. All of these details are important in providing optimal care for these complicated pregnancies.

References

Adams, RH, Gordon, J and Combes, B (1968) Hyperemesis gravidarum. I. Evidence of hepatic dysfunction. *Obstetrics and Gynecology*, **5**, 659–664

Adeniyi, FA and Olatunbosun, DA (1984) Origins and significance of the increased plasma alkaline phosphatase during normal pregnancy and pre-eclampsia. *British Journal of Obstetrics and Gynaecology*, **91**, 857–862

Adlercreutz, H, Svanborg, A and Anberg, A (1967) Recurrent jaundice in pregnancy. *American Journal of Medicine*, **42**, 335–347

Ammala, P and Kariniema, V (1981) Short-term variability of fetal heart rate in cholestasis of pregnancy. *American Journal of Obstetrics and Gynecology*, **141**, 217–220

Antia, FP, Bharadwaj, TP, Watsa, MC and Master, J (1958) Liver in normal pregnancy, pre-eclampsia and eclampsia. *Lancet*, **ii**, 776–778

Arevalo, JA and Washington, AE (1988) Cost-effectiveness of prenatal screening and immunization for hepatitis B virus. *Journal of the American Medical Association*, **259**, 365–369

Arias, F and Mancilla-Jimenez, R (1976) Hepatic fibrinogen deposits in pre-eclampsia. *New England Journal of Medicine*, **295**, 578–582

Baca, L and Gibbons, RB (1988) The HELLP syndrome: a serious complication of pregnancy with hemolysis, elevated levels of liver enzymes, and low platelet count. *American Journal of Medicine*, **85**, 590–591

Bal, V, Amin, SN, Rath, AS *et al.* (1987) Virological markers and antibody responses in fulminant viral hepatitis. *Journal of Medical Virology*, **23**, 75–82

Bean, WB, Cogswell, R, Dexter, M and Embick, JF (1949) Vascular changes of the skin in pregnancy. *Surgery, Gynecology and Obstetrics*, **88**, 739–752

Beasley, RP, Stevens, CE, Shiao, I-S and Meng, H-C (1975) Evidence against breast-feeding as a mechanism for vertical transmission of hepatitis B *Lancet*, **ii**, 740–741

Beasley, RP, Hwang, L-Y, Lin, C-C and Chien, C-S (1981) Hepatocellular carcinoma and hepatitis B virus. *Lancet*, **ii**, 1129–1133

Beasley, RP, Hwang, L-Y, Lee, GC-Y *et al.* (1983a) Prevention of perinatally transmitted hepatitis B virus infections with hepatitis B immune globulin and hepatitis B vaccine. *Lancet*, **ii**, 1099–1102

Beasley, RP, Hwang, L-Y, Stevens, CE *et al.* (1983b) Efficacy of hepatitis B immune globulin for prevention of perinatal transmission of the hepatitis B virus carrier state: final report of a randomized double-blind, placebo-controlled trial. *Hepatology*, **3**, 135–141

Berneau, J, Degott, C, Nouel, O *et al.* (1983) Non-fatal acute fatty liver of pregnancy. *Gut*, **24**, 340–344

Bis, KA and Waxman, B (1976) Rupture of the liver associated with pregnancy: a review of the literature and report of 2 cases. *Obstetrical and Gynecological Survey*, **31**, 763–772

Bornhanmanesh, F, Haghighi, P, Hekmat *et al.* (1973) Viral hepatitis during pregnancy. *Gastroenterology*, **64**, 304–312

Braverman, DZ, Johnson, ML and Kern, F (1980) Effects of pregnancy and contraceptive steroids on gallbladder function. *New England Journal of Medicine*, **302**, 362–364

Breen, KJ, Perkins, KW, Schenker, S *et al.* (1972) Uncomplicated subsequent pregnancy after idiopathic fatty liver of pregnancy. *Obstetrics and Gynecology*, **40**, 813–815

British Medical Journal Editorial (1976) Spontaneous rupture of the liver. *British Medical Journal*, **2**, 1278–1279

Britton, RC (1982) Pregnancy and esophageal varices. *American Journal of Surgery,* **143**, 421–425

Brown, MS, Reddy, KR, Hensley, GT *et al.* (1987) The initial presentation of fatty liver of pregnancy mimicking acute viral hepatitis. *American Journal of Gastroenterology*, **82**, 554–557

Burroughs, AK (1988) The management of bleeding due to portal hypertension. Part 1. The management of acute bleeding episodes. *Quarterly Journal of Medicine*, **67**, 447–458

Burroughs, AK, Seong, NH, Dojcinov, DM *et al.* (1982) Idiopathic acute fatty liver of pregnancy in 12 patients. *Quarterly Journal of Medicine*, **51**, 481–497

Campillo, B, Bernuau, J, Witz, M-O *et al.* (1986) Ultrasonography in acute fatty liver of pregnancy. *Annals of Internal Medicine*, **105**, 383–384

Centers for Disease Control (1985) Recommendations for protection against viral hepatitis. *Morbidity and Mortality Weekly Report*, **34**, 313–335

Cohen, L, Lewis, C and Arias, IM (1972) Pregnancy, oral contraceptives, and chronic familiar jaundice with predominantly conjugated hyperbilirubinaemia (Dubin–Johnson syndrome). *Gastroenterology*, **62**, 1182–1190

Cohen, S (1980) The sluggish gallbladder of pregnancy. *New England Journal of Medicine*, **302**, 397–398

Colonna, JO, Brems, JJ, Hiatt, JR *et al.* (1988) The quality of survival after liver transplantation. *Transplantation Proceedings*, **20**, 594–597

Combes, B, Shore, GM, Cunningham, FG *et al.* (1977) Serum glutamyl transpeptidase activity in viral hepatitis: suppression in pregnancy and by birth control pills. *Gastroenterology*, **72**, 271–274

Cuddihy, A and Whelton, MJ (1987) Infertility in chronic active hepatitis. *Hepatology*, **7**, 1146

Dacus, J and Muram, D (1987) Pruritus in pregnancy. *Southern Medical Journal*, **80**, 614–617

Dammann, HG, Hagemann, J, Runge, M and Kloppel, G (1982) In vivo diagnosis of massive hepatic infarction by computed tomography. *Digestive Diseases and Sciences*, **27**, 73–79

Davies, MH, Wilkinson, SP, Hanid, MA *et al.* (1980) Acute liver disease with encephalopathy and renal failure in late pregnancy and the early puerperium: a study of fourteen patients. *British Journal of Obstetrics and Gynaecology*, **87**, 1005–1014

De Pagter, AGF, Van Berge Henegouwen, GP, Ten Bokkel Huinink, JA and Brandt, K-H (1976) Familial benign recurrent intrahepatic cholestasis. *Gastroenterology*, **71**, 202–207

Dienstag, JL (1983) Non-A, non-B hepatitis. I. Recognition, epidemiology, and clinical features. *Gastroenterology*, **85**, 439–462

Ebert, EC, Sun, EA, Wright, SH *et al.* (1984) Does early diagnosis and delivery in acute fatty liver of pregnancy lead to improvement in maternal and infant survival? *Digestive Diseases and Sciences*, **29**, 453–455

Eisele, JW, Barker, EA and Smuckler, EA (1975) Lipid content in the liver of fatty metamorphosis of pregnancy. *American Journal of Pathology*, **81**, 545–560

Feller, A, Ugarte, G, Pino, ME *et al.* (1983) Acute fatty liver of pregnancy: a possible disorder of carnitine metabolism. *Gastroenterology*, **84**, 1150

Fulton, IC, Douglas, JG, Hutchon, DJR and Beckett, GJ (1983) Is normal pregnancy cholestatic? *Clinica Chimica Acta*, **130**, 171–176

Goudeau, A, Yvonnet, B, Lesage *et al.* (1983) Lack of anti-HBc IgM in neonates with HB$_s$Ag carrier mothers argues against transplacental transmission of hepatitis B virus infection. *Lancet*, **ii**, 1103–1104

Graham, DY and Smith, JL (1981) The course of patients after variceal haemorrhage. *Gastroenterology*, **80**, 800–809

Haemmerli, UP (1966) Jaundice during pregnancy with special emphasis on recurrent jaundice during pregnancy and its differential diagnosis. *Acta Medica Scandinavica*, (suppl 444) **179**, 1–98

Hague, WM, Fenton, DW and Duncan, SLB (1983) Acute fatty liver of pregnancy. *Journal of the Royal Society of Medicine*, **76**, 652–661

Hardison, WGM (1988) Gastrointestinal and liver disorders. In *Medical Counselling Before Pregnancy* (edited by DR Hollingsworth and R Resnik) pp. 511–523. New York: Churchill Livingstone

Henny, CP, Lim, AE, Brummelkamp, WH *et al.* (1983) A review of the importance of acute multi-disciplinary treatment following spontaneous rupture of the liver capsule during pregnancy. *Surgery, Gynecology and Obstetrics*, **156**, 593–598

Hiatt, JR, Hiatt, JCG, Williams, RA and Klein, SR (1986) Biliary disease in pregnancy: strategy for surgical management. *American Journal of Surgery*, **151**, 263–265

Hieber, JP, Dalton, D, Shorey, J and Combes, B (1977) Hepatitis and pregnancy. *Journal of Pediatrics*, **91**, 545–549

Holzbach, RT (1974) Acute fatty liver of pregnancy with disseminated intravascular coagulation. *Obstetrics and Gynecology*, **43**, 740–744

Holzbach, RT, Sivak, DA and Braun, WE (1983) Familial recurrent intrahepatic cholestasis of pregnancy: a genetic study providing evidence for transmission of a sex-limited, dominant trait. *Gastroenterology*, **85**, 175–179

Hou, SH, Levin, S, Ahola, S *et al.* (1984) Acute fatty liver of pregnancy. *Digestive Diseases and Sciences*, **29**, 449–452

Hoyumpa, AM, Desmond, PV, Avant, GR *et al.* (1979) Hepatic encephalopathy. *Gastroenterology*, **76**, 184–195

Infeld, DS, Borkowf, HI and Varma, RR (1979) Chronic-persistent hepatitis and pregnancy. *Gastroenterology*, **77**, 524–527

Ingerslev, M and Teilum, G (1946) Biopsy studies on the liver in pregnancy. *Acta Obstetrica et Gynecologica*, **25**, 339–375

Jonas, MM, Schiff, ER, O'Sullivan, MJ *et al.* (1987) Failure of centers for disease control criteria to identify hepatitis B infection in a large municipal obstetrical population. *Annals of Internal Medicine*, **107**, 335–337

Kaplan, MM (1985) Acute fatty liver of pregnancy. *New England Journal of Medicine*, **313**, 367–370

Kaushansky, A, Frydman, M, Kaufman, H and Homburg, R (1987) Endocrine studies of the ovulatory disturbances in Wilson's disease (hepatolenticular degeneration). *Fertility and Sterility*, **47**, 270–275

Kent, DR, Nissen, ED, Nissen, SE and Ziehm, DJ (1975) Effect of pregnancy on liver tumor associated with oral-contraceptives. *Obstetrics and Gynecology*, **51**, 148–151

Kern, F, Everson, GT, DeMark, B *et al.* (1981) Biliary lipids, bile acids, and gallbladder function in the human female. *Journal of Clinical Investigation*, **68**, 1229–1242

Kerr, MG, Scott, DB and Samuel, E (1964) Studies of the inferior vena cava in late pregnancy. *British Medical Journal*, **1**, 532–533

Khuroo, MS (1980) Study of an epidemic of non-A, non-B hepatitis. *American Journal of Medicine*, **68**, 818–824

Khuroo, MS and Datta, DV (1980) Budd–Chiari syndrome following pregnancy. *American Journal of Medicine*, **68**, 113–121

Khuroo, MS, Teli, MR, Skidmore, S *et al.* (1981) Incidence and severity of viral hepatitis in pregnancy. *American Journal of Medicine*, **70**, 252–255

Koff, RS and Galambos, JT (1987) Viral hepatitis. In *Diseases of the Liver* (edited by L Schiff and ER Schiff), pp. 457–581. Philadelphia: Lippincott

Krejs, GJ (1983) Jaundice during pregnancy. *Seminars in Liver Disease*, **3**, 73–82

Kumar, ML, Dawson, NV, McCullough, AJ *et al.* (1987) Should all pregnant women be screened for hepatitis B? *Annals of Internal Medicine*, **107**, 273–277

Kunelis, CT, Peters, RL and Edmondson, HA (1965) Fatty liver of pregnancy and its relationship to tetracycline therapy. *American Journal of Medicine*, **38**, 359–376

Kwast, BE and Stevens, JA (1987) Viral hepatitis as a major cause of maternal mortality in Addis Ababa, Ethiopia. *International Journal of Gynaecology and Obstetrics*, **25**, 99–106

Laatikainen, T and Ikonen, E (1977) Serum bile acids in cholestasis of pregnancy. *Obstetrics and Gynecology*, **50**, 313–318

Laatikainen, T and Tulenheimo, A (1984) Maternal serum bile acid levels and fetal distress in cholestasis of pregnancy. *International Journal of Gynaecology and Obstetrics*, **22**, 91–94

Larrey, D, Rueff, B, Feldmann, G *et al.* (1984) Recurrent jaundice caused by recurrent hyperemesis gravidarum. *Gut*, **25**, 1414–1415

Lee, KS, Lee, H, Moon, SJ *et al.* (1987) Hepatitis B vaccination of newborn infants: clinical study of new vaccine formulation and dose regimen. *Hepatology*, **7**, 941–945

Lee, S-D, Lo, K-J, Tsai, Y-T *et al.* (1988) Role of caesarean section in prevention of mother-infant transmissions of hepatitis B virus. *Lancet*, **ii**, 833–834

Liebman, HA, McGehee, WG, Patch, MJ and Feinstein, DI (1983) Severe depression of antithrombin III associated with disseminated intravascular coagulation in women with fatty liver of pregnancy. *Annals of Internal Medicine*, **98**, 330–333

Lin, H-H, Lee, T-Y, Chen, D-S *et al.* (1987) Transplacental leakage of HB$_e$Ag-positive maternal blood as the most likely route in causing intrauterine infection with hepatitis B virus. *Journal of Pediatrics*, **111**, 877–881

Lindheimer, MD and Katz, AI (1985) Current concepts: hypertension in pregnancy. *New England Journal of Medicine*, **313**, 675–680

Lunzer, M, Barnes, P, Byth, K and O'Hallaron, M (1986) Serum bile acid concentrations during pregnancy and their relationship to obstetric cholestasis. *Gastroenterology*, **91**, 825–829

McCormack, WM, George, H, Donner, A *et al.* (1977) Hepatotoxicity of erythromycin estolate during pregnancy. *Antimicrobial Agents and Chemotherapy*, **12**, 630–635

McKay, AJ, O'Neill, J and Imrie, CW (1980) Pancreatitis, pregnancy and gallstones. *British Journal of Obstetrics and Gynaecology*, **87**, 47–50

McKee, CM, Weir, PE, Foster, JH *et al.* (1986) Acute fatty liver of pregnancy and diagnosis by computed tomography. *British Medical Journal*, **292**, 291–292

McNair, RD and Jaynes, RV (1960) Alterations in liver function during normal pregnancy. *American Journal of Obstetrics and Gynecology* **84**, 62–67

Manas, KJ, Welsh, JD, Rankin, RA and Miller, DD (1985) Hepatic haemorrhage without rupture in pre-eclampsia. *New England Journal of Medicine*, **312**, 424–426

Minuk, GY, Liu, RC and Kelly, JK (1987) Rupture of the liver associated with acute fatty liver of pregnancy. *American Journal of Gastroenterology*, **82**, 457–460

Mitchell, MC, Boitnott, JK, Kaufman, S *et al.* (1982) Budd–Chiari syndrome: etiology, diagnosis and management. *Medicine*, **61**, 199–218

Munnell, EW and Taylor, HC (1947) Liver blood flow in pregnancy – hepatic vein catheterization. *Journal of Clinical Investigation*, **26**, 952–956

Newton, ER, Turksoy, N, Kaplan, M and Reinhold, R (1988) Pregnancy and liver transplantation. *Obstetrics and Gynecology*, **71**, 499–500

O'Neill, JP (1969) Surgical conditions complicating pregnancy. *Australian and New Zealand Journal of Obstetrics and Gynaecology*, **9**, 249–252

Pastorek, JG, Miller, JM and Summers, PR (1988) The effect of hepatitis B antigenemia on pregnancy outcome. *American Journal of Obstetrics and Gynecology*, **158**, 486–489

Perez, V, Gorodisch, S, Casavilla, F and Maruffo, C (1971) Ultrastructure of human liver at the end of normal pregnancy. *American Journal of Obstetrics and Gynecology*, **110**, 428–431

Pockros, PJ, Peters, RL and Reynolds, TB (1984) Idiopathic fatty liver of pregnancy: findings in ten cases. *Medicine*, **63**, 1–11

Potter, JM and Nestel, PJ (1979) The hyperlipidemia of pregnancy in normal and complicated pregnancies. *American Journal of Obstetrics and Gynecology*, **133**, 165–170

Powell-Jackson, PR, Melia, W, Canalese, J *et al.* (1982) Budd–Chiari syndrome: clinical patterns and therapy. *Quarterly Journal of Medicine*, **51**, 79–88

Ramalingaswami, V and Purcell, RH (1988) Waterborne non-A, non-B hepatitis. *Lancet*, **i**, 571–573

Reid, R, Ivey, KJ, Rencoret, RH and Storey, B (1976) Fetal complications of obstetric cholestasis. *British Medical Journal*, **1**, 870–872

Reyes, H (1982) The enigma of intrahepatic cholestasis of pregnancy: lessons from Chile. *Hepatology*, **2**, 87–96

Reyes, H, Ribalta, J, Gonzalez, MC *et al.* (1981) Sulfobromophthalein clearance tests before and after ethinyl estradiol administration, in women and men with familial history of intrahepatic cholestasis of pregnancy. *Gastroenterology*, **81**, 226 231

Reyes, H, Radrigan, ME, Gonzalez, MC *et al.* (1987) Steatorrhea in patients with intrahepatic cholestasis of pregnancy. *Gastroenterology*, **93**, 584–590

Riely, CA (1986) The liver in preeclampsia/eclampsia: the tip of the iceberg. *American Journal of Gastroenterology*, **81**, 1218–1219

Riely, CA, Latham, PS, Romero, R and Duffy, TP (1987) Acute fatty liver of pregnancy. *Annals of Internal Medicine*, **106**, 703–706

Rolfes, DB and Ishak, KG (1985) Acute fatty liver of pregnancy: a clinicopathologic study of 35 cases. *Hepatology*, **5**, 1149–1158

Rolfes, DB and Ishak, KG (1986a) Liver disease in pregnancy. *Histopathology*, **10**, 555–570

Rolfes, DB and Ishak, KG (1986b) Liver disease in toxemia of pregnancy. *American Journal of Gastroenterology*, **81**, 1138–1144

Rustgi, VK and Hoofnagle, JH (1987) Viral hepatitis during pregnancy. *Seminars in Liver Disease*, **7**, 40–46

Santangelo, WC, Dueno, MI, Estes, BL and Krejs, GJ (1988) Prophylactic sclerotherapy of large esophageal varices. *New England Journal of Medicine*, **310**, 814–818

Scheinberg, IH and Sternlieb, I (1975) Pregnancy in penicillamine-treated patients with Wilson's disease. *New England Journal of Medicine*, **293**, 1300–1302

Schreyer, P, Caspi, E, El-Hindi, JM and Eschar, J (1982) Cirrhosis – pregnancy and delivery: a review. *Obstetrical and Gynecological Survey*, **37**, 304–312

Schweitzer, IL, Dunn, AEG, Peters, RL and Spears, RL (1973) Viral hepatitis B in neonates and infants. *American Journal of Medicine*, **55**, 762–771

Scott, LD, Katz, AR, Duke, JH *et al.* (1984) Oral contraceptives, pregnancy, and focal nodular hyperplasia of the liver. *Journal of the American Medical Association*, **251**, 1461–1463

Scully, RE (1981) Case records of the Massachusetts General Hospital. *New England Journal of Medicine*, **304**, 216–224

Sheehan, HL (1940) The pathology of acute yellow atrophy and delayed chloroform poisoning. *Journal of Obstetrics and Gynaecology*, **47**, 49–62

Sibai, BM, Taslimi, MM, El-Nazer, A *et al.* (1986) Maternal–perinatal outcome associated with the syndrome of hemolysis, elevated liver enzymes, and low platelets in severe preeclampsia-eclampsia. *American Journal of Obstetrics and Gynecology*, **155**, 501–509

Siegel, M (1973) Congenital malformations following chickenpox, measles, mumps and hepatitis. *Journal of the American Medical Association*, **226**, 1521–1524

Snydman, DR (1985) Hepatitis in pregnancy. *New England Journal of Medicine*, **313**, 1398–1401

Stander, HJ and Cadden, JF (1934) Acute yellow atrophy of the liver in pregnancy. *American Journal of Obstetrics and Gynecology*, **28**, 61–69

Stauffer, RA, Adams, A, Wygal, J and Lavery, JP (1982) Gallbladder disease in pregnancy. *American Journal of Obstetrics and Gynecology*, **144**, 661–664

Steven, MM, Buckley, JD and Mackay, IR (1979) Pregnancy in chronic active hepatitis. *Quarterly Journal of Medicine*, **48**, 519–531

Stevens, CE, Beasley, RP, Tsui, J and Lee, W-C (1975) Vertical transmission of hepatitis B antigen in Taiwan. *New England Journal of Medicine*, **292**, 771–774

Stock, RJ, Labudovich, M and Ducatman, B (1985) Asymptomatic first-trimester liver cell adenoma: diagnosis by fine-needle aspiration cytology with cytochemical and ultrastructural study. *Obstetrics and Gynecology*, **66**, 287–290

Tong, MJ, Thursby, M, Rakela, J *et al.* (1981) Studies on the maternal-infant transmission of the viruses which cause acute hepatitis. *Gastroenterology*, **80**, 999–1004

Varma, RR, Michelsohn, NH, Borkowf, HI and Lewis, JD (1977) Pregnancy in cirrhotic and noncirrhotic portal hypertension. *Obstetrics and Gynecology*, **50**, 217–222

Varner, H and Rinderknecht, NK (1980) Acute fatty metamorphosis of pregnancy. A maternal mortality and literature review. *Journal of Reproductive Medicine*, **24**, 177–180

Vons, C, Smadja, C, Franco, D *et al.* (1984) Successful pregnancy after Budd–Chiari syndrome. *Lancet*, **ii**, 975

Vore, M (1987) Estrogen cholestasis. *Gastroenterology*, **93**, 643–647

Walker, FB, Hoblit, DL, Cunningham, FG and Combes, B (1974) Gamma glutamyl transpeptidase in normal pregnancy. *Obstetrics and Gynecology*, **43**, 745–749

Walshe, JM (1977) Pregnancy in Wilson's disease. *Quarterly Journal of Medicine*, **46**, 73–83

Waffarn, F, Carlisle, S, Pena, I *et al.* (1982) Fetal exposure to maternal hyperbilirubinemia. *American Journal of Diseases of Children,* **136**, 416–417

Weber, FL, Snodgrass, PJ, Powell, DE *et al.* (1979) Abnormalities of hepatic mitochondrial urea-cycle enzyme activities and hepatic ultrastructure in acute fatty liver of pregnancy. *Journal of Laboratory and Clinical Medicine*, **94**, 27–41

Weinstein, L (1982) Syndrome of hemolysis, elevated liver enzymes, and low platelet count: a severe consequence of hypertension in pregnancy. *American Journal of Obstetrics and Gynecology*, **142**, 159–167

Wong, VCW, Lee, AKY and Ip, HMH (1980) Transmission of hepatitis B antigens from symptom free carrier mothers to the fetus and the infant. *British Journal of Obstetrics and Gynaecology*, **87**, 958–965

Zanetti, AR, Feroni, P, Magliono, EM *et al.* (1982) Perinatal transmission of the hepatitis B virus and of the HBV-associated delta agent from mothers to offspring in Northern Italy. *Journal of Medical Virology*, **9**, 139–148

Zimmerman, HJ and Maddrey, WC (1987) Toxic and drug-induced hepatitis. In *Diseases of the Liver* (edited by L Schiff and ER Schiff) pp. 591–667. Philadelphia: Lippincott.

Chapter 7

Infection in pregnancy, including HIV

Frank D Johnstone, Jacqueline Mok and Ray P Brettle

HIV and other infections

Infections in pregnancy can cause serious morbidity or even be life-threatening for the woman, but may also cause death or long-term handicap of the fetus and newborn. This review is a selective one, and concentrates on infections found commonly in the developed world, particularly those where there are new data or renewed interest.

Susceptibility to infection and severity of disease in pregnancy

There is a widespread belief that immune function is to some extent impaired in human pregnancy, and that the pregnant woman is both more susceptible to a number of infections and at higher risk of complications. This belief has arisen partly because of anecdotal reports, for example the recent reports of maternal death from Group A streptococcal infection (Acharya, Lamont and Cooper, 1988; Kavi and Wise, 1988) and partly because of large studies of attack rates and complications. Many of these studies have been criticized, often because of the absence of a satisfactory non-pregnant control group. Pregnant women could also be over-represented in some studies because of their increased contact with health services. Even where higher complication rates are established in pregnant women, this may not necessarily reflect immune function: for example the higher rate of severe hepatitis observed in pregnant women in the tropics could be due to inadequate maternal nutrition (Sherlock, 1968). Nevertheless the totality of supporting evidence is impressive. This complicated subject has been excellently reviewed elsewhere (Lederman, 1984; Weinberg, 1984; Brabin, 1985).

Gestational changes in maternal immunity

Humoral immune response is probably similar in pregnant and non-pregnant women. Although there is a decrease in IgG concentrations with advancing gestation (Amino et al., 1978), the significance of this is uncertain and studies of vaccines in pregnancy have shown satisfactory antibody responses in pregnant women (Carvalho et al., 1977; Sumaya and Gibbs, 1979; Amstey, Insel and Pichichero, 1984; Brabin et al., 1984).

Cell mediated immunity does appear to be altered and probably mildly impaired in pregnancy. Most studies have found a decrease in T cells (Stelkauskas, Wilson and

Table 7.1.   Some infectious diseases that appear to be adversely affected by pregnancy

Infection	Clinical pattern (compared to non-pregnant woman)	References
Viruses		
Hepatitis A*	Increased attack rate	Morrow et al. (1968)
	More severe complications and death	Cruz et al. (1968); Borhanmanesh et al. (1973)
Hepatitis B*	Increased attack rate	Cossart (1977)
	Increased fulminant hepatitis	
Hepatitis Non-A, Non-B*	Increased attack rate	Khuroo et al. (1981)
	Increased fulminant hepatitis	
Papillomavirus	Increased spread of condylomata acuminata	Oriel (1971); Young, Acosta and Kaufman, (1973)
Influenza A	Increased mortality from pneumonia	Freeman and Barno (1959); Greenberg et al. (1958); Harris (1919)
Poliomyelitis	Increased attack rate	Siegel and Greenberg (1955)
	Higher incidence of residual paralysis	Weinstein, Aycock and Feenister (1951); Priddle et al. (1952)
Others		
Plasmodium falciparum	Increased parasitaemia	Brabin (1983)
	Increased complications	Gillies (1969); Watkinson and Rushton (1983); Diro and Beydoun (1982)
Entamoeba histolytica	More frequently fatal	Reinhardt (1980); Abioye (1973); Armon (1978); Lewis and Antia (1969)
Coccidiodomycosis	Higher incidence of dissemination	Drutz and Huppert (1983); Homer et al. (1961)
Candida albicans	Increased vaginal carriage	Ross (1980)
	Increased vaginitis	
Mycobacterium leprae	Increased reactivation	Duncan et al. (1981); Duncan and Pearson (1984); Duncan et al. (1982)
Listeria monocytogenes	Increased incidence	Campbell (1988); Lamont et al. (1988); Calman (1989)

Dray, 1975; Bulmer and Hancock, 1977; Sridama *et al.*, 1982) and within the T-cell subset a decrease in helper cells (Hirahara *et al.*, 1980; Sridama *et al.*, 1982). The tuberculin reaction, an example of T-cell-mediated immune reaction, may be reduced in pregnancy (Anderson, Ushijima and Larson, 1974). Morphological studies of lymph nodes from women in late pregnancy show reduced cell density and a depressed number of reaction centres. In addition, plasma from pregnant women appears to have immunosuppressive properties, with inhibition of the mixed lymphocyte reaction in lymphocytes from non-pregnant women (Björksten *et al.*, 1978; Bissenden, Ling and Mackintosh, 1980) and inhibition of phytohaemagglutinin stimulated lymphocyte cultures (Purtilo, Hallgren and Yunis, 1972; Valdimarsson *et al.*, 1983).

The effect of pregnancy on susceptibility to infection is perhaps best demonstrated in falciparum malaria, where there has been a detailed review (Brabin, 1983). Virtually all authors have shown that in endemic areas the concentration of malarial parasites is higher in the blood of pregnant women compared with non-pregnant women, that densities are highest in primigravidae with a progressive fall with parity, and that the maximum parasitaemia occurs in the second trimester with a reduction by term to non-pregnant levels. A small group of primigravidae followed longitudinally in Nigeria (Gillies, 1969) showed an increase in parasitaemia from 34 per cent before pregnancy to 79 per cent during pregnancy. In a similar way, carriage rates of *Candida albicans* are increased in pregnancy (Boyer and Kunik, 1982) although, on the contrary, cervical excretion of cytomegalovirus is suppressed in early pregnancy (Reynolds *et al.*, 1973).

Much other information concerns rates of clinical infection and complication (Table 7.1). An epidemic of non-A, non-B hepatitis that occurred in the Kashmir valley in 1978 was studied prospectively, the study being started within 2 weeks of the first report (Khuroo *et al.*, 1981). The incidence of viral hepatitis in pregnant women (17.3 per cent) was higher than that in non-pregnant women (2.1 per cent) and men (2.8 per cent), the incidence being higher in all trimesters. The rate of fulminant hepatic failure was higher in pregnant women (22.2 per cent) than in non-pregnant women (0 per cent) and men (2.8 per cent). All eight cases of fulminant hepatic failure were in the third trimester.

Although similar data for hepatitis have been reported for several different countries (D'Cruz, Balani and Iyer, 1968; Morrow *et al.*, 1968; Borhanmanesh *et al.*, 1973), factors such as nutrition may also be important, because studies in the developed world have not shown the course of viral hepatitis in pregnancy to be different from that in non-pregnant women (reviewed by Cossart, 1977).

Polio during pregnancy is associated with a greater attack rate of clinical infection and a greater frequency of paralytic illness than polio in non-pregnant subjects (Weinstein, Aycock and Feemster, 1951; Priddle *et al.*, 1952; Siegel and Greenberg, 1955). However in the last study the infection rate among pregnant patients was related to the number of children in the household, and it is possible that pregnant patients had more children than non-pregnant patients and were hence exposed to higher risk. Several studies have shown higher rates of pneumonia mortality in influenza epidemics in pregnant women (Harris, 1919; Greenberg *et al.*, 1958; Freeman and Barno, 1959).

Thus available evidence suggests that there is an alteration, and to some extent a mild impairment, of cell-mediated immunity in pregnancy. This has a slight, but definite, effect on susceptibility to some infections, and may contribute to the observed increase in virulence of others.

Human immunodeficiency virus

Human immunodeficiency virus 1 (HIV) is now one of the most common serious infections occurring in pregnancy. This, together with the profound potential effects of infection on mother and child, make it mandatory that all those involved in perinatal care are knowledgeable about this disease. There are recent reviews dealing with pregnancy (Feinkind and Minkoff, 1988; Johnstone and Mok, 1990).

Epidemiology and virology

The first cases of acquired immune deficiency syndrome (AIDS) were described in 1981. Since then the disease has become pandemic, with >150 000 cases reported from 149 countries throughout the world. Every continent has been affected, with the Americas accounting for almost 70 per cent of reports. In Europe, 30 countries reported about 21 000 cases, and in the United Kingdom 2228 AIDS cases had been notified to the Communicable Diseases Surveillance Centre by 30 April 1989 (AIDS News Supplement, 1989a); only 85 of these cases occurred in women. However, the number of cases of AIDS alone does not reveal the reservoir of infection and, in the UK, the total number of HIV positive reports exceed 10 000, with about 10 per cent female. Of these 1000 women, 83 per cent were aged between 15–44 years; 48.5 per cent were infected because of intravenous drug use whereas 28.4 per cent acquired HIV through heterosexual intercourse (AIDS News Supplement, 1989b).

HIV is transmitted primarily through sexual intercourse, exposure to blood and blood products, and from mother to child. Although first described among homosexual men, it is now known that on a global basis, heterosexual sex is the most common way of transmitting the virus (WHO, 1989). Sexual transmission of HIV occurs from men to women and from women to men. As yet, no clear difference has been demonstrated in the relative risk. In a multicentre European study (European Study Group, 1989), the rate of sexual transmission from an infected man to his female partner was greater where the man had full blown AIDS and CD4 lymphopenia, and where the woman had contracted a sexually transmitted disease within the previous five years. Anal intercourse was the only sexual practice clearly related to higher risk for the female partner. The transmission rate was 7 per cent when none of these three risk factors were present, rising to 67 per cent when two or more risk factors existed. An African study identified genital ulcer disease, *Chlamydia trachomatis* cervicitis, and the use of oral contraceptives as factors that may increase the susceptibility of women to HIV infection (Piot *et al.*, 1987).

A large Nairobi study has examined female-to-male transmission (Cameron *et al.*, 1989). The risk of acquiring HIV was much higher in uncircumcized men, and among men who acquired genital ulcer disease. A cumulative 43 per cent of uncircumcized men who acquired an ulcer seroconverted to HIV-1 after a single sexual exposure.

The virus responsible for AIDS was first discovered in 1983 (Barre-Sinoussi *et al.*, 1983). The term human immunodeficiency virus (HIV) was introduced in 1986 to replace previous terminology. With the discovery of a related human retrovirus in West Africa, the original AIDS virus is now known as HIV-1, while the West African virus is labelled HIV-2 (Coffin *et al.*, 1986). Both appear similar in transmission and clinical effects, although the pathogenesis of HIV-2 has been less well studied.

HIV belongs to the retrovirus family, characterized by the presence of reverse transcriptase, an enzyme that converts viral RNA to a complementary DNA copy, which is in turn inserted into the chromosomal DNA of the host cell (McClure and Weiss, 1987). The RNA, together with reverse transcriptase, is contained in the core and surrounded by an envelope which is derived from the membrane of the host cell. The bilayer envelope has two glycoprotein components – gp41 spans the membrane whereas gp 120 extends beyond it. The gp120 protein is most antigenic, containing the attachment site for CD4 receptors. The main target for HIV is the T4 lymphocyte, although any cell with the CD4 antigen (monocyte macrophages in the blood, brain and alveoli) is susceptible to viral invasion. HIV has also been found to infect follicular dendritic cells, neuroglial tissue, B lymphocytes and gastrointestinal epithelial cells (Dalgleish et al., 1984).

During infection, HIV is attached to the CD4 antigen, following which the virus particle is internalized. The mechanism is probably one of fusion of the viral envelope with the cell membrane, or endocytosis into an intracytoplasmic vesicle. In the cytoplasm, the virus is uncoated and a complementary DNA copy of viral DNA is made by reverse transcriptase. The double strand of viral DNA is then integrated into the host genome, and remains latent until activated. Several DNA viruses (herpes simplex type 1, polyoma viruses, varicella zoster virus, human herpes virus type 6 and cytomegalovirus) have been shown to activate HIV. The contribution of host and environmental factors to virus activation remain under study. The pathogenesis of HIV is not fully understood, and probably involves several mechanisms. Cell fusion occurs when the envelope glycoprotein (gp120) binds on to the CD4 antigen, and the resultant syncytia are cleared by the immune system. Free viral gp120 may bind to CD4 receptors of uninfected cells, leading to their destruction by the immune system, although the cells are not themselves infected by the virus. Infection with HIV may induce the formation of autoantibodies directed against gp120 and other HIV proteins. New virus particles that bud from the cell membrane also infect other cells. The immune responses that come into effect therefore also activate helper T cells that in turn result in increased viral replication and cell death. Death of CD4 cells leads to a progressive decline in immune functioning, and hence is the primary factor which determines the clinical course (Zagury et al., 1986).

Tests of diagnosis and prognosis

After primary infection with HIV, antibodies to core (p24) and envelope (gp120) proteins can usually be detected within 8 weeks, although some individuals take up to 6 months to seroconvert. Recently, however, work with the polymerase chain reaction (Ou et al., 1988) has suggested that infection in some cases may precede seroconversion by a much longer interval (Ranki et al., 1987; Imagawa et al., 1989; Pezzella et al., 1989), but this probably occurs in only 5 per cent of infected individuals (Horsburgh et al., 1989). The presence of antibody does not protect the individual from disease progression, and HIV can be isolated from antibody-positive patients. For screening purposes, enzyme-linked immunoassays (ELISA) are used. Two different ELISA techniques are needed to exclude false-positive results, and commonly used tests use an antiglobulin assay as well as a competitive binding assay. Some laboratories use Western blotting to analyse specific antibody responses. In adults, a positive antibody test is a specific and sensitive criterion for HIV infection. Maternal IgG antibody crosses the placenta, thereby limiting the usefulness of antibody testing for diagnosing HIV infection in the infant. Transplacentally acquired HIV antibody is cleared by around 18 months of age, although in exceptional circumstances children have been reported to clear maternal antibodies at 24 months. Antibody testing is therefore of limited value in young infants and testing for IgM antibody is not reliable in the presence of IgG. HIV antigen can be detected, either soon after infection or in the terminal stages of the disease, but most asymptomatic carriers are antigen negative.

The virus can also be cultured from peripheral blood lymphocytes and lymph nodes. The success of virus culture from lymphocytes is also correlated with disease progression, virus culture being positive in only 40 per cent of asymptomatic individuals. Again, the small sample size in paediatric patients limits the sensitivity of virus culture.

New laboratory tests are being evaluated, mainly to assess antibody negative patients who continue to engage in high risk activities, e.g. sexual contact where one partner is infected. The polymerase chain reaction technique of amplifying viral DNA shows promise in facilitating early diagnosis of HIV infection in children, as well as in evaluating latent infection in antibody negative patients (Ranki et al., 1987; Laure et al., 1988; Horsburgh et al., 1989; Imagawa et al., 1989; Pezzella et al., 1989). However, the false positive rate is high, and the long-term outcome is not yet known for individuals who are found to have viral DNA sequences in the genome, as this may not imply overt infection.

Immunological abnormalities reported in association with HIV infection are described with increasing frequency (Lane et al., 1983; Pinching et al., 1983; Aucouturier et al., 1986; Pinching and Weiss, 1986). In the early stages of infection, lymphocytosis occurs due to an increase in suppressor (CD8) cells. Subsequently, persistent destruction of CD4 cells leads to lymphopenia. With the fall in absolute numbers of CD4 cells, the helper:suppressor ratio drops below 2.0. A characteristic accompaniment is cutaneous anergy and a decreased lymphocyte proliferative response to mitogens. Although HIV infection was thought only to affect cell-mediated immunity, it is now recognized that the humoral immune system is also activated, and patients have polyclonal hypergammaglobulinaemia. Responses to specific antigens (e.g. tetanus and pneumococcal polysaccharides) have also been shown to be suboptimal.

The rate of progression from asymptomatic HIV infection to clinical disease is slow, and laboratory markers in combination with clinical disease are useful in predicting the onset of AIDS (Moss, 1988). Routine haematology may be useful, as normochromic anaemia, low white cell or platelet counts are important prognostic indicators of progression (Carne et al., 1987). At least five laboratory predictors have proved useful: these include the CD4 lymphocyte count, presence of p24 core antigen, decreasing titre of p24 antibody and rising levels of β_2-microglobulin and of neopterin (proteins which reflect monocyte-macrophage activation). In the San Francisco General Hospital cohort (Moss et al., 1988), β_2-microglobulin concentration was the most powerful predictor of progression to AIDS, but packed-cell volume, HIV p24 antigenaemia and the proportion and number of CD4 lymphocytes each independently predicted progression. Those subjects who were normal by all predictors had a 3-year progression rate of 7 per cent whereas those who were abnormal by two or more predictors had a progression rate of 57 per cent (Moss et al., 1988). These laboratory predictors are also being used to stratify subjects for therapeutic trials, and as measures of outcome.

Mother to child transmission of HIV

The first cases of paediatric AIDS were described in the infants of drug-addicted Haitian or sexually promiscuous mothers (Oleske *et al.*, 1983; Rubenstein *et al.*, 1983; Scott *et al.*, 1985) before it was apparent that the causative agent was a virus. Since then, HIV antigen has been demonstrated in amniotic fluid (Mundy *et al.*, 1987) and HIV has been isolated from fetal tissue at 16–20 weeks' gestation (Jovaisas *et al.*, 1985; Peutherer *et al.*, 1988) as well as from the thymus of an infant born at 28 weeks' gestation (Lapointe *et al.*, 1985) by caesarean section. Although it is difficult to exclude entirely the possibility of maternal contamination in these studies, a more recent report (Lyman *et al.*, 1988) of a 23-week fetus confirmed by DNA hybridization the presence of HIV within the nucleus of brain cells . There is thus no doubt that infection can occur transplacentally, and probably quite early in pregnancy. What remains to be discovered is the proportion of fetuses infected at different stages in pregnancy. It remains possible that some fetuses could be infected in late pregnancy or during delivery. Current laboratory tests do not distinguish intrauterine from intrapartum or postnatal infection.

The risk of HIV transmission from mother to child has not yet been quantified, although several studies are under way. Early reports suggested a transmission rate of at least 50 per cent, but were biased by the inclusion of children who presented with symptoms. Reliable estimates of the rate of infection can be obtained only by monitoring all infants born to HIV-positive women, instead of by following children with symptomatic disease. The European Collaborative Study is one such prospective study, and the minimum estimate of vertical transmission has been reported as 24 per cent (European Collaborative Study, 1988). The insensitivity of the tests currently available for diagnosing HIV infection in young infants means that higher rates may eventually be reported. Some antibody-negative children do appear to have evidence of HIV virus infection as judged by polymerase chain reaction (Laure *et al.*, 1988). Preliminary analysis of data from the European Collaborative Study suggested an association between clinical symptoms in the mother during pregnancy and the early onset of AIDS in infants (Mok *et al.*, 1987). This was not borne out when more data accumulated, but the later analysis used a different measure of outcome. Difficulties also arose in separating the effects of confounding variables, as the majority of mothers were intravenous drug users from socially deprived areas. The infants were therefore at risk of an increased perinatal morbidity and mortality, regardless of HIV status.

Whereas good evidence exists for transplacental infection, less is known about the role of breastfeeding in HIV transmission. HIV has been isolated from the acellular fraction of breast milk from HIV positive women, and case reports have described cases of postnatal transmission via breast milk (Ziegler *et al.*, 1985; Lepage *et al.*, 1987; Weinbreck *et al.*, 1988). However, the women in the reports were infected by blood transfusions given in the postnatal period, when they were likely to have been highly infectious owing to transient viraemia associated with seroconversion. It has been suggested that breast feeding by a mother who has been asymptomatic, albeit antibody positive throughout pregnancy might not confer an additional risk. For underdeveloped countries, where formula milk is not easily available and where poor standards of hygiene are used in constituting milk powder, breast feeding offers the infant optimum chances for survival under normal circumstances. Current recommendations for HIV-seropositive women not to breast-feed their infants should therefore apply only to developed countries where safe alternatives exist.

Effect of pregnancy on HIV disease

As discussed above, pregnancy is associated with a mild impairment of the immune system and both an increased maternal susceptibility and an enhanced virulence of some infections. For these reasons there have been concerns that pregnancy would adversely affect progression of HIV disease. Initial reports tended to confirm these concerns (Scott *et al.*, 1985; Minkoff *et al.*, 1987b). However, these studies were based on identification of mothers of children who had already developed AIDS, and who were themselves at particularly high risk. There are several studies in progress at present, but none has yet been reported in full. In the Edinburgh study (MacCallum *et al.*, 1988), women infected with HIV were compared according to whether or not they had had a pregnancy since seroconversion. The women who had had at least one pregnancy did not appear to have been adversely affected judging by clinical status, absolute CD_4 count or antigenaemia. Other reports using this type of analysis from Toulouse (Berrebi *et al.*, 1988) and from the Montefiore Medical Centre, New York (Schoenbaum *et al.*, 1989) have also suggested little or no increase in progression attributable to pregnancy. However, this type of analysis may be misleading, because the women who did not become pregnant may have differed in terms of duration of infection, presence of illness or drug-related behaviour: for instance, more women in Edinburgh who did not have a pregnancy continued to inject, and injection is itself associated with a decline in CD_4 count (Des Jarlais *et al.*, 1987). An alternative analysis involves tracking the decline in the CD_4 count in individual patients over years and assessing mathematically whether pregnancy increases the overall rate of decline. There is one preliminary report of such an analysis (Biggar *et al.*, 1989). This suggests that, compared with HIV-seronegative women with the same risk factors (drug abusers or Haitians), the loss of CD_4 cells was faster during pregnancy than during the postpartum period. The authors believed that the data were compatible with the hypothesis that pregnancy might mildly accelerate HIV-induced depletion of CD_4 lymphocytes, and could therefore increase the rate of progression of disease.

In short, conclusive evidence about the effect of pregnancy upon HIV disease is lacking. There does not appear to be a major adverse effect, although it seems possible that there may be a mild acceleration in the progressive loss of CD_4 lymphocytes and reports of clinical deterioration in pregnancy exist. However, there are also non-immunological ways in which pregnancy might affect HIV disease. Early symptoms of disease such as fatigue or dyspnoea might be attributed to pregnancy and indeed there are reports of maternal death when there may have been delay in diagnosis (Minkoff *et al.*, 1986). In addition, treatment may be withheld during pregnancy because of possible risks to the fetus. This applies particularly to azidothymidine (AZT), which will be much more widely used in asymptomatic individuals following the results of recent trials.

Effect of HIV on pregnancy outcome

Little is known about the factors influencing some HIV-infected women to avoid pregnancy, whereas others have single or repeated pregnancies. However, studies from Edinburgh and New York (Johnstone *et al.*, 1990; Selwyn *et al.*, 1989a) have shown that where pregnancy does occur, most infected women do not see HIV infection *per se* as a reason to terminate a wanted pregnancy. In the Edinburgh study, which compared seropositive and seronegative women tested for the same indications, the rate of induced abortion was high in both groups, but there was no statistically significant difference between them (Johnstone *et al.*, 1990). Thirty-one of 69 seropositive women chose termination (45 per cent) and 33 of 94 seronegative women did so (35 per cent). In a study from New York (Selwyn *et al.*, 1989a), 14 of 28 seropositive women (50 per cent) and 16 of 36 seronegative women (44 per cent) chose termination of pregnancy. In retrospective interviews, more of the HIV seropositive women, not surprisingly, were likely to have perceived their risk of perinatal transmission to be high; however, more important determinants were previous elective abortion, a negative emotional reaction to pregnancy and whether the pregnancy had been unplanned. Much remains to be explored in this area, as limitation of pregnancy is the only current method believed to reduce disease spread by vertical transmission.

In comparing delivery outcome, it is essential to have an adequate control group. Women infected with HIV are commonly injection drug users, may have adverse socioeconomic circumstances, and may abuse other substances (particularly cigarettes); thus there are reasons other than HIV infection for possible unfavourable pregnancy outcome. Three studies with satisfactory control groups (women who were tested for the same indications but were seronegative) have addressed this question. In the first, the incidences of preterm delivery, intrauterine growth retardation and low birth weight were 3–4 times higher in the study groups than in the background population, but there were no differences between the two study groups (Johnstone *et al.*, 1988). Similar data have been reported from centres in New York (Selwyn *et al*,. 1989b; Minkoff *et al.*, 1989).

Other studies (Minkoff *et al.*, 1987a; Gloeb, O'Sullivan and Efantis, 1988), without control groups, have reported high incidences of preterm labour and other obstetric problems.

In conclusion, although the numbers of patients in these studies are small, there does not appear to be a substantive overall effect of HIV infection upon pregnancy outcome. Nevertheless, there is a trend towards smaller babies, and infections of all types are more common in seropositive women. Clinical status is probably important, and although the effect of HIV infection may be minimal when the woman is well, it seems inevitable that there will be some detrimental effect when she becomes clinically ill.

Management of HIV-infected patients in pregnancy

The recognition of HIV-infected patients is important for optimal treatment of both mother and baby. Antenatal HIV counselling and testing has been well discussed (Holman *et al.*, 1989a, b) and the case for routinely offering HIV prenatal testing in high-risk areas has been argued (Minkoff and Landesman, 1988). It is part of the medical surveillance of HIV-infected patients to estimate the markers of progression of disease described above. This allows specific advice about risks, thus facilitating decisions about pregnancy termination, and also alerts clinicians to the likelihood of disease.

It is important to emphasize that HIV infection appears to be a relentlessly progressive immunological disorder. HIV-related disease includes many infections that do not come within the definition of AIDS and, indeed, in New York it is estimated that 50 per cent of deaths due to HIV disease never fulfil the surveillance definition for AIDS. Minkoff *et al.* (1990) reported 16 pregnant women with a CD_4 count of <300 cells/mm^3 at some time during their pregnancies: three developed opportunist infections, one had pneumonia and one had abscesses following caesarean section. There were no serious infections in the 40 HIV-seropositive women who had CD_4 counts consistently >300 cells/mm^3. Treatment should be started early in any infection in HIV-seropositive women, partly because infections may be more serious but also because activation of the immune system may be harmful in the progression of the disease.

The most common presentation of AIDS is *Pneumocystis carinii* pneumonia (PCP). This can present insidiously, with shortness of breath, or as an overwhelming infection. Deaths have been reported during pregnancy (Minkoff *et al.*, 1986) and a recent report identified a further 20 unpublished cases of women dying during pregnancy or within a year after termination of pregnancy (Koonin *et al.*, 1989). Each pregnancy had a complication, mostly preterm delivery, and most women died of PCP. The pregnant woman may be at more risk because of delay in diagnosis (symptoms put down to pregnancy) or inadequate treatment (because of concern about the fetus). The first line treatment of PCP is high dose sulphamethoxazole–trimethoprim (Septrin, Wellcome). Although trimethoprim is a folate antagonist and on theoretical grounds should not be used in pregnancy, adverse effects have not been established (Briggs *et al.*, 1983a). The main possible toxicity of sulphamethoxazole given close to delivery is neonatal jaundice. Although this complication is well described for long-acting sulphonamides, the risk with sulphamethoxazole appears low (Baskin, Law and Wenger, 1980). Sulphonamides compete with unconjugated bilirubin for binding to plasma albumin; unbound bilirubin, free to cross the blood–brain barrier, could result in kernicterus. This problem has been described when sulphonamides have been administered directly to the neonate, but never following exposure *in utero* (Briggs *et al.*, 1983b). Thus it seems clear that the risks of PCP far outweigh any possible risks of sulphamethoxazole–trimethoprim treatment. Pentamidine is also effective, but is usually used as second-line treatment. More recently, however, it has been used prophylactically in an aerosol preparation. There is no information about the safety of pentamidine in pregnancy, but as very little of an aerosol preparation is absorbed into the systemic circulation, aerosolized pentamidine may well prove to be safe.

Immunocompromised patients may also be at greater risk from cytomegalovirus and toxoplasmosis; measurement of baseline titres early in pregnancy is recommended. They may have more persistent episodes of genital herpes infections, and acyclovir may have to be considered close to delivery, although the safety of this drug in pregnancy has not been established. Clinical reactivation of hepatitis B infection in anti-HBs-positive patients has been reported (Vento *et al.*, 1989); as most pregnant HIV-seropositive women have markers of previous hepatitis infection, hepatitis B testing should be repeated shortly before delivery in order to identify babies requiring active and passive protection. Cervical intraepithelial neoplasia is a further problem in immune-compromised women, and colposcopy should be carried out (Spurrett, Jones and Stewart, 1988).

Azidothymidine (AZT) has now been shown to be of value not only in AIDS but also in asymptomatic individuals with low CD_4 counts (unpublished US trials). As this drug is therefore likely to be prescribed much more widely, safety in pregnancy will become a key issue. It is known to cross the placenta, but there is currently no published information about its use in human pregnancy.

There is at present no definite evidence that caesarean section protects against vertical transmission, but this has been suggested (Chiodo *et al.*, 1986) and more data are needed. At present, vaginal delivery should be planned. Fetal blood sampling and fetal scalp electrodes should not be used because of the possibility of infecting the fetus by inoculation with maternal cervical or vaginal secretions. Where a safe alternative exists, women should not breast feed.

Finally, care should be taken to prevent nosocomial spread of HIV. Health care workers are at very slight, but real, risk of acquiring infection; this has been discussed in detail recently (Mead, 1989). Other patients should not be at risk, but infection control procedures have to guarantee their safety also. Current procedures are designed to reduce risks for all patients by avoiding skin contact with body fluids. These should be standard procedures and not used simply for patients known to be infected or at high risk. Guidelines for obstetric practice have been suggested (RCOG, 1987).

Other viral diseases

Chickenpox

Varicella or chickenpox is an endemic and epidemic viral infection usually contracted in childhood. The initial primary infection is characterized by fever and an eruption. The eruption begins as a macule which progresses within 48 h through the stages of papule, vesicle, pustule and crust. The fever continues for about 5 days, during which time further viraemia produces fresh lesions individually or in crops.

Varicella then becomes a latent viral infection and reactivation may occur 40–50 years later in the form of varicella zoster, or shingles. This manifests itself usually by recurrence in the skin, although recurrence in motor nerves can also occur. A recurrence is characterized by the onset of severe pain and hyperaesthesia in the area affected together with malaise and slight fever. After 3–4 days the area affected develops an erythematous rash, which is followed by the appearance of closely grouped vesicles; these vesicles rapidly progress to pustules and crusts. There is usually an accompanying viraemia with sparse dissemination to other areas. In the immunocompromised, however, this viraemia may be prolonged or severe, producing disseminated varicella which looks the same as primary chickenpox.

Varicella zoster virus (VZV) does cross the placenta and may cause congenital or neonatal chickenpox, result in congenital malformations and produce an attack of varicella zoster or shingles in infancy without preceding chickenpox.

As a consequence of under-reporting, it is difficult to estimate the true incidence of chickenpox or herpes zoster in pregnancy but the attempts that have been made suggest rates of between one and five cases per 10 000 pregnancies, or around two pregnancies per 10 000 cases of chickenpox (Stagno and Whitley, 1985). Early reports suggested that chickenpox in pregnancy had a very high maternal mortality rate of 41 per cent of 17 pregnancies (Young, 1976), but this is artificially high because of over-reporting of serious cases. One prospective study revealed a mortality of 1/150 pregnancies whereas others suggested that only 9–14 per cent of cases of chickenpox in pregnancy developed pneumonia, with a 2–3 per cent mortality. These latter figures were no different from non-pregnant adult cases of chickenpox, in whom 11 per cent developed pneumonia (Young, 1976).

Transmission of virus from mother to fetus occurs in around 26 per cent of cases of maternal chickenpox but in probably very few, if any, cases of maternal shingles (Stagno and Whitley, 1985). The development of chickenpox in the first trimester of pregnancy is not associated with fetal death and its occurrence in the last trimester is not associated with either prematurity or fetal death (Siegel, Fuerst and Peress, 1966; Siegel and Fuerst, 1966).

The effects of VZV may include chromosomal abnormalities. In one case, a 2-year-old child whose mother suffered chickenpox during pregnancy showed a 26 per cent incidence of chromosomal breaks in peripheral blood leucocytes (Young, 1976). In a prospective study, two deaths from acute leukaemia occurred out of 270 children followed prospectively because of maternal chickenpox, representing a significant increase in incidence of leukaemia (Fine *et al.*, 1985).

Congenital malformations that have been associated with chickenpox during pregnancy include hypoplasia of limbs, limb deformity, cortical atrophy, ocular abnormalities and cicatricial skin lesions. Although it is difficult to prove a causal relationship because of the rarity of the condition, the consistency of the malformations is very suggestive of a specific syndrome associated with VZ virus (Srabstein *et al.*, 1974; Paryani and Arvin, 1986). A hypothesis has been advanced that seems to explain the constellation of abnormalities (Higa, Dan and Manabe, 1987).

Postnatal chickenpox (i.e. that occurring between days 10–28) is usually milder than congenital chickenpox and is rarely fatal; the mildness of this illness has been attributed to the presence of maternal antibody. By comparison, congenital chickenpox carries a significant mortality of 21 per cent if it occurs between the fifth and tenth postnatal day or 31 per cent if the maternal rash is within 4 days of delivery (Young, 1976).

There is no proven prophylactic regimen of treatment for VZV in pregnancy or in the neonatal period. VZV hyperimmune immunoglobulin appears indicated for children whose mothers develop chickenpox 4–5 days before delivery. Acyclovir is currently indicated only for primary VZV infections in immunocompromised patients. Acyclovir is not known to be teratogenic in animals. Although its use in human pregnancy has been reported, there is, as yet, no study detailing efficacy in preventing the congenital syndrome. Similarly, the efficacy of acyclovir in primary neonatal VZV infections has not yet been established.

Measles and mumps

Both infections are relatively rare in pregnancy. One study from Guinea-Bissau suggested a greatly increased perinatal mortality amongst children born to women exposed to measles in pregnancy, even without any obvious maternal infection (Aaby *et al.*, 1988). Mumps can cause abortion in early pregnancy, usually within 14 days of the onset of maternal illness (Siegel, Fuerst and Peress, 1966; Siegel and Fuerst, 1966) and there has been a suggested association between first trimester mumps, maternal infection and the subsequent development of diabetes (Fine *et al.*, 1985).

Rubella

Rubella is a mild infection of little consequence unless contracted during pregnancy. It occurs as endemic and epidemic infections and is characterized by malaise, headaches, conjunctivitis and fever. On the second day, a rash of rose-pink or macular spots appears in the face, spreads rapidly to the trunk and extremities and then fades within 1–3 days. There is accompanying lymphadenopathy. In adults, arthralgia may be a prominent feature of the illness.

The scope and extent of rubella embryopathy has been well documented since its description in the early 1940s. It is known that nearly 90 per cent of fetuses are infected when exposed *in utero* and over 80 per cent of congenitally infected infants suffer some damage (Alfort, 1976). A fetal viral infection occurs at least 2 weeks after maternal infection, persists for many months and produces changes slowly over time (Siegel, Fuerst and Peress, 1966). In a series of 200 infants with congenital rubella, 70 (35 per cent) had complicating thrombocytopenia (Cooper *et al.*, 1965). They presented with purpuric eruption within 24 h of delivery, the rash being most prominent on the face and upper trunk. Enlargement of the liver and spleen was noted in about 70 per cent of cases and lymphadenopathy occurred in about 20 per cent of cases.

The majority of effects occur on fetuses infected during the first trimester and any influence upon prematurity is confined to infections that have been acquired at this time (Miller, Cradock-Watson and Pollock, 1982). Late infections have little, if any, effect upon fetal mortality (Siegel and Fuerst, 1966). The earliest recorded effect of fetal infection occurred 12 days after the last menstrual period (Enders *et al.*, 1988). All pregnancies affected between 3 and 6 weeks after the menstrual period have resulted in fetal infection (Enders *et al.*, 1988). Despite immunization programmes, 3 per cent of pregnant women in the UK were found to be susceptible to rubella in late 1986 (Noah and Fowle, 1989) and Asian women are particularly at risk (Miller *et al.*, 1987). Currently about 20 rubella-damaged babies are born each year in the UK, although many more pregnancies are terminated because of rubella infection. It is hoped that the MMR (mumps, measles, rubella) vaccine, introduced in 1988, will eventually reduce this incidence.

It does appear that, very occasionally, fetal infection and damage can follow maternal reinfection with rubella. Best *et al* (1989) recently presented five cases of asymptomatic maternal reinfection with rubella that resulted in intrauterine infection. Two pregnancies were terminated, with virus being isolated from the products of conception. The three pregnancies that continued were each associated with a fetus showing congenital rubella syndrome and damage. Although the risks associated with reinfection are very small, all pregnant women who have contact with, or develop illnesses like, rubella should be tested, even if they have a history of rubella vaccination and have been reported previously to have rubella antibodies.

Hepatitis B (see also Chapter 6)

Type B hepatitis has a relatively long incubation period from 6 weeks to 6 months. The illness is not particularly different clinically from other forms of hepatitis except for, perhaps, a more severe prodrome. The acute illness may be complicated by rapid progression to liver failure and death. The infection may also be complicated by the eventual development of chronic liver disease or a chronic carrier state.

Hepatitis B carriage is common in parts of Asia and Africa, where in some communities the incidence may be as high as 30 per cent, and transmission is frequently by the maternal–fetal route. In most Western countries, <1 per cent of the general population are HBsAg carriers; populations with a high incidence of sexual promiscuity or drug abuse are at higher risk. Whether to carry out selective or universal screening in any geographic area depends upon prevalence and resources.

In the absence of treatment, about 90 per cent of infants will be infected where the mother is HBe and Ag positive (Beasley, Trepo and Stevens, 1977; Tong *et al.*, 1981; Lo *et al.*, 1985). If, in addition, the mother is serum HVB/DNA positive, then all infants will become chronic carriers (Lee *et al.*, 1986). Overall, about 90 per cent of infected babies become chronic carriers and, of these carriers, it is estimated that 25 per cent will die from primary hepatocellular carcinoma or cirrhosis of the liver

(Committee Report, 1989). These deaths occur between late childhood and early adulthood and are thus particularly devastating. Prevention of transmission is therefore of the greatest importance.

Where the mother is e-antigen or surface antigen positive, infants should receive hepatitis B immune globulin (HBIG) intramuscularly as soon as they are physiologically stable, preferably within 12 h of birth. Hepatitis B vaccine should also be given intramuscularly within 12 h of birth, at the same time as HBIG but at a different site. The second and third doses should be given 1 month and 6 months after the first, and it is recommended that testing for HBsAg and its antibody (antiHBs) should take place at 12–15 months of age in order to monitor the effectiveness of therapy (Committee Report, 1989). This approach will protect 85 per cent of babies (Beasley et al., 1983; Wong et al., 1984). Failures may be due to intrauterine transmission which, although uncommon, does occur in a few pregnancies; alternatively, Lee et al. (1989) suggest that some babies acquire infection during vaginal delivery, in cases where a very high HBV load is too great to be neutralized by HBIG given after birth. They present evidence to support their belief that infants born to carrier mothers with high serum HBV-DNA levels should not only be given combined passive and active immunization but should also be delivered by elective caesarean section. Serum HBV-DNA levels are not routinely measured at present and the place of caesarean section is, as yet, uncertain.

Although perinatal infection is most important, hepatitis B infection can also occur in the postnatal period. In longitudinal studies of hepatitis B in families, there is increasing frequency of previous or persistent infection in children (Mowat, 1980).

Cytomegalovirus

Cytomegalovirus (CMV) is a herpes virus with a propensity to latent and recurrent infections similar to that of other herpes viruses such as herpes simplex virus and varicella zoster virus. It is a ubiquitous organism, 90 per cent of adults having been exposed to the virus by the age of 60 years (Shurin, 1979).

Infection is usually subclinical or asymptomatic but in adults infection can be characterized by fever, lethargy, malaise, hepatosplenomegaly and transaminase abnormalities (Klemola, 1973; Starr, 1979). The haematological changes are similar to those of infectious mononucleosis except that the heterophile antibody responses are absent (Klemola, 1973); the virus is responsible for 50–76 per cent of non-Epstein–Barr Virus (non-EBV) mononucleosis (Starr, 1979). In the child, CMV infection is much more often associated with cervical lymphadenopathy and exudative tonsillitis (Pannuti et al., 1985).

Congenital CMV is now the commonest-known microbiological cause of brain damage in infancy (Lancet Editorial, 1989). It has been calculated that, as 3–4 babies per thousand deliveries in the UK are infected with CMV, and as 10 per cent of these babies sustain damage, there may be 235–310 CMV-damaged babies in the UK each year (Lancet Editorial, 1989). The clinical syndrome that may precede this damage consists of intrauterine growth retardation, jaundice, hepatosplenomegaly, microcephaly, choroidoretinitis, purpuric skin lesions, and thrombocytopenia or haemolytic anaemia (Starr, 1979). Only a small proportion of congenitally infected infants develop this acute illness (Peckham and Logan, 1988) but the outlook for these infants is poor: in one study (Pass et al., 1980) 34 symptomatic neonates had a mortality rate of 29 per cent; 70 per cent developed microcephaly, and only two of the original 34 were apparently normal at 2 years.

CMV may be transmitted in a variety of different ways to infants and the exact contribution of each method to the development of clinical disease is as yet obscure. The major risk is with primary maternal infection in pregnancy. Approximately 40 per cent of pregnant women are susceptible in the UK and of these, 1–2 per cent seroconvert during pregnancy (Stern and Tucker, 1973). Nearly all of these seroconversions, certainly more than 90 per cent, are asymptomatic. In such primary infections, the risk of fetal infection is approximately 20–50 per cent (Stern and Tucker, 1973; Grant, Edmond and Syme, 1981; Ahlfors *et al.*, 1982; Preece *et al.*, 1983), more in the last trimester (Preece *et al.*, 1983). Ten per cent of babies infected *in utero* have significant handicap (Peckham and Logan, 1988).

Reactivation of CMV occurs in 1–3 per cent and may account for one-quarter of congenital infections (Preece, Pearl and Peckham, 1984; Stern and Tucker, 1973). Maternal immunity does not seem to prevent congenital CMV infection but does seem to protect against serious complications. Some studies have suggested that damage can, very occasionally, result from recurrent infection (Ahlfors *et al.*, 1982; Preece, Pearl and Peckham, 1984; Rutter, Griffiths and Trompeter, 1985). Furthermore, there are occasional reports of congenital infection occurring in consecutive pregnancies, but the risk of a second child being damaged appears to be extremely low.

Viral replication in asymptomatic infected infants may persist well into childhood, and there have been suggestions that a proportion of this group, perhaps 10–20 per cent, will eventually develop late neurological sequelae, particularly sensorineural hearing loss and psychomotor retardation (Saigal *et al.*, 1982). As with varicella (another herpes virus infection), an increased incidence of malignancy has been noted following exposure to CMV *in utero* (Fine *et al.*, 1985).

Infants may also be infected via exposure to the virus in the birth canal. Cervical and urinary excretion of CMV in pregnancy varies from 2 to 28 per cent and depends on a number of factors (Hanshaw, 1976). The overall rate of CMV excretion in two groups of women, pregnant and non-pregnant, with similar demographic characteristics and CMV antibodies (89 per cent) was identical, at around 9 per cent (Stagno *et al.*, 1975). The lower prevalence of virus excretion (1.5 per cent) during the first trimester of pregnancy suggests that early pregnancy exerts a suppressive effect that wanes with advancing gestation. Increasing age also seems to reduce virus excretion, but multiparity seems to suppress virus excretion only at the cervix (Stagno *et al.*, 1975). Infection in the infant during the first 3 months of life correlates with cervical excretion at delivery and occurred in 40 per cent of infants born to mothers excreting CMV at delivery. Infection via breast milk has also been suggested as a route of transmission but the exact role of this route has not yet been determined. Viral excretion in infants begins between 30–60 days postnatally (Reynolds *et al.*, 1973).

Post-transfusion CMV infection can be another cause of neonatal CMV and occurred in 33 per cent of children having exchange transfusions for hyperbilirubinaemia, although few were symptomatic. Symptomatic post-transfusion CMV was associated with a seronegative mother, a birthweight of <1200g, a stay in an intensive care unit for >38 days and a transfusion of >50 ml blood (Simon, 1985).

CMV is a significant problem, with a number of affected babies similar to those with congenital rubella defects in non-epidemic years before the availability of immunization. A recent *Lancet* editorial (1989) has concluded that there is no logical basis for introducing a screening programme: there is no vaccine and there is no satisfactory anti-viral drug. CMV is therefore likely to remain an important cause of handicap for many years to come.

Herpes simplex virus (HSV)

Neonatal herpes simplex is an increasing problem because of the increasing frequency of genital herpes simplex. It has been estimated that between 1/2000 and 1/5000 deliveries may be affected each year in the USA (Stagno and Whitley, 1985). Maternal HSV infection can result in spontaneous abortion, premature labour, intrauterine growth retardation and congenital and perinatal infections of infants. Furthermore, although it is very rare, disseminated infection can occur in the mother and carries a mortality rate of 50 per cent. The problem may be over-emphasized if there are a significant number of asymptomatic cases but currently it is estimated that, unlike CMV, where only 5–10 per cent of those infected are symptomatic, 99 per cent of infants infected with HSV are symptomatic (Nahmias and Visintine, 1976). The untreated infant mortality of detected cases is between 40 and 60 per cent, with 50 per cent of the survivors having long term sequelae. The spectrum of clinical illness in the neonate can be divided into disseminated infection, with or without CNS involvement, and local infection of the skin or eyes. The majority of the mortality and morbidity associated with HSV occurs in the disseminated form or in CNS disease (Nahmias and Visintine, 1976). Although infection can occur *in utero* (Stone, 1986) and postnatally (more commonly), neonatal infection is thought to be contracted intrapartum in >80 per cent of cases. Caesarean section is thought to be protective if performed before, or shortly after, rupture of the membranes (Nahmias and Visintine, 1976), but the problem is to define those patients for whom caesarean section is necessary.

The major risk of neonatal infection occurs when vaginal delivery follows primary genital HSV infection in late pregnancy (Brown *et al.*, 1987). Although genital herpes is common in pregnancy, with an incidence of around 1 per cent, most of these episodes are recurrences. This poses much less risk to the neonate, partly because virus shedding lasts for an average of only 2–5 days compared with 3 weeks following primary infection (probably mainly because of much lower viral concentrations excreted) and partly because of high levels of transplacental neutralizing antibodies, which protect the infant.

A primary infection in pregnancy should generally be treated with acyclovir, although this is for the sake of the mother rather than for any proven benefit to the fetus. Where there is a history of genital herpes in her partner, a woman should be tested for herpes simplex antibody: if this is absent, she should be advised to abstain from intercourse during pregnancy.

When a woman has a history of recurrent genital herpes, screening for viral carriage close to delivery has been recommended in the past, but is not now considered to be indicated. Maternal cultures do not seem to predict accurately those infants who are at risk (Arvin *et al.*, 1986; Prober *et al.*, 1988). This is partly because of the short time during which shedding occurs, and also because the mothers of 70 per cent of infected neonates have no history of HSV and no lesions. The value of weekly viral cultures in women with a history of recurrent genital herpes was examined by Binkin, Koplan and Cates (1985): they calculated that only 25 per cent of women shedding virus at delivery would be identified, and that each case of neonatal herpes saved by screening would cost US$1.8 × 10^6. Although 30 cases of neonatal herpes per year could be prevented if the policy were carried out throughout the USA, this would be at a cost of 5700 unnecessary caesarean sections, resulting in three maternal deaths. Kelly (1988) described a practical approach to the problem based on clinical examination: caesarean section should be performed if a lesion suspicious of herpes were seen, and the membranes were intact or recently ruptured. Some would carry out this policy only if the infection were thought to be primary, as the risks in recurrent genital herpes are probably very low (Prober *et al.*, 1987). Infection rates have been shown to be similar following vaginal delivery or caesarean section if the membranes have been ruptured for ≥4 h (Marshall and Peckham, 1983). Acyclovir can improve the prognosis for infected babies and Kelly has suggested that this drug should be given to the baby if neonatal cultures are positive, if the mother's infection is primary or if the baby's condition gives cause for concern. The position could change rapidly if more specific assessment of the individual were possible, for example if there were more rapid diagnostic tests for the presence of herpes excretion that could be used on the labour ward, or if high titres of maternal antibody could be shown definitively to protect the newborn from HSV infection.

Parvovirus and erythema infectiosum

The first human infection with parvovirus was reported by Cossart *et al.* (1975). During the screening of blood donors' sera for hepatitis B, nine donors were noted to have a particular antigen in their sera which was distinct from hepatitis B and had the morphology and density of a parvovirus.

In 1981 it was demonstrated that antibodies to this particular antigen were usually acquired between the ages of 4 and 10 years and that 61 per cent of adults had antibodies (Edwards *et al.*, 1981; Cohen, Mortimer and Pereira, 1983); at that time the only known clinical illness associated with parvovirus was the mild febrile illness that had been noted in two soldiers following tattooing in Africa (Shneerson, Mortimer and Vandervelde, 1980). Between 1981 and 1983 it was noted that acute infection with parvovirus was the principal cause of acute anaemic episodes during chronic haemolytic anaemias such as those associated with sickle cell disease, hereditary spherocytosis and pyruvate kinase deficiency (Serjeant *et al.*, 1981; Duncan *et al.*, 1983; Kelleher *et al.*, 1983). Laboratory studies demonstrated that the pathophysiology was inhibition of colony formation but the common childhood presentation remained unknown (Mortimer *et al.*, 1983). In 1983 outbreaks of erythema infectiosum or fifth disease were associated with acute parvovirus in outbreaks that occurred in London (Anderson *et al.*, 1983). The clinical picture in these outbreaks was of a mild febrile illness associated with headaches, anorexia, arthralgia and a rash. There might be a characteristic slapped appearance, followed by a maculopapular eruption on the trunk and extremities coinciding with the appearance of antibodies (Anderson *et al.*, 1983; Cohen, 1984).

Infection with parvovirus during pregnancy has been shown to be associated with spontaneous abortion in the first trimester and with aplastic crises, resulting in hydrops fetalis and causing intrauterine death, mid-trimester abortion or stillbirth (Cossart *et al.*, 1975; Anand *et al.*, 1987; Carrington *et al.*, 1987; Gray, Davidson and Anand, 1987). As in chronic anaemias, the disorder appears to be related to shortened red cell survival and hyperplastic erythropoiesis. In this situation the erythroid progenitor cells seem to be particularly vulnerable to agents such as parvovirus (Gray, Davidson and Anand, 1987).

A total of 36 fetal deaths have now been reported but >130 normal pregnancies have been shown to be unaffected by an acute maternal infection. As with many rare conditions, the reporting of severe cases may distort the apparent attack rate. Prospective studies are required, but on published cases of acute parvovirus infections of pregnancy the fetus is affected in around 20–30 per cent of cases (Anand *et al.*, 1987; Carrington *et al.*, 1987). However, among women unselected for exposure to parvovirus it is an uncommon infection during pregnancy and rarely, if ever, produces congenital anomalies. In a recent review Brown (1989) concludes that at least 80 per cent of pregnancies in which parvovirus B19 infections occur result in normal livebirths, and emphasizes that the threat of parvovirus B19 infection to the fetus is still being assessed. The monitoring of maternal serum alphafetoprotein levels and the use of serial ultrasound examinations have been recommended to detect developing hydrops fetalis (Carrington *et al.*, 1987).

Bacterial infections in pregnancy

Group B streptococcal infection

The group B streptococcus (GBS) is one of the most frequent causes of life-threatening infection in the neonate (Boyer and Gotoff, 1988). Early onset disease has an incidence of approximately 1–4/1000 births and a mortality rate of 20–80 per cent. Late onset disease has an incidence of one-half that of early onset, and a lower mortality. The main risk factors are prematurity and low birthweight, prolonged rupture of membranes, and intrapartum fever (Boyer *et al.*, 1983a).

As infection is transmitted intrapartum, and as the reservoir of GBS is the mother's vaginal or anorectal flora, much attention has been paid to antenatal screening and treatment. Maternal carriage rates vary from 8 to 31 per cent (Ancona, Ferrieri and Williams, 1980; Anthony *et al.*, 1981) and nearly 70 per cent of women with GBS in early pregnancy remain colonized at delivery (Boyer *et al.*, 1983b). Treatment of these women does not appear to reduce the carriage rate at delivery (Hall *et al.*, 1976; Anthony, Okada and Hobel, 1978) and, even if their sexual partners are also treated, 60 per cent of women still carry GBS in labour (Gardner *et al.*, 1979).

Intrapartum chemoprophylaxis is effective in reducing colonization of the baby and greatly reduces the incidence of early onset disease (Boyer *et al.*, 1983c; Boyer and Gotoff, 1986). Penicillin G is the drug of choice, with ampicillin also useful, and erythromycin is known to be effective in penicillin-sensitive individuals.

Postpartum prophylaxis for the neonate has the great advantage that penicillins appear virtually free of toxicity in neonates, whereas there is a definite, although very small, risk of acute anaphylaxis and death from shock in adults. Such chemo-prophylaxis can reduce the incidence of neonatal colonization and may help to suppress early onset infections (Siegel *et al.*, 1982). However, most severe and potentially fatal infections are in babies already displaying symptoms at birth, and, particularly in the very preterm infant, postpartum treatment may be too late.

The dilemma of which chemotherapeutic strategy to use is that because such a high proportion of women carry GBS it is inappropriate to treat them all; but because most cases of life-threatening infection present at birth, intrapartum prophylaxis is essential for certain individuals. This dilemma of selection of cases has been very clearly and carefully considered by Boyer and Gotoff in an excellent review (Boyer and Gotoff, 1988) and a series of earlier papers. These authors carried out antenatal screening of all patients and paid particular attention to the three main risk factors of prematurity/low birthweight, prolonged rupture of membranes and intrapartum fever. In women who carried GBS, and with risk factors, one in 25 of the babies had group B disease, and this included 4.6 per cent of the population. Sixty per cent of women neither had risk factors nor had been shown to carry GBS and the incidence of group B disease in their babies was only 1:3300. Boyer and Gotoff recommended treating women with GBS carriage and risk factors during labour, and suggested that giving penicillin at birth to babies from women colonized but without risk factors might also be helpful (Siegel *et al.*, 1982). They argued that such a scheme would be cost effective (Boyer and Gotoff, 1988) and it is certainly logical. Where a routine screen is not carried out during pregnancy, management will have to depend on Gram staining of vaginal swabs in the labour ward, and a high degree of readiness to treat on clinical grounds, especially where preterm delivery is likely.

Listeriosis

Listeria monocytogenes is a Gram-positive, non-acid fast, non spore-forming coryne-form bacterium that can produce human, animal and especially fetal infections (Bojsen-Moller, 1972; Lamont, Postlethwaite and Macgowan, 1988). It is widely distributed in the environment and is usually a sporadic infection but it can produce both nosocomial and community outbreaks (Bojsen-Moller, 1972; Lamont, Postlethwaite and Macgowan, 1988). The incidence of listeriosis in both animals and humans is increasing and between 1975 and 1985 the increase in England and Wales in humans was nearly 400 per cent (Lamont, Postlethwaite and Macgowan, 1988). The peak incidence of infection is in the spring for animals and the autumn for humans. The exact source of many infections is unknown but asymptomatic carriage in the pharynx, vagina and gastrointestinal tract does occur (Bojsen-Moller, 1972; Lamont, Postlethwaite and Macgowan, 1988). Thus the infection may be airborne, may be sexually-transmitted or may be ingested from contaminated food.

Outbreaks have occurred in association with unpasteurized milk or cheese as a consequence of mastitis in cattle. However, it has been shown that the organisms can proliferate at $\geqslant 6°C$ and above and this is the likely cause for the majority of outbreaks connected with food (Bojsen-Moller, 1972; Calman, 1989): for instance, the method of preparation of soft ripened cheese allows the organism to multiply to levels as high as $10^4/g$; in addition, a recent survey revealed contamination at low bacterial counts of rapidly chilled cooked convenience foods, of 12 per cent of pre-cooked poultry and of 18 per cent of cooked-chill meals or ready-to-eat salads. Incorrect storage or reheating could boost these levels however and as a consequence the government recently issued a circular to all doctors warning of the hazards for susceptible groups such as pregnant women (Calman, 1989).

Only 10–30 per cent of infections in humans are associated with no obvious immunological deficiency: the majority of infections are associated with defects of cell-mediated immunity, the elderly debilitated patient or pregnancy. Examples of defective immunological states include leukaemias, malignancies, iatrogenic immunosuppression and alcoholic liver disease. Common presentations include meningitis, primary bacteraemias, endocarditis and non-meningeal central nervous system infections. Uncommon presentations include pneumonia, adult respiratory distress syndrome, hepatitis and peritonitis (Bojsen-Moller, 1972; Lamont, Postlethwaite and Macgowan, 1988).

In 1988 there were 35 reported cases of listeriosis in Scotland, 63 per cent associated with pregnancy (Campbell, 1988). The maternal infection may be silent or may present as a 'flu-like illness associated with fever, rigors, generalized pain, pharyngitis, diarrhoea and urinary tract symptoms but sterile urine, or as a meningo-encephalitis. Of the cases reported by Campbell (1988) 54 per cent resulted in intrauterine or neonatal death. Much of this was due to very preterm labour together with intrauterine infection, with septicaemia, pneumonia or later meningitis. A characteristic feature seems to be the presence of meconium staining despite the prematurity. The late neonatal infections occur from the third to the 35th day and present as meningitis or septicaemia, with no associated maternal infection, and are acquired via passage through the birth canal or from attendants (Bojsen-Moller, 1972; Lamont, Postlethwaite and Macgowan, 1988).

Treatment of listeriosis with high dose ampicillin therapy (6–8 g/day in adults) has prevented perinatal listeriosis (Evans *et al.*, 1985). However, as Spencer (Spencer, 1987) concludes: 'Success in managing this condition depends not so much on considering the diagnosis but more on the degree of fetal or neonatal infection at the time of presentation'.

Chlamydial infections

The genus *Chlamydia* contains two species, *C. trachomatis* and *C. psittaci*. *C. psittaci* is responsible for a wide variety of respiratory, urogenital and systemic infections in animals and man is only incidentally infected. Infection with avian strains usually produces a respiratory infection of varying severity but the frequent failure to identify avian sources has led to suggestions that the infections may be acquired from animal sources, or even spread from man to man. Human infections with mammalian strains have been reported in association with bovine chlamydiosis in California and France.

Enzootic abortion of ewes is an important cause of stillbirth, abortion or the delivery of weak lambs, and is caused by certain mammalian strains of *C. psittaci*. In what was previously the Federal Republic of Germany up to 60 per cent of abortions in sheep are caused by the disease, while in the UK it is widespread, is increasing and has been estimated to cause up to 30 per cent of abortions in sheep. Recently attention has been drawn to the dangers for women exposed to the organism during pregnancy. Infection can occur from contact with infected products of conception, from infected pastures or from clothes and those at risk include farmers' wives, veterinary surgeons and others having contact with farms. The illness begins with a short febrile prodrome of up to 4 days accompanied by vomiting and chest or abdominal pains, or by severe headache with meningism. Of six reported cases, four had evidence of disseminated intravascular coagulation, three had mild renal or hepatic dysfunction and four had myocardial abnormalities. The patients were usually found to have severe septicaemia, with five requiring intensive care and one mother dying. Early delivery appeared to be beneficial for the mother in three cases. As in other cases of serious infection in pregnancy, the outlook is serious for the fetus, with only one surviving in the cases reported. In the presence of an appropriate history, 'atypical' organisms must not be overlooked in cases of serious sepsis of pregnancy and treatment with erythromycin, tetracycline or rifampicin should be considered (McKinlay *et al.*, 1985).

Lyme disease

Lyme disease is a tick-borne infection caused by the spirochaete *Borrelia burgdorferi* and characterized by a distinctive skin lesion called erythema chronicum migrans, by arthritis, by neurological disorders and by cardiac conduction abnormalities. It is the commonest tick-borne illness in the United States of America and has also been described in Europe and the UK.

Lyme disease during pregnancy has been associated in five patients with fetal death in the second trimester, prematurity and cortical blindness. In two other cases, transmission of spirochaetes from mother to fetus was demonstrated and was associated with cardiac abnormalities and intrauterine or perinatal death (MacDonald, Benach and Burgdorfer, 1987).

Other infections

Toxoplasmosis

Toxoplasmosis is a common cause of abortions in animals especially sheep. Human congenital toxoplasmosis was first described in the 1930s although retrospective diagnoses have been made as far back as the early 1900s (Remington and Desmonts, 1976).

The incidence of congenital toxoplasmosis varies according to the background prevalence of the disease which ranges from 5 per cent in Navajo Indians to 95 per cent in Parisian women (Remington and Desmonts, 1976). The variations are probably caused by eating habits: women in countries such as France and Austria, with a very high prevalence, may eat more raw meat containing oocytes of *Toxoplasma gondii*. Oocytes in cat faeces represent an alternative source of infection.

The toxoplasma cysts cross the placenta and produce a lymphocytic response in fetal tissues. Necrosis of brain parenchyma and cortex occurs. Periventricular vasculitis can result in necrosis of brain tissue, which sloughs off into the ventricles and may cause obstructive hydrocephalus. Destruction of the retinal layers can cause eventual optic and choroid atrophy. As with many other infections, the risk of congenital infection is greatest for infections acquired during the first two trimesters of pregnancy (Desmonts and Coevreur, 1974; Remington and Desmonts, 1976). The infection rate in neonates has been reported as between 30 and 40 per cent as a consequence of maternal infections, but severe congenital toxoplasmosis resulting in death or CNS or occular involvement occurred only following maternal infection within the first two trimesters (Desmonts and Coevreur, 1974; Remington and Desmonts, 1976) and in only about 15 per cent of infected babies overall. Treatment with spiramycin (similar to erythromycin) is thought to decrease the number of affected offspring, probably by treating the infection in the placenta, as the drug is not thought to cross the placenta in significant amounts (Desmonts and Coevreur, 1974).

The need for screening is determined by prevalence of infection in the community. In Paris, where the infection is very common, 95 per cent of women are immune by the age of 34 years (Remington and Desmonts, 1976) and >80 per cent of pregnant women have antibodies. It is easy to follow up the remaining small number of non-immune women, and these women are at high risk. In the UK the prevalence of the infection is lower: thus, only 20 per cent of pregnant women in Scotland are immune (Williams, Scott and MacFarlane, 1981) and 34 per cent of women in London have immunity by the age of 34 years (Remington and Desmonts, 1976). Screening would result in following up the majority of pregnant women, with very low risks of seroconversion. In two studies, one from London (Ruoss and Bourne, 1972) and the other from Glasgow (Williams, Scott and MacFarlane, 1981), 10 677 susceptible women were shown to have only 28 definite seroconversions (0.25 per cent). In the 7471 babies studied, there were only three definite congenital infections

(0.05 per cent) but no major morbidity or sequelae. Thus although screening is worth while in France and is a routine part of antenatal care, serious problems due to toxoplasmosis are rare in the UK and routine screening does not appear to be indicated at present.

Coccidioidomycoses

This illness is caused by the fungus *Coccidioides immitis* and is endemic in the South West of the USA. It is transmitted by the inhalation of fungal spores and consequently the incidence is greatest in the drier months when it is dustborne. About 30–50 per cent of those exposed develop symptoms, after an incubation period of 1–3 weeks. Initially, symptoms are very non-specific and include anorexia, headache, cough and fever, however, after an interval of as much as several months, approximately 0.2 per cent of those exposed will develop a disseminated disease which, before the use of amphotericin B was fatal in 50 per cent of cases. Dissemination is ten times commoner in the dark skinned and is also common in males (Harris, 1966).

As yet, it is not clear whether dissemination is commoner in pregnancy, because as usual the more severe forms are more often reported; the mortality rate, however, is much higher, 91 per cent instead of 50 per cent, if dissemination occurs during pregnancy (Drutz and Huppert, 1983). The illness has no effect on fertility and no fetal involvement has been noted. The infection does, however, involve the placenta and, as with other serious infections, there is a high fetal mortality of nearly 50 per cent. The treatment, as with non-pregnant disseminated cases is with amphotericin, which does not seem to affect the fetus but does produce appreciable side effects for the mother (Harris, 1966).

Other infections in pregnancy

This review, of necessity, focuses on a few infections only. It does not deal with many sexually transmitted infections. There is no discussion of malaria, a major cause of maternal mortality in endemic areas (reviewed by Brabin, 1983) and many other infections important in the developing world. Finally, it does not discuss infectious problems of major importance in obstetrics, such as pyelonephritis, septic abortion, chorioamnionitis or postpartum sepsis. This is not a reflection of lack of appreciation of the significance of these problems but simply the constraints of space and the overall plan of discussing organisms rather than disease presentation.

Update

This chapter was submitted in 1989. Since then there have been a number of important developments. A further report from the European Collaborative Study (*Lancet*, 1991, **1**, 253–260) showed a vertical transmission rate, based on 372 children born at least eighteen months before the analysis, of only 12.9 per cent. A further 2.5 per cent of children had persistent virus isolation but lost antibody and were clinically well. Overall transmission rate may be less than previously believed. It has also become clearer that vertical transmission is different in different populations of women and some of the factors influencing transmission have been elucidated.

References

Aaby, P, Bukh, J, Lisse, IM *et al.* (1988) Increased perinatal mortality among children of mothers exposed to measles during pregnancy. *Lancet*, **i**, 516

Abioye, AA (1973) Fatal amoebic colitis in pregnancy and puerperium: a new clinico-pathological entity. *Journal of Tropical Medicine and Hygiene*, **76**, 97–100

Acharya, U, Lamont, CAR and Cooper, K (1988) Group A beta-haemolytic streptococcus causing disseminated intravascular coagulation and maternal death. *Lancet*, **i**, 595 (letter)

Ahlfors, K, Ivarsson, SA, Johnsson, T and Svanberg, L (1982) Primary and secondary maternal cytomegalovirus infections and their relation to congenital infections. Analysis of maternal sera. *Acta Paediatrica Scandinavica*, **71**, 109–113

AIDS News Supplement (1989a) CDS weekly report. **6 May** (CDS 81/18)

AIDS News Supplement (1989b) CDS weekly report. **15 July** (CDS 89/28)

Alfort, CA (1976) Rubella. In *Infectious Diseases of the Fetus and the Newborn Infant* (edited by JS Remington and JO Klein) Philadelphia: WB Saunders

Amino, N, Tanizawa, O, Kiyoshi, M *et al.* (1978) Changes of serum immunoglobulins IgG, IgA, IgM and IgE during pregnancy. *Obstetrics and Gynecology*, **52**, 415–420

Amstey, MS, Insel, RA and Pichichero, ME (1984) Neonatal passive immunization by maternal vaccination. *Obstetrics and Gynecology*, **63**, 105–109

Anand, A, Gray, ES, Brown, T *et al.* (1987) Human parvovirus infection in pregnancy and hydrops fetalis. *New England Journal of Medicine*, **316**, 183–186

Ancona, RJ, Ferrieri, P and Williams, PP (1980) Maternal factors that enhance the acquisition of group B streptococci by newborn infants. *Journal of Medical Microbiology*, **13**, 272–280

Anderson, FD, Ushijima, RN and Larson, CL (1974) Recurrent herpes genitalis. Treatment with mycobacterium bovis (BCG). *Obstetrics and Gynecology*, **43**, 797–805

Anderson, MJ, Jones, SE, Fisher-Hoch, SP *et al.* (1983) Human parvovirus, the cause of erythema infectiosum (fifth disease)? *Lancet*, **i**, 1378

Anthony, BF, Okada, DM and Hobel, CJ (1978) Epidemiology of group B streptococcus: longitudinal observations during pregnancy. *Journal of Infectious Diseases*, **137**, 524–530

Anthony, BF, Eisenstadt, R, Carter, J *et al.* (1981) Genital and intestinal carriage of group B streptococci by newborn infants. *Journal of Medical Microbiology*, **13**, 272

Armon, PJ (1978) Amoebiasis in pregnancy and the puerperium. *British Journal of Obstetrics and Gynaecology*, **85**, 264–269

Arvin, AM, Hensleigh, PA, Prober, CG *et al.* (1986) Failure of antepartum maternal cultures to predict the infants' risk of exposure to herpes simplex virus at delivery. *New England Journal of Medicine*, **315**, 796–800

Aucouturier, P, Conderc, LJ, Gouet, D *et al.* (1986) Serum immunoglobulin G subclass dysbalances in the lymphadenopathy syndrome and acquired immune deficiency syndrome. *Clinical and Experimental Immunology*, **63**, 234–240

Barre-Sinoussi, F, Chermann, JC, Rey, F *et al. et al.* (1983) Isolation of a T-lymphotropic retrovirus from a patient at risk for acquired immune deficiency syndrome (AIDS). *Science*, **220**, 868–871

Baskin, CG, Law, S and Wenger, NK (1980) Sulfadiazine rheumatic fever prophylaxis during pregnancy: does it increase the risk of kernicterus in the newborn? *Cardiology*, **65**, 222–225

Beasley, RP, Trepo, C and Stevens, W (1977) The e antigen and vertical transmission of hepatitis B surface antigen. *American Journal of Epidemiology*, **105**, 94–98

Beasley, RP, Hwang, L and Stevens, CE (1983) Efficacy of hepatitis B immune globulin for prevention of perinatal transmission of hepatitis B virus carrier state: final report of a randomized double-blind, placebo controlled trial. *Hepatology*, **3**, 135–141

Berrebi, A, Puel, J, Tricoire, J *et al.* (1988) The influence of pregnancy on the evolution of HIV infection. *IV International Conference on AIDS*, **Abstract No. 4041, Book 1**, 270

Best, JM, Banatvala, JE, Morgan-Capner, P, and Miller, E (1989) Fetal infection after maternal reinfection with rubella: criteria for defining reinfection. *British Medical Journal*, **299**, 773–775

Biggar, BJ, Minkoff, HL, Willoughby, A *et al.* (1989) The effect of pregnancy on immune status in HIV(+) and HIV (−) women. *Society of Perinatal Obstetricians 9th Annual Meeting*, **Abstract No. 390**, 400

Binkin, NJ, Koplan, JP and Cates, W (1985) Preventing neonatal herpes: the value of weekly viral cultures in pregnant women with recurrent genital herpes. *Journal of the American Medical Association*, **251**, 2816–2821

Bissenden, JG, Ling, NR and Mackintosh, P (1980) Suppression of mixed lymphocyte reactions by pregnancy serum. *Clinical and Experimental Immunology*, **39**, 195–202

Björksten, B, Soderstrom, T, Damber, M-G, von Schoultz, B and Stigbrand, T (1978) Polymorphonuclear leucocyte function during pregnancy. *Scandinavian Journal of Immunology*, **8**, 257–262

Bojsen-Moller, J (1972) Human listeriosis. *Acta Pathologica et Microbiologica Scandinavica*, **Suppl 229**

Borhanmanesh, F, Haghighi, P, Hekmat, K *et al.* (1973) Viral hepatitis during pregnancy. *Gastroenterology*, **64**, 304–313

Boyer, KM and Gotoff, SP (1986) Prevention of early-onset neonatal group B streptococcal disease with selective intrapartum chemoprophylaxis. *New England Journal of Medicine*, **314**, 1665–1669

Boyer, KM and Gotoff, SP (1988) Antimicrobial prophylaxis of neonatal group B streptococcal sepsis. *Clinics in Perinatology*, **15**, 831–850

Boyer, KM and Kunik, L (1982) Changes in the vaginal flora of women with various clinical presentations. *Developments in Industrial Microbiology*, **23**, 521–525

Boyer, KM, Gadzala, CA, Burd, LI *et al.* (1983a) Selective intrapartum chemoprophylaxis of neonatal group B streptococcal early-onset disease: I. Epidemiologic rationale. *Journal of Infectious Diseases*, **148**, 795–801

Boyer, KM, Gadzala, CA, Kelly, PD *et al.* (1983b) Selective intrapartum chemoprophylaxis of neonatal group B streptococcal early-onset disease: II. Predictive value of prenatal cultures. *Journal of Infectious Diseases*, **148**, 802

Boyer, KM, Gadzala, CA, Kelly, PD and Gotoff, SP (1983c) Selective intrapartum chemoprophylaxis of group B streptococcal early-onset disease: III Interruption of mother-to-infant transmission. *Journal of Infectious Diseases*, **148**, 810–816

Brabin, BJ (1983) An analysis of malaria in pregnancy in Africa. *Bulletin of the World Health Organization*, **61**, 1005–1016

Brabin, BJ (1985) Epidemiology of infection in pregnancy. *Reviews of Infectious Diseases*, **7**, 579–603

Brabin, BJ, Nagel, J, Hagenaars, AM *et al.* (1984) The influence of malaria and gestation on the immune response to one and two doses of adsorbed tetanus toxoid in pregnancy. *Bulletin of the World Health Organization*, **62**, 919–930

Briggs, GG, Bodendorfer, TW, Freeman, RK and Yaffe, SJ (1983a) In *Drugs in Pregnancy and Lactation*, 1st edn, pp. 365–366. Baltimore:Williams and Wilkins

Brown, KE (1989) What threat is human parvovirus B$_{19}$ to the fetus? *British Journal of Obstetrics and Gynaecology*, **96**, 764–767

Brown, ZA, Vontver, LA, Benedetti, J *et al.* (1987) Effects on infants of a first episode of genital herpes during pregnancy. *New England Journal of Medicine*, **317**, 1246–1251

Bulmer, R and Hancock, KW (1977) Depletion of circulating T lymphocytes in pregnancy. *Clinical and Experimental Immunology*, **28**, 302–305

Calman, KC (1989) Listeriosis and food. *Scottish Home and Health Department*, **SHHD/CAMO (89)** 1

Cameron, DW, Simonsen, JN, D'Costa, LJ *et al.* (1989) Female to male transmission of human immunodeficiency virus type 1: risk factors for seroconversion in men. *Lancet*, **ii**, 403–407

Campbell, DM (1988) Listeriosis in Scotland 1988. *Communicable Diseases Report (Scotland)*, **89/17**, 6–7

Carne, CA, Weller, IVD, Loveday, C and Adler, MW (1987) From persistent generalised lymphadenopathy to AIDS: who will progress? *British Medical Journal*, **294**, 868–869

Carrington, D, Gilmore, DH, Whittle, MJ *et al.* (1987) Maternal serum alpha-fetoprotein – a marker of fetal aplastic crisis during intrauterine human parvovirus infection. *Lancet*, **i**, 433–435

Carvalho, AA, Giampaglia, CMS, Kimura, H *et al.* (1977) Maternal and infant antibody response to meningococcal vaccination in pregnancy. *Lancet*, **ii**, 809–811

Chiodo, F, Ricchi, E, Costigliola, P *et al.* (1986) Vertical transmission of HTLVIII *Lancet*, **i**, 739 (letter)

Coffin, J, Haase, A, Levy, JA *et al.* (1986) What to call the AIDS virus? (letter) *Nature*, **321**, 10

Cohen, BJ (1984) Update on the human parvovirus. *Communicable Diseases Report (Scotland)*, **84/10a**, VII–VIX

Cohen, BJ, Mortimer, PP and Pereira, MS (1983) Diagnostic assays with monoclonal antibodies for the human serum parvovirus-like virus (SPLV). *Journal of Hygiene*, **91**, 113–130

Committee Report (1989) Prevention of perinatal transmission of hepatitis B virus: prenatal screening of all pregnant women for hepatitis B surface antigen. *New York State Journal of Medicine*, **89**, 352–354

Cooper, LZ, Green, RH, Krugman, S *et al.* (1965) Neonatal thrombocytopenic purpura and other manifestations of rubella contracted in utero. *American Journal of Diseases of Children*, **110**, 416–427

Cossart, YE (1977) The outcome of hepatitis B virus infection in pregnancy. *Postgraduate Medical Journal*, **53**, 610–613

Cossart, YE, Field, AM, Cant, B and Widdows, D (1975) Parvovirus-like particles in human sera. *Lancet*, **i**, 72–73

Dalgleish, AG, Beverley, PCL, Clapham, PR *et al.* (1984) The CD4 (T4) antigen is an essential component of the receptor for the AIDS retrovirus. *Nature*, **312**, 763–767

D'Cruz, IA, Balani, SG and Iyer, LS (1968) Infectious hepatitis and pregnancy. *Obstetrics and Gynecology*, **31**, 449–455

Desmonts, G and Couvreur, J (1974) Congenital toxoplasmosis, a prospective study of 378 pregnancies. *New England Journal of Medicine*, **290**, 1110–1116

Diro, M and Beydoun, SN (1982) Malaria in pregnancy. *Southern Medical Journal*, **75**, 959–962

Des Jarlais, DC, Friedman, SR, Marmor, M *et al.* (1987) Development of AIDS, HIV seroconversion, and potential co-factors for T4 cell loss in a cohort of intravenous drug users. *AIDS*, **1**, 105–111

Drutz, DJ and Huppert, M (1983) Coccidioidomycosis: factors affecting the host–parasite interaction. *Journal of Infectious Diseases*, **147**, 372–390

Duncan, ME and Pearson, JMH (1984) The association of pregnancy and leprosy. III Erythema nodosum leprosum in pregnancy and lactation. *Leprosy Review*, **55**, 129–142

Duncan, ME, Melsom, R, Pearson, JMH and Ridley, DS (1981) The association of pregnancy and leprosy. 1. New cases, relapse of cured patients and detrioration in patients on treatment during pregnancy and lactation – results of a prospective study of 154 pregnancies in 147 Ethiopian women. *Leprosy Review*, **52**, 245–262

Duncan, ME, Pearson, JMH, Ridley, DS *et al.* (1982) Pregnancy and leprosy: the consequences of alterations of cell-mediated and humoral immunity during pregnancy and lactation. *International Journal of Leprosy*, **50**, 425–435

Duncan, JR, Potter, CB, Cappellini, MD *et al.* (1983) Aplastic crisis due to parvovirus infection in pyruvate kinase deficiency. *Lancet*, **ii**, 14–16

Edwards, JMB, Kessel, I, Gardner, SD *et al.* (1981) A search for a characteristic illness in children with serological evidence of viral or toxoplasma infection. *Journal of Infection*, **3**, 316–323

Enders, G, Nickerl-Pacher, U, Miller, E and Cradock-Watson, JE (1988) Outcome of confirmed periconceptional maternal rubella. *Lancet*, **i**, 1445–1447

European Collaborative Study (1988) Mother to child transmission of HIV infection. *Lancet*, **ii**, 1039–1042

European Study Group (1989) Risk factors for male to female transmission of HIV *British Medical Journal*, **298**, 411–415

Evans, JR, Allen, AC, Stinson, DA *et al.* (1985) Perinatal listeriosis: report of an outbreak. *Pediatric Infectious Disease Journal*, **4**, 237–241

Feinkind, L and Minkoff, ML (1988) HIV in pregnancy. *Clinics in Perinatology*, **15**, 189–202

Fine, PEM, Adelstein, AM, Snowman, J *et al.* (1985) Long term effects of exposure to viral infections in utero. *British Medical Journal*, **290**, 509–511

Freeman, DW and Barno, A (1959) Deaths from Asian influenza associated with pregnancy. *American Journal of Obstetrics and Gynecology*, **78**, 1172–1175

Gardner, SE, Yow, MD, Leeds, LJ *et al.* (1979) Failure of penicillin to eradicate group B streptococcal colonization in the pregnant woman. A couple study. *American Journal of Obstetrics and Gynecology*, **135**, 1062–1065

Gillies, MM (1969) Malaria, anaemia and pregnancy. *Annals of Tropical Medicine and Parasitology*, **63**, 245–263

Gloeb, DJ, O'Sullivan, MJ and Efantis, J (1988) Human immunodeficiency virus infection in women 1. The effects of human immunodeficiency virus on pregnancy. *American Journal of Obstetrics and Gynecology*, **159**, 756–761

Grant, S, Edmond, E and Syme, J (1981) A prospective study of cytomegalovirus infection in pregnancy—1. Laboratory evidence of congenital infection following maternal primary and reactivated infection. *Journal of Infections*, **3**, 24–31

Gray, ES, Davidson, RJD and Anand, A (1987) Human parvovirus and fetal anaemia. *Lancet*, **i**, 1144

Greenberg, M, Jacobziner, H, Pakter, J and Weisl, BAG (1958) Maternal mortality in the epidemic of Asian influenza, New York City, 1957. *American Journal of Obstetrics and Gynecology*, **76**, 897–902

Hall, RT, Barnes, W, Krishnan, I et al. (1976) Antibiotic treatment of parturient women colonized with group B streptococci. *American Journal of Obstetrics and Gynecology*, **124**, 630–634

Hanshaw, JB (1976) Cytomegalovirus. In *Infectious Diseases of the Fetus and the Newborn Infant* (edited by JS Remington and JO Klein) Philadelphia: WB Saunders

Harris, JW (1919) Influenza occurring in pregnant women. *Journal of the American Medical Associaton*, **72**, 978–980

Harris, RE (1966) Coccidioidomycosis complicating pregnancy. *Obstetrics and Gynecology*, **28**, 401–405

Higa, K, Dan, K and Manabe, H (1987) Varicella-zoster virus infection during pregnancy: hypothesis concerning the mechanisms of congenital malformations. *Obstetrics and Gynecology*, **69**, 214–222

Hirahara, F, Gorai, I, Tanaka, K et al. (1980) Cellular immunity in pregnancy: subpopulations of T lymphocytes bearing Fc receptors for IgG and IgM in pregnant women. *Clinical and Experimental Immunology*, **41**, 353–357

Holman, S, Berhaud, M, Sunderland, A et al. (1989a) Women infected with human immunodeficiency virus: counseling and testing during pregnancy. *Seminars in Perinatology*, **13**, 7–15

Holman, S, Sunderland, A, Berthaud, M et al. (1989b) Prenatal HIV counseling and testing. Clinical *Obstetrics and Gynecology*, **32**, 445–455

Homer, RS, McNall, EG, Oura, M and Golino, M (1961) Natural resistance to infectious diseases during pregnancy: possible relationship to serum properdin concentration. *American Journal of Obstetrics and Gynecology*, **81**, 29–41

Horsburgh, CR Jr, Ou, CY, Jason, J et al. (1989) Duration of human immunodeficiency virus infection before detection of antibody. *Lancet*, **ii**, 637–640

Imagawa, DT, Lee, MM, Wolinsky, SM et al. (1989) Human immunodeficiency virus type 1 infection in homosexual men who remain seronegative for prolonged periods. *New England Journal of Medicine*, **320**, 1458–1462

Johnstone, FD and Mok, J (1990) HIV infection. In *Infection in Obstetrics and Gynaecology* (edited by AB Maclean) pp. 72–94. Oxford: Blackwell

Johnstone, FD, MacCallum, L, Brettle, R et al. (1988) Does infection with HIV affect the outcome of pregnancy? *British Medical Journal*, **296**, 467

Johnstone, FD, Brettle, RP, MacCallum, LR et al. (1990) Women's knowledge of their HIV antibody state: its effect on their decision whether to continue the pregnancy. *British Medical Journal*, **300**, 23–24

Jovaisas, E, Koch, MA, Schafer, A et al. (1985) LAV/HTLV III in a 20 week fetus. *Lancet*, **ii**, 1129

Kavi, J and Wise, R (1988) Group A beta-haemolytic streptococcus causing disseminated intravascular coagulation and maternal death. *Lancet*, **i**, 993–994 (letter)

Kelleher, JF, Luban, NL, Mortimer, PP and Kamimura, T (1983) Human serum 'parvovirus': a specific cause of aplastic crisis in children with hereditary spherocytosis. *Journal of Pediatrics*, **102**, 720–722

Kelly, J (1988) Genital herpes during pregnancy. (Editorial) *British Medical Journal*, **297**, 1146–1147

Khuroo, MS, Teli, MR, Skidmore, S et al. (1981) Incidence and severity of viral hepatitis in pregnancy. *American Journal of Medicine*, **70**, 252–255

Klemola, E (1973) Cytomegalovirus infection in previously healthy adults. *Annals of Internal Medicine*, **79**, 267–268

Koonin, LM, Ellerbrock, TV, Atrash, HK et al. (1989) Pregnancy associated deaths due to AIDS in the United States. *Journal of the American Medical Association*, **261**, 1306–1309

Lamont, RJ, Postlethwaite, R and Macgowan, AP (1988) Listeria monocytogenes and its role in human infection. *Journal of Infection*, **17**, 7–28

Lancet Editorial (1989) Screening for congenital CMV. *Lancet*, **ii**, 599–600

Lane, HC, Masur, H, Edgar, LC et al. (1983) Abnormalities of B cell activation and immunoregulation in patients with the acquired immunodeficiency syndrome. *New England Journal of Medicine*, **309**, 453–458

Lapointe, N, Michaud, J, Pekovic, D, Chausseau, JP and Dupuy, JM (1985) Transplacental transmission of HTLV III virus. *New England Journal of Medicine*, **312**, 1325–1326

Laure, F, Lourgnaud, V, Rouziouz, C et al. (1988) Detection of HIV-1 DNA in infants and children by means of the polymerase chain reaction. *Lancet*, **ii**, 538–540

Lederman, MM (1984) Cell-mediated immunity and pregnancy. *Chest*, **86**, 7(s)–9(s)

Lee, SD, Lo, KJ, Wu, JC *et al.* (1986) Prevention of maternal–infant hepatitis B virus transmission to immunization: the role of serum hepatitis B virus DNA. *Hepatology*, **6**, 369–373

Lee, SD, Lo, KJ, Tsai, YT *et al.* (1989) Role of caesarean section in prevention of mother–infant transmission of hepatitis B virus. *Lancet*, **ii**, 833–834

Lepage, P, Van de Perre, P, Carael, M *et al.* (1987) Postnatal transmission of HIV from mother to child. *Lancet*, **ii**, 400

Lewis, EA and Antia, AV (1969) Amoebic colitis: review of 295 cases. *Transactions of the Royal Society of Tropical Medicine and Hygiene*, **63**, 633–638

Lo, KJ, Tsai, YT, Lee, SD *et al.* (1985) Immunoprophylaxis of infection with hepatitis B virus in infants born to hepatitis B surface antigen-positive carrier mothers. *Journal of Infectious Diseases*, **152**, 817–822

Lyman, WA, Kress, Y, Rubinstein, A *et al.* (1988) Evidence of human immunodeficiency virus infection in human fetal tissues. *Annals of the New York Academy of Sciences*, **549**, 258–259

McClure, MO and Weiss, RA (1987) Human immunodeficiency virus and related viruses. In *Current Topics in AIDS* (edited by MS Gottlieb, DJ Jeffries, D Mildvan, AJ Pinching, TC Quinn and RA Weiss) pp. 95–117. Chichester: John Wiley

MacCallum, LR, France, AJ, Jones, ME *et al.* (1988) The effects of pregnancy on the progression of HIV infection. In *IV International Conference on AIDS* (Stockholm), **Book 1, Abstract No. 4032**, 267

MacDonald, AB, Benach, JL and Burgdorfer, W (1987) Stillbirth following maternal Lyme disease. *New York State Journal of Medicine*, **7**, 615–616

McKinlay, AW, White, N, Buxton, D *et al.* (1985) Severe chlamydia psittaci sepsis in pregnancy. *Quarterly Journal of Medicine*, **New Series 57**, 689–696

Marshall, WC and Peckham, CS (1983) The management of herpes simplex in pregnant women and neonates. *Journal of Infection*, **6 (suppl 1)**, 23–29

Mead, PB (1989) AIDS: risk to the health profession. *Clinical Obstetrics and Gynaecology*, **32**, 485–496

Miller, E, Cradock-Watson, JE and Pollock, TM (1982) Consequences of confirmed maternal rubella at successive stages of pregnancy. *Lancet*, **ii**, 781–784

Miller, E, Nicoll, A, Rousseau, SA *et al.* (1987) Congenital rubella in babies of South Asian women in England and Wales: an excess and its causes. *British Medical Journal*, **294**, 737–739

Minkoff, H and Landesman, SH (1988) The case for routinely offering prenatal testing for human immunodeficiency virus. *American Journal of Obstetrics and Gynecology*, **159**, 793–796

Minkoff, H, de Regt, RH, Landesman, S *et al.* (1986) Pneumocystis carinii pneumonia associated with acquired immunodeficiency syndrome in pregnancy: a report of three maternal deaths. *Obstetrics and Gynecology*, **67**, 284–287

Minkoff, H, Nanda, D, Menez, R and Fikrig, S (1987a) Pregnancies resulting in infants with acquired immunodeficiency syndrome or AIDS related complex. *Obstetrics and Gynecology*, **69**, 285–287

Minkoff, H, Nanda, D, Mendez, R and Fikrig, S (1987b) Pregnancies resulting in infants with acquired immunodeficiency syndrome or AIDS related complex: follow-up mothers, children, and subsequently born siblings. *Obstetrics and Gynecology*, **69**, 288–291

Minkoff, HL, Gail, M, Willoughby, A *et al.* (1989) The effect of HIV infection on the course and short term outcome of pregnancy. *Society of Perinatal Obstetricians, 9th Annual Meeting*, **Abstract No. 391**, 401

Minkoff, HL, Willoughby, A, Mendez, H *et al.* (1990) Serious infections during pregnancy among women with advanced human immunodeficiency virus infection. *American Journal of Obstetrics and Gynecology*, **162**, 30–34

Mok, JQ, Giaquinto, C, De Rossi, A *et al.* (1987) Infants born to HIV sero-positive mothers – preliminary findings from a multicentre European study. *Lancet*, **i**, 1164–1168

Morrow, RH Jr, Smetana, HF, Sai, FT and Edgcomb, JH (1968) Unusual features of viral hepatitis in Accra, Ghana. *Annals of Internal Medicine*, **68**, 1250–1264

Mortimer, PP, Humphries, RK, Moore, JG *et al.* (1983) A human parvovirus like virus inhibits haematopoietic colony formation in vitro. *Nature*, **302**, 426–429

Moss, AR (1988) Predicting who will progress to AIDS *British Medical Journal*, **297**, 1067–1068

Moss, AR, Bacchetti, P, Osmond, D *et al.* (1988) Seropositivity for HIV and the development of AIDS or AIDS related condition: three year follow up of the San Francisco General Hospital Cohort. *British Medical Journal*, **296**, 745–750

Mowat, AP (1980) Viral hepatitis in infancy and childhood. *Clinics in Gastroenterology*, **9**, 191–212

Mundy, D, Schinazi, RF, Gerber, AR *et al.* (1987) Human immunodeficiency virus isolated from amniotic fluid. *Lancet*, **ii**, 459–460

Nahmias, AJ and Visintine, AM (1976) Herpes simplex. In *Infectious Diseases of the Fetus and the Newborn Infant* (edited by JS Remington and JO Klein) Philadelphia: WB Saunders

Newman, RG (1983) The need to redefine 'addiction'. *New England Journal of Medicine*, **308**, 1096–1098

Noah, ND and Fowle, SE (1989) Immunity to rubella in women of childbearing age in the United Kingdom. *British Medical Journal*, **297**, 1301–1304

Oleske, J, Minnefor, A, Cooper, R *et al.* (1983) Immune deficiency syndrome in children. *Journal of the American Medical Association*, **249**, 2345–2349

Oriel, JD (1971) Natural history of genital warts. *British Journal of Venereal Diseases*, **47**, 1–13

Ou, CY, Kwok, S, Mitchell, SW *et al.* (1988) DNA amplification for direct detection of HIV 1 in DNA of peripheral blood mononuclear cells. *Science*, **239**, 295–297

Pannuti, CS, Vilas Boas, LS, Angelo, MJ *et al.* (1985) Cytomegalovirus mononucleosis in children and adults: differences in clinical presentation. *Scandinavian Journal of Infectious Diseases*, **17**, 153–156

Paryani, SG and Arvin, AM (1986) Intrauterine infection with varicella-zoster virus after maternal varicella. *New England Journal of Medicine*, **314**, 1542–1545

Pass, RF, Stagno, S, Myers, GJ and Alford, CA (1980) Outcome of symptomatic congenital cytomegalovirus infection results of long-term longitudinal follow-up. *Pediatrics*, **66**, 758–762

Peckham, CS and Logan, S (1988) Cytomegalovirus infection in pregnancy. In *Proceedings of the 11th European Congress of Perinatal Medicine* (Chur, Switzerland) (edited by EV Cosmi and GC DiRenzo) pp. 255–260. Switzerland: Harwood

Peutherer, JF, Rebus, S, Aw, D *et al.* (1988) Detection of HIV in the fetus: a study of six cases. *Proceedings of IV International Conference on AIDS*, **Book 1**, 436

Pezzella, M, Rossi, P, Lombardi, V *et al.* (1989) HIV viral sequences in serogative people at risk detected by in situ hybridization and polymerase chain reaction. *British Medical Journal*, **298**, 713–716

Pinching, AJ and Weiss, RA (1986) AIDS and the spectrum of HTLV III/LAV infection. *International Review of Experimental Pathology*, **28**, 1–44

Pinching, AJ, McManus, TJ, Jeffries, DJ *et al.* (1983) Studies of cellular immunity in male homosexuals in London. *Lancet*, **ii**, 126–130

Piot, P, Kreiss, JK, Ndinya-Achola, JO *et al.* (1987) Heterosexual transmission of HIV. *AIDS*, **4**, 199–206

Preece, PM, Blount, JM, Glover, J *et al.* (1983) The consequences of primary cytomegalovirus infection in pregnancy. *Archives of Disease in Childhood*, **58**, 970–975

Preece, PM, Pearl, KN and Peckham, CS (1984) Congenital cytomegalovirus infection. *Archives of Disease in Childhood*, **59**, 1120–1126

Priddle, HD, Lenz, WR, Young, DC and Stevenson, CS (1952) Poliomyelitis in pregnancy and the puerperium. *American Journal of Obstetrics and Gynecolgy*, **63**, 408–413

Prober, CG, Sullender, WM, Yasukawa, LL, Au DS, Yeager, AS and Arvin, AM (1987) Low risk of herpes simplex virus infections in neonates exposed to the virus at the time of vaginal delivery to mothers with recurrent genital herpes simplex virus infections. *New England Journal of Medicine*, **316**, 240–244

Prober, CG, Hensleigh, PA, Boucher, FD *et al* (1988) Use of routine viral cultures at delivery to identify neonates exposed to herpes simplex virus. *New England Journal of Medicine*, **318**, 887–891

Purtilo, DT, Hallgren, HM and Yunis, EJ (1972) Depressed maternal lymphocyte response to phytohaemagglutinin in human pregnancy. *Lancet*, **i**, 769–771

Ranki, A, Valle, SL, Krohn, M *et al.* (1987) Long latency precedes overt seroconversion in sexually transmitted human immunodeficiency virus infection. *Lancet*, **ii**, 589–593

RCOG (1987) *Report of the Royal College of Obstetricians and Gynaecologists Sub-committee on Problems Associated with AIDS in Relation to Obstetrics and Gynaecology*. London: RCOG

Reinhardt, MC (1980) Effects of parasitic infections in pregnant women. *Ciba Foundation Symposium*, **77 (New Series)**, 149–170

Remington, JS and Desmonts, G (1976) Toxoplasmosis. In *Infectious Diseases of the Fetus and the Newborn Infant* (edited by JS Remington and JD Klein) Philadelphia: WB Saunders

Reynolds, DW, Stagno, S, Hosty, TS, Tiller, M and Alford, CA (1973) Maternal cytomegalovirus excretion and perinatal infection. *New England Journal of Medicine*, **289**, 1–5

Ross, JM (1980) Perinatal implications of the lower genital tract flora. *CIBA Foundation Symposium, Amsterdam*, **77**, 69–83

Rubenstein, A, Sicklick, M, Gupta, A *et al.* (1983) Acquired immunodeficiency with reversed T4/T8 ratios in infants born to promiscuous and drug addicted mothers. *Journal of the American Medical Association*, **249**, 2350–2356

Ruoss, CF and Bourne, GL (1972) Toxoplasmosis in pregnancy. *Journal of Obstetrics and Gynaecology of the British Commonwealth*, **79**, 1115

Rutter, D, Griffiths, P and Trompeter, RS (1985) Cytomegalic inclusion disease after recurrent maternal infection. *Lancet*, **ii**, 1182

Saigal, S, Lunyk, O, Larke, RPB and Chernesky, MA (1982) The outcome in children with congenital cytomegalovirus infection. *American Journal of Diseases of Children,* **136**, 896–901

Schoenbaum, EE, Davenny, K, Selwyn, PA *et al.* (1989) The effect of pregnancy on progression of HIV related disease. *5th International Conference on AIDS*, Montreal, Abstract MBP8

Scott, GB, Fischl, MA, Klimas, N *et al.* (1985) Mothers of infants with the acquired immunodeficiency syndrome. Evidence for both symptomatic and asymptomatic carriers. *Journal of the American Medical Association*, **253**, 363–366

Selwyn, PA, Schoenbaum, EE, Davenny, K *et al.* (1989b) Prospective study of human immunodeficiency virus infection and pregnancy outcomes in intravenous drug users. *Journal of the American Medical Association*, **261**, 1289–1294

Selwyn, PA, Carter, RJ, Schoenbaum, EE *et al.* (1989) Knowledge of HIV antibody status and decision to continue or terminate pregnancy among intravenous drug users. *Journal of the American Medical Association*, **261**, 3567–3571

Serjeant, GR, Topley, JM, Mason, K *et al.* (1981) Outbreak of aplastic crises in sickle cell anaemia associated with parvovirus like agent. *Lancet*, **ii**, 595–597

Sherlock, S (1968) Jaundice in pregnancy. *British Medical Bulletin*, **24**, 39–43

Shneerson, JM, Mortimer, PP and Vandervelde, EM (1980) Febrile illness due to a parvovirus. *British Medical Journal*, **2**, 1580

Shurin, SB (1979) Infectious mononucleosis. *Pediatric Clinics of North America*, **26**, 315–326

Siegel, M and Fuerst, HT (1966) Low birth weight and maternal virus disease. *Journal of the American Medical Association,* **197**, 680–684

Siegel, M and Greenberg, M (1955) Incidence of poliomyelitis in pregnancy. *New England Journal of Medicine*, **253**, 841–847

Siegel, M, Fuerst, HT and Peress, NS (1966) Comparative fetal mortality in maternal virus diseases. *New England Journal of Medicine*, **274**, 768–771

Siegel, JD, McCracken, GH, Threlkeld, N *et al.* (1982) Single-dose pencillin prophylaxis of neonatal group B streptococcal disease. Conclusion of a 41 month controlled study. *Lancet*, **i**, 1426–1430

Simon, TL (1985) Cytomegaloviruses and blood transfusion. *Plasma Therapy and Transfusion Technology*, **6**, 69–79

Spencer, JAD (1987) Perinatal listeriosis (Editorial). *British Medical Journal*, **295**, 349

Spurrett, B, Jones, DS and Stewart, G (1988) Cervical dysplasia and HIV infection. *Lancet*, **i**, 237

Srabstein, JC, Morris, N, Bryce Larke, RP *et al.* (1974) Is there a congenital varicella syndrome? *Journal of Pediatrics*, **84**, 239–243

Sridama, V, Pacini, F, Yang, SL *et al.* (1982) Decreased levels of helper T-cells – a possible cause of immunodeficiency in pregnancy. *New England Journal of Medicine*, **307**, 352–356

Stagno, S and Whitley, RJ (1985) Herpes virus infections of pregnancy. Part II: herpes simplex and varicella-zoster virus infections. *New England Journal of Medicine*, **313**, 1327–1329

Stagno, S, Reynolds, D, Tsiantos, A *et al.* (1975) Cervical cytomegalovirus excretion in pregnant and nonpregnant women: suppression in early gestation. *Journal of Infectious Diseases*, **131**, 522–527

Starr, SE (1979) Cytomegalovirus. *Pediatric Clinics of North America*, **26**, 283–293

Stelkauskas, AJ, Wilson, BS and Dray, S (1975) Inversion of levels of human T and B cells in early pregnancy. *Nature*, **258**, 331–332

Stern, H and Tucker, SM (1973) Prospective study of cytomegalovirus infections in pregnancy. *British Medical Journal*, **2**, 268–270

Stone, KM (1986) Current considerations in the obstetric and gynaecological management of herpes simplex virus infection. *Journal of Reproductive Medicine*, **31**, 452

Sumaya, CV and Gibbs, RS (1979) Immunization of pregnant women with influenza A/New Jersey/76 virus vaccine: reactogenicity and immunogenicity in mother and infant. *Journal of Infectious Diseases*, **140**, 141–146

Tong, MJ, Thursby, MW, Lin, JH *et al.* (1981) Studies on the maternal infant transmission of the hepatitis B virus and HBV infection within families. *Progress in Medical Virology*, **27**, 137–147

Valdimarsson, H, Mulholland, C, Fridiksdottir, V and Coleman, DV (1983) A longitudinal study of leucocyte blood counts and lymphocyte responses in pregnancy: a marked early increase of monocyte–lymphocyte ratio. *Clinical and Experimental Immunology*, **53**, 437–443

Vento, S, Perri, GDi., Luzzati, R *et al.* (1989) Clinical reactivation of hepatitis B in anti-HBs positive patients with AIDS. *Lancet*, **i**, 332–333

Watkinson, M and Rushton, DI (1983) Plasmodial pigmentation of placenta and outcome of pregnancy in West African mothers. *British Medical Journal*, **287**, 251–254

Weinberg, ED (1984) Pregnancy-associated depression of cell-mediated immunity. *Reviews of Infectious Diseases*, **6**, 814–831

Weinbreck, P, Loustaud, V, Denis, F *et al.* (1988) Postnatal transmission of HIV infection. *Lancet*, **i**, 482

Weinstein, L, Aycock, WL and Feemster, RF (1951) The relation of sex, pregnancy and menstruation to susceptibility in poliomyelitis. *New England Journal of Medicine*, **245**, 54–58

WHO (1989) Global programme on AIDS and programme of STD. *Consensus Statement from Consultation on Sexually Transmitted Diseases as a Risk Factor for HIV Transmission. Geneva 4–6 January*, **WHO/GPA/INF/89.1**

Williams, KAB, Scott, JM and MacFarlane, DE (1981) Congenital toxoplasmosis; a prospective survey in the West of Scotland. *Journal of Infection*, **3**, 219–229

Wong, VC, Reesink, HW and Ip, HMM *et al.* (1984) Prevention of the HB$_s$Ag carrier state in newborn infants of mothers who are chronic carriers of HB$_s$Ag and HB$_e$Ag by administration of hepatitis B vaccine and hepatitis B immunoglobulin. *Lancet*, **i**, 921–926

Young, NA (1976) Chicken pox, measles and mumps. In *Infectious Diseases of the Fetus and the Newborn Infant* (edited by JS Remington and JO Klein) Philadelphia: WB Saunders

Young, RL, Acosta, AA and Kaufman, RH (1973) The treatment of large condylomata acuminata complicating pregnancy. *Obstetrics and Gynecology*, **41**, 65–73

Zagury, D, Bernard, J, Leonard, R *et al.* (1986) Longterm cultures of HTLV-III infected T cells: a model of cytopathology of T cell depletion in AIDS. *Science*, **231**, 850–853

Ziegler, JB, Cooper, DA, Johnson, RO and Gold, J (1985) Postnatal transmission of AIDS associated retrovirus from mother to infant. *Lancet*, **i**, 896–898

Socially related disorders: drug addiction, maternal smoking and alcohol consumption

M Hepburn

Introduction

Drugs, prescribed or non-prescribed, legal or illegal and including tobacco and alcohol, are all potentially harmful to health. When they are used by a pregnant woman, there is also a risk to the baby's health. The term 'drugs', as commonly used, does not include tobacco or alcohol but only those drugs subject to 'misuse'. There are many alternative terms used to describe this kind of drug-taking including drug abuse, drug misuse, problem drug use and inappropriate drug use; the term 'drug misuse' was the one adopted by the Home Office Review on the Misuse of Drugs which defined it as: (1) the non-medical use of drugs intended for use only as part of a proper course of medical treatment, and (2) the illicit use of drugs which have no generally accepted medical purpose (Ministerial Group on the Misuse of Drugs, 1988).

The accuracy of prevalence data relating to the use of drugs, tobacco and alcohol is variable and depends on a number of factors including the legality and social acceptability of the three types of substance which in turn may influence the honesty with which people describe their habits.

Patterns of use

Drug misuse

Because the drugs that are commonly misused either are illegal to possess or (equally commonly) have been illegally obtained, few people willingly volunteer the information that they use such drugs. This information is, therefore, often indirectly obtained, coming to light only when people using drugs present, for example with related legal or medical problems. Home Office notifications provide another source of data but these numbers are much less than the actual number of addicts. The discrepancy is not simply due to undernotification but also to the increasingly wide range of drugs used, most of which are not included in the list of controlled drugs that require Home Office notification and many of which are prescribable or prescribed. Nevertheless, such direct and indirect information as does exist suggests that the level of drug misuse continues to increase, albeit in an irregular manner, with a particularly large and rapid rise in the late 1960s and early 1970s and again in the early 1980s (Ministerial Group on the Misuse of Drugs, 1988). As noted, the drugs that are misused have changed, the major changes being a decrease in heroin use (partly due to difficulties in obtaining sufficient supplies of sufficient purity), an increase in use of pharmaceutical preparations, and a move towards polydrug use, including a wide range of pharmaceutical products not previously considered in the context of drug misuse. In Scotland, the move towards pharmaceutical preparations has been particularly marked and the major drugs encountered in obstetric practice in Glasgow are buprenorphine (Temgesic) and benzodiazepines (principally Temazepam). In Britain, as in Europe as a whole, there has also been evidence of increasing availability of cocaine but as yet no evidence of a dramatic increase in the use of cocaine or alkaloidal cocaine ('crack'), which remains slight in comparison to the size of the problem in the USA.

There has also been a change in the population who use drugs in terms of age, sex and social class. Home Office notifications have been highest in the under-25s and, whereas drug misuse was previously very much commoner in males, it appears there has been a disproportionately large increase in the number of women who use drugs, to a level now approaching or equalling that in men.

The Home Office report (Ministerial Group on the Misuse of Drugs, 1988) notes that from being associated with 'an alternative youth sub-culture mainly centred in London', drug misuse has spread to all social classes in all parts of the country. It quotes the Medical Advisory Council on the Misuse of Drugs (ACMD) in its report on treatment and rehabilitation as stating that 'the majority (of drug users) are relatively stable individuals who have more in common with the general population than with any essentially pathological sub-group'. It is true that drug users are no different from non drug-using members of their community. It is also true that drug misuse occurs in all social classes but the spread is uneven with the problem being greatest in the lower socioeconomic groups, where it differs in a number of respects from the problem in the higher socioeconomic groups. In Scotland, this polarization of drug misuse is particularly marked with a pattern of drug misuse which correlates strongly with the pattern of deprivation. Thus in Glasgow it has been demonstrated that the vast majority of identified users live in the poorer areas of the city [Standard Committee of Drug Abuse (SCODA), 1985] but within these areas they have no particular characteristics that distinguish them from other people living there.

Cigarette smoking

Nicotine is also a highly addictive substance and in fact is rated by many drug users as much more difficult to give up than heroin. Unlike heroin, however, its use is legal although there has been a change in recent years in its social acceptability. Thus, the increasing pressures on smokers to stop smoking make many reluctant to give accurate information, either about whether they smoke at all or about their exact level of consumption; therefore data regarding smoking habits, although more accurate than data regarding drug misuse, are nevertheless subject to inaccuracies and under-reporting (Campbell, 1988).

Although a higher proportion of men than women smoke, smoking rates for both sexes have shown a decline in recent years [*General Household Survey* (GHS); Office of Population Censuses and Surveys, 1986]. Although the rates for women are reported to be declining more slowly than those for men, this may simply be a reflection of the number of men switching to pipes or cigars (Office of Population Censuses and Surveys, 1986). Among women, prevalence rates have fallen more slowly in the younger age groups and in 1984 the figures showed a higher percentage of girls than boys smoking in the 16–19 years age group. After rising in the 1970s, average cigarette consumption by men and women has been falling during the 1980s; consumption levels for women, however, have fallen more slowly and remain higher than those recorded in the early 1970s. The prevalence of cigarette smoking is higher in Scotland than in England, and in the whole of the UK is higher in the lower socioeconomic groups, and particularly in the unemployed. The proportion of women who smoke in the unskilled manual group started to fall later than that in other groups. Among women, smoking is also higher among those who are widowed, divorced or separated, compared with those who are single, married or co-habiting.

Thus, in 1984, one in three women smoked, and it remains a particular problem among the young aged <19 years and those in the lower socioeconomic groups. The problem of smoking is particularly great in Scotland where in 1984, lung cancer became the leading cause of death from cancer in women.

Alcohol consumption

Alcohol is legal, on the whole socially acceptable, and consumed at some time or other by the majority of the population. In 1984 in Great Britain among people aged 18 years or more, only 7 per cent of men and 13 per cent of women considered themselves 'abstainers', defined as people who never drank or who had consumed no alcohol in the previous 12 months (Office of Population Censuses and Surveys, 1984).

Alcohol consumption usually causes problems only when it becomes 'excessive' or 'uncontrolled' and in such a situation can be very damaging socially, mentally and physically. The limits implied by these terms, however, are totally arbitrary, different for men and women, variable between individuals and in different circumstances for the same individual, and almost completely unmeasurable.

Most information on drinking habits is self-reported, and such social surveys have consistently recorded lower levels of alcohol consumption than would be expected from alcohol sales (GHS, 1984). In the 1984 GHS, comparison of people's self-image of their drinking habits with their self reported quantity and frequency of drinking showed an increasingly weak correspondence as consumption levels rose, suggesting an unwillingness to face facts realistically.

Fewer women than men drink; those that do, drink less and there are fewer heavy drinkers among women (Office of Population Censuses and Surveys, 1984). It should be pointed out, however, that safe limits for alcohol consumption for women are lower than those for men; moreover, the methods for assessing alcohol consumption used in the GHS have inaccuracies that may lead to underestimation of the problem, particularly in women.

Nevertheless, the 1984 GHS reports an increase in alcohol consumption between 1978 and 1984 among women of all ages; similarly, a survey of drinking habits in Scotland showed increased consumption between 1976 and 1984 among women of all ages (Goddard, 1986). Further evidence of relative or absolute increases in alcohol consumption among women comes from the increased death rate in women from liver cirrhosis and the increases in drink-related convictions among women. The increase in drink-related mental hospital admissions for women demonstrates the increasing problem for women as a group and in comparison to men; the male:female ratio for such admissions was 4:1 in 1971 but 2:1 in 1982.

In the GHS of 1984, consumption levels were higher among younger women but lower among women with young dependent children; men's levels of consumption did not appear to be affected in this way by the presence of dependent children. Men in the lower socioeconomic groups were more likely to be in the heavy drinking category, whereas women in the unskilled manual group were more likely to be abstainers or occasional drinkers.

Thus, in summary, despite the differences in legal status and social acceptability of drugs, cigarettes and alcohol, there are similarities in the difficulties in obtaining accurate data regarding prevalence of use and consumption levels. Use of all three substances or groups of substances is increasing in women relative to men and, with the exception of cigarettes there is also an absolute increase in levels of use in women; in the case of all three it is consumption in the younger women that is particularly worrying.

Drug use and cigarette smoking both show correlations with socioeconomic status, higher consumption occurring in the lower groups. Alcohol consumption, on the other hand, shows no such correlation and if anything, the reverse trend is evident. However, although there is a greater proportion of abstainers among women in the manual group, with higher drinking rates in the higher socioeconomic groups, there is evidence that among heavy drinkers there is a subgroup of socially disadvantaged women, also likely to be smokers (Heller *et al.*, 1988).

Drug-taking in pregnancy

General effects on maternal health

Many of the problems experienced by pregnant women who use drugs are a consequence of their background of socioeconomic deprivation, compounded, for those who have a heavy or chaotic habit, by the consequent effects on their lifestyle. Thus they may experience an extensive range of domestic and economic problems causing, among other things, housing difficulties and social isolation. For those with a heavy habit, there are additional problems as a consequence of self-neglect and poor diet; where that habit is financed by shoplifting or prostitution there are legal repercussions and, in the case of prostitution, the risk of sexually transmitted diseases including hepatitis B and HIV infection.

Intravenous drug use *per se* involves the risk of overdosage (often as a result of variable purity of street drugs), thrombophlebitis and thrombosis of peripheral veins as well as infection, both locally at the injection site and systemically, including hepatitis B and HIV.

It must be emphasized, however, that many drug users (and probably the great majority) do not have a chaotic habit and are able to maintain a normal lifestyle. Nevertheless, they remain exposed to the risks of maintaining and practising their habit and they experience problems in common with other women from deprived environments.

Effects of drug use on pregnancy

Studies on effects of maternal drug-taking during pregnancy have centred largely on use of opiate drugs, either heroin or methadone prescribed as a heroin substitute. Most of the early large volume of published work came from the USA. There is, nevertheless, a considerable volume of data on use of other drugs in other countries, including Britain. Interpretation of all available data must take into account the cultural and ethnic differences of different countries and communities and is subject to the limitations already mentioned, the principal one being the difficulty in knowing which drug or drugs have been consumed, at what time and in what quantity. Many of these studies involve small samples examined retrospectively. Polydrug use makes it difficult to draw firm conclusions about the effects of a specific drug and especially to relate those effects to any dosage pattern. Many of the postulated harmful effects are multifactorial and may result from other associated factors such as smoking, socioeconomic deprivation, or secondary effects of drug misuse on the parents' lifestyle or the mother's general health, as already described.

Opiates

Heroin use may interfere with reproduction at a very early stage by causing reduced gonadotrophin production, secondary amenorrhoea (Bai et al., 1974; Perlmutter, 1974), anovulation, and thus infertility. Conversely, it has also been claimed that opiate use increases circulating gonadotrophin levels which in turn is associated with an increased incidence of multiple births (Rementeria, Janakammal and Hollander, 1975). Although amenorrhoea is commonly seen, infertility seems largely a theoretical problem, presumably because the supply and purity of drugs are usually variable and consumption levels effectively intermittent. The amenorrhoea however, causes difficulties in accurate dating of pregnancy compounded by the frequency with which drug-using women attend late for antenatal care; this, in turn, makes it difficult to monitor fetal growth accurately or to be precise about the gestation at delivery.

Congenital abnormalities in children of opiate-using mothers have been reported irregularly but there is no evidence that the incidence is increased in comparison with the general population (Harper et al., 1974; Perlmutter, 1974; Rothstein and Gould, 1974, and no proof of teratogenicity of either heroin or methadone (Stauber, Schwerdt and Tylden, 1982). Increased spontaneous abortion rates are sometimes quoted (Perlmutter, 1974) but are difficult to verify.

There are reports of increased rates of a number of antenatal complications including antepartum haemorrhage (due both to placenta praevia and abruptio placentae), pregnancy-induced hypertension and breech presentation (Pelosi et al., 1975; Finnegan, 1982) but again, these are very inconsistent and would appear to relate more to problems of the women's general health and social circumstances and the amount of antenatal care received than to any specific opiate effects; it is repeatedly observed that women who use drugs tend, for one reason or another, to receive very little antenatal care and, in fact, are often first seen when admitted in labour (Perlmutter, 1974). In such circumstances it is difficult to identify the aetiology of complications with any precision.

A constant observation, however, is an increased rate of low birthweight (Perlmutter, 1974; Pelosi et al., 1975; Fricker and Segal, 1978; Klenka, 1986), with greater numbers of both small-for-gestational-age and preterm babies (the latter possibly the explanation for reports of an increase in breech deliveries). Consequently, most studies report increased rates of fetal loss substantially related to low birthweight and preterm delivery with increased rates of intrauterine death and premature stillbirth, and neonatal deaths among preterm babies (Blinick, Jerez and Wallach, 1973; Harper et al., 1974; Perlmutter, 1974; Pelosi et al., 1975; Blinick et al., 1976; Connaughton et al., 1977; Fricker and Segal, 1978; Finnegan, 1982; Stauber, Schwerdt and Tylden, 1982; Bolton, 1987). The high reported rates of intrauterine death and preterm delivery are often attributed to repeated episodes of fetal withdrawal, resulting from erratic maternal drug consumption. This, in turn, is postulated to cause intrauterine hypoxia and increased uterine activity leading to preterm labour. In support of this hypothesis are quoted reports of reduced rates of stillbirth, preterm delivery and low birthweight in women maintained during pregnancy on a constant dose of methadone (Strauss *et al.*, 1974; Bolton, 1987).

Fluctuations in maternal drug levels no doubt make a significant contribution but the precise cause of the poor fetal growth is uncertain. Naeye *et al.* (1973) have reported that the growth retardation is due to a reduced cell number; that it is a specific opiate effect has been suggested by reports of a higher rate of low birthweight in opiate-addicted women receiving no antenatal care, compared with non-drug-using women with no antenatal care (Connaughton *et al.*, 1977). Such hypotheses are, however, largely conjectural and many other factors undoubtedly contribute, including the general health and nutrition of the mother as well as her social and economic circumstances. Polydrug use is common: drug-using women almost always smoke cigarettes and a number also drink alcohol.

The observed effects of adequate antenatal care (Strauss *et al.*, 1974; Deren, 1986) and regular methadone administration in such women are variable, possibly owing in part to the fact that prescription of methadone does not always stop the use of other drugs.

Labour and delivery

No particular problems are encountered in labour although the finding of meconium-stained liquor has been frequently reported (Blinick, Jerez and Wallach, 1973; Perlmutter, 1974; Blinick *et al.*, 1976; Fricker and Segal, 1978; Stauber, Schwerdt and Tylden, 1982). This has been interpreted as indicating not acute fetal distress in labour but, rather, recurrent episodes of antenatal stress caused by repeated fetal drug withdrawals as a result of irregular drug supplies (already implicated as a cause of fetal morbidity).

Difficulty in establishing venous access due to thrombosis of the peripheral veins is a real and extremely common problem. Elective induction of labour has been suggested by some as a solution to this, as well as to a number of other problems. As many drug-using women deliver, if not preterm, then certainly before 40 weeks' gestation, this is often an impractical solution; not only do they usually labour spontaneously by term, but they commonly labour quickly and uneventfully and there is no need for intervention unless the development of obstetric complications justifies it. Although their babies may be at greater risk of problems, including intrapartum fetal distress, intervention is not often necessary.

The question of analgesia in labour is the subject of much debate. There is an argument for avoiding opioid analgesics: much higher doses would be needed by women still using drugs while their use in women successful in remaining drug free might theoretically jeopardize their success, while liberal use of epidural or spinal anaesthesia may be preferable, but whatever is deemed appropriate, it is important to ensure that the woman is not deprived of adequate analgesia.

The neonate

Where the mother has been using drugs, either illicit heroin or prescribed methadone, near the time of delivery, there is a significant chance that the baby will exhibit signs of drug withdrawal. It was originally claimed that methadone maintenance therapy for the mother did not cause withdrawal symptoms in the baby; it has subsequently been shown, however, that not only does methadone cause withdrawal symptoms in the neonate but that these are often more severe and more prolonged than those attributable to heroin, although later in onset (Cohen and Neumann, 1973; Perlmutter, 1974; Strauss *et al.*, 1974; Newman, Bashkow and Calko, 1975; Blinick *et al.*, 1976; Stimmel and Adamsons, 1976; Harper *et al.*, 1977).

In the majority of cases withdrawal symptoms appear within the first 24–48 h after birth; those due to methadone, however, may not appear until later, however, perhaps as long as 6 days after birth (Perlmutter, 1974). It has been reported that the onset of symptoms may even be delayed until possibly as late as 2–4 weeks after birth but it seems that, in such cases, earlier mild symptoms of withdrawal are present and that these infants are exhibiting either prolonged withdrawals or a later exacerbation of symptoms rather than a truly delayed onset. Variations in reported incidence, severity and timing of the onset of withdrawal symptoms may well simply reflect observer variations (Zelson, 1973; Strauss *et al.*, 1974; Stimmel and Adamsons, 1976).

The infant exhibiting drug withdrawal is typically irritable: this may range from hyperactivity through hypertonus, to twitching and ultimately convulsions. Such babies have a disturbed sleep pattern, a characteristic high-pitched cry and, although hungry, they do not feed well.

There is lack of agreement on the incidence of jaundice in babies of drug-using mothers: it is variously reported as increased (Pelosi *et al.*, 1975), decreased (Perlmutter, 1974), and unchanged (Fricker and Segal, 1978); it has also been reported as being commoner and more severe where the mother used methadone compared with heroin (Zelson, Lee and Casalino, 1973). Respiratory distress syndrome has been reported as decreased (Glass, Rajegowda and Evans, 1971; Perlmutter, 1974; Pelosi *et al.*, 1975), unchanged (Connaughton *et al.*, 1977) and decreased with heroin but not methadone (Zelson, Lee and Casalino, 1973); in support of a reduction is cited the observation of accelerated lung maturation, as measured by lecithin:sphingo-myelin ratios (Gluck and Kulovich, 1973) and increases in cord prolactin levels (Parekh *et al.*, 1981) in babies of drug-using women.

Disturbances of respiratory control *in utero* have been demonstrated in the babies of women on methadone maintenance (Richardson, O'Grady and Olsen, 1984) and after birth these abnormalities persist (Ward *et al.*, 1986). It has been suggested that such abnormalities might contribute to the reported increase of sudden infant death syndrome (SIDS) in such babies, an increase which is reported to be even greater in babies of mothers maintained on methadone (Cohen and Neumann, 1973).

The range of severity of the symptoms exhibited is wide: many babies are simply described as rather 'jittery' or have a high-pitched cry but require no specific treatment, whereas at the other end of the spectrum a number of babies are extremely sick requiring intensive care with sedation and prolonged supportive therapy.

Attempts have been made to correlate the timing of onset, severity and duration of withdrawal symptoms with patterns of maternal drug use. It has been suggested that the time of onset of withdrawals depends on the maternal dose of drug, the duration of addiction and the time since the last dose (Zelson, 1973; Strauss *et al.*, 1974). On the other hand there is disagreement about a relationship between the severity of fetal withdrawal symptoms and these features of maternal drug use, a correlation being observed by some (Harper *et al.*, 1977) but not by others (Fricker and Segal, 1978). Overall, there are no clear-cut associations and it is not possible to predict accurately, from a history of the mother's drug use during the antenatal period, which babies will develop withdrawal symptoms or when they will start and to what degree of severity they will develop. This is, no doubt, attributable in part to the already observed fact that there is no way of establishing with any degree of accuracy which drugs are being taken by the mother and in what quantity. Even where methadone is prescribed, it may be taken in association with other drugs or sold to allow purchase of different drugs. Nevertheless, even allowing for these uncertainties, no simple relationship has been shown, in mothers maintained on methadone between methadone levels in the neonate and the severity of withdrawals (Blinick *et al.*, 1975).

Methadone maintenance

Concern for the fetus strongly motivates pregnant women to give up drugs; pregnancy, therefore, affords a unique opportunity to achieve the changes in lifestyle necessary for long-term success in remaining drug free. There are, however, anxieties about the risks to the fetus of detoxification during pregnancy. Detoxification of the mother must inevitably result in detoxification of the fetus; that this is stressful for the fetus is supported by the finding of increased amniotic fluid catecholamines during maternal drug withdrawal (Zuspan *et al.*, 1975). Fetal death during maternal detoxification, widely reported, is held to be a consequence of this stress (Rementeria and Nunag, 1973; Perlmutter, 1974; Fraser, 1976; Vaille, 1985). For this reason, maternal detoxification during pregnancy is considered by many to be unjustifiably hazardous for the fetus and, for many years, methadone maintenance throughout pregnancy has been widely advocated as the management of choice.

Initially, methadone maintenance was considered to have minimal effects on, or risks for, the fetus, and was reported not to result in withdrawal symptoms in the neonate (Wallach, Jerez and Blinick, 1969). Subsequently, however, methadone has been shown to have the same range of effects as heroin and these are often observed to be more severe (Cohen and Neumann, 1973; Zelson, Lee and Casalino, 1973; Perlmutter, 1974). The scope for accurate comparison is limited by lack of data on dosage, but the need for caution has been emphasized with the suggestion that methadone dosage should be carefully controlled at levels as low as possible. Debate on the role of methadone maintenance in pregnancy has been complicated by the advent of HIV infection and the need to reduce high-risk behaviour, in particular the intravenous injection of drugs.

The role of methadone in combating the spread of HIV infection is not the same as its role in the treatment of drug misuse and indeed, there is a degree of conflict between the two. In both situations the benefits of methadone maintenance derive mainly from the fact that the drug is legal, prescribed and oral, the oral route of administration being of obvious importance in trying to limit spread of HIV infection. There is the potential for stabilizing both the dose of drug and the lifestyle of the user and this is an opportunity for establishing contact and thus the provision of routine health care. The disadvantages are that, as noted, methadone is just as harmful to the fetus, just as addictive (if not more so) to mother and baby, and has an increasingly limited role, as the use of heroin is being increasingly replaced by polydrug use with a wide range of drugs in the management of which methadone has little or no relevance. A further disadvantage is that the prescription of maintenance methadone does not prevent the use of other drugs, in particular by the intravenous route. In the treatment of drug misuse in pregnancy the alternative – antenatal detoxification – as already noted, is claimed to be unacceptably hazardous to the fetus. In Glasgow, this has not been our experience of antenatal detoxification, and promising initial results (Hepburn and Forrest, 1988) have been maintained in an increasingly large series of women. To what extent these results are attributable to good contact with the pregnant drug users, allowing more effective provision of antenatal care (already identified as a factor of great importance) is impossible to tell. It is, however, the management requested by many of the women and, regardless of the mechanism of success, these results confirm it is justifiable to include detoxification in the range of options offered to pregnant drug-using women. Methadone maintenance will be appropriate in some cases but it should not be seen as the only possible form of management. It is essential that each woman be assessed individually and her management tailored to meet her particular needs and wishes. There is not one uniform method of management suitable or applicable to all.

Long-term prognosis for children
Good data on long-term effects on children of maternal drug use during pregnancy are virtually non-existent. Such information as exists is sparse, conflicting and often based on small study groups. The absence of accurate drug histories and the presence of other social problems makes firm conclusions difficult (Kaltenbach and Finnegan, 1984). There is, as yet, no definite evidence about long-term effects of the withdrawal syndrome itself. Among the children of drug-using mothers, the possibility of long-term minimal cerebral dysfunction in association with growth retardation has been suggested by a number of reports (Blinick *et al.*, 1976). Physical and behavioural development have been reported to be adversely affected and these abnormalities have been reported to persist even when the children are in foster care (Hill and Tennyson, 1986). Behavioural problems in the absence of developmental abnormalities have also been reported (Wilson, Desmond and Verniaud, 1973). Treatment with methadone maintenance has been claimed to have no long-term effect on babies and to result in normal long-term follow-up (Blinick, Jerez and Wallach, 1973; Newman, 1976). The possible contribution to such outcomes of the socially stabilizing effects of methadone is evident.

Although reports of long-term harm do exist, it is the lack of evidence of significant sequelae that is more compelling (Stimmel and Adamsons, 1976). It is possible that the most deleterious effects may prove to be not a direct consequence of drug use in pregnancy *per se* but, rather, to result from the numerous social problems predisposing to, and arising from, drug misuse. The importance of the therapeutic relationship with staff providing antenatal care (Stauber, Schwerdt and Tylden, 1982), the importance of dealing with other social problems (Rothstein and Gould, 1974) and the importance of offering treatment to the family as a whole (Lief, 1985) cannot be overemphasized.

Other drugs

Other drugs used in Britain at present include cocaine (with the prospect of alkaloidal cocaine or 'crack' in the near future), amphetamines, cannabis and benzodiazepines. There is a much smaller volume of literature on effects on pregnancy of these drugs compared with opiates. From what does exist, the most striking feature is not the differences in effect but rather the similarities, albeit with different underlying mechanisms: thus there is no convincing evidence of teratogenesis but there are increased rates of small babies with increased rates of consequent problems.

Cocaine
Until recently, there was very little information regarding the effects of cocaine use in pregnancy but this is now growing with increasing use of cocaine and particularly 'crack' in the United States. The evidence from such reports is conflicting, however.

Cocaine is a powerful vasoconstrictor, which has been reportedly associated with increased rates of maternal hypertension, spontaneous abortion and placental abruption (Chasnoff et al., 1985; Smith and Deitch, 1987), although the association with maternal hypertension and abruption has not been a constant observation (Chouteau, Namerow and Leppert, 1988). Necrotizing enterocolitis in the newborn has been attributed to ischaemic infarction of the bowel (Telsey, Merrit and Dixon, 1988). There are reports of increased rates of fetal abnormality but on the whole the evidence is poor. Whereas some report increased rates of low birthweight due to both growth retardation and preterm deliveries (Cherukuri et al., 1988; Chouteau, Namerow and Leppert, 1988), others report no such effect (Chasnoff et al., 1985). An increased incidence of small-for-gestational-age babies has been attributed to cocaine's appetite-suppressant effect (Riley, 1987). There is lack of agreement on whether cocaine results in a neonatal withdrawal syndrome and, if so, its precise features. Neonatal behavioural abnormalities have been reported (Chasnoff et al., 1985), although not always to a significant extent (Cherukuri et al., 1988), and others have failed to note any such effects (Madden, Payne and Miller, 1986).

Amphetamines
Although amphetamine use by pregnant women is not uncommon, it is often used together with other drugs, and information regarding its specific effects in pregnancy is sparse. Again, there is evidence both for and against an association with increased rates of fetal abnormality (Little, Snell and Gilstrap, 1988) but, on the whole, it seems unlikely that there is any major relationship. Again the only adverse effect reported is an increase in small babies, both small for gestational age and preterm (Oro and Dixon, 1987), with the suggestion of behavioural alterations.

Marijuana
There is considerable research evidence that marijuana use affects reproductive and sexual function in both men and women (Smith and Deitch, 1987). Marijuana is most commonly taken together with the other drugs, particularly tobacco and alcohol, so that specific effects of its use in pregnancy are difficult to identify. It is variably reported to result in an increase in small babies, both small for gestational age and preterm, to have no effect on fetal growth, to potentiate the effect of alcohol in causing fetal alcohol syndrome, or even to cause a similar syndrome itself, and to result in behavioural abnormalities in neonates (Hill and Tennyson, 1986). Such reports demonstrate that the precise effects of marijuana use upon pregnancy outcome remain uncertain.

Benzodiazepines
Surveys of drug-taking among pregnant women in Edinburgh from 1963 to 1965 and in Glasgow from 1982 to 1984 suggested that 5 per cent and 2 per cent of women, respectively, used anxiolytics/sedatives/hypnotics (Rubin et al., 1986). Despite this low self-reported level of use, growing concern over the level of benzodiazepine dependence in Britain led the Committee on Safety of Medicines (1988) to recommend limitations on their use.

Benzodiazepines are now the most commonly prescribed drugs in Britain (Institute for the Study of Drug Dependence, 1988): 40×10^6 temazepam capsules are prescribed each month in the UK. Although many people become dependent on benzodiazepines as a result of prescribed therapy, many more do not, and considerable quantities of illegally obtained temazepam are now available on the streets.

There is very little information regarding use of temazepam in pregnancy but there is clearly little concern over low-dose use as it is routinely prescribed in many maternity hospitals!

The use of diazepam in very early pregnancy has been implicated as a cause of increased rates of cleft palate, and, in maternal doses >30 mg/day, of a withdrawal syndrome in the baby (Harrison, 1986): this syndrome is described as including neonatal hypotonia, hypothermia, hyperbilirubinaemia, feeding difficulties with poor sucking, and respiratory difficulties with apnoea (Hill and Tennyson, 1986). The effects of benzodiazepine use on the fetus have not, however, been studied or documented to any great extent. The effects of use at therapeutic levels are clearly not comparable with the effects of illicit street use at dosage levels several hundred times the therapeutic dose. It is information regarding use at these higher levels that is required and, given the widespread use of benzodiazepines in Britain today, further study is clearly necessary.

A greater awareness of any demonstrable risks to mother and baby, together with a more responsible attitude to prescribing, will help, but not solve, the problem of illicit use.

Smoking in pregnancy

Although the number of people who smoke is decreasing, the relative proportion of smokers who are women is increasing, and particularly women in the lower socio-economic groups. It has been reported that 25–35 per cent of pregnant women smoke throughout pregnancy, of whom one-quarter smoke >20 cigarettes per day (Condon, 1986). There is also a strong association between smoking and drinking. In one series, however, it was reported that 100 per cent of women who drank alcohol made a successful attempt to reduce their alcohol consumption during pregnancy; on the other hand, of the women who smoked, only 57 per cent successfully reduced their habit whereas 40 per cent tried but failed (Condon and Hilton, 1988). Although many of the drinkers would not have a problem, the vast majority of the smokers would be dependent on a drug, the addictive power of which is well known. That so many succeeded in reducing their habit by themselves – a trend consistently observed (Rubin et al., 1986; Johnson, McCarter and Ferencz, 1987; Kleinman and Kopstein, 1987) – emphasizes the unique opportunity for behavioural modification that pregnancy affords.

Effects on early pregnancy

As with the drugs of abuse already discussed, tobacco is reported to affect many different stages of reproduction. Although there are reports to the contrary (De Mouzon, Spira and Schwartz, 1988), there is a considerable volume of data suggesting an association between smoking and reduced female fertility, with a probable causal relationship (Stillman, Rosenberg and Sachs, 1986) and dose-related response. It has been suggested that some of the effects occur only in heavier smokers (Howe et al., 1985). It seems likely that these adverse effects operate throughout the entire process of reproduction and may include an effect on male fertility (Lincoln, 1986). Increased rates of spontaneous abortion of chromosomally normal fetuses have been reported, but no significant increase in the incidence of fetal malformations (King and Fabro, 1983; Lincoln, 1986; Stillman, Rosenberg and Sachs,

1986). It has been suggested that fetuses with trisomy 21 are more susceptible to the harmful effects of cigarette smoking, resulting in a disproportionately large early pregnancy loss of these fetuses in smokers. This, in turn, is held to be the explanation for the reduced incidence of live Down's syndrome births among smokers (Hook and Cross, 1984; Shiono, Klebanoff and Berendes, 1986). A racial difference with a more marked reduction in Black women has been attributed to a greater vulnerability to cigarette smoke of trisomy fetuses in such women (Hook and Cross, 1988). It has been reported that maternal serum alphafetoprotein (MSAFP) levels are higher in smokers than in non-smokers (Thomsen et al., 1983), the explanation given being that smoking results in increased permeability of the placental barrier, with leakage of the AFP molecule to the maternal circulation. Although there was obviously no suggestion of an increased incidence of neural tube defects, confirmation of these higher levels would be of significance in the interpretation of MSAFP measurements; a subsequent study has failed to confirm these findings (Haddow et al., 1984).

Effects on later pregnancy

Cigarette smoking produces both acute and chronic effects on mother and fetus and it has been suggested that the acute effects on the woman are no different, whether or not she is pregnant. Despite the opportunities for studying the effects of cigarette smoking upon the mother and fetus, and the technological advances to assist in doing so, there remains a lack of consensus and considerable uncertainty about the precise mechanisms by which adverse effects on the fetus are produced. There are a number of possibilities, however. Nicotine is a vasoconstrictor that stimulates the adrenergic system and crosses the placenta easily; there are thus a number of ways in which it could produce haemodynamic changes in mother and fetus. Carbon monoxide, produced during smoking, binds to haemoglobin, producing high levels of carboxy-haemoglobin in both maternal and fetal blood, with consequent reduction in the ability to transport oxygen resulting in fetal hypoxia. There are also a number of other products of cigarette smoking that could have a direct toxic effect.

Smoking produces a rise in maternal heart rate and blood pressure, shortly followed by a rise in fetal heart rate demonstrated in most (Sontag and Wallace, 1935; Quigley et al., 1979; Kelly, Mathews and O'Conor, 1984; Morrow, Ritchie and Bull, 1988) but not all (Lehtovirta et al., 1983) studies, with a decrease in fetal heart rate baseline variability and fetal movements (Kelly, Mathews and O'Conor, 1984). It has been suggested that nicotine, by causing vasoconstriction, results in reduced uterine perfusion (Quigley et al., 1979), and decreased placental intervillous blood flow has been observed during cigarette smoking (Lehtovirta et al., 1983). These effects on the uteroplacental blood flow have been attributed to the effects of nicotine on the maternal circulation of the placenta. Other studies have shown no significant change in uterine-artery vascular resistance but changes suggestive of a direct increase in the vascular resistance of the placenta from the fetal side which might affect placental oxygen exchange. The fetoplacental circulatory changes were similar to those seen in intrauterine growth retardation (Morrow, Ritchie and Bull, 1988).

Whatever the acute haemodynamic effects of maternal smoking on the fetus, there is no doubt that regular smoking by the mother leads to chronic effects on placental function which adversely affect the fetus. On histological examination of the placentae of smokers, the lesions seen are characteristic of underperfusion, probably of a periodic rather than a continuous nature (Naeye, 1978).

Among smokers there is evidence of premature placental calcification, taken to indicate premature ageing of the placenta and suggested to have a relationship with intrauterine growth retardation (Brown *et al.*, 1988). Although this study showed an increase in placental calcification in smokers, it failed to show an increased incidence of small-for-gestational-age babies.

Babies of smokers

Among the babies of women who smoke there are reports of increased perinatal mortality and morbidity (Butler and Bonham, 1963; US Department of Health and Human Services, 1983), although an increased death rate is not invariably reported (Underwood *et al.*, 1967). There is an adverse effect on fetal growth (Meyer, Jonas and Tonascia, 1976), with smoking causing a dose-related reduction in birthweight (Kline, Stein and Hutzler, 1987); there is a suggestion that this effect is greater with increasing maternal age (Cnattingius *et al.*, 1985). This reduction in birthweight is variously reported to be increased when maternal weight gain is low (Davies *et al.*, 1976) and to be independent of maternal dietary intake and nutritional status (Naeye, 1981). Maternal weight gain has been reported to be the same in smokers and non-smokers (Meyer, 1978); it has also been claimed that poor maternal weight gain in the third trimester, if it occurs, is likely to be an effect, not a cause, of poor fetal growth (Stillman, Rosenberg and Sachs, 1986).

Although smoking is closely associated with a number of adverse social factors, it has been claimed that the effects of maternal smoking on fetal weight are independent, not only of maternal body size but also of parity, socioeconomic status and the amount of antenatal care provided (as judged by the number of antenatal visits) (Hoff *et al.*, 1986). It has been shown that the effect of smoking on birthweight will be reduced if the woman stops smoking. The earlier in pregnancy she stops smoking, the greater the benefit, and it has been suggested that women who stop smoking before 16 weeks' gestation have babies with birthweights similar to those of babies of non-smokers (MacArthur and Knox, 1988).

There is lack of agreement on the contribution of prematurity to the increased rate of low birthweight. Increased rates of premature deliveries (Meyer, Jonas and Tonascia, 1976; Pirani, 1978; US Department of Health and Human Services, 1983) and premature rupture of membranes (PROM) are reported (Underwood *et al.*, 1967), but other studies suggest that there is no increase in preterm deliveries (Lowe, 1959) and that the increase in low birthweight is entirely due to inappropriately grown babies. However, in addition to an increased incidence of PROM, there are reports of higher rates of antepartum haemorrhage due to placenta praevia, abruptio placentae and bleeding with no apparent cause, all of which might lead to increased rates of preterm delivery (US Department of Health and Human Services, 1983).

Not surprisingly, as smoking constitutes a state of chronic stress for the fetus, there is a decreased incidence of respiratory distress syndrome (Curet *et al.*, 1983). The incidence of pregnancy-induced hypertension is also reduced (Murphy *et al.*, 1980) but when it does occur, the prognosis for the fetus is much worse (King and Fabro, 1983).

Long-term prognosis for children

There is considerable debate on whether smoking by a woman during pregnancy has long-term effects on the development, physical or mental, of her child. Smoking is associated with many other adverse social factors including drinking, low socio-economic status, poverty and poor diet, all of which contribute to long-term disadvantage for a child. It is, consequently, very difficult to assess how much of any effect on the development of children is attributable solely to maternal smoking.

There are reports that although smoking results in reduced birthweight, its effect on infant size is not long term and, in fact, is no longer evident by the age of 8 months (Barr *et al.*, 1984). Other studies have suggested that whereas the growth of such children in terms of weight and head circumference does catch up to some extent during the first year of life, there remains a permanent deficit (Russell, Taylor and Law, 1968): there is evidence to suggest a long-term effect not only on growth but also on development (Butler and Goldstein, 1973) with some delay still apparent at 10 years of age. Intellectual impairment may be accompanied by behavioural abnormalities including hyperactivity (Naeye and Peters, 1984).

It appears that children of women who smoke have a higher incidence of lower respiratory tract illness but it is also reported that this may be due, not so much to passive smoking after birth, but rather to some effect of smoking during pregnancy (Taylor and Wadsworth, 1987). A higher incidence of sudden infant death syndrome (SIDS) has been reported in a number of studies (King and Fabro, 1983). There have been suggestions of an increased risk of childhood malignancy in the children of smokers (Stjernfeld *et al.*, 1986) and finally, completing the circle, a suggestion – unsubstantiated – of increased infertility among the offspring of smoking women (Baird and Wilcox, 1986).

Alcohol consumption in pregnancy

There has long been recognition of the potential risk to the fetus of maternal drinking in pregnancy: a spectrum of abnormalities in the babies of women who drank was described in 1968 (Lemoine *et al.*, 1968) and the term 'fetal alcohol syndrome' was introduced in 1973 (Jones and Smith, 1973). Many women drink before and during pregnancy but, of these, only a few drink heavily or have a drinking habit that constitutes a problem. Although the confirmation of pregnancy may motivate many women to reduce their alcohol intake or to stop drinking completely, many will be drinking before and around the time of conception, a period held by some to be of critical importance (Hanson, Streissguth and Smith, 1978). There is, however, considerable debate about the dangers of drinking at different times relative to pregnancy, about the forms of alcohol which are most harmful, about the importance of dose, frequency and pattern of drinking, and about the effect of changing drinking habits at different stages of the pregnancy.

Effects on conception and early pregnancy

High levels of alcohol consumption, acute and chronic, affect reproductive endocrinology and sexual function in men. There is possibly an effect, to a lesser extent, on reproductive endocrinology in women, with menstrual disorders and infertility reported to occur (Smith and Asch, 1987), but there is no evidence of any significant effect with moderate levels of consumption.

It has been reported that alcohol consumption in pregnancy results in increased rates of spontaneous abortion. In one study there was an increased miscarriage rate at a drinking level at or above one ounce of absolute alcohol twice a week (Kline *et al.*, 1980); another (Harlap and Shiono, 1980) reported an increased rate of second-trimester spontaneous abortions among women who drank 1–2 drinks per day compared with those who drank less. These increased rates, however, are an inconsistent finding (Grisso *et al.*, 1984).

Effects on later pregnancy

Some studies have suggested an increased incidence of placental abruption and consequently of stillbirths (Marbury *et al.*, 1983), but there is no conclusive evidence of increased death rates, and certainly not in women with only moderate levels of alcohol consumption.

Alcohol is known to have a suppressant effect on uterine contractility and because of this tocolytic action has, in fact, been used in the past in the treatment of preterm labour. In association with maternal drinking there have been reported increased rates of both preterm and post-term delivery (Ouellette *et al.*, 1977) but an effect on gestational length is not consistently observed (Mills *et al.*, 1984). What is a consistent finding, however, is an increased rate of low birthweight, particularly due to small-for-gestational-age babies. Other findings are reduced placental weights, infections and meconium staining of the liquor (Sokal, Miller and Reed, 1980). In addition to the effect on its growth, the fetus may exhibit facial and other anomalies as well as abnormalities of neurological development; these effects in combination constitute the much publicized 'fetal alcohol syndrome' (Jones and Smith, 1973).

Effect on the fetus

Fetal alcohol syndrome (FAS)
This 'syndrome', which was first given the title in 1973, has in recent years been the centre of much attention and debate. Criteria for diagnosis have been described by the Fetal Alcohol Study Group and many variations of these have been published. Essentially these babies have reduced growth pre- and/or postnatally, neurological abnormalities, and facial and other anomalies. It has been suggested that this combination of defects is unique to alcohol, with the claim that it has never been seen in a child whose mother is not an alcoholic (Hill and Tennyson, 1986): although a similar picture may be produced by other toxins, that attributable to alcohol can, it is said, be distinguished (Hadi, Hill and Castillo, 1987). Conversely, there is a suggestion that this syndrome is not specifically caused by alcohol, that it is seen in other situations and is thus a non-specific effect that may be produced by the action of any of a number of possible agents acting at a critical stage in pregnancy (Zuckerman and Hingson, 1986).

The growth retardation of FAS as described by Jones and Smith (1973) affects all parameters of growth – weight, length and head circumference – and forms a continuum extending from the antenatal period into early life. It is reported that such children show no postnatal catch-up in growth, and they are often described as exhibiting a failure to thrive. Endocrine studies are normal, and a reduction in fetal cell numbers as a toxic effect of antenatal alcohol consumption has been postulated as a cause for the growth retardation (Hadi, Hill and Castillo, 1987).

The reduced head circumference, which may amount to microcephaly, must inevitably be accompanied by abnormal brain growth and development. Thus, although neurological abnormalities including irritability, disturbed sleeping, hypertonicity and poor sucking may be seen in the neonatal period and later (Hanson, Streissguth and Smith, 1978), with evidence of developmental delay, the most important effect of central nervous system dysfunction is mental retardation.

The facial abnormalities vary but include shortened palpebral fissures, possibly related to reduced growth of the eyes, an underdeveloped or absent philtrum, a thin upper lip and/or hypoplastic maxilla resulting in a broad, flat mid-face. FAS as described, however, is rare, even in comparison with the number of women who drink heavily in pregnancy. The incidence of FAS has been reported to be higher in older mothers and lower socioeconomic groups (Streissguth, 1978), although there is no doubt that it is also seen in middle class women (Little, 1977). Nevertheless, these and other factors such as smoking and the use of other drugs, as well as variations in susceptibility, must be of importance in determining the incidence of FAS.

Reduced fetal growth

The combination of features covered by the term FAS is, as already noted, very rare; a much more commonly described effect associated with alcohol consumption during pregnancy is growth retardation, which may be seen in the absence of other abnormalities. Whereas FAS is associated only with very heavy maternal drinking, growth retardation is also attributed to the effects of lower, 'moderate' levels of consumption. There is, however, considerable debate about the risks of different levels of intake and what, if any, is the safe upper limit. There is also uncertainty about the risks of drinking at different stages of pregnancy and about the effects on birthweight of altering drinking habits before or during pregnancy.

Patterns and levels of drinking

The effect on birthweight of moderate drinking in pregnancy is uncertain: there are a number of studies reporting reduction in fetal weight with levels of alcohol consumption of 1–2 drinks per day (Mills *et al.*, 1984), whereas others suggest no effect with 30 g of ethanol per week (Halmesmäki, Raivio and Ylikorkala, 1987). A doubling of the low birthweight rate was noted with levels of 100 g/week compared with 50 g/week (Wright *et al.*, 1983), although another study showed no effect with consumption of <100 g/week (Sulaiman *et al.*, 1988). Little (1977) noted an effect on birthweight with consumption of 1 ounce of absolute alcohol per day, the effect being present with drinking before pregnancy, greater with drinking in late pregnancy, but absent with drinking in early and mid-pregnancy. Marbury *et al.* (1983) showed no association between alcohol consumption and reduction in birthweight.

These and many other studies have compared the effects of different levels of alcohol consumption in an attempt to establish a safe level of drinking in relation to pregnancy. Such an exercise, however, is extremely difficult because of the difficulties in establishing alcohol intake accurately. Such data are usually obtained retrospectively, so that inaccuracies due to the already-discussed under-reporting are compounded by faulty recall. The contributory effect of other variables may also account for the lack of consensus. The *General Household Survey* (Office of Population Censuses and Surveys, 1984) reported increased rates of abstinence and low consumption among women whose partners are in the lower socioeconomic groups. Wright *et al.* (1983) reported increased numbers of heavy drinkers in social classes I and II. Although another British study of pregnant women (Heller *et al.*, 1988) confirmed that drinking rates were higher in higher socioeconomic groups, it also showed that among heavy drinkers there was a small group of socially disadvantaged women who were also likely to be smokers. Heavy drinking and smoking are associated and are reported to have both separate and additive effects on fetal growth (Little, 1977; Wright *et al.*, 1983).

The various studies and their methodological problems are reviewed by Zucker-man and Hingson (1986). Reduction of heavy drinking (Ouellette *et al.*, 1977) in mid-pregnancy, has been suggested to improve fetal growth (Rosett *et al.*, 1983). Conversely, an increased rate of small-for-gestational-age babies has been noted among alcoholic mothers who abstained during pregnancy (Little *et al.*, 1980). There is uncertainty regarding whether 'binge' drinking is more or less harmful than regular drinking with a lower maximum maternal blood level of alcohol (Ouellette *et al.*, 1977). There have been suggestions that beer may be more harmful to the baby (Kaminski *et al.*, 1981; Kline, Stein and Hutzler, 1987; Sulaiman *et al.*, 1988) but the evidence is conflicting (Marbury *et al.*, 1983) and the question remains unresolved.

Mechanism of fetal damage

The precise mechanism by which alcohol affects fetal growth and/or development is unknown: it may be a direct toxic effect or an effect mediated by the alcohol metabolite acetaldehyde (Veghely and Osztovics, 1978). There is an increased rate of zinc excretion in association with alcohol consumption and consequently, lowered serum zinc levels are seen; a possible aetiological link with reduced birthweight due to drinking has been considered (King and Fabro, 1983; Zuckerman and Hingson, 1986).

Long-term prognosis

The reduced size associated with alcohol consumption during pregnancy is reported to persist into childhood. Follow-up of children to the age of 8 months showed that, unlike the growth retardation due to cigarette smoking, which is, to some extent, compensated for by increased postnatal growth, that due to alcohol persists and therefore becomes, with time, relatively more significant than that attributable to smoking (Barr *et al.*, 1984). These children also showed lower mental and motor development (Streissguth *et al.*, 1980).

Overall risk

There seems little doubt that high levels of maternal drinking during pregnancy are harmful to the fetus. The combination of effects known as the 'fetal alcohol syn-drome' may be seen in some of these infants, although many babies of mothers who drink heavily are perfectly normal. Whether this 'syndrome' is specific to alcohol or represents a more general toxic effect is uncertain. What is even more uncertain is the effect on the fetus of 'moderate' levels of alcohol consumption. The definition of 'moderate', the problems in obtaining an accurate drinking history and the presence of numerous confounding factors no doubt contribute to the varying results of the numerous studies carried out: thus, such studies have produced conflicting evidence on the effects of dosage and timing of drinking and of changing drinking habits before or during pregnancy.

Reactions to such uncertainty vary. The weight of evidence currently suggests that 'moderate' or 'social' levels of consumption do not harm the fetus. There are however reports that even low levels of drinking may carry some risk. The US

Surgeon General (1981) recommended total abstinence during pregnancy as did the Royal College of Psychiatrists (1982). The Scientific Advisory Committee on Consumption of Alcohol in Pregnancy (Royal College of Obstetricians and Gynaecologists, 1985) suggested that, as alcohol is potentially damaging to the developing fetus, it is advisable for women to stop drinking during pregnancy; it pointed out, however, the lack of evidence that the occasional drink is dangerous. In the absence of absolute proof, a recommendation of total abstinence gives the only guarantee of safety; nevertheless, as indicated by the RCOG, this is a general recommendation and for the individual it is probably reasonable to take the view that alcohol consumption in pregnancy, provided that it is kept at low levels, does not constitute an unacceptable risk for the fetus. Many women will already have drunk alcohol around the time of conception and during early pregnancy before the pregnancy is confirmed; by then, advice regarding abstinence at that time will be not only irrelevant but potentially harmful. Such equivocal data should be interpreted sensibly to maintain a balance between giving advice to ensure optimum health of the fetus and avoiding causing unnecessary and unhelpful anxiety and feelings of guilt in the mother.

Summary

Drugs, alcohol and tobacco all have the potential for a wide range of harmful effects on the whole process of reproduction and, in particular, on the growth and development of the unborn baby. The precise effects on the baby of each of the three types of substance have not yet been established. Many of the effects attributed to them are inconsistently reported and non-specific, with the exception of that group of features collectively referred to as the 'fetal alcohol syndrome'. That too, however, may be not a specific effect of alcohol but simply another non-specific effect of an insult to fetal development at a particular stage of pregnancy. One consistently observed feature, however, is that all three, by whatever mechanism, may result in an increased incidence of low birthweight and may be associated with increased fetal morbidity and mortality; these effects would appear to be dose related.

All three types of substance have addictive properties and in the case of all three there is a wide spectrum of level of use. At the lower end of the spectrum, the effects on the pregnancy may be minimal and use can be controlled by the individual; at the other end of the spectrum the fetus may suffer more severe harm and addiction can be a serious problem. Although considerable efforts have been devoted to the study of the harmful effects on the pregnancy and the mechanisms by which these are produced, considerably less effort has been directed towards the study of ways of helping pregnant women to stop using these substances. The attitude is prevalent that the responsibility of those caring for pregnant women is simply to provide the information that these substances can be harmful and that responsibility for behavioural change thereafter lies entirely with the women. There is clearly a need for provision of such information, because many women are apparently ignorant of either the possible dangers of smoking and drinking or the levels of consumption associated with such risks. Ignorance or misunderstanding were reported in a number of studies to be higher among those who smoked or drank substantial amounts of alcohol (Little et al., 1981; Ashford, Gerlis and Johnson, 1986; Buist and Yu, 1987; McKnight and Merrett, 1987). Although it is possible that these women continued to smoke and drink because they were unaware of the dangers, it is also possible that they received as much information as the abstainers, but did not believe it, or subconsciously did not want to acknowledge it.

The attitude that the provision of information should be sufficient is inappropriate for several reasons. First, it ignores the importance of the addictive power of these substances. Some writers express surprise that pregnant women continue to smoke, drink or use drugs, despite knowledge of the possible dangers to the fetus; what is perhaps more surprising is that this knowledge produces a consistent response by the women, albeit with varying degrees of success, in reducing or stopping their use of these substances (Streissguth et al., 1983; Fried, Barnes and Drake, 1985; Johnson, McCarter and Ferencz, 1987). Unfortunately, these successes are often not maintained post partum. This appears particularly to be the case where addiction is greater, as in cigarette smoking and heavy alcohol consumption compared with light drinking. Thus, pregnancy produces the impetus for reducing consumption or stopping altogether, but other measures are necessary for long-term success.

Second, provision of information alone is ineffective in persuading pregnant women to stop smoking, drinking or using drugs. Whether the information is given verbally alone, or with the additional provision of written information in the form of a booklet that can be read later, makes little or no difference (Subcommittee of the Research Committee of the British Thoracic Society, 1983; Campbell, Hansford and Prescott, 1986). Self-help programmes and teaching of behavioural skills appear to improve success rates (Nowicki et al., 1984; Windsor et al., 1985; Lilley and Forster, 1986) but these remain disappointingly low.

The provision of information alone is also inadequate because it fails to recognize the importance of social factors, including level of education, expectations of health and living standards, lifestyle and cultural factors, as well as socioeconomic status. The correlation between success in giving up smoking during pregnancy and length of women's education has been noted (Kleinman and Kopstein, 1987); the level of education will also be relevant because of its social implications. It has been suggested that greater degrees of maternal attachment to the fetus are associated with greater success in giving up drinking during pregnancy but the absence of such a correlation with stopping smoking is attributed to the overriding addictive power of smoking (Condon and Hilton, 1988). It has been suggested that the degree of 'pregnancy wantedness' might influence such maternal behaviour; however, although higher rates of giving up smoking have been reported where the pregnancy is planned, not surprisingly, this effect is very small (Weller, Eberstein and Bailey, 1987). For long-term success in giving up smoking, drinking and drugs, a change in lifestyle is necessary and, in a follow-up of heroin addicts, those who achieved and sustained abstinence showed the greatest changes in lifestyle (Oppenheimer, Stimson and Thorley, 1979).

Use of cigarettes and/or drugs has a strong association with socioeconomic deprivation. Although this is less so with alcohol consumption, it may be relevant for a small group of women who drink heavily. Social problems are not only of great importance in the use of addictive substances, but may be central to the whole problem. Any attempt to deal with problems of addiction must therefore address these social issues if it is to have any hope of success. Not only must attention be given to all of the woman's problems, but it is important to consider her not in isolation, but as part of a family unit, the whole of which requires treatment and help (Lief, 1985).

The delivery of such a service is of great importance. Lack of self-confidence and self-esteem are often underlying problems in the use of addictive substances. To be successful in changing their behaviour, women must have confidence in their ability to succeed (Godin and Lepage, 1988) and it is vital that help is provided in a supportive and non-judgemental way.

Objectives should be realistic: although total abstinence is obviously the ideal, it will often be unattainable. The knowledge that this is likely to be so may discourage many women, particularly if they perceive an attitude among staff that total abstinence is the only acceptable option; any reduction in levels of use is worth while, however, and such lesser degrees of success should be encouraged and viewed positively, particularly when accompanied by other measures that improve social stability.

The actual information that is given to women is important. Use of the concept of relative risk is often unhelpful. Thus for example, although the Froggatt Report (Independent Scientific Committee on Smoking and Health, 1988) observed a 28 per cent increase in perinatal mortality rates (and thus a much higher relative risk to the fetus) in association with smoking, the absolute risk to the individual baby is still very low. Information must, therefore, be realistic if it is not to be ignored, either because it is too frightening or makes the problem appear insurmountable or because it appears to be simply untrue. From their own observations the women are aware of the low absolute risk to the individual and will disregard any unduly alarmist information or advice.

Thus, in summary, there is no doubt that use of drugs, tobacco and alcohol by pregnant women can be harmful to the fetus. Although it is important to establish precisely the nature and mechanism of such effects, it is, perhaps, of even greater importance to study ways of helping women to stop using such substances.

Pregnancy produces a unique stimulus and a powerful motivation for change. Its effect in producing behaviour modification is impressive and such an opportunity for intervention should not be wasted. The information given to women, and the objectives of any management, must be realistic. Women should be viewed in the wider family context and social issues addressed; social problems often underlie, and predispose to, the use of addictive substances. The problem is not simply one of stopping the use of these substances but of maintaining abstinence in the long term. This in turn requires changes in lifestyle. The responsibility for such change does not lie solely with the women but also with those involved in the provision of health care and social support to pregnant women.

As with many other health care issues, the use of drugs, tobacco and alcohol is not confined to pregnancy. The problem has much wider relevance and management should ideally be directed more towards prevention. Failing this, pregnancy affords a unique opportunity for intervention with the possibility of much longer-term benefit.

References

Ashford, A, Gerlis, R and Johnson, P (1986) Smoking in pregnancy: is the message getting through? *Journal of the Royal College of General Practitioners*, **36**, 494–495

Bai, J, Greenwald, E, Caterini, H and Kaminetzky, H (1974) Drug-related menstrual aberrations. *Obstetrics and Gynecology*, **44**, 713–719

Baird, DD and Wilcox, AJ (1986) Future fertility after perinatal exposure to cigarette smoke. *Fertility and Sterility*, **46**, 368–371

Barr, HM, Streissguth, AP, Martin, DC and Herman, CS (1984) Infant size at eight months of age; relationship to maternal use of alcohol, nicotine and caffeine during pregnancy. *Pediatrics*, **74**, 336–341

Blinick, G, Jerez, E and Wallach, RC (1973) Methadone maintenance, pregnancy and progeny. *Journal of the American Medical Association*, **225**, 477–479

Blinick, G, Inturrisi, CE, Jerez, E and Wallach, RC (1975) Methadone assays in pregnant women and progeny. *American Journal of Obstetrics and Gynecology*, **121**, 617–621

Blinick, G, Wallach, RC, Jerez, E and Ackerman, BD (1976) Drug addiction in pregnancy and the neonate. *American Journal of Obstetrics and Gynecology*, **125**, 135–142

Bolton, PJ (1987) Drugs of abuse. In *Drugs and Pregnancy. Human Teratogenesis and Related Problems* (edited by DF Hawkins) pp. 180–210. Edinburgh: Churchill Livingstone

Brown, HL, Miller, JM, Khawli, O and Gabert, HA (1988) Premature placental calcification in maternal cigarette smokers. *Obstetrics and Gynecology*, **71**, 914–917

Buist, A and Yu, D (1987) Smoking and pregnancy: awareness, attitudes and habit changes. *Health Bulletin*, **45/4 July**, 179–184

Butler, NR and Bonham, DG (1963) *Perinatal Mortality: The First Report of the 1958 British Perinatal Mortality Survey*. Edinburgh: E and S Livingstone

Butler, NR and Goldstein, H (1973) Smoking in pregnancy and subsequent child development. *British Medical Journal*, **4**, 573–575

Campbell, IA (1988) Stopping patients smoking. *British Journal of Diseases of the Chest*, **82**, 9–15

Campbell, IA, Hansford, M and Prescott, RJ (1986) Effect of a 'stop smoking' booklet on smokers attending for chest radiography: a controlled study. *Thorax*, **41**, 369–371

Chasnoff, IJ, Burns, WJ, Schnoll, SH and Burns, KA (1985) Cocaine use in pregnancy. *New England Journal of Medicine*, **313**, 666–669

Cherukuri, R, Minkoff, H, Feldman, J *et al.* (1988) A cohort study of alkaloidal cocaine ('crack') in pregnancy. *Obstetrics and Gynecology*, **72**, 147–151

Chouteau, M, Namerow, PB and Leppert, P (1988) The effect of cocaine abuse on birthweight and gestational age. *Obstetrics and Gynecology*, **72**, 351–354

Cnattingius, S, Axelsson, O, Eklund, G and Lindmark, G (1985) Smoking, maternal age and fetal growth. *Obstetrics and Gynecology*, **66**, 449–452

Cohen, SN and Neumann, LL (1973) Methadone maintenance during pregnancy. *American Journal of Diseases of Children*, **126**, 445–446

Committee on Safety of Medicines (1988) *Current Problems, No. 21*

Condon, JT (1986) The spectrum of fetal abuse in pregnant women. *Journal of Nervous and Mental Disease*, **174**, 509–516

Condon, JT and Hilton, CA (1988) A comparison of smoking and drinking behaviours in pregnant women: who abstains and why. *Medical Journal of Australia*, **148**, 381–385

Connaughton, JF, Reeser, D, Schut, J and Finnegan, LP (1977) Perinatal addiction: outcome and management. *American Journal of Obstetrics and Gynecology*, **129**, 679–686

Curet, LB, Rao, AV, Zachman, RD *et al.* (1983) Maternal smoking and respiratory distress syndrome. *American Journal of Obstetrics and Gynecology*, **147**, 446–450

Davies, DP, Gray, OP, Ellwood, PC and Abernathy, M (1976) Cigarette smoking in pregnancy: association with maternal weight gain and fetal growth. *Lancet*, **i**, 385–387

De Mouzon, J, Spira, A and Schwartz, D (1988) A prospective study of the relation between smoking and fertility. *International Journal of Epidemiology*, **17**, 378–384

Deren, S (1986) Children of substance abusers: a review of the literature. *Journal of Substance Abuse Treatment*, **3**, 77–94

Finnegan, LP (1982) Outcome of children born to women dependent on narcotics. In *The Effects of Maternal Alcohol and Drug Abuse on the New Born* (edited by B Stimmel) pp. 55–102. New York: Haworth Press

Fraser, AC (1976) Drug addiction in pregnancy. *Lancet*, **ii**, 896–899

Fricker, HS and Segal, S (1978) Narcotic addiction, pregnancy and the newborn. *American Journal of Diseases of Children*, **123**, 360–366

Fried, PA, Barnes, MV and Drake, ER (1985) Soft drug use after pregnancy compared to use before and during pregnancy. *American Journal of Obstetrics and Gynecology*, **151**, 787–792

Glass, L, Rajegowda, BK and Evans, HE (1971) Absence of respiratory distress syndrome in premature infants of heroin addicted mothers. *Lancet*, **ii**, 685–686

Gluck, L and Kulovich, MV (1973) Lecithin/sphingomyelin ratios in amniotic fluid in normal and abnormal pregnancy. *American Journal of Obstetrics and Gynecology*, **115**, 539–546

Goddard, E (1986) *Drinking and Attitudes to Licensing in Scotland*. Edinburgh: HMSO

Godin, G and Lepage, L (1988) Understanding the intentions of pregnant nullipara to not smoke cigarettes after childbirth. *Journal of Drug Education*, **18**, 115–124

Grisso, JA, Roman, E, Inskip, H *et al.* (1984) Alcohol consumption and outcome of pregnancy. *Journal of Epidemiology and Community Health*, **38**, 232–235

Haddow, JE, Palomaki, G, Kloza, EM *et al.* (1984) Does smoking influence serum alpha-fetoprotein levels in mid trimester pregnancies? *British Journal of Obstetrics and Gynaecology*, **91**, 1188–1191

Hadi, HA, Hill, JA and Castillo, RA (1987) Alcohol and reproductive function: a review. *Obstetrical and Gynecological Survey*, **42**, 69–74

Halmesmäki, E, Raivio, KO and Ylikorkala, AO (1987) Patterns of alcohol consumption during pregnancy. *Obstetrics and Gynecology*, **69**, 594–597

Hanson, JW, Streissguth, AP and Smith, DW (1978) The effects of moderate alcohol consumption during pregnancy on fetal growth and morphogenesis. *Journal of Pediatrics*, **92**, 457–460

Harlap, S and Shiono, PH (1980) Alcohol, smoking and incidence of spontaneous abortions in the first and second trimester. *Lancet*, **ii**, 173–176

Harper, RG, Solish, GI, Purow, HM *et al.* (1974) The effect of a methadone treatment program upon pregnant heroin addicts and their newborn infants. *Pediatrics*, **54**, 300–305

Harper, RG, Solish, G, Feingold, E *et al.* (1977) Maternal ingested methadone, body fluid methadone and the neonatal withdrawal syndrome. *American Journal of Obstetrics and Gynecology*, **129**, 417–424

Harrison, R (1986) The use of non essential drugs, alcohol and cigarettes during pregnancy. *Irish Medical Journal*, **79**, 338–341

Heller, J, Anderson, HR, Bland, JM *et al.* (1988) Alcohol in pregnancy: Patterns and associations with socioeconomic, psychological and behavioural factors. *British Journal of Addiction*, **83**, 541–551

Hepburn, M and Forrest, CA (1988) Does infection with HIV affect the outcome of pregnancy? *British Medical Journal*, **296**, 934

Hill, RM and Tennyson, LM (1986) Maternal drug therapy: effect on fetal and neonatal growth and neurobehaviour. *Neurotoxicology*, **7**, 121–140

Hoff, C, Wertelecki, W, Blackburn, WR *et al.* (1986) Trend associations of smoking with maternal fetal and neonatal morbidity. *Obstetrics and Gynecology*, **68**, 317–320

Hook, EB and Cross, PK (1984) Cigarette smoking and Down's syndrome. *American Journal of Human Genetics*, **37**, 1216–1224

Hook, EB and Cross, PK (1988) Maternal cigarette smoking, Down's syndrome in live births and infant race. *American Journal of Human Genetics*, **42**, 482–489

Howe, G, Westhoff, C, Vessey, M and Yeates, D (1985) Effects of age, cigarette smoking and other factors on fertility: findings in a large prospective study. *British Medical Journal*, **290**, 1697–1700

Independent Scientific Committee on Smoking and Health (1988) Chairman Sir Peter Froggatt. *Report*. London: HMSO

Institute for the Study of Drug Dependence (1988) *Drug Abuse Briefing*, 3rd edn, **p. 7**. London: ISDD

Johnson, SF, McCarter, RJ and Ferencz, C (1987) Changes in alcohol, cigarette and recreational drug use during pregnancy – implications for interventions. *American Journal of Epidemiology*, **126**, 695–702

Jones, KL and Smith, DW (1973) Recognition of the fetal alcohol syndrome in early infancy. *Lancet*, **ii**, 999–1001

Kaltenbach, K and Finnegan, LP (1984) Developmental outcome of children born to methadone maintained women: a review of longitudinal studies. *Neurobehavioural Toxicology and Teratology*, **6**, 271–275

Kaminski, M, Franc, M, Le Bouvier, M *et al.* (1981) Moderate alcohol use and pregnancy outcome. *Neurobehavioural Toxicology and Teratology*, **3**, 173–181

Kelly, J, Mathews, KA and O'Conor, M (1984) Smoking in pregnancy: effects on mother and fetus. *British Journal of Obstetrics and Gynaecology*, **91**, 111–117

King, JC and Fabro, S (1983) Alcohol consumption and cigarette smoking. Effect on pregnancy. *Clinical Obstetrics and Gynecology*, **26**, 437–448

Kleinman, JC and Kopstein, A (1987) Smoking during pregnancy 1967–80. *American Journal of Public Health*, **77**, 823–825

Klenka, HM (1986) Babies born in a district general hospital to mothers taking heroin. *British Medical Journal*, **293**, 745–746

Kline, J, Stein, Z and Hutzler, M (1987) Cigarettes, alcohol and marijuana: varying associations with birthweight. *International Journal of Epidemiology*, **16**, 44–51

Kline, J, Stein, Z, Shrout, P *et al.* (1980) Drinking during pregnancy and spontaneous abortion. *Lancet*, **ii**, 176–180

Lehtovirta, P, Forss, M, Kariniemi, V and Rauramo, I (1983) Acute effects of smoking on fetal heart rate variability. *British Journal of Obstetrics and Gynaecology*, **90**, 3–6

Lemoine, P, Harrousseau, H, Borteyru, J-P and Menuet, J-C (1968) Les enfants de parents alcooliques, anomalies observées. A propos de 127 cas. *Ouest-Medical*, **25**, 476–482

Lief, NR (1985) The drug user as a parent. *International Journal of the Addictions*, **20**, 63–97

Lilley, J and Forster, DP (1986) A randomized controlled trial of individual counselling of smokers in pregnancy. *Public Health*, **100**, 309–315

Lincoln, R (1986) Smoking and reproduction. *Family Planning Perspectives*, **18**, 79–84

Little, BB, Snell, LM and Gilstrap, LC (1988) Methamphetamine abuse during pregnancy: outcome and fetal effects. *Obstetrics and Gynecology*, **72**, 541–544

Little, RE (1977) Moderate alcohol use during pregnancy and decreased infant birthweight. *American Journal of Public Health*, **67**, 1154–1156

Little, RE, Streissguth, AP, Barr, HM and Herman, CS (1980) Decreased birthweight in infants of alcoholic women who abstained during pregnancy. *Journal of Pediatrics*, **96**, 974–977

Little, RE, Grathwohl, HL, Streissguth, AP and McIntyre, C (1981) Public awareness and knowledge about the risks of drinking during pregnancy in Multnomah County, Oregan. *American Journal of Public Health*, **71**, 312–314

Lowe, CR (1959) Effect of mother's smoking habits on birthweight of her children. *British Medical Journal*, **2**, 673–676

MacArthur, C and Knox, EG (1988) Smoking in pregnancy and effects of stopping at different stages. *British Journal of Obstetrics and Gynaecology*, **95**, 551–555

McKnight, A and Merrett, D (1987) Alcohol consumption in pregnancy – a health education problem. *Journal of the Royal College of General Practitioners*, **37**, 73–76

Madden, JD, Payne, TF and Miller, S (1986) Maternal cocaine abuse and effect on the newborn. *Pediatrics*, **77**, 209–211

Marbury, MC, Linn, S, Monson, R *et al.* (1983) The association of alcohol consumption with outcome of pregnancy. *American Journal of Public Health*, **73**, 1165–1168

Meyer, MB (1978) How does maternal smoking affect birthweight and maternal weight gain? Evidence from the Ontario Perinatal Mortality Study. *American Journal of Obstetrics and Gynecology*, **131**, 888–893

Meyer, MB, Jonas, BS and Tonascia, JA (1976) Perinatal events associated with maternal smoking during pregnancy. *American Journal of Epidemiology*, **103**, 464–476

Mills, JL, Graubard, GI, Harley, EE *et al.* (1984) Maternal alcohol consumption and birthweight. How much drinking during pregnancy is safe? *Journal of the American Medical Association*, **252**, 1875–1879

Ministerial Group on the Misuse of Drugs (1988) *Tackling Drug Misuse: A Summary of the Government's Strategy*, 3rd edn. Home Office, London

Morrow, RJ, Ritchie, JWK and Bull, SB (1988) Maternal cigarette smoking: the effects on umbilical and uterine blood flow velocity. *American Journal of Obstetrics and Gynecology*, **159**, 1069–1071

Murphy, JF, Drumm, JE, Mulcahy, R and Daly, L (1980) Maternal smoking on fetal birthweight and on growth of the fetal biparietal diameter. *British Journal of Obstetrics and Gynaecology*, **87**, 462–466

Naeye, RL (1978) Effects of maternal cigarette smoking on the fetus and placenta. *British Journal of Obstetrics and Gynaecology*, **85**, 732–737

Naeye, RL (1981) Influence of maternal cigarette smoking during pregnancy on fetal and childhood growth. *Obstetrics and Gynecology*, **57**, 18–21

Naeye, NL and Peters, EC (1984) Mental development of children whose mothers smoked during pregnancy. *Obstetrics and Gynecology*, **64**, 601–617

Naeye, RL, Blanc, W, Le Blanc, W and Khatamec, MD (1973) Fetal complications of maternal heroin addiction: abnormal growth, infections and episodes of stress. *Journal of Pediatrics*, **83**, 1055–1061

Newman, RG (1976) Methadone maintenance: it ain't what it used to be. *British Journal of Addiction*, **71**, 183–186

Newman, RG, Bashkow, S and Calko, D (1975) Results of 313 consecutive live births of infants delivered to patients in the New York City Methadone Maintenance Treatment Program. *American Journal of Obstetrics and Gynecology*, **121**, 233–237

Nowicki, P, Gintzig, L, Hebel, JR *et al.* (1984) Effective smoking intervention during pregnancy. *Birth*, **11**, 217–224

Office of Population Censuses and Surveys: Social Survey Division (1984) *General Household Survey*. London: HMSO

Office of Population Censuses and Surveys: Social Survey Division (1986) *General Household Survey*. London: HMSO

Oppenheimer, E, Stimson, GV and Thorley, A (1979) Seven-year follow-up of heroin addicts: abstinence and continued use compared. *British Medical Journal*, **2**, 627–630

Oro, AS and Dixon, SP (1987) Perinatal cocaine and methamphetamine exposure: maternal and neonatal correlates. *New England Journal of Medicine*, **297**, 528–530

Ovellette, EM, Rosett, HL, Rosman, NP and Weiner, L (1977) Adverse effects on offspring of maternal alcohol abuse during pregnancy. *New England Journal of Medicine*, **297**, 528–530

Parekh, A, Mukherjee, TK, Jhaveri, R *et al.* (1981) Intrauterine exposure to narcotics and cord blood prolactin levels. *Obstetrics and Gynecology*, **57**, 447–449

Pelosi, MA, Frattarda, M, Apuzzio, J *et al.* (1975) Pregnancy complicated by heroin addiction. *Obstetrics and Gynecology*, **45**, 512–515

Perlmutter, J (1974) Heroin addiction and pregnancy. *Obstetrical and Gynecological Survey*, **29**, 439–446

Pirani, BBK (1978) Smoking during pregnancy. *Obstetrical and Gynecological Survey*, **33**, 1–13

Quigley, ME, Sheehan, KL, Wilkes, MM and Yen, SSC (1979) Effects of maternal smoking on circulating catecholamine levels and fetal heart rates. *American Journal of Obstetrics and Gynecology*, **133**, 685–690

Rementeria, JL and Nunag, NN (1973) Narcotic withdrawal in pregnancy. Stillbirth incidence with a case report. *American Journal of Obstetrics and Gynecology*, **116**, 1152–1156

Rementeria, JL, Janakammal, S and Hollander, M (1975) Multiple births in drug addicted women. *American Journal of Obstetrics and Gynecology*, **122**, 958–960

Richardson, BS, O'Grady, JP and Olsen, GD (1984) Fetal breathing movements and response to carbon dioxide in patients on methadone maintenance. *American Journal of Obstetrics and Gynecology*, **150**, 400–405

Riley, D (1987) The management of the pregnant drug addict. *Bulletin of the Royal College of Psychiatrists*, **11**, 362–365

Rosett, HL, Weiner, L, Lee, A *et al.* (1983) Patterns of alcohol consumption and fetal development. *Obstetrics and Gynecology*, **61**, 539–546

Rothstein, P and Gould, JB (1974) Born with a habit. Infants of drug addicted mothers. *Pediatric Clinics of North America*, **21**, 307–321

Royal College of Obstetricians and Gynaecologists (1985) *Statement of Scientific Advisory Committee on alcohol consumption in pregnancy*, London: RCOG

Royal College of Psychiatrists (1982) Alcohol and alcoholism. *Bulletin of Royal College of Psychiatrists*, **6**, 69

Rubin, PC, Craig, GF, Gavin, K and Sumner, D (1986) Prospective survey of use of therapeutic drugs, alcohol and cigarettes during pregnancy. *British Medical Journal*, **292**, 81–83

Russell, CS, Taylor, R and Law, CE (1968) Smoking in pregnancy, maternal blood pressure, pregnancy outcome, baby weight and growth and other related factors. A prospective study. *British Journal of Preventive and Social Medicine*, **22**, 119–126

Shiono, PH, Klebanoff, MA and Berendes, HW (1986) Congenital malformations and maternal smoking during pregnancy. *Teratology*, **34**, 65–71

Smith, CG and Asch, RH (1987) Drug abuse and reproduction. *Fertility and Sterility*, **48**, 355–373

Smith, JE and Deitch, KV (1987) Cocaine: a maternal, fetal and neonatal risk. *Journal of Pediatric Health Care*, **1**, 120–124

Sokal, RJ, Miller, SI and Reed, G (1980) Alcohol abuse during pregnancy: an epidemiological model. *Alcoholism*, **4**, 134–145

Sontag, LW and Wallace, RF (1935) The effects of cigarette smoking during pregnancy upon the fetal heart rate. *American Journal of Obstetrics and Gynecology*, **29**, 77–83

Standing Committee on Drug Abuse (SCODA) (1985) *Drug Problems in Greater Glasgow*: Report of the SCODA Fieldwork Survey in Greater Glasgow Health Board, London: Chameleon Press

Stauber, M, Schwerdt, M and Tylden, E (1982) Pregnancy birth and puerperium in women suffering from heroin addiction. *Journal of Psychosomatic Obstetrics and Gynaecology*, 128–138

Stillman, RJ, Rosenberg, MJ and Sachs, BP (1986) Smoking and reproduction. *Fertility and Sterility*, **46**, 545–565

Stimmel, B and Adamsons, K (1976) Narcotic dependency in pregnancy. Methadone maintenance compared to use of street drugs. *Journal of the American Medical Association*, **235**, 1121–1124

Stjernfeld, M, Berglund, K, Lindsten, J and Ludvigsson, J (1986) Maternal smoking during pregnancy and risk of childhood cancer. *Lancet*, **i**, 1350–1352

Strauss, ME, Andresko, M, Stryker, JC *et al.* (1974) Methadone maintenance during pregnancy. Pregnancy, birth and neonate characteristics. *American Journal of Obstetrics and Gynecology*, **120**, 895–900

Streissguth, AP (1978) Fetal alcohol syndrome: an epidemiological perspective. *American Journal of Epidemiology*, **107**, 467–478

Streissguth, AP, Barr, HM, Martin, DC and Herman, CS (1980) Effects of maternal alcohol, nicotine and caffeine use during pregnancy on infant mental and motor development at eight months. *Alcoholism: Clinical and Experimental Research*, **4**, 152–164

Streissguth, AP, Denby, BL, Barr, HM *et al.* (1983) Comparison of drinking and smoking patterns during pregnancy over a six-year interval. *American Journal of Obstetrics and Gynecology*, **145**, 716–724

Subcommittee of the Research Committee of the British Thoracic Society (1983) Comparison of four methods of smoking withdrawal in patients with smoking related diseases. *British Medical Journal*, **286**, 595–597

Sulaiman, ND, Florey, C du V, Taylor, DJ and Ogston, SA (1988) Alcohol consumption in Dundee primigravidas and its effects on outcome of pregnancy. *British Medical Journal*, **296**, 1500–1503

Taylor, B and Wadsworth, J (1987) Maternal smoking during pregnancy and lower respiratory tract illness in early life. *Archives of Disease in Childhood*, **62**, 786–791

Telsey, AM, Merrit, A and Dixon, SD (1988) Cocaine exposure in a term neonate: necrotizing enterocolitis as a complication. *Clinical Pediatrics*, **27**, 547–550

Thomsen, SG, Isager-Sally, L, Lange, AP *et al.* (1983) Smoking habits and maternal serum alpha-fetoprotein levels during the second trimester of pregnancy. *British Journal of Obstetrics and Gynaecology*, **90**, 716–717

Underwood, PB, Kesler, KF, O'Lane, JM and Callaghan, DA (1967) Perinatal smoking empirically related to pregnancy outcome. *Obstetrics and Gynecology*, **29**, 1–8

US Department of Health and Human Services (1983) *The Health Consequences of Smoking for Women: A Report of the Surgeon General*. Washington DC: US Government Printing Office

US Surgeon General (1981) Advisory on alcohol and pregnancy. *FDA Drug Bulletin*, **11**, 9–10

Vaille, C (1985) Risks incurred by children of drug-addicted women: some medical and legal aspects. *Bulletin on Narcotics*, **37**, 149–156

Veghely, PV and Osztovics, M (1978) The alcohol syndrome, the intrarecombigenic effect of acetaldehyde. *Separatum Experientia*, **34**, 195–196

Wallach, RC, Jerez, E and Blinick, G (1969) Pregnancy and menstrual function in narcotics addicts treated with methadone. *American Journal of Obstetrics and Gynecology*, **105**, 1226–1229

Ward, SLD, Schuetz, S, Krishna, V *et al.* (1986) Abnormal sleeping ventilatory pattern in infants of substance abusing mothers. *American Journal of Diseases of Children*, **140**, 1015–1020

Weller, RH, Eberstein, IW and Bailey, M (1987) Pregnancy wantedness and maternal behaviour during pregnancy. *Demography*, **24**, 407–412

Wilson, GS, Desmond, MM and Verniaud, WM (1973) Early development of infants of heroin-addicted mothers. *American Journal of Diseases of Childhood*, **126**, 457–462

Windsor, RA, Cutter, G, Morris, J *et al.* (1985) The effectiveness of smoking cessation methods for smokers in public health maternity clinics – a randomized trial. *American Journal of Public Health*, **75**, 1389–1392

Wright, JT, Waterson, EJ, Barrison, IG. *et al.* (1983) Alcohol consumption: pregnancy and low birth-weight. Lancet, **i**, 663–665

Zelson, C (1973) Current concepts. Infant of the addicted mother. *New England Journal of Medicine*, **289**, 1393–1395

Zelson, C, Lee, SJ and Casalino, M (1973) Neonatal narcotic addiction, comparative effects of maternal intake of heroin and methadone. *New England Journal of Medicine*, **289**, 1216–1220

Zuckerman, BS and Hingson, R (1986) Alcohol consumption during pregnancy: a critical review. *Developmental Medicine and Child Neurology*, **28**, 649–661

Zuspan, FP, Gumpel, JA, Mejia-Zelaya, A *et al.* (1975) Fetal stress from methadone withdrawal. *American Journal of Obstetrics and Gynecology*, **122**, 43–46

Part Two

Fetal Problems

Chapter 9

Diagnosis and management of pregnancies complicated by fetal abnormality

Stephen A Walkinshaw and John Burn

Introduction

Fetal abnormalities have become a major issue in obstetric practice for three reasons. First, progressive improvement in the health of pregnant women has had the result that an increasing proportion of fetal and infant mortality and morbidity are accounted for by malformations and genetic defects: collectively these disorders account for three-quarters of severe handicap, up to 50 per cent of clinically recognized first trimester loss and 20 per cent of perinatal deaths (Northern Regional Health Authority, 1988). Second, parental awareness of the potential for fetal abnormality has increased: concerns over the effects of medications and trisomy 21 in the offspring of older couples are two examples. Third, advances in prenatal diagnostic techniques have greatly increased the scope for intervention.

IDENTIFICATION OF PREGNANCIES AT RISK

In obstetric practice, it is essential to be aware of the potential for prenatal diagnosis of fetal abnormality and to be aware of circumstances where such abnormalities are more likely. Thus some pregnancies will be *predictably* at high risk of fetal abnormality whereas, in others, systematic screening will lead to the identification of *unpredictable* fetal abnormalities.

The predictable high risk pregnancy

Risk predictable before pregnancy

A clinical history and examination may make possible the identification of a high-risk pregnancy. Typically, clues will emerge at the booking interview where attention is given to the maternal medical history, parental family history or examination of immediate family members. With the evolution of first-trimester diagnosis for chromosomal and single gene disorders, the diagnostic process will need to move to the preconception period in order that appropriate investigations of other family member and preparation for specialized analyses during pregnancy may be arranged.

Structural abnormality in a preceding child is a typical starting point for such assessments. These abnormalities may be divided into three major categories:

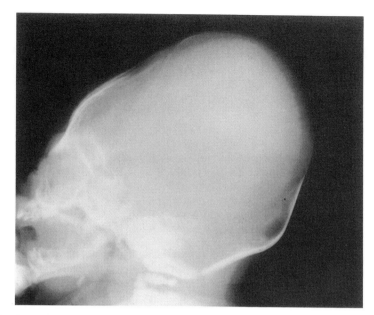

Figure 9.1. Lateral skull radiograph of an infant with cranial moulding in one horn of a bicornuate uterus. The child was labelled 'microcephalic' when, in fact, cranial volume and subsequent development were normal

deformation, disruption and malformation. The term malformation should be reserved for those cases where the fault is thought to be inherent in the zygote and most abnormalities encountered in obstetric practice fall into this category; the other categories are dealt with first.

Deformation

Deformation caused by mechanical compression usually arises as an unpredictable defect due to oligohydramnios secondary to prolonged premature rupture of the membranes or severe renal tract anomaly. A relatively rare predictable deformation is that attributable to uterine malformation. The child shown in Figure 9.1 was labelled microcephalic, when, in fact, the cranial volume was normal. The head circumference had been reduced dramatically by moulding in one horn of a bicornuate uterus. A history of a previously deformed child or of urogenital abnormality in the mother would have identified this pregnancy as being at high risk.

Disruption

The term disruption is applied to abnormalities generally thought to be acquired, rather than being due to genetic abnormality. The most common of these, mechanical disruptions by amniotic bands, are regarded as unpredictable. Figure 9.2 demonstrates the hand of a neonate with this abnormality. Excision of the skin bridge between the abnormal fingers allowed the normally formed middle finger to be restored to its normal position. Chemical disruption, on the other hand, may be predictable and identification of mothers at risk is possible in early pregnancy and prepregnancy.

DRUG EXPOSURE

A number of women will enter pregnancy with co-existing health problems requiring long-term medication. Ideally, such women should be counselled before becoming pregnant about the teratogenic risks of their current therapy and, if a safer alternative is available, alterations to treatment and stabilization of new treatment should be considered before embarking on a pregnancy.

The true role of drugs in the aetiology of fetal abnormality is not clear. Fetal susceptibility, maternal age, and maternal nutritional status are important. Even thalidomide was associated with malformation in only 25 per cent of pregnancies exposed at the appropriate gestation. Drugs rarely give rise to specific syndromes, and their effects may be dependent on timing, the same drug causing a spectrum of abnormalities.

Evidence of teratogenicity has been described in very few instances: cytotoxic agents, anticonvulsants, warfarin, lithium and high-dose quinine are those most likely to be encountered in obstetric practice. There is some concern over trimethoprim, pyrimethamine (an antimalarial) and higher doses of oestrogens or progestational agents.

Epidemiological evidence for a lack of teratogenic effect is available for very few drugs. Most commonly used antihypertensive drugs appear to be safe, as are oral contraceptive steroids (Royal College of General Practitioners, 1975). The list of drugs implicated in studies is large, and comprehensive evaluation is beyond the scope of this chapter. Drugs commonly encountered and the abnormalities detectable by ultrasound are shown in Table 9.1 (for a fuller listing, refer to Koren, Edwards and Miskin, 1987).

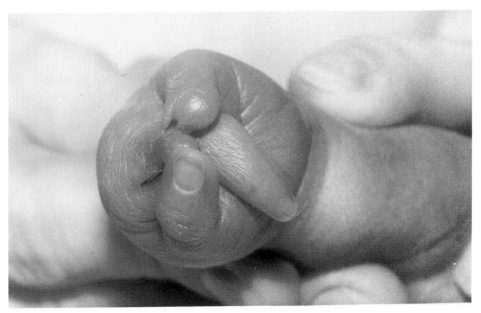

Figure 9.2.   Severe digital disruption by amniotic bands, a remnant of which is visible beside the thumb. The terminal portion of three digits is missing. The normal fourth finger was held in across the palm by the skin bridge between the bases of the third and fifth digits

Table 9.1.   Drugs in pregnancy associated with detectable fetal abnormality

Drug	Detectable abnormality[a]
Amitryptyline	Micrognathia, limb reduction
Antithyroid drugs	Fetal goitre
Carbemazepine	NTD, ASD, hypertelorism, clefting
Chloroquine (high dose)	Polydactyly, hemi-hypertrophy
Chlorpropamide	Microcephaly, hand/foot anomalies
Clomiphene	? NTD
Codeine	? Hydrocephaly/skeletal/cardiac
Cotrimoxazole	? NTD
Diazepam	Clefting, ? cardiac
Danazol	Virilization, ? NTD/cardiac
Diphenhydramine	? Clefting
Imipramine	Exencephaly
Isoniazid	NTD
Lithium	Cardiac (Ebstein's anomaly), NTD
Oestrogens (high dose)	Virilization, ? cardiac/limb reduction
Phenytoin	Microcephaly, IUGR, craniofacial
Phenothiazines	? Microcephaly
Primidone	As for phenytoin
Progestagens (high dose)	Virilization, ? NTD/cardiac
Quinine (high dose)	Hydrocephaly, cardiac, facial, dysmelias
Tolbutamide	Hand anomalies
Valproate	NTD, cardiac, trigoncephaly
Warfarin	Nasal hypoplasia, skeletal

[a] NTD, neural tube defect; ASD, atrial septal defect; IUGR, intrauterine growth retardation;?, mainly case reports and not substantiated by larger studies. Based on Koren, Edwards and Miskin (1987)

MATERNAL DISEASE

A number of maternal diseases carry a predictable risk of detectable fetal abnormality.

Figure 9.3 shows a baby who required a pacemaker in infancy because of congenital heart block. The mother had systemic lupus erythematosus. This disease imparts a risk of cardiac abnormality, mainly conduction defects, but including other structural anomalies. The risk appears limited to those women with serological evidence of the anti-Ro (SS-A) antibody (Taylor *et al.*, 1986). Such women require detailed fetal echocardiography on a regular basis. The same mother subsequently had a healthy child despite the persistence of antibody.

Other maternal disorders associated with a predictable risk of fetal abnormality are listed in Table 9.2.

The maternal disease predominantly associated with fetal abnormality is diabetes mellitus (see also Chapter 1). The rate of all abnormalities is two to three times that of the non-diabetic population (Cousins, 1983) and is thought to be related to poor periconceptional control (Miller *et al.*, 1981), although the precise aetiology is obscure. Groups achieving tight diabetic control at prepregnancy clinics have seen reductions of malformation rates towards normal (Fuhrmann *et al.*, 1984). Skeletal, cardiac, neural tube, gastrointestinal and (less frequently) renal abnormalities are the defects most commonly encountered. Our experience over 10 years in a combined obstetric–diabetic clinic reflects this: cardiac anomalies were 7.5 times, skeletal anomalies 3.7 times, gastrointestinal anomalies 3.1 times and neural tube defects 2.3 times as common as in the pregnancies of non-diabetic women.

With this type of information, it is possible to plan ultrasound examinations for the

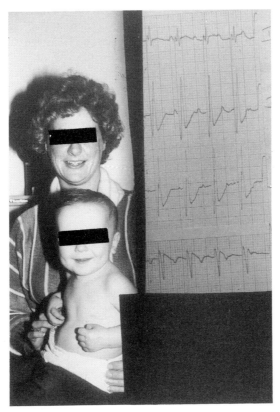

Figure 9.3. A child with complete heart block, following implantation of a pacemaker. The mother had systemic lupus erythematosus. The electrocardiographic trace shows the paced rhythm with dissociation of the p waves. Anti Ro antibodies are thought to have crossed the placenta and damaged the fetal cardiac conducting system. A subsequent pregnancy resulted in a healthy child with normal conduction despite persistence of the maternal antibody

detection of these anomalies. Our practice for pregnancies complicated by insulin-dependent diabetes is as follows:

1. Scan at 12–14 weeks for anencephaly and major skeletal defects
2. Serum AFP at 16 weeks
3. Anomaly screen at 18–19 weeks

Table 9.2   Maternal disease associated with detectable fetal abnormality

Condition	Detectable anomaly
Diabetes mellitus	Skeletal, neural tube, cardiac, renal, gastrointestinal
Graves' disease	Fetal goitre, hydrops, tachyarrhythmia
Allo-immune thrombocytopenia	Hydrocephaly, cystic cerebral lesions
Congenital adrenal hyperplasia	Virilization
Hypoparathyroidism	Skeletal anomalies
Myotonic dystrophy	Polyhydramnios
Haemoglobinopathies	Hydrops fetalis
Systemic lupus erythematosus	Hydrops fetalis, bradycardia, structural cardiac lesions

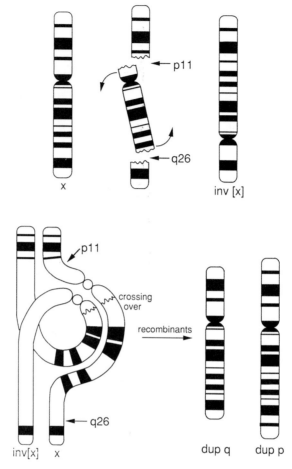

Figure 9.4. A large pericentric (breaks on opposite sides of the centromere) inversion has occurred in one of the X chromosomes in this female. The abnormal chromosome (inv X) must form a loop during meiosis in order to pair correctly with the normal X. If a crossover occurs within the loop the resultant pair of chromosomes will be abnormal. One will have a piece of short arm in place of the end of the long arm (dup p) and the other will have a piece of long arm at both ends (dup q)

4. Fetal echocardiography at 20 weeks
5. Scan at 26–28 weeks for anomaly and growth

Similar ultrasound protocols can be designed for other conditions.

Chromosomal aneuploidy
Aneuploidy, literally translated, means 'not good set', and refers to any departure from the normal pattern of 44 autosomes and two sex chromosomes. The best recognized form of aneuploidy is trisomy, particularly trisomy 21 (Down's syndrome). Two groups are at predictable risk of trisomy: those who have had a previous trisomic child (with an empirical or observed recurrence risk of approximately 1 per cent) and older mothers.

Older mothers constitute the largest group of pregnancies predictably at risk. Risk estimates based on maternal age are crude, the risk of trisomy 21 at 16 weeks at age 35 years being 0.35 per cent and at age 40 years 1.23 per cent [see Ferguson-Smith and Yates (1984) and Hook and Chamber (1983) for precise estimates based on age]. Maternal perception of abnormality and termination of pregnancy, society's perception of abnormality and the availability of resources (both medical and laboratory), all have a role in determining the uptake of prenatal diagnosis in this group of pregnancies.

Evidence has accumulated that assessment of risk for trisomy based on age alone is not an efficient method for detecting these abnormalities (Wald and Cuckle, 1987). In the Northern Region of England, as determined by the Regional Fetal Abnormality Survey 1984–1987, only 10 per cent of trisomy 21 pregnancies were detected prenatally. Serum screening using various additional parameters appears to offer a greater likelihood of increasing the rate of detection without increasing procedure-related pregnancy loss and this is discussed later.

The other major category of chromosome abnormalities associated with a predictable risk are those where a parent has a chromosomal rearrangement, such as inversion, Robertsonian translocation or reciprocal translocation. In each case, incorrect repair of two or more breaks may lead to disturbance of normal chromosome structure. An inversion involves two breaks in a chromosome with subsequent reversal of the broken segment and is described as pericentric if the centromere is involved or paracentric if the segment is confined within the long or short arm of the chromosome. At gamete formation, the affected chromosomes must form a circular pattern or loop to permit pairing with their normal partners prior to separation during meiosis. Crossovers may occur within the loop and the resultant chromosomes will be abnormal, with duplication of one segment and loss of another (see Figure 9.4). The frequency of viable but abnormal offspring is dependent upon the size of the inversion. Small inversions rarely result in viable abnormal offspring, as crossovers produce a major imbalance. Large inversions, on the other hand, result in frequent crossovers within the loop, with much smaller trisomic and monosomic segments: recurrent malformed fetuses are therefore a regular outcome.

In Robertsonian translocation two chromosomes become attached end-to-end, the 14:21 translocation being a typical example. The balanced carrier appears to have 45 chromosomes and is normal. At meiosis the free 21 chromosome is liable to enter the gamete together with its partner attached to the number 14 chromosome, resulting in trisomy 21. A female carrier of such a rearrangement has approximately a 10 per cent risk of a trisomy 21 child following each conception. Transmission of an unbalanced karyotype from the male is rare and a risk of 1 per cent has been observed.

Reciprocal translocation involves the exchange of fragments between two chromosomes. In the example shown (Figure 9.5) the normal number 8 chromosome was transmitted in the sperm together with a number 4 chromosome carrying the tip of the short arm of 8 attached to its short arm. The child was thus trisomic for the tip of chromosome 8 and monosomic for a small piece of the short arm of chromosome 4. The child had the typical clinical appearance of Wolf, or 4p−, syndrome. The risk of abnormal but viable offspring is influenced by the size of the fragment and may be predicted to some extent by the mode of presentation. For example, the detection of the abnormality following recurrent miscarriage implies that the condition is rarely associated with viability, the empirical risk for an abnormal live child being 5 per cent. Recognition following the birth of an abnormal child, on the other hand, carries a risk of close to 20 per cent.

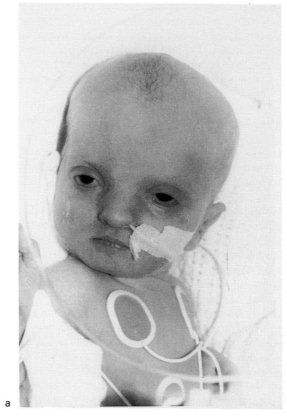

a

Figure 9.5. (a) A child with the typical 'Greek helmet' profile of Wolf syndrome due to deletion of the terminal short arm of chromosome 4. (b) The chromosome spread was reported normal initially by one cytogenetics unit. The two number 4 chromosomes appeared normal but closer examination of the terminal portions of the number 4 chromosomes (arrowed) showed one to stain slightly abnormally. Parental karyotypes revealed a translocation in the father between chromosome 4 and 8. The number 4 transmitted to the child from father was the derivative chromosome with the terminal portion of 4 replaced by the terminal portion of 8. The sperm also contained the normal number 8 with the result that the child was monosomic for the tip of 4 and trisomic for the tip of chromosome 8

Syndromes and simple gene defects

A large and increasing number of fetal abnormalities has been described in which a single gene defect or a small deletion, beyond the resolution of current microscopic techniques, has resulted in disordered development. Pedigree analysis may reveal the typical patterns of autosomal recessive, autosomal dominant or X-linked transmission. In isolated cases of abnormality, a high risk of recurrence may be predicted on the basis of a recognizable pattern or syndrome. Over 1500 syndromes have now been documented. In addition to reference texts such as *Smith's Recognisable Patterns of Human Malformation* (Jones, 1988), computerized databases have been constructed and these are invaluable in the identification of rarer disorders. The London Dysmorphology database (Winter, Baraitser and Douglas, 1984) is a good example of such a system.

The actual risk of recurrence for particular abnormalities may vary considerably.

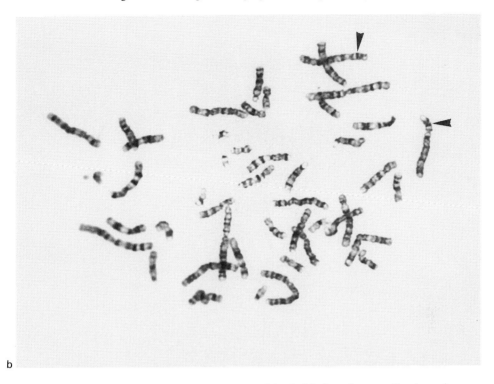

b

Clinical geneticists frequently quote an empirical risk for abnormality based upon overall experience of that abnormality (Table 9.3) but it is important to remember that most, if not all, malformations are heterogeneous and occasional families will be at high risk of recurrence.

Figure 9.6 shows a stillborn infant with Fraser syndrome (cryptophthalmos, renal agenesis, heart defects, imperforate anus, syndactyly) referred to a specialist clinic during the antenatal period with growth retardation and oligohydramnios. This is an autosomal recessive disorder. The parents were first cousins, consanguinity being associated with a tenfold increase in the risk of recessive disorders. They were,

Table 9.3. Empirical risks for common malformations

	Empirical risk (%)		
Anomaly	Siblings	Offspring	Reference
Anencephaly/spina bifida	2	4	Wald and Cuckle, 1984
Cardiac[a]	1–5	4–10	Burn, 1987
Renal agenesiss	3		Carter, Evans and Pescia, 1979
Oesophageal atresia/fistula	<1	<1	Warren, Evans and Carter, 1980
Exomphalos	1	<1	Walkinshaw (unpublished data)
Gastroschisis	negligible	negligible	Walkinshaw (unpublished data)
Diaphragmatic hernia	<1	<1	David and Illingworth, 1976
Clefting	1.8	3	
Isolated palate			
Lip/palate	4	4.3	Harper, 1984

[a] Individual risk rigures dependent upon structural defect

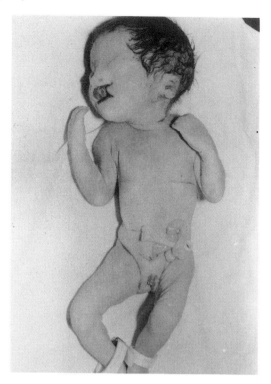

Figure 9.6. A stillborn female infant born of consanguineous parents with the typical features of autosomal dominant Fraser syndrome: skin-covered eyes (cryptophthalmos), syndactyly and facial cleft-ing. There was vaginal and external auditory atresia. Death was due to pulmonary hypoplasia secondary to oligohydramnios due to bilateral renal agenesis

therefore, predictably at risk. Sadly, their next child had renal agenesis without the other features of the syndrome. Had this been the presenting child, then an empirical risk of 3 per cent based on family studies (Carter, Evans and Pescia, 1979) would have been offered, masking the higher 25 per cent risk actually involved.

The textbook assertion that malformations are multifactorial, postulating that multiple additive genes with or without environmental factors result in the crossing by some individuals of a disease threshold, has been validated in only a few clinical conditions. Dominant genes in particular, influenced by chance factors and other genes, may show variable penetrance, mimicking a 'disease threshold' model. Figure 9.7a shows the typical ultrasonographic appearances of cystic renal dysplasia in the second child of a couple whose first child succumbed to the same anomaly. The father was found to have an absent kidney and his sister gave birth to a child shown prenatally to have unilateral cystic renal dysplasia (Figure 9.7b). Acceptance of the concept of single-gene defects with incomplete penetrance is important as molecular studies become feasible to seek comparable defects within the family.

The third example demonstrates an X-linked disorder. Typically, these are charac-terized by affected males connected by phenotypically normal females and by an absence of male-to-male transmission. It must be remembered that carrier females may be affected in any X-linked disorder, though usually less severely, due to the

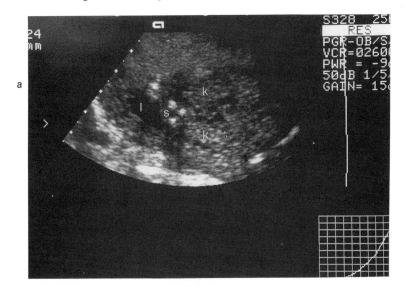

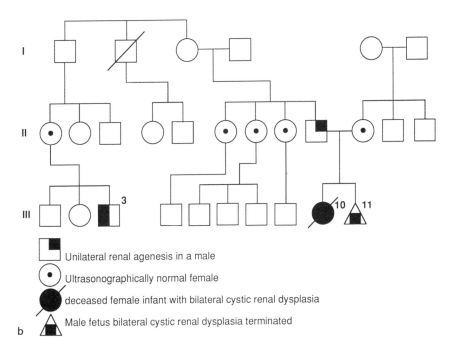

Figure 9.7. (a) Sonogram performed at 24 weeks' gestation. There is severe oligohydramnios and ultrasound appearances are consistent with bilateral cystic renal dysplasia (k, kidney; s, spine; l, liquor); (b) family tree from the infant described above. The inheritance pattern suggests autosomal dominant renal adysplasia with variable penetrance

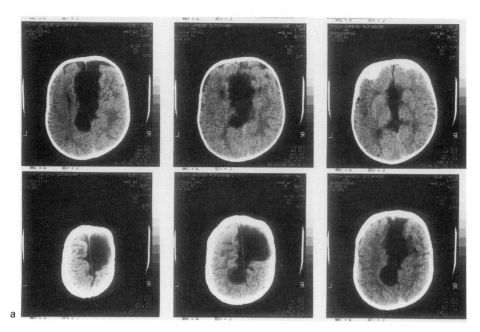

a

Figure 9.8.   (a) Intracerebral findings in OFD type 1 syndrome. The computed tomogram was carried out following identification of multiple cystic areas in the fetal cerebrum on antenatal ultrasound; (b) face of infant with OFD type 1 syndrome showing midline pseudocleft and hamartoma in oral cavity; (c) oral cavity of mother of above infant examined after delivery. There is a midline pseudocleft in the upper lip. She had a gap in her lower dentition associated with an abnormal frenulum, lobulation of the tongue and had had an oral hamartoma removed in childhood

vagaries of X inactivation. The orofaciodigital syndrome (OFD) type I is such a condition and illustrates the general need for examination of parents, sibs and sometimes other relatives for minor features of genetic disease. Figure 9.8a shows cranial computed tomography from a neonate with OFD I. Investigation was prompted by detection of intracranial cysts on prenatal ultrasound. The mother (Figure 9.8c) shared with her daughter (Figure 9.8b) the midline pseudocleft of the upper lip, multiple frenulae and lobulated tongue typical of the condition and had had oral haematomata removed as a child. These features were noted only after birth.

As the list of syndromes and genetic disorders detectable by prenatal ultrasound is now lengthy, it is important to assess each couple individually. As in any aspect of medicine, a detailed history is essential. Previous ultrasound findings, autopsy descriptions, previous genetic counselling and any other relevant details should all be ascertained. Consultation with clinical geneticists may be essential to establish the range of severity of particular disorders and consultation with obstetric ultrasonologists will be necessary to determine the feasibility of prenatal diagnosis and the timing of ultrasound examinations. Thereafter, the couple can be realistically counselled as to what can be offered and when, and their feelings towards prenatal diagnosis and termination of pregnancy assessed.

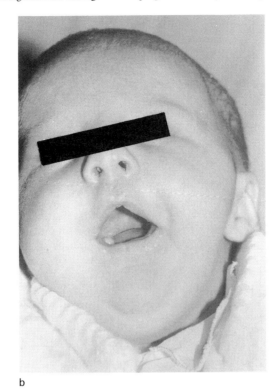

b

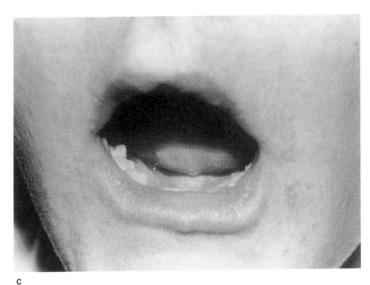

c

Risk predictable from coincidental events in pregnancy
A number of problems may arise by chance during any pregnancy which will predictably increase the risk of fetal abnormality in that pregnancy. These are, by definition, disruptive events.

Maternal infection

In general terms, a congenital syndrome resulting from fetal viral infection in early pregnancy has been described for most common viral infections. As a rule, the earlier the infection, the more likely it is to be teratogenic. Although many of the problems associated with these infections may be reduced by new approaches to immunization, it has been estimated that 3 per cent of all fetal abnormality is due to maternal infection; this is likely to be an underestimate. It is, therefore, important to be aware of the possible effects of such infection, especially during local outbreaks.

Figure 9.9 shows a fetus with isolated ascites detected at routine ultrasound examination at 19 weeks. A TORCH (toxoplasmosis, rubella, cytomegalovirus, herpes) screen was performed and maternal antibodies to human cytomegalovirus were markedly elevated. CMV was isolated from amniotic fluid and therapeutic termination requested and performed.

Table 9.4 lists the likelihood of fetal abnormality following proven maternal infection (derived from multiple sources) and those abnormalities likely to be detectable by ultrasound. For many viral infections, data are incomplete or scanty. It is therefore vital that any fetus with detectable abnormality, either prenatally or at birth, is fully screened to exclude congenital infection as a cause. It must be stressed that many of the effects of congenital infection do not produce structural anomaly and that such screening forms only part of the assessment of these pregnancies.

Radiation exposure

Women may undergo radiological investigation during pregnancy, either inadvertently or for concurrent acute illness. In rare instances, radiation therapy may be instituted for malignant disease in the presence of a pregnancy.

In late pregnancy, the major concern has been directed at the effects of such exposure on the development of childhood malignancies (Knox *et al.*, 1987). In early

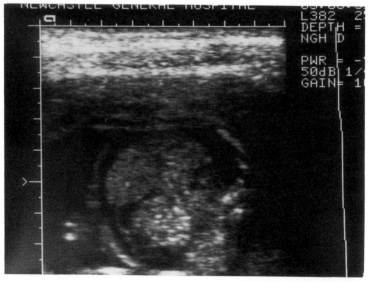

Figure 9.9. Sonogram of fetus at 20 weeks' gestation. Isolated ascites noted. Human CMV isolated from amniotic fluid

pregnancy, concern has been expressed regarding teratogenesis and it is not unusual for termination to be requested on the grounds of radiological exposure.

At the pre-blastocyst stage, the embryo is relatively insensitive to teratogenesis but is sensitive to the lethal effects of radiation. During early organogenesis there is sensitivity to both its teratogenic and lethal effects in addition to sensitivity to its growth-retarding effects. In the early fetal period, there is a reduction in teratogenic sensitivity except for the central nervous system. If exposure is high enough in these later stages, permanent cell depletion of various organ systems can occur and this may result in hypoplasia (Table 9.5).

It is not generally felt that exposures of <5 rad (0.05 Gy) confer any additional risk of fetal abnormality, although the current radiobiological view is that it is unlikely that there is a definitive threshold. The most recent analyses of Japanese data suggest that this risk should be increased by a factor of three. The main ultrasonically detectable abnormalities are microcephaly and microphthalmia; it appears that other abnormalities are extremely rare in the absence of these. Detection of microcephaly should, however, prompt a detailed search for other anomalies.

These doses must be compared with those likely to pertain to modern radiological exposures, which are shown in Table 9.6.

Table 9.4.   Detectable fetal abnormality associated with maternal infection

Virus	Risk of abnormality	Detectable abnormality
Rubella	81% at <10 weeks. Minimal for detectable anomaly >13 weeks	Cardiac (PDA, pulmonary stenosis), microcephaly, microphthalmia
Human CMV	4% severe congenital CMV at birth. Anomaly risk in 1st trimester unknown but <1.5%. May be small risk in 2nd trimester	Hydrops, microcephaly, microphthalmia, cardiac, exomphalos, oesophageal atresia
HSV	Unquantified but small risk below 20 weeks	Hydranencephaly, microcephaly, microphthalmia, short digits
Varicella	1st trimester <1%; 2nd trimester, sporadic but few data	Limb hypoplasia, small digits, microphthalmia, hydramnios, skin lesions, microcephaly, cerebellar lesions
EBV	<1%. Very rare	Micrognathia, cardiac, cerebral, microphthalmia, hydrops (myocarditis)
Coxsackie	Risk of cardiac defect twice normal for B3/B4. Risk of urogenital defects for types B2/B4	Cardiac, hydrops/tachyarrhythmia, hypo- or epispadias
Influenza	Overal increase in abnormality rates of ×2–2.5	Neural tube defects, cardiac commonest but no syndrome
Mumps	2%	Left cardiac outflow obstruction due to endocardial fibroelastosis
Parvovirus	At <18 weeks at least 5%; still risk in later pregnancy; overall risk may be higher	Hydrops secondary to aplastic crisis
HIV	Rare embryopathy	–
Toxoplasmosis	1.8% at <16 weeks. Risk of minor calcification may be higher in later pregnancy	Ascites, unilateral or bilateral hydrocephaly, intracranial intrahepatic calcification

Table 9.5.   Fetal risks associated with maternal exposure to radiation

Menstrual age (weeks)	Minimum dose for severe retardation (rad)	Minimum dose for malformation (rad)
4.5–6	20–50	20
7–15	50	50

Drug exposure and substance abuse
In addition to those women entering pregnancy on drug therapy, a number of women will ingest drugs in early pregnancy for simple complaints, or for medical conditions presenting in pregnancy (see Table 9.1).

Within this category come the substances of abuse: opiates, cannabis, cocaine and alcohol (see also Chapter 8). It is difficult in many instances to separate the effects of these substances from the social and nutritional conditions associated with these women.

The fetal alcohol syndrome is well described (see Figure 9.10) (Poskitt, 1984). Alcohol consumption in excess of 50 g/day carries a 40 per cent risk of the syndrome, with consumption of 30–50 g carrying a 10 per cent risk. Consumption of smaller amounts may be associated with some manifestations of the syndrome, although the precise relationship has not been established. Many of the features of the syndrome are difficult to delineate with any certainty by ultrasound, but cardiac anomalies, intrauterine growth retardation, microcephaly, craniofacial anomalies, some skeletal manifestations and clefting should be detectable.

Opiate and amphetamine abuse do not appear to carry an excess risk of abnormality. Recent large studies confirm that marijuana also carries no risk (Zuckerman *et al.*, 1989). The position for cocaine is less clear. Zuckerman *et al.* (1989) have suggested that there is a slight increase in fetal anomalies, without any identifiable pattern, in cocaine abusers, even after removal of confounding factors. Confirmation of this increased risk associated with cocaine abuse has come from Chavez, Mulinare and Cordero (1989), who found a consistent increase in urogenital anomalies.

Risk predictable by pregnancy complication
A number of complications of pregnancy are associated with the finding of fetal malformations.

Table 9.6.   Doses to uterus from routine radiological procedures

Radiographs	Number of films (mean)	Dose to uterus (mSv)
Chest	1.3	< 0.01
Lumbar spine	3.4	3.16
Abdomen	1.4	2.57
Pelvis	1.1	1.68
IVU	8.2	3.58
Barium meal	7.8	3.6
Barium enema	8.8	16.0
Cholangiography	8.0	0.8
Cholecystography	4.5	0.4
Pelvic CT		50–100

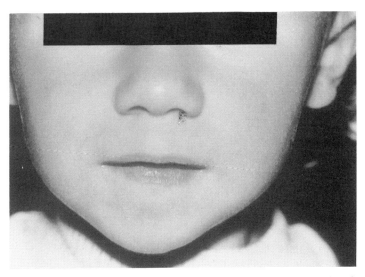

Figure 9.10.   Face of child with fetal alcohol syndrome. Height and weight were below the 3rd centile. Short palpebral fissures and a poorly developed philtrum (flat upper lip) are illustrated

Small for gestational age

Three per cent of cases of severe intrauterine growth retardation have chromosomal abnormalities (Cook and Young, 1986) and as many as 5–15 per cent of infants born showing signs of intrauterine growth retardation (IUGR) may have evidence of chromosomal disorder or genetic disease. The precise incidence of non-chromosomal fetal abnormality among fetuses suspected of IUGR is unknown. Growth failure in the second trimester carries the highest risk of abnormality and karyotypic abnormalities are common in this group, especially triploidy (Crane, Bever and Cheung 1985). The possibility of viral infection and associated abnormalities should be considered. Skeletal dysplasias are often identified at this stage.

Data in the third trimester, when most pregnancies complicated by IUGR are diagnosed, are more controversial. Severe symmetrical IUGR should raise the question of cytogenetic abnormality or of severe cardiac anomaly. Whether fetuses with less severe growth failure, symmetrical or asymmetrical, are at risk is more questionable. Detailed ultrasound examination should be carried out but the frequency of detectable abnormality should not be overstated. Our own experience in prospective trials of fetal monitoring in suspected IUGR identified during the third trimester, involving over 100 consecutive fetuses with an estimated fetal weight of less than the 5th centile for gestational age, suggests that this risk is <1 per cent.

Fetal Doppler studies may identify unsuspected abnormalities, especially chromosomal trisomies (Trudinger and Cook, 1985) and abnormal findings on continuous wave equipment should result in a detailed abnormality screen.

Oligohydramnios

Abnormality should always be suspected in the presence of oligohydramnios; this is especially true during the second trimester. Ultrasound examination can be

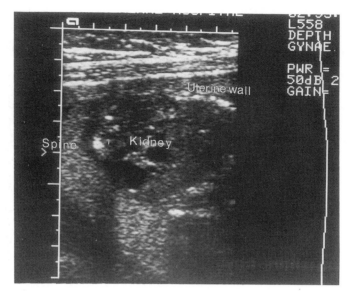

Figure 9.11.   Sonogram of fetus at 19 weeks' gestation. There is severe oligohydramnios and cystic renal dysplasia, in this case secondary to outlet obstruction with a fused single kidney

extremely difficult and karyotyping may require expertise in late chorion villus sampling or fetal blood sampling.

Over 50 per cent of consecutive referrals to the Fetal Assessment Clinic in our unit over the last 12 months with severe oligohydramnios before 22 weeks' gestation had

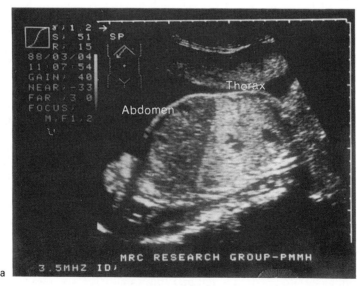

Figure 9.12.   (a) Sonogram of fetus at 28 weeks' gestation. There is polyhydramnios secondary to cystic adenomatoid malformation of the right lung; (b) sonogram of a fetus at 34 weeks' gestation with marked polyhydramnios. The left hand exhibits arthrogryposis and there is micrognathia; (c) similar view in the neonatal period. The neonate required ventilatory support for poor respiratory effort. A diagnosis of fetal akinesia syndrome was made and support was withdrawn

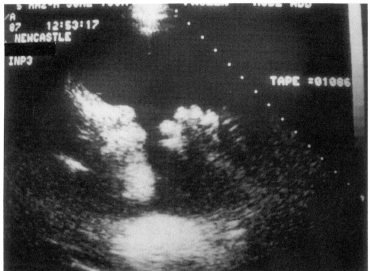

b

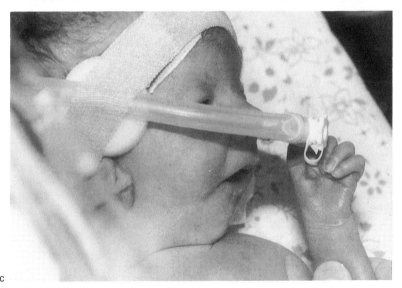

c

demonstrable abnormality. Renal outflow obstruction, renal aplasia or dysplasia and cytogenetic abnormalities are common. Figure 9.11 shows one of these cases, a fetus of 19 weeks gestation with anhydramnios due to a fused dysplastic kidney.

Detailed and often repeated examination of these fetuses is necessary and karyotyping is mandatory.

Polyhydramnios
Figures 9.12a–c relate to two fetuses referred for ultrasound examination with severe polyhydramnios. The fetus in Figure 9.12a has a structural defect, cystic adenomatoid malformation of the lung, the lesion occupying almost the entire thorax. The fetus in Figures 9.12b and 9.12c has more subtle abnormalities, with

Table 9.7.   Detectable fetal abnormality associated with polyhydramnios

Obstructive:	Head and neck	Tumours of neck, oral cavity
	Thorax	Tumours, skeletal dysplasia, diaphragmatic hernia
	Gastrointestinal	Atresia, especially oesophageal and duodenal
Open lesion		Neural tube defect
		Anterior abdominal wall defect
		Bladder extrophy
Neurogenic		Anencephaly
	Neuromuscular	Myotonic dystrophy
		Degenerative
Tumours:	Teratoma	Thyroid, sacrococcygeal
Cardiac decompensation		Anaemia
		Cardiac anomaly
		Tachyarrhythmia
		Non-immune hydrops

questionable micrognathia and arthrogryposis of the hand. A prenatal diagnosis was not made on this fetus, who had Pina Shokeir syndrome type 1, a degenerative disease of the anterior horn cells. This is one subgroup of fetal akinesia syndrome, in which deficient fetal movement results in diminished swallowing with resultant polyhydramnios.

Chamberlain, Manning and Morrison, (1984), using a definition of liquor pool >8 cm as polyhydramnios, noted a malformation rate of 4.0 per cent, eight times that of pregnancies with normal liquor volume, although traditional teaching has suggested higher rates. The range of abnormalities is wider, the main groups being as shown in Table 9.7. In addition to mainly structural anomalies, conditions causing non-immune hydrops or a number of neuromuscular diseases must be recognized. Ultrasound examination must, therefore, include assessment of fetal activity.

Multiple pregnancy
Most studies demonstrate that twin pregnancy carries a risk of fetal abnormality (Little and Bryan, 1986) approximately twice that of singleton pregnancy. In part, this is due to those abnormalities specific to twin pregnancies, namely conjoined twins, acardia and anomalies secondary to early intrauterine death of a co-twin. Some other groups of abnormalities are commoner in twin pregnancies: hydrocephalus, oesophageal atresia, tracheo-oesophageal fistula and cardiac defects are the most important (Bryan, Little and Burn, 1987).

Repeated daily anomaly scanning is required in these pregnancies.

Severe proteinuric hypertension
Early severe pre-eclampsia should raise the question of non-immune fetal hydrops and ultrasound examination should be performed before a decision about delivery (Robertson *et al.*, 1985).

Breech presentation
It is well recognized that a fetus presenting by the breech is more likely to have congenital malformation than a fetus in which the presentation is cephalic. The abnormality rate is approximately threefold (Brenner, Bruce and Hendricks, 1974), with hydrocephaly, neural tube defects, neuromuscular disorders and autosomal trisomies the commonest anomalies.

Detailed examination by ultrasound should form part of the assessment of a breech presentation.

The unpredictable high-risk pregnancy

The previous sections describe the identification of pregnancies where fetal abnormality might be suspected. However, increasing numbers of prenatally diagnosed abnormalities are detected as a result of deliberate screening of ostensibly normal pregnancies.

Before considering the role of screening, it is important to outline the techniques available for prenatal diagnosis.

Available techniques

Ultrasound
Diagnostic ultrasound remains the workhorse of prenatal detection of fetal abnormality. Technical developments in ultrasound in the 1970s and early 1980s resulted in considerable improvements in imaging quality within a short time, the result being rapid obsolescence of most diagnostic equipment. This pace of development has slackened and modern real-time scan equipment gives a high resolution image.

Until recently, the focus of early obstetric ultrasound was upon accurate estimation of gestation age and this remains an important function of ultrasound examination during the first half of pregnancy. However, the availability of resources and the increasing importance of fetal abnormality as a cause of perinatally related loss has made it essential that optimum use be made of the routine scan. It is recommended that the maximum information can be obtained by offering examination at 18–20 weeks' gestation (Members of the Joint Study Group on Fetal Abnormalities, 1989).

Such a change in emphasis requires that the highest quality ultrasound equipment should be available for routine obstetric scanning. This, allied to adequate training of ultrasonographers, clear guidelines as to what constitutes an adequate anomaly screen and clear lines of command to experienced and available medical ultrasonologists, forms the basis of a good service for the detection of fetal abnormality.

Newer techniques in diagnostic imaging are being evaluated. Vaginal ultrasound is currently being assessed for prenatal diagnosis (Rottem *et al.*, 1989). The role of magnetic resonance imaging (MRI) is under review.

Invasive techniques
Screening for genetic and chromosomal disorders and for structural abnormality requires the availability of invasive techniques in order to obtain samples for cytogenetic analysis, DNA diagnosis and biochemical studies. Figure 9.13 demonstrates the techniques available.

AMNIOCENTESIS
Amniocentesis remains the standard technique. With improvements in cell culture techniques, samples obtained between 10 and 40 weeks' gestation can be used for cytogenetic analysis. Although a procedure-related loss rate of 1 per cent is generally quoted (Tabor *et al.*, 1986), experienced operators using good ultrasound equipment and (preferably) scanning during the procedure may obtain loss rates of less than this. The possibility of culture failure (1–1.5 per cent of samples) or mosaicism (0.25 per cent) must be taken into account and repeat amniocentesis, placental biopsy or fetal blood sampling should be available as a back-up procedure.

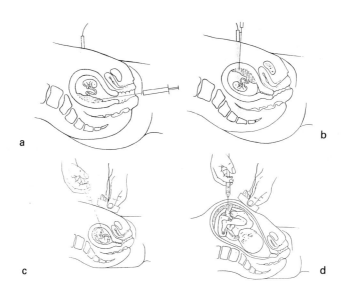

Figure 9.13. Invasive techniques for biopsy of fetal material: (a) transcervical chorion villus sampling; (b) transabdominal chorion villus sampling; (c) amniocentesis; (d) percutaneous fetal blood sampling

CHORION VILLUS SAMPLING

This allows early and rapid karyotype diagnosis. There is now extensive experience using both transcervical and transabdominal routes. Transcervical sampling is generally carried out at 9–11 weeks' gestation, the loss rates outside this narrow window being considerably higher. Fetal loss rates in transcervical sampling are closely related to the frequency with which the procedure is performed and the number of attempts required to obtain a sample, being on average 3.34 per cent in centres with extensive experience (Jackson, 1988). Transabdominal sampling can be carried out from 8 weeks onwards. Initial concern over its feasibility beyond 28 weeks (Pijpers *et al.*, 1988) appear to have been unfounded and we have successfully obtained results from placental biopsy using direct preparations up to 36 weeks' gestation. Loss rates using the transabdominal approach appear to be similar to those from transcervical sampling (Jackson, 1988) although several groups have reported loss rates of <2 per cent (Lilford *et al.*, 1987; Nicolaides, Soothill and Roseavar, 1987); furthermore, the learning curve may be more acceptable. Mosaicism is a major problem in chorion villus samples, being between 2.3 and 3 per cent, and in the case of reported trisomies, the fetuses are likely to be normal (Schulz and Miller, 1986). Choice of route is dependent upon personal experience and, ideally, both routes should be available.

FETAL CORD BLOOD SAMPLING

Fetal cord blood sampling is now performed under direct ultrasound guidance, without fetoscopic visualization (Daffos, Capella-Pavlovsky and Forestier, 1985). This technique is technically more demanding than early diagnostic techniques and can be carried out from about 18 weeks to give rapid cytogenetic analysis. The loss rates attributable to the procedure are not well described, but overall appear to be around 7 per cent, equally distributed before and after 28 weeks' gestation (Whittle,

1989). This high loss rate may partly reflect the indications for which the procedure is being carried out for others have suggested loss rates of 1 per cent (Daffos, Capella-Pavlovsky and Forestier, 1985). In addition, emergency delivery as a consequence of the procedure may be required in up to 12.5 per cent of cases (Chueh and Golbus, 1989). It is, therefore, a technique that should be performed in a limited number of centres.

Biochemical techniques
Maternal screening by serum alphafetoprotein (AFP) for open neural tube defects is now well established (Wald and Cuckle, 1984), the risk being dependent upon the incidence of the condition within a given population. Raised serum AFP may also allow detection of anterior abdominal wall defects by use of scanning densitometry of amniotic fluid acetylcholinesterase (AChE), with anterior wall defects having the less dense band (Peat and Brock, 1984).

Other refinements include adjustment of serum AFP for maternal weight and for estimated gestation by biparietal diameter (Wald and Cuckle, 1987), which may reduce the false-positive rate. Similarly, it is now appreciated that Afro-Caribbean women appear to produce relatively elevated levels of AFP, and Asian women reduced levels.

Recent studies have demonstrated an association between low maternal serum AFP and fetal trisomy, the geometric mean of AFP levels in affected pregnancies being 0.75 multiples of the median (Wald and Cuckle, 1987). This phenomenon has been confirmed by similar findings in AFP levels in both amniotic fluid and fetal serum. The overlap between levels in trisomy and the normal population is greater than that in neural tube defects.

Unconjugated oestriols appear to be lower in the serum of pregnancies with trisomy (Wald *et al.*, 1988). Levels of β-HCG (human chorionic gonadotrophin) in maternal serum are elevated in pregnancies with trisomy (Bogart, Pandian and Jones, 1987).

These markers function independently of each other and of age, and combinations of age and serum markers are being introduced to compute a risk of trisomy for an individual pregnancy: this is the concept of isorisk. The object of such complex analyses is to improve the detection rate of autosomal trisomy without increasing the loss of normal pregnancies through an increase in the amniocentesis rate.

Identification of fetuses at risk by serum screening

Neural tube defects
Standard protocols now exist in most areas offering serum screening for neural tube defects in order to identify pregnancies at risk. Current controversy revolves around whether high-resolution ultrasound or amniocentesis should be used for diagnosis. Description of specific cranial findings in open defects (Nicolaides *et al.*, 1986) has polarized these arguments (see Figure 9.14).

Amniocentesis following a raised maternal serum AFP will detect 98 per cent of anencephaly and 98 per cent of open neural tube defects (Wald and Cuckle, 1984, 1987). For every five defects detected, one pregnancy will be lost because of a false–positive result or as a direct consequence of amniocentesis. Selective ultrasound following a finding of raised maternal serum AFP should detect all anencephaly and has a sensitivity of 80–90 per cent for open spina bifida, with a false-positive rate of 0.3–3 per cent (Hashimoto *et al.*, 1985; Nicolaides and Campbell, 1987). There

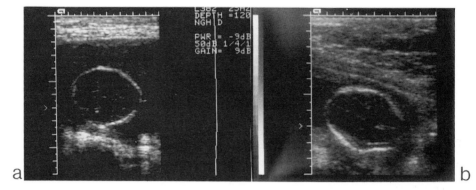

Figure 9.14. Cranial ultrasonography in open neural tube defects: (a) sonogram of normal cranial outline in a fetus at 18 weeks' gestation; (b) sonogram demonstrating the 'lemon sign' in a fetus at 18 weeks' gestation with open lumbar spina bifida

are few data on the detection rates obtainable by ultrasound screening alone. Data from the Northern region of the UK from 1984 to 1987, which has a low rate of serum screening, shows that 90 of 92 anencephalic fetuses were identified by ultrasound but that only 36 of 82 open defects were detected where ultrasound examination was performed between 16 and 24 weeks. A combination of serum screening followed by level 2 or 3 ultrasound examination in the first instance may prove satisfactory, provided that amniocentesis is used where ultrasound examination is unsatisfactory or inconclusive.

Even allowing for the apparent reduction in the prevalence of neural tube defects over the last decade, it would appear that screening has resulted in a 40 per cent reduction in the birth incidence of open neural tube defects (Carstairs and Cole, 1984).

Autosomal trisomy
With an age cut-off of 35 years and complete uptake, it should be possible to detect 35 per cent of trisomy 21 fetuses. In practice, detection rates are closer to 10–15 per cent (Northern Regional data). With use of isorisk estimates based on serum AFP and age, 40 per cent of these fetuses would be detectable for the same false-positive rate (Cuckle, Wald and Thompson, 1987). Age and β-HCG appear to be the best simple combination, with a detection rate of 50 per cent associated with an amniocentesis rate of 5 per cent (Wald *et al.*, 1988b). More complex formulae using a combination of age, AFP, β-HCG and oestriols could detect 60 per cent of trisomy 21 fetuses without any increase in the rate of amniocentesis (Wald *et al.*, 1988a). Other refinements, such as the use of ratios (White, Papiha and Magnay, 1989) may improve discrimination further.

Ultrasound screening
Most prenatally detected anomalies come to light as a result of ultrasound examination, now generally performed at 18–20 weeks' gestation. A large number of anomalies are detectable at this stage in pregnancy; however, the ability to detect anomalies in the setting of busy antenatal clinics and routine scanning sessions should not be compared with the data quoted from tertiary referral units. Table 9.8 shows the detection rates from the Northern Regional Fetal Abnormality Survey for 1986 (unpublished data). As an example of a specific abnormality, during the five years of

Table 9.8.   Diagnoses made prenatally in the Northern region of England during 1986 as a proportion of all cases coming to specialist attention within one year of birth

Diagnosis	Proportion
Unilateral renal damage treated by nephrectomy	7/7
Obstruction of the pelvic ureteric junction treated by pyeloplasty	14/14
Bladder outlet obstruction	7/8
Bilateral renal agenesis or lethal dysplasia	9/13
Anencephaly	25/27
Open neural tube defects	23/46
Isolated hydrocephalus	10/12
Anterior abdominal wall defects	11/16
Tracheo-oesophageal fistula/atresia	1/10
Duodenal atresia	1/5
Lower gut atresia	0/13
Diaphragmatic hernia	1/16
Lethal skeletal dysplasia	0/4
Non-immune hydrops	4/6

this Survey (1984–1988), the detection rate for anterior abdominal wall defects when ultrasound examination took place between 16 and 22 weeks was only 59 per cent (Walkinshaw et al., in press). Such data cover a wide range of ultrasound equipment and expertise and emphasize what is realistically achievable in current practice.

For certain defects, detection rates are even poorer. Prenatal detection of major cardiac malformations remains low, being <10 per cent between 1984 and 1987. An understanding of the value of a simple four-chamber view of the heart (Allan et al., 1986) should result in the detection of most significant lesions.

A detailed ultrasound examination should, at minimum, include comments on the following: femur length, biparietal diameter; skull shape, ventricular size, cerebellar shape; facial appearance; spine, all limbs, hands and feet; four-chamber view of heart; thorax, diaphragm; anterior abdominal wall, insertion umbilical cord; stomach bubble, abdominal contents; kidneys and bladder; position and attitude of fetus, fetal activity; liquor volume, and placental site. Figure 9.15 demonstrates the type of detail that can be achieved. It cannot be overemphasized that such results are possible only if adequate time and facilities are available.

MANAGEMENT OF ANTENATALLY DIAGNOSED FETAL ABNORMALITY

The aims of prenatal diagnosis of fetal abnormality are threefold. First, the identification at an early gestation of abnormalities incompatible with survival or associated with severe handicap will make available the option of therapeutic termination. Second, prenatal diagnosis will identify some fetuses who would benefit from intervention during the antenatal period or from early alerting of paediatric services. Finally, there is a group of fetuses in whom antenatal identification may result in changes in timing, site or mode of delivery.

The multidisciplinary approach

The key to successful management of prenatally diagnosed fetal abnormality lies in the coordination of the activities of a number of specialities. Even the most apparently straightforward detectable abnormality, open neural tube defect, will involve several different specialists – obstetrician, radiologist, clinical geneticist and paediatrician, all of whom will have a role in the management of the pregnancy and in counselling the couple.

Ideally, centres should be available where this coordinated approach is more formally organized. Many areas in the UK are developing multidisciplinary fetal assessment clinics to offer such advice and expertise. Such a clinic may be able to offer infrequently required practical skills, such as fetal cord blood sampling, but more importantly the group will be exposed to rare and difficult problems on a regular basis and may be able to examine different management approaches.

The core of such a team will consist of specialists in fetal medicine, neonatology, radiology, clinical genetics and paediatric surgery but close links with paediatric cardiology, nephrology, neurology and pathology will need to be developed. Ideally such a group should meet to review its diagnostic abilities and management strategies on a regular basis.

Counselling before diagnosis

Predictable risk

Counselling before diagnosis is an essential part of the management of pregnancies where there is a predictable risk of fetal abnormality. Where the possibility of

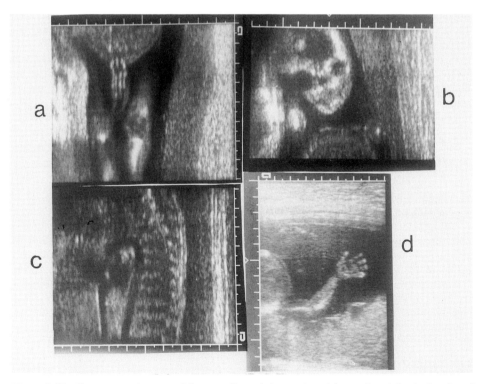

Figure 9.15. Sonograms of a normal fetus at 19 weeks' gestation: (a) anterior abdominal wall and umbilical cord insertion; (b) face; (c) aortic arch; (d) forearm and digits

abnormality is predictable before pregnancy, formal genetic counselling should have been carried out and, if not, should be offered early in pregnancy. Couples should be aware of the risks of abnormality, the ability to detect particular anomalies and the limitations of prenatal diagnosis. Their views on termination of pregnancy should be explored at this stage.

It is important that counselling includes a realistic appraisal of the feasibility of prenatal diagnosis and the aim of prenatal diagnosis in each case. Where the risk of abnormality arises through a coincidental event during early pregnancy, the couple must be counselled about the precise risk, if known. It needs to be emphasized that not all of the effects of particular teratogens will be detectable. In most cases reassurance will have a central role.

It remains debatable whether the issue of fetal abnormality should be raised before diagnosis where the indication for ultrasound is a pregnancy complication. In our experience many women suspect this, especially if repeated ultrasound examinations by increasingly senior ultrasonographers are being performed. If no counselling is to be performed before scanning, it should be mandatory that the couple are counselled, however briefly, immediately after the diagnosis is confirmed. This requires the availability of senior medical staff during all routine ultrasound sessions.

Counselling for routine screening

If screening for fetal abnormality and autosomal trisomy is to be expanded, it is essential that women booking for antenatal care are fully informed of the types of screening offered, the problems and limitations associated with the screening techniques and the sequence of events that will follow the identification of a potential problem. Ideally, women should opt in to screening protocols after consideration of their own views on abnormality and termination. It appears that the community as a whole still requires the availability of prenatal diagnosis and therapeutic termination for abnormality during the second trimester (Pickworth and Burn, 1988).

Assessment of the abnormality

The management of fetal abnormality resolves itself into a series of questions:

1. What is the precise diagnosis and how confident is that diagnosis?
2. What do we know of the aetiology and natural history of the abnormality?
3. Are there any other structural or cytogenetic abnormalities associated with these findings?
4. What is the prognosis?
5. Should therapeutic termination or non-intervention be considered?
6. Can we modify the outcome by treatment *in utero*?
7. How, where and when should the baby be delivered?
8. Who needs to know?

Diagnostic accuracy

The crucial initial question would seem self-evident: what is the diagnosis? It is important to remember that reliable prenatal diagnosis on a national scale is a very recent phenomenon. There are few data on the false–positive and false-negative rates for anomaly scanning; erroneous or incomplete diagnoses may be made.

Although the organ system may be correctly diagnosed, the diagnostic accuracy within that system remains suspect. Scott and Renwick (1988), studying cases of urinary tract abnormality notified to the Northern Regional Fetal Abnormality Survey between 1984 and 1986 (unpublished data), found that not only were 22 per cent of notified cases normal on postnatal examination but that the diagnosis in those in whom uropathy was confirmed postnatally was inaccurate in 33 of 74 perinatal survivors.

Even in very skilled hands, the false-negative rate for major cardiac abnormalities in a referral population was 8.5 per cent (Crawford, Chita and Allan, 1988), although the false-positive rate was only 1.3 per cent. Our own data for anterior abdominal wall defects demonstrates a true false-positive diagnosis rate of 5 per cent and in those confirmed postnatally the category of diagnosis was incorrect in 15 per cent (Walkinshaw *et al.*, in press). As the prognosis of gastroschisis and exomphalos are markedly different, erroneous diagnosis may have important clinical implications.

When counselling couples where a fetal anomaly is suspected, great care is required where it is known that there is risk of false-positive or imprecise diagnoses.

Natural history of fetal abnormalities

Before offering advice following a diagnosis of fetal abnormality, it is necessary to understand what the course of that condition is likely to be. In the initial stages of prenatal diagnosis, understanding of the progression of these abnormalities relied heavily upon the paediatric literature. However, it is now clear that abnormalities diagnosed prenatally may represent a different group from those surviving and presenting to paediatricians.

It has been suggested that, for some abnormalities, the outlook is poorer in those diagnosed before delivery than for those not detected. The most compelling evidence for this is in the case of diaphragmatic hernia. Adzick *et al.* (1985) demonstrated that only 20 per cent of prenatally diagnosed cases survived, in comparison with the figure normally quoted from the paediatric surgical literature of 50 per cent. Our own experience with this condition supports this observation. Cardiac defects diagnosed prenatally also appear to have a poor prognosis (Crawford, Chita and Allan, 1988), as these are a selected group of severe defects. It is not known whether prenatally diagnosed isolated hydrocephaly has a poorer long-term outcome than the conditions detected in the neonatal period. Definitive advice is therefore not always possible even after wide consultation.

It is not clear whether this apparently poor prognosis for antenatal diagnosis represents a phase in prenatal diagnosis, i.e. that we are currently diagnosing only severe abnormalities and that, as the rate of prenatal diagnosis improves, then apparent prognosis will improve.

Associated abnormality

Abnormalities are rarely isolated. The findings of a particular anomaly on scan, particularly during routine screening, should result in further specific assessment, either locally or if necessary in a unit with expertise in fetal medicine. Detailed knowledge of the literature is required for such examinations and such specialists as paediatricians and clinical geneticists may be invaluable. The commonest problem is that of associated chromosomal risk. Information on the precise risk for many abnormalities is incomplete or reflects the experience of tertiary centres.

Specific abnormalities such as non-immune hydrops, duodenal atresia, cysts of the posterior cranial fossa, cystic hygromas, and holoprosencephaly have well-recognized associations with autosomal trisomy and X monosomy. Exomphalos but not gastroschisis is associated with trisomy 13 and 18, with 18 per cent being affected (unpublished data). It is now clear that cardiac lesions diagnosed prenatally have a very marked association with autosomal trisomy (Crawford, Chita and Allan, 1988). Figure 9.16 shows a neonate with trisomy 13 diagnosed prenatally using percutaneous umbilical cord sampling following the identification of cardiac abnormalities in a small-for-gestational-age fetus. The cardiac anomaly itself would have been potentially operable, but the diagnosis of trisomy fundamentally altered the subsequent management of the pregnancy.

Antenatally diagnosed diaphragmatic hernia (Adzick *et al.*, 1985) and renal tract anomalies (Rodeck and Nicolaides, 1983) may also carry an increased risk of abnormality. Of more concern is the finding that the choroid plexus cyst previously considered benign, when persistent beyond 22 weeks, can be associated with trisomy (Chitkara *et al.*, 1988).

It is clear that, in the diagnosis of many anomalies, careful consideration must be given to cytogenetic analysis. The timing of diagnosis and the effect that such a diagnosis will have upon the obstetric management will largely determine the method by which samples are obtained, but access to all methods will be required.

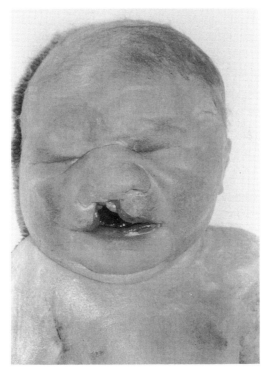

Figure 9.16.   Facial appearance of a neonate with trisomy 13. Prenatal diagnosis was made by percutaneous fetal cord blood sampling prompted by the finding of a major cardiac malformation in a small-for-gestational-age fetus at 34 weeks' gestation

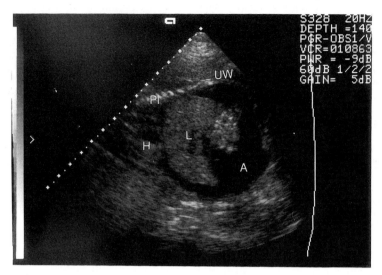

Figure 9.17. Sonogram of fetus at 19 weeks' gestation. There is oligohydramnios, hydrothorax and ascites. These findings persisted until 22 weeks and investigations were all normal. By 28 weeks the fetus was anatomically normal with normal liquor volume. A normal infant was delivered at term. (UW, uterine wall; Pl, pleural fluid; H, heart; L, liver; A, ascites)

Care must be taken not to subject the mother to unnecessary invasive procedures if the information is going to result in no change of management.

Termination of pregnancy

Views on prognosis in prenatal diagnosis are intimately bound up with perceptions of what is a lethal abnormality or one that would lead to severe handicap. This has led to prenatal diagnosis being regarded as a tool to identify pregnancies where therapeutic termination should be offered: the 'seek and destroy' approach.

There are many diagnoses where there is little doubt that therapeutic termination is a reasonable management: anencephaly, left heart hypoplasia, severe bilateral renal cystic dysplasia, severe generalized lymphangiectasia, holoprosencephaly, trisomies 13 and 18, than tophoric skeletal dysplasia are examples. However, there are many instances where the prognosis is less certain. Figure 9.17 shows the ultrasound appearances of massive ascites and oligohydramnios in a fetus of 20 weeks' gestation. All investigations, including karyotype analysis, were normal. On the basis of the persistent ultrasound findings, in particular severe oligohydramnios at this gestation, therapeutic termination was offered to the couple: they declined. On ultrasound examination 8 weeks later, the fetus was normal, with normal liquor volume. Subsequently a normal baby was delivered, with no apparent structural or developmental problems to date.

Conservative management may, however, also lead to problems. Figure 9.18a shows the initial scan of the femur on a fetus referred with the suspicion of lethal skeletal dysplasia, appearing to confirm the diagnosis. A definitive diagnosis could not be made on radiological grounds alone and the pregnancy continued. At birth the femora were adjudged clinically to be normal, although radiography (Figure 9.18b) shows the slight residual angulation of femoral shafts and the epimetaphyseal

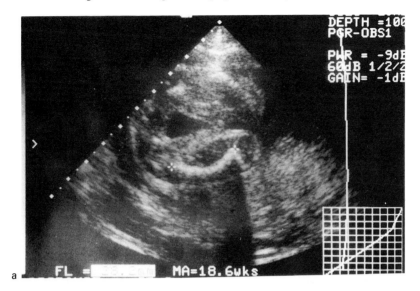

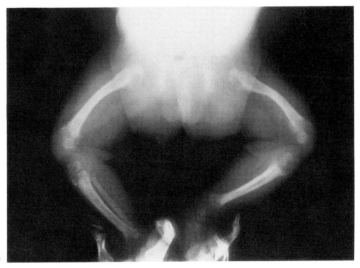

Figure 9.18. (a) Acute angulation of the femur was identified on routine scanning in the second trimester; the parents decided to proceed with the pregnancy. On subsequent scanning the femora became progressively straighter with the result that at birth the mild angulation seen radiographically (b) was not recognized clinically. The epimetaphyseal changes are the result of the underlying disorder, autosomal dominant hypophosphatasia. The mother and two male sibs showed minor features of this variable disorder

changes of hypophosphatasia. In contrast, Figure 9.19 shows the ultrasound findings in a fetus at 20 and 30 weeks' gestation in a family at risk of infantile polycystic disease. The difficulties in making a clear-cut diagnosis in this condition are well described (Luthy and Hirsch, 1985). In this case, the findings at 20 weeks were inconclusive, and the consensus advice from the multidisciplinary team was to continue the pregnancy; by 30 weeks the diagnosis was clear and the pregnancy ended in a neonatal death.

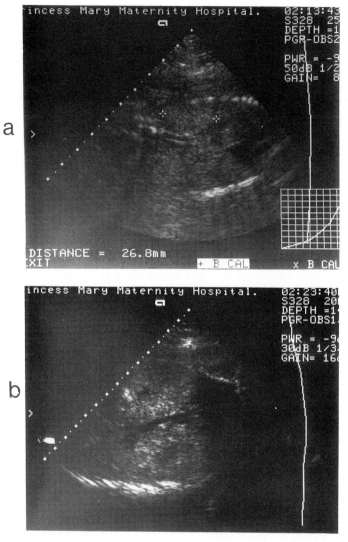

Figure 9.19.   (a) Sonogram of fetus at 19 weeks at risk of infantile polycystic disease. The right kidney is shown in longitudinal section. Renal length is normal although there is a slight increase in echogenicity. Liquor volume is marginally reduced; (b) the same fetus at 28 weeks. Both kidneys are markedly enlarged with marked echogenicity characteristic of infantile polycystic disease

These cases remind us that termination of pregnancy is not the automatic answer to the diagnosis of abnormality and that sensitive and informed counselling is required. Couples must understand the uncertainties and have realistic hopes and expectations. Similarly, ill-informed advice may result in termination for potentially salvageable babies. Examining anterior abdominal wall defects diagnosed between 1984 and 1988, we identified two cases of exomphalos without associated abnormality and one of gastroschisis where therapeutic termination was carried out on the grounds of fetal abnormality.

Increasingly, many couples have opted to continue pregnancies in the face of severe defects, resulting in either intrauterine death or early neonatal death. Many have expressed the view that they found it easier to cope with grief having seen and held their child. The psychological effects of termination for an abnormal fetus should not be underestimated, and parental peace of mind should not be sacrificed on the altar of perinatal mortality statistics. Given some of the uncertainties of diagnostic accuracy and natural history, it may be more appropriate to support couples through these pregnancies. This approach is most easily sustained in cases of lethal malformation. For many couples the major fear is of a surviving child with severe handicap and yet many commentators would argue that therapeutic termination is most easily justified in cases of lethal anomaly.

Treatment of fetal abnormality

Surgical treatment

With the increasing diagnosis of abnormalities correctable postnatally, attention has been directed to the potential of surgery *in utero*. The main candidates for such therapy are fetuses with anomalies involving abnormal collections of fluid amenable to drainage or continuous shunting, such as obstructive uropathy, hydrocephalus, hydrothorax, ascites and pericardial effusion. These techniques and the indications for their use remain experimental and controversial.

Selection of appropriate cases remains the key. Other major structural abnormalities and karyotypic abnormalities are very common in all of these conditions (Chervenak *et al.*, 1985; Reuss *et al.*, 1988; Rodeck *et al.*, 1988) and intervention in the presence of other major anomalies may be contraindicated. Detailed examination and karyotyping are mandatory before considering fetal therapy.

Animal experimental work (Flake and Harrison, 1989) has established that fetal shunting procedures can be effective. However, results from human fetal shunt procedures remain disappointing (Manning *et al.*, 1986). This is attributable in part to the presence of other undiagnosed anomalies (Chervenak *et al.*, 1985) and in part to the dearth of information on the natural history of these abnormalities.

HYDROCEPHALUS

Experience to date suggests that shunting *in utero* for isolated fetal ventriculomegaly offers no clear benefit to the fetus (Manning *et al.*, 1986). Although more infants survive, more of them have major handicaps. It is likely that there will be fetuses who would benefit from intrauterine shunting but it has not been possible so far to identify these accurately. Much more information is required on the long-term outcome of isolated fetal ventriculomegaly.

OBSTRUCTIVE UROPATHY

This remains one of the most controversial areas of fetal medicine. Data from the International Fetal Surgery Register (Manning *et al.*, 1986) has suggested that intrauterine shunting may be of value, especially in fetuses with posterior urethral valves. Other groups have reported equally good outcomes in untreated fetuses (Reuss *et al.*, 1988). The development of aggressive neonatal treatment of renal failure with early neonatal renal transplantation has brought the conflict between the 'invasive' and 'expectant' groups into sharp relief. Although intrauterine shunting may prevent pulmonary hypoplasia by restoration of normal amniotic fluid volume, this does not necessarily mean that renal function will be normal. The last three cases of fetuses who underwent intrauterine shunting procedures after referral from our region demonstrate the difficulties. All survived the neonatal period but all developed severe renal failure during that time: one has subsequently died, one has had a renal transplant and one is maintained on multiple drug therapy; whether this constitutes success is debatable.

Current investigation attempts to determine more accurately which fetuses might benefit from treatment *in utero*. It would appear that obstructive uropathy and severe oligohydramnios diagnosed before 20 weeks' gestation carry a very poor prognosis (Harrison *et al.*, 1982). Ultrasound renal appearances of increased echogenicity or cortical cysts have poor prognostic significance (Mahoney *et al.*, 1984). Fetal urine production can be measured by bladder assessment (McFadyen, Wigglesworth and Dillon, 1983; Mahoney *et al.*, 1984), or assessment of amniotic fluid accumulation following placement of shunts, the absence of re-accumulation being a grave sign. Biochemical assessment of urine offers the best possibility, with loss of concentrating ability, reflected by high urinary sodium, being indicative of severe renal compromise (Gollbus *et al.*, 1985; Nicolaides and Rodeck, 1985); unfortunately, low urinary sodium does not necessarily indicate good renal function (Wilkins *et al.*, 1987). Serial sampling may select fetuses with deteriorating function who may benefit from early intervention. However, even ultrasound appearances that would be regarded as favourable i.e. reasonable renal tissue and liquor volume within normal limits, do not guarantee a good outcome. The fetus in Figure 9.20, delivered at 38 weeks' gestation following conservative management, required dialysis from day 2.

The current view in the UK is clearly shifting towards conservative management (White, 1989). Ultimately, only a well-designed trial of fetal surgery versus active paediatric management is likely to answer the question of whether intervention *in utero* is of benefit.

HYDROTHORAX

Fetal hydrothorax, isolated or in association with fetal hydrops, carries a poor prognosis due largely to intrathoracic compression of the developing lung resulting in pulmonary hypoplasia (Castillo *et al.*, 1987). Repeated aspiration and intrauterine pleuro–amniotic shunts have been utilized in the treatment of this abnormality (Rodeck *et al.*, 1988). These pregnancies require detailed investigation including karyotyping, especially in the presence of hydrops. Spontaneous resolution of isolated hydrothorax can occur.

medical therapy

Currently, only a few abnormalities can be treated by medical means, the commonest being hydrops secondary to fetal tachyarrhythmias (Maxwell *et al.*, 1988). Structural heart disease must be excluded by fetal echocardiography. Digoxin remains the drug of first choice, although other antiarrhythmic agents have been used in refractory cases (Wladimiroff, Stewart and Reuss, 1989). The prognosis is largely dependent upon the gestation at diagnosis and the degree of associated hydrops and hydramnios. Treatment in the absence of effusions may not be indicated, especially as spontaneous resolution can occur (Figure 9.21).

Other medical treatments include maternal dexamethasone treatment to prevent virilization in congenital adrenal hyperplasia (White, New and Dupont 1987), transfusion of fetuses with non-immune hydrops (Nicolaides *et al.*, 1985), and platelet infusion in allo-immune thrombocytopenia (Daffos *et al.*, 1988). There have also been anecdotal reports of treatment *in utero* of metabolic disorders. The most promising new development in fetal medical treatment is that of fetal bone marrow transplant for immune deficiency syndromes and storage disorders (Chueh and Golbus, 1989).

Delivery: where, when and how?

Where?

Having identified and investigated a potentially treatable abnormality, the question arises as to where best to deliver the abnormal child. Considerable stress has already been generated by the diagnosis and it is important not to accentuate this by unnecessary transfer of care to central units.

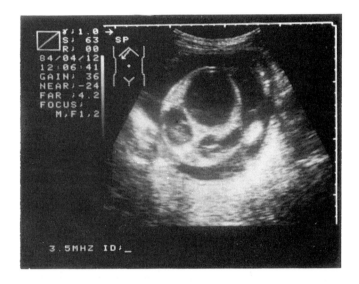

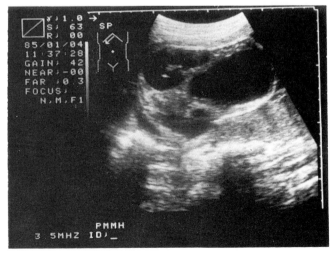

Figure 9.20. Sonograms of a fetus at 30 weeks' gestation: there is megacystis with bilateral hydronephrosis; liquor volume is normal; following delivery dialysis was required

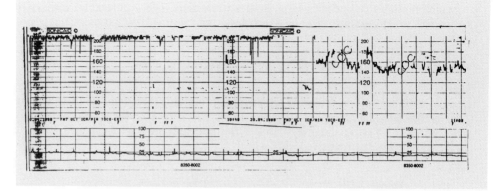

Figure 9.21. Antenatal fetal heart recording in a fetus at 32 weeks' gestation with supraventricular tachycardia. The heart was structurally normal and no hydrops was evident. During this particular recording spontaneous resolution occurred, the fetus remaining in normal rhythm thereafter

The main category of fetuses who may benefit from transfer *in utero* are those where (1) immediate surgery is required, e.g. anterior wall defects, intrathoracic space-occupying lesions, tumours, or (2) neonatal intensive care is required, e.g. hydrops, the fetus at risk of pulmonary hypoplasia, duct-dependent cardiac lesions. Most other abnormalities, unless being delivered prematurely, rarely need immediate intensive management, e.g. most cardiac lesions, unilateral hydronephrosis, and hydrocephalus. Delivery should therefore take place locally, with close liaison with the regional neonatal, paediatric, cardiological and surgical units about the timing of postnatal transfer.

When?

Many of these defects require the expertise of a number of specialists and the availability of intensive care facilities. It should be the responsibility of the multidisciplinary team to coordinate the timing of delivery so that all necessary personnel are available. This will mean that in many of these pregnancies, labour will be induced on a set day, for example to link with a neonatal surgical operating session.

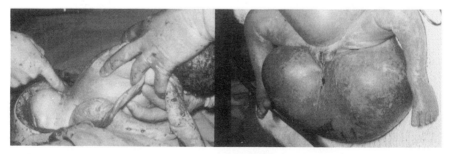

Figure 9.22. Delivery by elective caesarean section at 34 weeks of a fetus with a large sacrococcygeal teratoma, initially detected at 18 weeks' gestation. Delivery was precipitated by reduction in the fetal growth velocity and the rapidly increasing size of the tumour

Few abnormalities benefit from premature delivery, worsening non-immune hydrops, some fetal tumours and hydrocephalus being the most common exceptions. Figure 9.22 shows the delivery of a fetus at 35 weeks' gestation with a massive sacrococcygeal teratoma, delivered in view of impaired fetal growth and increasing polyhydramnios. Discussion within a fetal medicine team should lay the ground rules for timing of delivery for the commoner abnormalities.

How?
There is little evidence to suggest that abdominal delivery is indicated for fetal abnormality alone. Exceptions to this are teratomas, which may be traumatized leading to haemorrhage during delivery, and hydrocephalaus, where vaginal delivery may not be feasible. Under some circumstances, hydropic fetuses or those where the abdomen is markedly distended (as in meconium perforation) abdominal delivery may be safer. There is not convincing evidence that abdominal delivery is needed for fetuses with anterior abdominal wall defects.

AUDIT AND COUNSELLING

Audit

Following delivery, stillbirth or termination, it is vital that the prenatal diagnosis is confirmed. Consent for pathological examination should be sought in all cases and where consent is refused, permission for limited system examination or postmortem radiological examination should be explored. These examinations should be carried out by the regional perinatal pathologist. Diagnosis and counselling are meaningless unless accurate. In surviving babies, confirmation by radiology, clinical examination or surgery will be obtained.

It is also vital that this information is fed back to the prenatal diagnostic group in order that they may audit the diagnosis and advice given for that pregnancy. Any group involved in the diagnosis of fetal abnormality should have an easily accessed index system, preferably computerized, into which prenatal findings, investigations, counselling information, outcome and postnatal or postmortem findings can be entered. Ready access to ultrasound photography and/or videotapes of all suspected anomalies should exist for review. Ideally, regular audit meetings of such a group should be held in order to review current developments in each field, to review ultimate diagnoses and to consider alterations in policies in the light of continuing experience.

It is of equal importance that such information is fed back to the referring units and that new developments or management plans are communicated to referring consultants.

Post-delivery counselling

Following delivery of a fetus or child with an abnormality and full assessment and confirmation of the diagnosis, couples will require considerable support.

Whatever the outcome, firm arrangements must be in hand for long-term counselling. The nature of this, and the most appropriate person to carry out this counselling, will vary, depending on the abnormality, the outcome and the future implications. In units developing fetal medicine expertise within a multidisciplinary group, discussion about the most appropriate counsellor for each case can be decided in advance, avoiding multiple follow-up apapointments for different specialities.

Conclusion

Fetal abnormalities have, in recent years, assumed a major status as a cause of preventable or avoidable morbidity and mortality. Their sensible and sensitive management will pose a major challenge for many years to come.

References

Adzick, NS, Harrison, MR, Glock, PL *et al*. (1985) Diaphragmatic hernia in the fetus: prenatal diagnosis and outcome in 94 cases. *Journal of Paediatric Surgery*, **20**, 357–362

Allan, LD, Tynan, MJ, Campbell, S *et al*. (1986) Echocardiographic and anatomical correlates in the fetus. *British Heart Journal*, **44**, 444–451

Bogart, MH, Pandian, MR and Jones, DW (1987) Abnormal maternal serum chorionic gonadotrophin levels with fetal chromosome abnormalities. *Prenatal Diagnosis*, **7**, 623–630

Brenner, WE, Bruce, RD and Hendricks, CH (1974) The characteristics and perils of breech presentation. *American Journal of Obstetrics and Gynecology*, **118**, 700–712

Bryan, E, Little, J and Burn, J (1987) Congenital anomalaies in twins. *Clinical Obstetrics and Gynaecology*, **1**, 697–721

Burn, J (1987) The aetiology of congenital heart disease. In *Paediatric Cardiology* (edited by RH Anderson, FJ Macartney, EA Shinebourne and M Tynan) pp. 15–37. Edinburgh: Churchill Livingstone

Carstairs, V and Cole, S (1984) Spina bifida and anencephaly in Scotland. *British Medical Journal*, **289**, 1182–1184

Carter, CD, Evans, K and Pescia, G (1979) A family study of renal agenesis. *Journal of Medical Genetics*, **16**, 176–188

Castillo, RA, Devoe, LD, Falls, G *et al.*, (1987) Pleural effusions and pulmonary hypoplasia. *American Journal of Obstetrics and Gynecology*, **157**, 1252–1255

Chamberlain, PF, Manning, FA and Morrison, I (1984) Ultrasound evaluation of amniotic fluid volume. II The relationship of increased amniotic fluid volume to perinatal outcome. *American Journal of Obstetrics and Gynecology*, **150**, 250–258

Chavez, GF, Mulinare, JM and Cordero, JS (1989) Maternal cocaine use during early pregnancy as a risk factor for congenital urogenital anomalies. *Journal of the American Medical Association*, **262**, 795–798

Chervenak, FA, Berkowitz, RL, Tortora, M *et al.* (1985) The management of fetal hydrocephalus. *American Journal of Obstetrics and Gynecology*, **151**, 933–942

Chitkara, U, Congwell, C, Norton, J *et al.* (1988) Choroid plexus cysts in the fetus a benign anatomic variant or pathologic entity? Report of 41 cases and review of the literature. *Obstetrics and Gynecology*, **72**, 185–189

Chueh, J and Golbus, MS (1989) Diagnosis and management of the abnormal fetus. *Fetal Medicine Review*, **1**, 61–78

Cook, JP and Young, ID (1986) Second trimester chorionic villus (placental) biopsy. *Lancet*, **i**, 969

Cousins, L (1983) Congenital anomalies among infants of diabetic mothers: etiology, prevention, prenatal diagnosis. *American Journal of Obstetrics and Gynecology*, **147**, 333–338

Crane, JJP, Bever, HA and Cheung, SW (1985) Antenatal ultrasound findings in fetal triploidy syndrome. *Journal of Ultrasound in Medicine*, **4**, 519–524

Crawford, DC, Chita, SK and Allan, LD (1988) Prenatal detection of congenital heart disease: factors affecting obstetric management and survival. *American Journal of Obstetrics and Gynecology*, **159**, 352–356

Cuckle, HS, Wald, NJ and Thompson, SG (1987) Estimating a woman's risk of having pregnancy associated with Down's syndrome using her age and maternal serum alpha-fetoprotein level. *British Journal of Obstetrics and Gynaecology*, **94**, 387–402

Daffos, F., Capella-Pavlovsky, M and Forestier, F (1985) Fetal blood sampling during pregnancy with the use of a needle guided by ultrasound: a study of 606 consecutive cases. *American Journal of Obstetrics and Gynecology*, **153**, 655–660

Daffos, F, Forestier, F, Kaplan, C and Cox, W (1988) Prenatal diagnosis and management of bleeding disorders with fetal blood sampling. *American Journal of Obstetrics and Gynecology*, **158**, 939–946

David, TJ and Illingworth, CA (1976) Diaphragmatic hernia in the South-West of England. *Journal of Medical Genetics*, **13**, 253–262

Ferguson-Smith, MA and Yates, JRW (1984) Maternal age specific rates for chromosome aberrations and factors influencing them: report of a collaborative European study on 52,965 amniocenteses. *Prenatal Diagnosis*, **4**, 5–44

Flake, AW and Harrison, MR (1989) Experimental malformations and their correction. In *Fetal Medicine 1* (edited by C. Rodeck) pp. 90–117. Oxford: Blackwell

Fuhrmann, K., Reiher, H, Semmler, K and Glockner, E (1984) The effect of intensified conventional insulin therapy before and during pregnancy on the malformation rate in offspring of diabetic mothers. *Experimental Clinical Endocrinology*, **83**, 173–177

Golbus, MS, Filly, RA, Callen, P *et al.* (1985) Fetal urinary tract obstruction: management and selection for treatment. *Seminars in Perinatology*, **9**, 91–97

Harper, P (1984) In *Practical Genetic Counselling* (edited by P Harper) p. 201. Oxford: Wright

Harrison, MR, Golbus, MS, Filly, RA *et al.* (1982) Management of the fetus with congenital hydronephrosis. *Journal of Paediatric Surgery*, **17**, 728–742

Hashimoto, BE, Mahoney, BS, Filly, RA *et al.* (1985) Sonography, a complementary examination to alphafetoprotein testing for fetal neural tube defect. *Journal of Ultrasound in Medicine*, **4**, 307–310

Hook, EB and Chamber, PK (1983) Chromosome abnormality rates at amniocentesis and in live born infants. *Journal of the American Medical Association*, **249**, 2034–2038

Jackson, L (1988) *CVS Newsletter*, Philadelphia. Feb 1–8

Knox, EC, Stewart, AM, Kneale, GW and Filman, EA (1987) Prenatal irradiation and childhood cancer. *Journal of the Society for Radiological Protection*, **7**, 3–15

Koren, G, Edwards, MB and Miskin, M (1987) Antenatal sonography of fetal malformations associated with drugs and chemicals. A guide. *American Journal of Obstetrics and Gynecology*, **176**, 79–85

Lilford, RJ, Irving, JC, Linton, G and Mason, MK (1987) Transabdominal chorion villus sampling: 100 consecutive cases. *Lancet*, **i**, 1415

Little, J and Bryan, E (1986) Congenital anomalies in twins. *Seminars in Perinatology*, **10**, 50–64

Luthy, DA and Hirsch, JH (1986) Infantile polycystic disease: observations from attempts at prenatal diagnosis. *American Journal of Medical Genetics*, **20**, 505–517

McFadyen, IR, Wigglesworth, JS and Dillon, MJ (1983) Fetal urinary tract obstruction: is active intervention before delivery indicated? *British Journal of Obstetrics and Gynaecology*, **90**, 342–349

Mahoney, BS, Filly, FA, Callen, PW *et al.* (1984) Sonographic evaluation of renal dysplasia. *Radiology*, **152**, 143–146

Manning, FA, Harrison, MR, Rodeck, CH *et al.* (1986) Catheter shunts for fetal hydronephrosis and hydrocephalus. Report of the International Fetal Surgery Registry. *New England Journal of Medicine*, **315**, 336–340

Maxwell, DJ, Crawford, DC, Curry, PV *et al.* (1988) Obstetric importance diagnosis and management of fetal tachycardias. *British Medical Journal*, **287**, 107–110

Members of the Joint Study Group on Fetal Abnormalities (1989) Recognition and management of fetal abnormalities. *Archives of Disease in Childhood*, **64**, 971–976

Miller, E, Hare, JW, Cloherty, JP *et al.* (1981) Elevated maternal haemoglobin A_{1c} in early pregnancy and major congenital abnormalities in infants of diabetic mothers. *New England Journal of Medicine*, **304**, 1331–1334

Nicolaides, KH and Campbell, S (1987) Diagnosis of fetal abnormalities by ultrasound. *Clinical Obstetrics and Gynecology*, **1**, 591–622

Nicolaides, KH and Rodeck, CH (1985) Fetal therapy. In *Progress in Obstetrics and Gynaecology Vol 5* (edited by J. Studd) pp. 40–57. Edinburgh: Churchill Livingstone

Nicolaides, KH, Soothill, PW and Roseavar, SK (1987) Transabdominal placental biopsy. *Lancet*, **ii**, 855

Nicolaides, KH, Rodeck, CH, Lange, I. *et al*. (1985) Fetoscopy in the assessment of unexplained fetal hydrops. *British Journal of Obstetrics and Gynaecology*, **92**, 671–678

Nicolaides, KH, Gabbe, SG, Guidetti, R *et al*. (1986) Ultrasound screening for spina bifida: cranial and cerebellar signs. *Lancet*, **i**, 72

Northern Regional Health Authority *Collaborative Survey of Perinatal, Neonatal and Late Neonatal Deaths in the Northern Region, 1981–1988.*

Peat, D and Brock, DJH (1984) Quantitative estimation of the density ratios of esterase bands in human amniotic fluids. *Clinical Chimica Acta*, **138**, 319–324

Pickworth, J and Burn, J (1988) Late abortion and the law. *British Medical Journal*, **296**, 715

Pijpers, L, Jahoda, MGJ, Wladimiroff, JW *et al*. (1988) Transabdominal chorion villus biopsy in second and third trimesters of pregnancy to determine fetal karyotype. *Lancet*, **ii**, 822–823

Poskitt, EME (1984) Foetal alcohol syndrome. *Alcohol and Alcoholism*, **19**, 159–168

Royal College of General Practitioners (1975) Morbidity and drugs in pregnancy. *Journal of the Royal College of General Practitioners*, **25**, 631–645

Reuss, A, Stewart, PA, Wladimiroff, JW and Scholtmeijer, RJ (1988) Non-invasive management of fetal obstructive uropathy. *Lancet*, **ii**, 949–951

Robertson, L, Ott, A, Mack, L *et al*. (1985) Sonographically documented disappearance of nonimmune hydrops fetalis associated with maternal hypertension. *Western Journal of Medicine*, **143**, 382–386

Rodeck, CH and Nicolaides, KH (1983) Ultrasound guided invasive procedures in obstetrics. *Clinical Obstetrics and Gynecology*, **10**, 515–539

Rodeck, CH, Fisk, NM, Fraser, DI and Nicolini, U (1988) Long-term in utero drainage of fetal hydrothorax. *New England Journal of Medicine*, **319**, 1135–1138

Rottem, S, Bronshtein, M, Thaler, I and Brandes, JM (1989) First trimester transvaginal sonographic diagnosis of fetal anomalies. *Lancet*, **i**, 444–445

Schulze, B and Miller, K (1986) Chromosomal mosaicism and maternal cell contamination in chorionic villi cultures. *Clinical Genetics*, **30**, 239–240

Scott, JES and Renwick, M (1988) Antenatal diagnosis of congenital abnormalities in the urinary tract. Results from the Northern Region Fetal Abnormality Survey. *British Journal of Urology*, **62**, 295–300

Tabor, A, Masden, M, Obel, EB *et al*. (1986) Randomized controlled trial of genetic amniocentesis in 4606 low risk women. *Lancet*, **ii**, 1287–1293

Taylor, PV, Scott, JS, Gerlis, LM, Esscher, E and Scott, O (1986) Maternal antibodies against fetal cardiac antigens in congenital complete heart block. *New England Journal of Medicine*, **315**, 667–672

Trudinger, BJ and Cook, CM (1985) Umbilical and uterine arterial flow velocity waveforms in pregnancies associated with major fetal abnormality. *British Journal of Obstetrics and Gynaecology*, **92**, 666–670

Wald, NJ and Cuckle, HS (1984) Open neural tube defects. In *Antenatal and Neonatal Screening for Disease* (edited by NJ Wald) pp. 25–73. Oxford: Oxford University Press

Wald, NJ and Cuckle, HS (1987) Recent advances in screening for neural tube defects and Down's syndrome. *Clinical Obstetrics and Gynecology* **1**, 649–676

Wald, NJ, Cuckle, HS, Densen, JW *et al*. (1988a) Maternal serum unconjugated oestriol as an antenatal screening test for Down's syndrome. *British Journal of Obstetrics and Gynaecology*, **95**, 334–341

Wald, NJ, Cuckle, HS, Densen, JW *et al*. (1988b) Maternal serum screening for Down's syndrome in early pregnancy. *British Medical Journal*, **297**, 883–887

Walkinshaw, SA, Renwick, M, Hehisch, G and Hey, EN (1991) How good is ultrasound in the detection and evaluation of anterior abdominal wall defects? *British Journal of Radiology*, in press

Warren, J, Evans, K and Carter, CO (1980) Offspring of patients with tracheo-oesophageal fistula. *Journal of Medical Genetics*, **16**, 338–340

White, I., Papiha, SS and Magnay, D (1989) Improving methods of screening for Down's syndrome. *New England Journal of Medicine*, **320**, 401–402

White, PC, New, MI and Dupont, B (1987) Congenital adrenal hyperplasia. *New England Journal of Medicine*, **316**, (i) 1519–1525; (ii) 1580–1586

White, RHR (1989) Fetal uropathy. Conservative management is best. *British Medical Journal*, **298**, 1408–1409

Whittle, MJ (1989) Cordocentesis. *British Journal of Obstetrics and Gynaecology*, **96**, 262–264

Wilkins, IA, Chitkara, U, Lynch, L *et al.* (1987) The nonpredictive value of fetal urinary electrolytes: preliminary report of outcomes and correlations with pathologic diagnosis. *American Journal of Obstetrics and Gynecology*, **157**, 694–698

Winter, RM, Baraitser, M and Douglas, T (1984) A computerized data base for the diagnosis of rare dysmorphic syndromes. *Journal of Medical Genetics*, **21**, 121–123

Wladimiroff, JW, Stewart, PA and Reuss, A (1989) Medical treatment of the fetus. In *Fetal Medicine 1* (edited by CH Rodeck) pp. 154–176. Oxford: Blackwell

Zuckerman, B, Frank, DA, Hingson, R *et al.* (1989) Effect of maternal marijuana and cocaine use on fetal growth. *New England Journal of Medicine*, **320**, 762–768

Chapter 10

Prematurity

HL Halliday

Introduction

Prematurity remains one of the world's major health problems. Mary Ellen Avery from Boston has said that of the 11×10^6 premature babies born each year throughout the world, only 1×10^6 survive. Mortality rates in developing countries are much greater than those in the developed world, because of malnutrition, infection, economic factors and limited medical services (Joseph, 1989). These factors are also associated with intrauterine growth retardation so that, world wide, there were about 21×10^6 low-birthweight (<2500 g) babies born in 1979, representing an overall incidence of 17 per cent of all births that year. Those born in developing countries make up >90 per cent of the total (World Health Organization, 1980). There is a close link between improvement in infant mortality rates and the ratio of government expenditure on health and defence: as the ratio increases in favour of defence spending, the improvement in infant mortality declines (Joseph, 1989).

Surviving premature infants may suffer respiratory and neurological disabilities with recurrent illness throughout childhood. The aetiology of prematurity is diverse, with prenatal and perinatal factors often determining the eventual outcome for the baby. Management plans should be tailored to suit individual women with premature delivery, taking into account mortality and morbidity risks and being aware of the ethical dilemmas that arise in assessment of cost:benefit ratio for the very premature baby.

Definitions

Until quite recently, *prematurity* was defined as a baby whose birthweight was <2501 g. This definition was based upon the facts that birthweight was the most frequently and reliably recorded measurement at birth and that outcome was closely related to size. Babies of <2501 g are now termed *low birthweight* (LBW) and form a heterogeneous group containing both preterm and growth-retarded babies, who have different neonatal problems and long-term outcomes.

A *preterm* baby is one who is born following a pregnancy of <259 days (37 completed weeks) (World Health Organization, 1977). WHO recommends calculating gestational age in days from the start of the last menstrual period but a potential drawback is the overestimation of gestational age if the menstrual cycle is irregular or there is post-pill amenorrhoea (Hall *et al.*, 1985). If the gestational age is overestimated, the incidence of preterm birth will be underestimated. Gestational age assessment should be based upon the best clinical estimate, which may involve maternal history, ultrasound scanning and neonatal examination.

This classification, which separates preterm and low birthweight, is not completely satisfactory in that it involves two distinct cut-off points, namely gestation and weight, which do not delineate major steps in physiological maturation or fetal survival. Indeed, in Sweden about one-half of all preterm babies weigh >2500 g and are therefore not low birthweight (Ericson *et al.*, 1984). These appropriately grown, slightly immature babies have only minor problems in the neonatal period and show no increase in mortality. The definition of a preterm baby thus spans a wide range from 22 weeks (equivalent to a birthweight of 500 g) to 36 weeks (2500 g) with vast differences in early neonatal problems and long-term outcome.

More recently, definitions have been developed to take into account the improved survival of very small preterm babies and to separate them into groups. *Very low birthweight* (VLBW) babies are defined as those weighing ≤1500 g at birth and *extremely low birthweight* (ELBW) as ≤1000 g. Others have defined the *very immature* infant as one born before 28 weeks of gestation (Macfarlane *et al.*, 1988).

Growth retardation must also be taken into account and this means that birthweight should be related to gestational age by means of appropriate growth charts (Keen and Pearse, 1985; Lucas, Cole and Gandy, 1986) that have been derived from relatively uncomplicated pregnancies (Figure 10.1). *Small for gestational age* (SGA) can be defined as a birthweight below the 10th centile (sometimes the 3rd or even the 5th centile) for gestational age, and *large for gestational age* as birthweight above the 90th centile for gestational age. Assessment of abnormal growth is much easier after birth than prenatally despite improved techniques of ultrasound imaging and the development of mathematical models to predict fetal growth (Deter *et al.*, 1986).

Incidence

In developed countries, the incidence of low birthweight is between 3 and 7 per cent (Villar and Belizan, 1982). Developing countries have an incidence of low birthweight about four times higher than those of developed countries, ranging from 10 to 43 per cent (Villar and Belizan, 1982). Growth retardation accounts for about 50 per cent of low birthweight in developed countries compared with more than 75 per cent in developing countries. When the incidence of low birthweight is >10 per cent, as it is in nearly all developing countries, the excess is almost entirely due to growth-retarded babies. The proportion of preterm babies is constant in most countries at about 5–7 per cent, with any excess of low birthweight due to growth-retarded babies at term.

In developed countries, very-low-birthweight babies account for about 1 per cent of births. In the UK in 1983, 1.3 per cent of all births in the Northern Region of England were between 24 and 31 weeks' gestation (Wariyar, Richmond and Hey, 1989). In the USA in 1979, babies of under 28 weeks' gestation accounted for 0.6 per cent of all live births, and those of 28–32 weeks for 1.0 per cent (van den Berg and Oeschli, 1984).

Preterm birth rates have fallen in Haguenau (France) from 8.2 per cent in 1972 to 5.6 per cent in 1981 (Papiernik *et al.*, 1985) and in Aberdeen from 9.3 per cent in 1951–1955 to 6.8 per cent in 1976–1980 (Hall, 1985), but other regions have shown little change. For very immature babies with gestational ages <28 weeks, however,

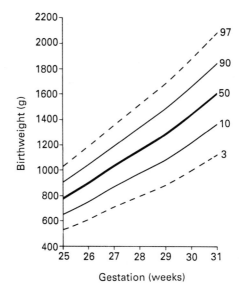

Figure 10.1. Birthweight percentiles for babies of gestational ages 25–31 weeks

there has been an increase in incidence over the past decade to 0.26 per cent, which probably reflects increased reporting (Macfarlane *et al.*, 1988) but may be associated with increased use of assisted fertilization (Lancaster, 1986): this author found a 24 per cent rate of preterm delivery after fertilization *in vitro*.

Epidemiology

Four circumstances may lead to the birth of a preterm baby (Rush *et al.*, 1976; Halliday, 1988; Wariyar, Richmond and Hey, 1989): these are uncomplicated spontaneous preterm labour, premature rupture of the membranes, complicated emergency delivery and elective preterm delivery (Table 10.1) (Ritchie and McClure, 1979).

Table 10.1.   Studies showing factors associated with preterm delivery

Source	Rush *et al.*, 1976	Halliday, 1988	Wariyar, Richmond and Hey, 1989
Place	Oxford	Belfast	Northern Region of England
Years of study	1973–1974	1981–1985	1983
Type of study	Hospital	Hospital	Regional
Criteria	<37 weeks	<1500 g	23–31 weeks
Numbers of liveborn	429	423	267
Distribution (%)			
Uncomplicated			
Spontaneous	38[a]	28	40
Premature rupture of membranes	?	21	18
Complicated emergency	24	23	26
Elective delivery	28	28	16
Total	90[a]	100	100

[a]10% multiple pregnancy

Complications preceding emergency delivery are placental abruption, maternal infection, rhesus isoimmunization, eclampsia and prolapsed cord, whereas elective preterm delivery is usually the result of severe pre-eclampsia, maternal renal disease or intrauterine growth retardation. Spontaneous preterm labour accounts for 28–40 per cent of preterm births, with the lower figure in the more selected hospital-based population (Table 10.1). Premature rupture of the membranes is an antecedent in about 20 per cent of preterm labours, and complicated or emergency deliveries occur in about 25 per cent of cases. The rate of elective preterm delivery was 16 per cent in the Northern Regional Study (Wariyar, Richmond and Hey, 1989) and 28 per cent in both the Belfast hospital (Halliday, 1988) and the Oxford hospital studies (Rush *et al.*, 1976).

Outcome is determined by both gestational age and the circumstances which precipitated preterm delivery rather than the mode of delivery (Halliday, 1988; Wariyar, Richmond and Hey, 1989) (Table 10.2). Babies born after elective delivery have the best outcome and lowest handicap rates (most intact survivors). There are a number of reasons for this, including more advanced gestation, experienced and well-prepared resuscitation team, increased use of antenatal corticosteroids and proximity of intensive care facilities. The selected hospital-based population with elective preterm delivery has the best outcome for these reasons. The poorest outcome is found in the groups with uncomplicated spontaneous preterm labour and complicated emergency delivery for different reasons. The spontaneous preterm labour group are of lower gestational age, and the complicated group, following antepartum haemorrhage, eclampsia or rhesus isoimmunization, are more likely to be in poor condition at birth (Halliday, 1988). The outcome for the group with premature rupture of the membranes appeared better in the hospital study than in the regional study but, once infection occurred, the Belfast babies were classed as complicated and labour was induced or accelerated on this account (Halliday, 1988). Provided that the duration of membrane rupture is short (48 h to 7 days) maturation of the fetal lungs may occur (Worthington, Maloney and Smith, 1977; Wennergren *et al.*, 1986) rather than pulmonary hypoplasia, which is associated with membrane rupture before 20 weeks' gestation (Wigglesworth, Desai and Guerrini, 1981). The distinction between spontaneous, complicated and elective preterm delivery is important to enable effective preventive measures to be taken, to allow obstetricians to intervene appropriately and to counsel prospective parents properly.

Physiology and preterm labour

Usually, the initiation of labour is triggered by the fetus when it is sufficiently mature to survive when breathing air (Thorburn, 1986). A number of trigger mechanisms for the initiation of labour have been proposed, including a shift in the balance of oestrogen/progesterone effects towards oestrogen, release of oxytocin and increased uterine synthesis of prostaglandins (Rice, Jenkin and Thorburn, 1987). The actual mechanism in humans is not completely understood, although there does appear to be a common biochemical end-point of an increase in the biosynthesis of prostaglandins (Mitchell, 1984). A full understanding of the mechanisms by which preterm labour may be initiated will only be gained when the mechanism of the onset of labour at term is more fully understood (Bennett and Elder, 1988).

Prostaglandins are probably also important in preterm labour and plasma concentrations in women during preterm labour are higher than those in women of similar

Table 10.2.   Outcome of liveborn preterm babies by antecedents of delivery

Delivery	Rush et al. (Oxford)		Halliday, 1988 (Belfast)		Wariyar, Richmond and Hey, 1989 (Northern Region of England)	
	Survival (%)	Intact Survival	Survival (%)	Intact Survival	Survival (%)	Intact Survival
Uncomplicated spontaneous	92[a]	ND	68	60	67	57
Premature rupture of membranes	?	ND	90	88	62	58
Complicated emergency	90	ND	60	53	68	62
Elective delivery	97	ND	93	91	79	77
Total	92	ND	78	73	68	62

[a] Excludes multiple pregnancies; ND, no data

gestational age who are not in labour (Dubin *et al.*, 1980). Furthermore, prostaglandin synthetase inhibitors are effective in delaying preterm labour (Niebyl, Blake and White, 1980) but they should not be used in clinical practice because of their effects on the ductus arteriosus of the fetus. Prostaglandins are produced by the fetal membranes or decidua but stimuli releasing them have not been established. Bacterial infection of the genital tract is a common antecedent of preterm labour (Minkoff, 1983; Toth *et al.*, 1988); when amnion cells in tissue culture are exposed to bacteria, their output of prostaglandin E increases considerably, with the response varying according to the organism (Lamont, Rose and Elder, 1985). Bacteria possess phospholipase activity (Bejar *et al.*, 1981) and it is likely that release of this enzyme by genital tract pathogens stimulates prostaglandin synthesis in the fetal membranes to initiate preterm labour (Bennett and Elder, 1988). Apart from bacterial infection, such as chorioamnionitis or urinary tract infection, there are other possible triggers for prostaglandin production: these include over-distension of the uterus in polyhydramnios or multiple pregnancy and perhaps distortion of the fetal membranes in cases of cervical incompetence.

Once the mechanism of the onset of labour in humans has become fully understood it may be possible more reliably to predict, and subsequently to prevent, preterm labour.

Prediction of preterm birth

A large number of risk factors associated with preterm delivery have been identified (Table 10.3). Scoring systems have been derived from retrospective analyses of populations using some form of 'weighting' of factors found to correlate best with preterm delivery. These systems must then be tested prospectively in different populations so that they can be validated (Creasy, Gummer and Liggins, 1980). The validity of any scoring system depends upon its sensitivity and specificity (Lumley, 1987): sensitivity is the proportion of women who have been designated as high risk and go on to have a preterm birth. Specificity is the proportion of women having a term birth who were correctly identified as low risk. A scoring system that is not sensitive enough (fails to predict most of the preterm births) can be improved by changing the cut-off point but this will reduce its specificity (more people are labelled as high risk) (Guzick, Daikoku and Kaltreider, 1984). For example, a scoring system set to identify 13 per cent of pregnant women as high risk by the second trimester had a sensitivity of 64 per cent, correctly predicting that proportion of preterm births. When the cut-off point was changed to include 32 per cent of the women as high risk, the sensitivity increased to 80 per cent but the specificity was reduced from 90 to 71 per cent (Creasy, Gummer and Liggins, 1980). Another scoring system which identified 26 per cent of mothers as high risk, predicted 64 per cent of preterm births and 67 per cent of neonatal deaths (Halliday, Jones and Jones, 1980).

Although calculation of the sensitivity and specificity of a scoring system is necessary in order to establish validity, from a practical point of view the positive predictive value of the test is more important: this is the proportion of women in the high-risk group who go on to have a preterm birth. In the study mentioned above this was 30 per cent with the high cut-off point and 15 per cent with the low cut-off point (Creasy, Gummer and Liggins, 1980). The negative predictive value is the proportion of women with a low-risk score who have a term delivery and this was about 98 per cent in both high and low cut-off groups.

Table 10.3. Risk factors associated with preterm delivery

Type	Factors
Maternal	
General	Small stature and low weight
	Diabetes mellitus
	Renal disease
	Chronic hypertension
	Low socioeconomic status
	Smoking and alcohol
	Grand multiparity
	Previous mid-trimester abortion
	Previous preterm labour
	History of infertility
	Use of intrauterine contraceptive device
Current pregnancy	Febrile illness
	Urinary tract infection
	Isoimmunization
	Anaemia
	Pre-eclampsia
	Appendicitis
Uterine anomalies	Congenital uterine malformations
	Uterine fibroids
	Cervical incompetence
Placental and membrane	Polyhydramnios
	Oligohydramnios
	Premature rupture of the membranes
	Chorioamnionitis
	Threatened abortion
	Placental abruption
	Placenta praevia
Fetal	Congenital anomalies
	Multiple pregnancy
Iatrogenic	Elective induction of labour; repeat caesarean section

In general, prediction of preterm delivery is poor for primigravid patients and better for multiparae, in whom studies indicate that it is possible to predict about 75 per cent of preterm births by identifying 15–20 per cent of the population as high risk (Creasy, Gummer and Liggins, 1980). However, the positive predictive value of being high risk, even in multiparae, is low with 85 per cent of these women delivering at term. Repeating the assessment as pregnancy progresses allows complications that develop to be included in the score and improves the predictive value (Hobel, 1982). However, the later the assessment is made, the less the time for intervention. In general, scoring systems are unpopular with obstetricians (Main and Gabbe, 1987), although their use may remind less experienced clinicians to look for and record relevant features of past obstetric and social histories (Hall and Chang, 1982). The educational value of risk scoring systems should not be overlooked, although there is a possible danger of the clinician being falsely reassured by a low score.

Other methods of trying to predict preterm labour include assessment of uterine activity using a tocodynamometer, assessment of the cervix, which is often applied in multiple pregnancies, and ultrasound examination for fetal breathing movements.

Tocodynamometer

This is an instrument that non-invasively monitors uterine activity (Newman et al., 1987) and it has been used to predict the onset of preterm labour in women at high risk. Enthusiasm for this technique, often applied to women in their own homes monitored by telephone, mushroomed in California (Newman et al., 1987) until a randomized controlled trial showed it to be ineffective (Iams et al., 1987). In this prospective study there were no differences in the rate of preterm birth, incidence of preterm labour or mean birthweight, suggesting that the beneficial effects previously attributed to home monitoring of uterine contractions were due to the frequent nurse contact and recognition of early symptoms of preterm labour (Iams et al., 1987).

Cervical assessment

Cervical dilatation in the second and third trimesters is associated with preterm labour: if the internal os is dilated $\geqslant 1$ cm, the risk of preterm labour is increased fourfold (Papiernik et al., 1986); if dilated $\geqslant 2$ cm, then the risk is increased 15-fold (Leveno, Cox and Roark, 1986), but the sensitivity and specificity of this investigation is low, even when combined with standardized risk scoring systems (Main and Gabbe, 1987).

Fetal breathing movements

Women in suspected preterm labour who have absent fetal breathing movements usually progress to delivery within 48 h, whereas those with fetal breathing do not (Castle and Turnbull, 1983), unless the membranes have ruptured or chorioamnionitis is present (Agustsson and Patel, 1987). One study, however, has shown that absence of fetal breathing movements is a reliable indicator of imminent preterm delivery, irrespective of fetal membrane rupture (Besinger, Compton and Hayashi, 1987).

In general, however, none of these methods has gained widespread acceptance because of poor predictive value and the time necessary to screen large populations of women at risk.

Prevention of preterm birth

The difficulties in preventing preterm birth lie in the poor predictability of risk scoring systems and the lack of a reliable test of early preterm labour. Prevention of preterm birth encompasses both prevention of preterm labour and delay or inhibition of preterm labour.

Prevention of preterm labour

Attempts to prevent preterm labour have been made using cervical cerclage, vigilant antenatal care, bed rest, progestogens and tocolytic drugs.

Cervical cerclage
Cervical incompetence is probably an uncommon condition that may arise from trauma to the cervix during labour or at dilatation of the cervix (Dunn, 1976; Lumley, 1986), or after cone biopsy (Jones, Sweetman and Hibbard, 1979). It may

also occur in association with structural uterine abnormalities or as an isolated structural congenital anomaly. The use of cervical cerclage depends upon obstetricians' views of the prevalence of cervical incompetence and this varies from <1/1000 to 80/1000 pregnancies (Grant, Chalmers and Enkin, 1982). Three recent randomized controlled trials of cervical cerclage have shown it to be ineffective in prolonging pregnancy (Dor *et al.*, 1982; Lazar *et al.*, 1984; Rush *et al.*, 1984). A larger trial of 905 pregnant women showed a very modest benefit of cervical cerclage in reducing deliveries before 33 weeks from 18 to 13 per cent (MRC/RCOG Working Party on Cervical Cerclage, 1988). The results of this trial suggest that the operation had a beneficial effect in about 1 in 25 patients, but puerperal pyrexia was twice as common, which is in keeping with a previous study that suggested an increased incidence of chorioamnionitis in treated women (Rush *et al.*, 1984). The subgroup of women with previous early deliveries may benefit the most (MRC/RCOG Working Party, 1988). Women who demonstrate bulging of the membranes through a partially dilated cervical os on ultrasound may be at highest risk and benefit from cervical cerclage (Vaalamo and Kivikoski, 1983) but further studies are needed before clear guidelines can be given.

Antenatal care
Provision of increased antenatal care to women with risk factors formed the basis of the Haguenau perinatal study (Papiernik *et al.*, 1985), which showed a reduction in preterm deliveries during a 12-year period. The reduction was greatest (50 per cent) for births before 34 weeks' gestation but no effect was found in high-risk cases (previous preterm delivery, maternal age <22 years or >35 years, bleeding during pregnancy or no antenatal care by an obstetrician). The Haguenau programme included educating pregnant women about their own risks of preterm delivery, and improvements were more marked in women of lower social class who had fewer years of schooling (Papiernik, Bouyer and Dreyfus, 1985). Studies from France and the USA have shown that antenatal home visiting by nurses and midwives failed to reduce the incidence of preterm birth (Spira *et al.*, 1981; Olds *et al.*, 1986) but, although designed on a randomized basis, these trials were too small to be conclusive.

Bed rest
Bed rest has been included in preterm prevention programmes, particularly in France (Spira *et al.*, 1981; Papiernik, 1984) but this form of treatment is usually reserved for twin pregnancies. Two controlled trials have shown that bed rest in hospital from 29 weeks and 32 weeks respectively for twin pregnancies is ineffective in decreasing preterm deliveries (Hartikainen-Sorri and Jouppila, 1984; Saunders *et al.*, 1985); indeed, these studies from Finland and Zimbabwe suggested that bed rest increased the number of very-low-birthweight babies. Bed rest at home rather than in hospital has not been studied.

Progestogens
The rationale for using progestogens is that they reduce uterine activity, but there is no evidence of progesterone deficiency in human preterm labour. Trials of progesterone in the prevention of preterm labour are unsatisfactory and show conflicting results. It seems unlikely that any significant benefit is derived from the use of progestogens in this situation.

Tocolytic drugs

These drugs, usually β-mimetics, have been used to prevent or to inhibit preterm labour (Keirse, 1984a, b). Prophylactic use has been tested in a randomized trial of multiple pregnancies, showing no difference in duration of gestation or birthweight (Gummerus and Halonen, 1987). Because these drugs have very short half-lives it is unlikely that oral administration would achieve serum levels adequate to be effective in prevention of preterm delivery, even in high-risk groups.

Inhibition of preterm labour

Studies of drugs to inhibit preterm labour are bedevilled by the difficulty in making a diagnosis of preterm labour. The usual definition is of regular, painful uterine contractions associated with progressive cervical dilatation and effacement occurring before 37 completed weeks of gestation (Huddleston, 1982); however, in some women, dilatation of the cervix can occur in the absence of regular painful contractions and not all women with regular contractions go on to deliver in a few days. Absence of fetal breathing movements increases the chances of progressive preterm labour (Castle and Turnbull, 1983; Agustsson and Patel, 1987; Besinger, Compton and Hayashi, 1987).

Studies of tocolytic drugs should always be controlled because >50 per cent of women treated with placebo remain undelivered a week after admission to such trials (Anderson and Turnbull, 1982). Other problems arise with recruitment to these studies, as many women have contraindications to treatment and in others it is not possible to keep either the subject or the obstetrician blind to the treatment group, because of effects such as increase in maternal heart rate. It has been estimated that as few as 10–20 per cent of women presenting in preterm labour are candidates for long-term tocolytic therapy (Spellacy *et al.*, 1979; Creasy and Herron, 1981). It is possible that this figure can be increased by the use of preterm birth-prevention programmes (Herron, Katz and Creasy, 1982; Konte, Creasy and Laros, 1988). This type of programme uses a scoring system to identify women with abnormal past obstetric histories and social problems, who form a high-risk group for preterm labour. They are then educated to recognize the early signs and symptoms of preterm labour, such as palpable uterine contractions, low backache, diarrhoea, abdominal cramps, and increase in vaginal discharge. This, combined with a weekly cervical examination, means that 84 per cent of women present at a time when tocolytic drugs are said to have a high chance of arresting preterm uterine activity and prolonging pregnancy (Herron, Katz and Creasy, 1982). A later study using the same prevention programme increased the eligibility for tocolytic treatment from 44 to 57 per cent but did not significantly alter the spontaneous preterm labour rate or the incidence of preterm birth (Konte, Creasy and Laros, 1988).

Drugs used to inhibit preterm labour include β-mimetics, ethanol, prostaglandin inhibitors and magnesium sulphate.

β-Mimetic drugs

β-Mimetic drugs currently have the most widespread usage (Keirse, 1984b). In 1985 a meta-analysis of all the placebo-controlled trials of β-mimetic drugs (King *et al.*, 1985) showed that they were effective in delaying delivery for at least 24 h and in reducing the numbers of babies born preterm. There was no evidence, however, that treatment was associated with a reduction in neonatal morbidity or mortality. This study concluded that β-mimetics might have a place in delaying labour long enough

Table 10.4.   Side effects of β-mimetic drugs used to inhibit preterm labour

Type	Effect
Cardiovascular	Maternal tachycardia
	Inotropic effect
	Increased cardiac output
	Decreased diastolic blood pressure
	Arrhythmias
	Pulmonary oedema
	Fetal tachycardia
	Maternal death
Metabolic	Hyperglycaemia
	Hypokalaemia
	Lipolysis
Other	Restlessness and agitation
	Tremor
	Nausea and vomiting
	Bronchodilatation
	Thrombocytopenia

to allow transfer of the mother to a Regional Perinatal Centre and to allow administration of betamethasone to promote pulmonary maturation (King *et al.*, 1985). The same authors have updated their experience to include 16 randomized controlled trials and their conclusions are the same (King *et al.*, 1988). Adverse maternal effects affecting the cardiovascular system such, as tachycardia, palpitations, dysrhythmias and even death (Table 10.4), will probably limit the widespread use of these drugs until more information on their efficacy has been obtained. Two studies of long-term outcome of children exposed to ritodrine *in utero* suggest impaired school performance (Polowczyk *et al.*, 1984; Hadders-Algra, Touwen and Huisjes, 1986).

Ethanol
Ethanol was used to inhibit preterm labour before β-mimetics were tried (Fuchs and Fuchs, 1981) but the major drawbacks are that quite high blood alcohol levels are necessary before this treatment is effective, and that the mortality rate of babies delivered within 6 h of treatment is higher than that of controls.

Prostaglandin synthetase inhibitors
These may be effective in inhibiting preterm labour, although this has not been conclusively proved (Niebyl, Blake and White, 1980). The major contraindication to their use is constriction of the fetal ductus arteriosus which may cause persistent pulmonary hypertension in the newborn.

Magnesium sulphate
This drug can be used to prevent preterm labour (Spisso, Harbert and Thiagarajah, 1982; Valenzuela and Cline, 1982) because of its effect on relaxing smooth muscle. There are, however, no controlled trials of its use nor of calcium-channel-blocking drugs, which may have similar effects (Forman, Anderson and Ulmsten, 1981).

There is a need for more randomized controlled clinical trials of existing, let alone new, interventions to prevent or inhibit preterm labour (Chalmers, 1984; Milner, Enkin and Mohide, 1984). To ensure adequate sample sizes, these trials will have to be multicentred, and their outcome measures should report not just gestation at delivery but neonatal mortality and morbidity data. In Dublin there has been an improved perinatal mortality rate secondary to a reduction in spontaneous preterm labour without the use of tocolytic drugs (Boylan and O'Driscoll, 1983).

Obstetric management

Strategies for management will differ according to the clinical antecedents of pre-term birth (Table 10.1). These may be classified as follows: (1) management of spontaneous, uncomplicated preterm labour; (2) management of premature rupture of the membranes; (3) management of complicated preterm labour or delivery; (4) elective preterm delivery.

Management of spontaneous, uncomplicated preterm labour (Table 10.5)

The first step is to make a diagnosis of preterm labour, which is not always easy: if one relies upon the presence of contractions alone, the diagnosis will be wrong about 50 per cent of the time; however, if the obstetrician waits for dilatation and effacement of the cervix before making a firm diagnosis it may be too late to use tocolytic drugs (Downey and Martin, 1983). Most obstetricians who use tocolytic drugs would treat on the basis of frequent, regular painful contractions (see above). The second step is to assess gestational age accurately and to estimate fetal weight. Gestational age is a better predictor of outcome than fetal weight (Verloove-Vanhorick et al., 1986; Patterson and Halliday, 1988) and survival rates based upon gestational age have been published (Herschel et al., 1982; Verloove-Vanhorick et al., 1986; Yu et al., 1986; Halliday, 1988). Figure 10.2 shows survival rates for babies from 23 to 32 weeks' gestation born at Royal Maternity Hospital, Belfast, from 1981 to 1985 (Halliday, 1988). These survival rates apply to all babies of <1500 g, including those electively delivered who have a better outcome. Both paediatricians (Clyman et al., 1979) and obstetricians (Goldenberg et al., 1982) often fail to appreciate the true survival rates in their own hospitals, which is disappointing as the obstetrician's perception of viability is a major factor in determining neonatal outcome (Golden-berg et al., 1982).

The decisions to use tocolytic drugs, to use corticosteroids to mature the fetal lungs, and to intervene to expedite delivery will all be based upon the obstetrician's view of viability and his faith in the abilities of his paediatric colleagues (Bowes, 1981). Before initiating drug treatment, attempts to exclude chorioamnionitis and maternal and fetal infection should be made. The risks of infection will be increased in the presence of ruptured membranes (see below), but potential pathogens have been isolated from amniotic fluid of women in preterm labour with intact mem-branes. Pre-existing intrauterine infection may predispose to preterm labour, as a

Table 10.5. Obstetric management of spontaneous, uncomplicated preterm labour

Diagnosis of preterm labour
Assessment of gestational age
Estimation of fetal weight
Exclusion of infection
Consideration of tocolytic drugs
Corticosteroids to mature fetal lungs
Decision on mode of delivery

Table 10.6.   Contraindications to use of
β-mimetic drugs in inhibition of preterm labour

Maternal cardiac disease
Severe maternal hypertension
Intrauterine infection
Severe congenital malformation
Antepartum haemorrhage
Poorly controlled diabetes mellitus

history of pelvic inflammatory disease, the use of intrauterine contraceptive devices and multiple sex partners are associated both with preterm rupture of membranes and with chorioamnionitis (Toth *et al.*, 1988). Vaginal and rectal swabs should be taken from all women in preterm labour so that infection with group B streptococci, *Listeria monocytogenes or Haemophilus influenzae* may be excluded (Dornan and Halliday, 1988). Urine should also be examined directly and sent for culture. Unfortunately, clinical signs of intrauterine infection occur late, and routine laboratory measurements of erythrocyte sedimentation rate, white blood cell count and differential are of limited use, being variably affected by pregnancy, labour and corticosteroid administration (Gibbs, 1977). An elevated serum C-reactive protein level has been used as an early indicator of infection in preterm rupture of the membranes (Evans *et al.*, 1980); if a cut-off level of 30 mg/l is used this test is reasonably specific and sensitive (Fisk *et al.*, 1987). Uterine tenderness, maternal pyrexia, or fetal tachycardia should be taken as signs of intrauterine infection and warrant further investigation, consideration of antibiotic cover and acceleration of labour (see below).

Tocolytic therapy combined with corticosteroids should be considered for all uncomplicated preterm labours from 24 to 32 weeks' gestation (Dornan and Halliday, 1988). The contraindications to β-mimetic treatment are shown in Table 10.6. Corticosteroids are not effective before 24 weeks but should be used from 24 weeks to 32 weeks (Liggins and Howie, 1972) as there is now convincing evidence, from a number of randomized controlled trials, of their efficacy in reducing the incidence and severity of respiratory distress syndrome and improving survival (Crowley, 1989). The primary aim of tocolytic therapy is to delay labour for at least 48 h in order to allow fetal lung maturation (Collaborative Group on Antenatal Steroid Therapy, 1981). Secondary aims are to increase gestational age significantly so that both neonatal mortality (Figure 10.2) and the costs of intensive care are reduced (Pomerance, Schifrin and Meredith, 1980). In Los Angeles the average cost of hospital care fell by US$5400/week between 29 and 34 weeks' gestation, based upon 1977 prices (Pomerance, Schifrin and Meredith, 1980).

If tocolytic treatment fails, or if gestational age is >32 weeks in preterm labour when the vertex is presenting, the obstetrician must decide upon the best method of delivery. The aim should be to minimize intrapartum asphyxia and birth trauma. In uncomplicated preterm labour, vaginal delivery is both permissible and desirable (Dornan and Halliday, 1988). It is essential that labour should proceed in a hospital with appropriate facilities for neonatal resuscitation, stabilization and aftercare. Transfer of the mother with the baby *in utero*, with or without intravenous tocolytic therapy, is preferable to transfer of the baby after birth, because survival without handicap is greater after maternal transfer (Blake, Pollitzer and Reynolds, 1979; Cordero, Backes and Zuspan, 1982; Halliday *et al.*, 1986).

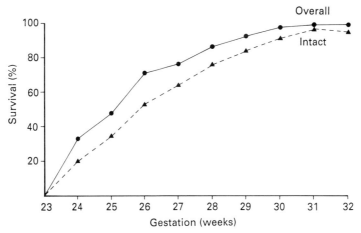

Figure 10.2. Percentage survival by gestational age for babies <1500 g birthweight and <33 weeks' gestation, born in Royal Maternity Hospital, Belfast from 1981 to 1985. Overall survival refers to babies alive at hospital discharge and intact survival means the absence of major handicap at a minimum age of 2 years

Continuous electronic fetal heart rate monitoring and intermittent fetal scalp pH determinations should be available and used if time permits. Routine forceps delivery is no longer recommended, but a large episiotomy is essential, with good control of the fetal head at crowning. Although the incidence of intraventricular haemorrhage (diagnosed by ultrasound) in babies weighing <1250 g delivered by caesarean section is less than those born after vaginal delivery (both vertex and breech presentations) the clinical significance of these findings is unknown (Szymonowicz, Yu and Wilson, 1984). Studies showing reduced neonatal mortality and morbidity rates after caesarean section compared with vaginal delivery (Haesslein and Goodlin, 1979; Fairweather, 1981) are almost equally balanced by studies showing no effect on outcome by method of delivery (Peacock and Hirata, 1981; Yu et al., 1984a; Anderson et al., 1988). Intraventricular haemorrhage within 1 h after birth has been reported to be increased in babies of women who had been in active labour regardless of the route of delivery (Anderson et al., 1988). These studies were not, however, designed as randomized trials and what is needed is a prospective clinical trial with proper randomization, but allowing caesarean section for specific indications that might develop in the group randomized to vaginal delivery. Analysis of the data would have to be by intention to treat. Until this study has been carried out, uncomplicated vertex-presenting preterm babies should be delivered vaginally (Healy, 1987; Dornan and Halliday, 1988).

Analgesia is needed less often in preterm labour because it is less painful and more rapid than term labour. Opiate analgesia should be avoided because of central respiratory depression of the baby as a result of the prolonged half-life. If pain relief is needed, epidural analgesia is preferred because it does not cause fetal respiratory depression.

If fetal distress occurs in labour, caesarean section should be performed unless the fetus has been deemed non-viable, for example if the gestational age is <24–25 weeks and the estimated fetal weight is <600–700 g (Bowes, 1981; Dornan and Halliday, 1988; Hack and Fanaroff, 1988). In labour it is often possible to perform a lower segment transverse incision during caesarean section and this is to be preferred to a classic incision, as maternal morbidity is less (Halperin, Moore and Hannah, 1988).

Premature rupture of the membranes

This is defined as rupture of the membranes before the onset of regular uterine contractions. It occurs in about 10 per cent of all pregnancies, but in >30 per cent of preterm deliveries (Mead, 1983). The aetiology is unknown but may include intrauterine infection, trauma, cervical incompetence and abnormal tensile strength of the membranes (Artal, Sokal and Neuman, 1976). The diagnosis of premature rupture of the membranes may be suggested by maternal history and confirmed by finding amniotic fluid in the vagina on sterile speculum examination (see Figure 10.3). The fluid should be collected for culture and phospholipid analysis to predict fetal lung maturity (Goldstein et al., 1980; Stedman et al., 1981). Sometimes the diagnosis is in doubt and the use of the nitrazine test or of 'ferning' may be helpful (Dornan and Halliday, 1988); the absence of amniotic fluid on ultrasound scan is also very suggestive.

Management of preterm pregnancy complicated by premature rupture of the membranes is based upon the balance between the risks of intrauterine infection on the one hand and the risks of prematurity on the other (Veille, 1988). It seems that the incidence of chorioamnionitis does not increase with increasing duration of membrane rupture (Schreiber and Benedetti, 1980; Johnson et al., 1981). These and other studies confirm that the risks of fetal infection in prolonged rupture of the membranes are insignificant compared with the risks of preterm delivery (Daikoku et al., 1981; Johnson et al., 1981). The compelling evidence that immaturity presents the greatest risk in preterm pregnancy complicated by ruptured membranes means that every effort should be made to prolong pregnancy and to prevent respiratory distress syndrome in this group of patients.

Nevertheless, it is important to detect signs of chorioamnionitis at an early stage so that appropriate intervention can be made. Maternal pyrexia, maternal and fetal tachycardia, leucocytosis, uterine tenderness and purulent or foul-smelling vaginal discharge are late signs of chorioamnionitis. In the absence of maternal pyrexia, Gram staining and culture of amniotic fluid are the only reliable predictors of occult or early chorioamnionitis (Miller et al., 1980; Mead, 1983). Whenever possible, amniocentesis should be included in the evaluation of preterm rupture of membranes where delay in delivery is being considered as part of the management, but it is successful in only 50 per cent of cases (Garite et al., 1979). With evidence of frank or occult infection, management should include parenteral antibiotic treatment and early delivery. If labour begins spontaneously after rupture of the membranes, tocolytic drugs should not be used to suppress it.

For pregnancies >33 weeks' gestation, or those where fetal lung maturity has been confirmed, there is probably little to be gained from conservative management and delivery should be effected, preferably by the vaginal route (Wennergren et al., 1986). If the fetal lungs are immature, controversy exists as to whether or not corticosteroids should be given. Only one study has demonstrated an increase in maternal and neonatal infections following corticosteroids, but this occurred only if the membranes were ruptured for >48 h (Taeusch et al., 1979). Reduction in the incidence of respiratory distress syndrome after the use of maternal corticosteroids in prolonged rupture of membranes has been demonstrated in two studies (Mead and Clapp, 1977; Young et al., 1980), but not in others (see Mead, 1983). Expectant management alone probably carries less risk of infection but if combined with corticosteroids the risk of sepsis increases after 48 h. Gestational age may thus become an important determinant in the decision to use corticosteroids, in the presence of ruptured membranes. As a general rule, if tocolytic drugs are indicated, then corticosteroids are also, unless the fetal lungs can be demonstrated to be mature (Crowley, 1989).

The risk of group B streptococcal sepsis increases in pregnancies complicated by premature rupture of the membranes and infection with this organism might even stimulate membrane rupture and subsequent premature labour (Regan, Chao and Jones, 1981). As antenatal screening is ineffective in identifying high risk mothers, it is important to obtain a vaginal swab at the time of admission from all mothers with premature rupture of the membranes. This will identify nearly all the women colonized with this organism whose infants subsequently become infected (Pasnick, Mead and Philip, 1980). In these circumstances, intrapartum treatment with large doses of ampicillin reduces both the incidence of transmission of the organism (Yow et al., 1979) and the incidence of streptococcal infection of the newborn (Boyer and Gotoff, 1986). Long-term antibiotic prophylaxis is unhelpful, however, as it will mask the early signs of intrauterine infection and encourage resistant strains of bacteria to emerge.

A plan of management based upon gestational age, pulmonary maturity and suspected infection is shown in Figure 10.3.

Complicated preterm delivery

Included in this group are antepartum haemorrhage, maternal infection, erythroblastosis, eclampsia, prolapsed cord, malpresentation and some cases of multiple pregnancy. In many of these circumstances, delivery is an emergency rather than an elective procedure.

Antepartum haemorrhage
Placental abruption occurring preterm may cause severe fetal hypoxia and, in general, a significant antepartum haemorrhage is an indication for delivery, often by emergency caesarean section. Tocolytic drugs are usually contraindicated, as they may exacerbate uterine bleeding by relaxation of smooth muscle. Placenta praevia is more difficult to diagnose preterm, but if bleeding is marked or fetal hypoxia is present, it is an indication for emergency caesarean section. Classical caesarean section may be needed when the lower uterine segment has not formed. Puerperal fever is increased after classical section and in subsequent pregnancies the scar is more likely to be abnormal and to show dehiscence (Halperin, Moore and Hannah, 1988).

Erythroblastosis, eclampsia and prolapsed cord are uncommon causes of emergency delivery preterm, but each is associated with poor neonatal outcome due to acute or chronic hypoxia.

Breech presentation
The mode of delivery for the preterm breech fetus is a controversial issue. Advice favouring caesarean section is invariably based upon retrospective studies of outcome (Duenhoelter et al., 1979; Smith, Spencer and Hull, 1980; Kauppila et al., 1981; Cox, Kendall and Hommers, 1982). Mortality and morbidity (asphyxia, trauma and intracranial haemorrhage) are lower in abdominally delivered preterm breech babies but control infants may not be precisely matched in these studies

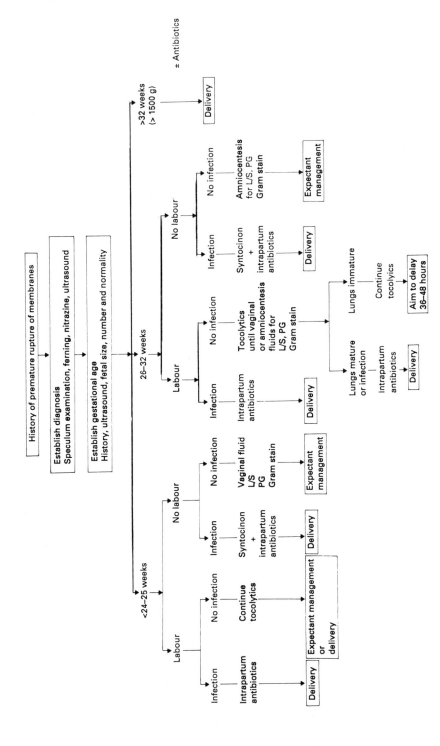

Figure 10.3.   Flow chart for the management of suspected preterm rupture of the membranes: LS = lecithin/sphingomyelin ratio; PG = phosphatidylglycerol

(Duenhoelter *et al.*, 1979; Kauppila *et al.*, 1981). Cervical entrapment and cord prolapse appear to be the most deleterious events in the course of the vaginal preterm breech delivery. Duenhoelter *et al.* (1979) went as far as to recommend caesarean section for all babies with an estimated weight of between 1000 and 2500 g until a prospective controlled randomized study showed evidence to the contrary. Smith, Spencer and Hull (1980) advised caesarean section, whenever possible, for preterm babies of 26–34 weeks' gestation presenting by breech with more cautious advice from Kauppila *et al.* (1981) who justified vaginal delivery from 32 weeks' gestation, provided that the estimated fetal weight was at least 1500 g and that careful electronic fetal monitoring was used. The same authors recommended primary caesarean section for footling breech presentation or obstetric complications such as pre-eclampsia, diabetes or intrauterine growth retardation (Kauppila *et al.*, 1981). Similar advice has been given by others (Yu *et al.*, 1984b) who have noted the reduction in long term neurological morbidity reported after caesarean section for preterm breech presentations (Ingemarsson, Westgrin and Svenningsen, al., 1978).

Multiple pregnancy
About one-half of twin pregnancies deliver preterm and the problems that arise are often associated with malpresentation and difficulty in assessing the health of the second twin before or during labour. Multiple pregnancy rates are increasing as a result of more widespread use of drugs to stimulate ovulation and of techniques of *in vitro* fertilization (Wood *et al.*, 1984). Bed rest and tocolytic treatment are ineffective in reducing preterm delivery rates in multiple pregnancy.

Corticosteroids should be used as for singleton pregnancy and vaginal delivery contemplated only if the first twin is a vertex presentation (Healy, 1987; Traub, McClure and Reid, 1988).

Elective preterm delivery

This accounts for up to one quarter of preterm deliveries and the incidence has increased recently as neonatal intensive care and neonatal outcome have improved. Elective preterm delivery usually originates from severe pre-eclampsia, maternal hypertension and intrauterine growth retardation (Halliday, 1988). These babies have better survival rates than those of the other three groups (Rush *et al.*, 1976; Yu *et al.*, 1984a; Halliday, 1988; Wariyar, Richmond and Hey, 1989).

Neonatal care

This should take place in a neonatal unit within a maternity hospital that is staffed and equipped to provide an appropriate level of care (Royal College of Physicians of London, 1988). This may entail transport of the mother before delivery or of the baby after birth (Blake, Pollitzer and Reynolds, 1979). Properly equipped ambulances with nursing and medical staff in attendance should be available for these transfers (Blake *et al.*, 1975).

Meta-analysis of 19 non-randomized studies of neonatal outcome shows improvement for inborn babies compared with outborn when birthweight is between 1000 and 2000 g (Ozminkowski, Wortman and Roloff, 1988).

Resuscitation and stabilization

The prevention of asphyxia or its early detection is of vital importance, as asphyxia is a major determinant of neonatal outcome in very low birthweight babies. When the 5-min Apgar score is <4, the mortality rate of babies <1500 g is about 60 per cent, whereas only 15 per cent of these babies die when the Apgar score at 5 min is from 4 to 10 (Yu, Zhao and Bajuk, 1982). Asphyxia also predisposes to respiratory distress syndrome, periventricular haemorrhage and necrotizing enterocolitis (Yu and Wood, 1978; Szymonowicz, Yu and Wilson, 1984; Halliday, McClure and Reid, 1989).

No matter the mode of delivery, the most experienced obstetrician or paediatrician available should supervise the delivery and resuscitation of the very preterm baby (Halliday, 1988). One study has demonstrated improved outcome in babies of <31 weeks' gestation who were electively intubated at birth (Drew, 1982). Survival rate increased from 51 to 77 per cent in the babies who were immediately intubated and given continuous positive airway pressure in the labour ward. The decision to resuscitate the very immature baby should be taken by a senior paediatrician, if possible after discussion with the parents during labour. The wishes of the parents are important but their views are often based upon the information provided for them by paediatricians (Wilson *et al.*, 1983) or obstetricians (Goldenberg *et al.*, 1982) and they may underestimate the prognosis of preterm babies and the limit of viability, which is now about 22–23 weeks' gestation (Bowes, 1981; Hack and Fanaroff, 1988). If any doubt exists, the baby should be resuscitated first and discussion with parents and senior medical staff can take place later. For babies born by elective preterm delivery, resuscitation of all babies is the rule unless an obvious congenital abnormality, such as myelomeningocele or Potter's syndrome, is recognizable at birth.

As outcome relates better to gestational age than to birthweight (Verloove-Vanhorick *et al.*, 1986; Patterson and Halliday, 1988), hospitals should not set weight limits as criteria for non-resuscitation. For the last two years, our hospital has discharged as alive and well, babies with birthweights <500 g. Assessment at birth must therefore include an estimation of gestational age, especially if there are any doubts about dates or an ultrasound scan has not been performed between 14 and 20 weeks. Marked bruising, very thin, shiny skin and fusion of the eyelids suggest extreme prematurity and reduced likelihood of survival, but these signs are by no means absolute (Cross, Becker and Congdon, 1985; Halliday, 1988).

The Apgar score is the traditional method of assessment of a baby's condition at birth but its application to the very preterm baby is less well established (Catlin *et al.*, 1986). For the preterm baby, heart rate and respiratory effort are the most important components of the Apgar score, and colour the least helpful. The preterm baby will often have reduced muscle tone, respiratory efforts and reflex activity at birth and consequently have lower Apgar scores (Catlin *et al.*, 1986). Apgar score at 1 min or earlier is probably the best method for determining the need for intubation, whereas the 5- or 10-min score is an indication of how well resuscitation is proceeding and of the long-term prognosis (Halliday, 1988). The method of resuscitation for preterm babies is similar to that of term babies and has been described elsewhere (Ostheimer, 1982; Halliday, 1988).

Temperature control

The maintenance of normal body temperature is very important during resuscitation and aftercare of the preterm baby. Prevention of heat loss from evaporation and radiation is important, as cooling increases metabolic rate and oxygen consumption, causing acidosis, hypoglycaemia and coagulation disorders. The newborn should be carefully dried with a warm towel and nursed initially under a radiant warmer (Halliday, 1988). Prolonged use of a radiant warmer, however, is associated with increased insensible water losses (Weldon and Rutter, 1982; Hull and Chellappah, 1983), and increased oxygen consumption (Le Blanc, 1982). Preterm babies can be kept warm in double-walled incubators which reduce radiant and total heat losses (Marks *et al.*, 1981), by covering them with a thin plastic blanket (Baumgart, Fox and Polin, 1982) or using high humidity which decreases evaporative water loss and cooling (Harpin and Rutter, 1985). The use of an incubator is therefore preferred to a radiant warmer after the initial period of stabilization. Air mode control results in a more stable thermal environment than body (or skin) temperature servo-control in modern incubators (Ducker *et al.*, 1985).

Problems of the preterm baby

Apart from asphyxia and poor temperature control, preterm babies may have problems related to immaturity of virtually every body system (Table 10.7). Immaturity of the respiratory system is probably the most important determinant of the need for neonatal intensive care and long-term outcome (Patterson and Halliday, 1988).

Respiratory problems

Respiratory distress syndrome (RDS) or surfactant deficiency is the commonest cause of respiratory failure in the preterm infant and is the major reason for mechanical ventilation of the newborn, accounting for 75 per cent of the total. RDS may present at birth as apnoea in the very preterm baby, or later with signs of respiratory distress – grunting, indrawing, tachypnoea and cyanosis. Mechanical ventilation is used to treat respiratory failure (Table 10.8). The techniques of mechanical ventilation of the newborn have been described elsewhere (Roberton, 1983; Tarnow-Mordi, 1988).

Surfactant replacement treatment has recently been shown to be very effective in improving the outcome of preterm infants. Two major types of surfactant have been used: a synthetic one consisting of dipalmitoylphosphatidylcholine (DPPC) and phosphatidyglycerol (PG) has been given prophylactically to babies of <30 weeks' gestation at birth (Ten Centre Study Group, 1987); natural ones prepared from animal lungs or amniotic fluid, which contain a mixture of phospholipids and proteins have been used both as prophylaxis (Enhorning *et al.*, 1985; Merritt *et al.*, 1986) and as treatment for established RDS (Collaborative European Multicentre Group, 1988; Halliday, 1989a). Prophylaxis with DPPC and PG has been shown to reduce mortality and complications such as pneumothorax and pulmonary interstitial emphysema without increasing the incidence of patent ductus arteriosus (Ten Centre Study Group, 1987). Natural surfactants used in prophylaxis studies reduce mortality and pneumothorax rates by about 50 per cent without altering the incidence of patent ductus arteriosus (Halliday, 1989a); the number of surviving infants without bronchopulmonary dysplasia is doubled. In the treatment of severe RDS, natural

Table 10.7.   Immaturity of body systems related to problems of the preterm baby

Body system	Clinical problem
Central nervous	Intraventricular haemorrhage Apnoea of prematurity Poor suck and swallow
Respiratory	Respiratory distress syndrome Pneumonia Pneumothorax Bronchopulmonary dysplasia
Cardiovascular	Persistent ductus arteriosus Hypotension
Gastrointestinal	Poor gastric emptying Abdominal distension Malnutrition Necrotizing enterocolitis
Hepatic	Jaundice of prematurity Persistent jaundice
Renal	Fluid and electrolyte imbalance Glycosuria
Endocrine/metabolic	Hypocalcaemia Transient hypothyroidism Hypo- and hyperglycaemia Hypothermia Rickets and osteopenia
Skin	High insensible water losses Bruising, abrasions

Host defence	Infections
	    bacterial
	    fungal
	    viral

Eyes	Retinopathy of prematurity
Haematological	Anaemia Coagulation disorders
Psychosocial	Parental bonding difficulties

surfactants reduce mortality by >40 per cent, pneumothorax by about 70 per cent, intraventricular haemorrhage by about 25 per cent and bronchopulmonary dysplasia by about 35 per cent (Halliday, 1989a); survival without bronchopulmonary dysplasia is increased by 40 per cent. There is no doubt that the introduction of surfactant replacement as a method of treating the preterm baby has revolutionized neonatal care and its widespread use based upon commercial preparations is on the horizon (Halliday, 1990).

Table 10.8   Respiratory failure: indications for mechanical ventilation of the preterm baby

1. Apnoea at birth

2. Respiratory acidosis:
    pH <7.20 when $P_{a,CO2}$ >9 kPa

3. Hypoxaemia:
    P_{aO2} <6 kPa in >80% oxygen ± CPAP

Outcome for the preterm baby

Neurodevelopmental outcome for the smallest survivors of neonatal intensive care has improved dramatically. Before 1960, major developmental problems were found in 60–70 per cent of surviving preterm babies (Lubchenco *et al.*, 1963; Drillien, 1967). Now, even in babies who needed mechanical ventilation for RDS, the risk of permanent brain injury is low unless there is associated severe asphyxia or large intracranial haemorrhage (Fitzhardinge, 1978; Markestad and Fitzhardinge, 1981).

Currently, the best results are achieved in regional perinatal centres where inborn babies weighing <1500 g at birth have handicap rates of <10 per cent (Stewart and Reynolds, 1974; Stewart, Turcan and Rawlings, 1977; Kitchen *et al.*, 1982).

For analysis of changes in survival over time and for comparisons between hospitals and regions a knowledge of birthweight-specific mortality rates is necessary (Goldenberg *et al.*, 1985). Alternatively, survival by gestational age may be used (Figure 10.2). Survival rate increases in a sigmoid fashion with advancing gestational age, and the 50 per cent survival point is reached at between 25 and 26 weeks. One geographical study has shown that handicap, unlike mortality, was apparently unrelated to gestational age or birthweight (van Zeben-Van der Aa *et al.*, 1989). Others have shown that handicap rates increase as birthweight decreases, so that 33 per cent of babies weighing <600 g have major disability, 15 per cent of those weighing 600–699 g and 10 per cent of those weighing 700–799 g (Yu, 1987). Handicap rates of babies born at 24–28 weeks were 24 per cent (Yu *et al.*, 1984b) and 21 per cent, respectively (Milligan, Shennan and Hoskins, 1984), and in neither study did babies born at 24–26 weeks' gestation have a significantly higher handicap rate than those born at 27–28 weeks.

The age of follow-up is important as many babies diagnosed as having cerebral palsy at 1 year seem to outgrow their 'disability' and have no motor deficit at 7 years (Nelson and Ellenberg, 1982). Two to three years is the best time to assess children for major disability (*Lancet* Editorial, 1980). School learning problems, however, may be quite common in children who were very preterm (Nickel, Bennett and Lawson, 1982; Hirata *et al.*, 1983; Hack and Fanaroff, 1988).

The most important perinatal factor affecting outcome in preterm babies is the availability of intensive care before, during and after birth. There are significant differences in outcome between inborn and outborn babies (Cordero, Backes and Zuspan, 1982; Kitchen *et al.*, 1984; Halliday *et al.*, 1986; Ozminkowski, Wortman and Roloff, 1988). Gestational age, 5-min Apgar score and the presence of respiratory distress within 1 h of birth can be used to predict 94 per cent of neonatal survivors and 53 per cent of deaths (Patterson and Halliday, 1988). Shennan, Milligan and Hoskins (1985) added hypotension, infection and intraventricular haemorrhage as significant factors in predicting poor outcome. These authors showed that factors associated with improved survival included preterm labour preceding delivery, antenatal corticosteroid treatment of >36 h, female sex and early diuresis (Shennan, Milligan and Hoskins, 1985). In another study, handicaps were associated with antepartum haemorrhage, absence of antenatal corticosteroid treatment and multiple pregnancy (Kitchen *et al.*, 1985). Maternal social class is also related to subsequent handicap rate (Escalona, 1982), as is poor postnatal head growth (Hack and Breslau, 1986).

Advances in the understanding of the aetiology of preterm birth and improvements in perinatal care have been associated with improved survival of preterm babies. The development of perinatology as a field where obstetricians and paediatricians meet to form a partnership has led to better understanding of each others' problems and a realistic assessment of what is possible with optimal perinatal care (McClure and Scott, 1988). The objective of perinatal care is not merely to improve survival of preterm babies but to reduce handicaps in survivors. To this end it is important for obstetricians and paediatricians alike to monitor carefully all new treatments that they introduce by using controlled clinical trials if possible and by including both short- and long-term outcomes in these studies.

References

Agustsson, P and Patel, NE (1987) The predictive value of fetal breathing movements in the diagnosis of preterm labour. *British Journal of Obstetrics and Gynaecology*, **94**, 860–863

Anderson, ABM and Turnbull, AC (1982) Effect of oestrogens, progesterones and betamimetics in pregnancy. In *Effectiveness and Satisfaction in Antenatal Care* (edited by MW Enkin and I Chalmers) pp. 161–181. London: Heinemann

Anderson, GD, Boda, HS, Sibai, BM *et al.* (1988) The relationship between labor and route of delivery in the preterm infant. *American Journal of Obstetrics and Gynecology*, **158**, 1382–1390

Artal, R, Sokal, RJ and Neuman, M (1976) The mechanical properties of prematurely and non-prematurely ruptured membranes. Methods and preliminary results. *American Journal of Obstetrics and Gynecology*, **125**, 655–659

Baumgart, S, Fox, WW and Polin, RA (1982) Physiologic implications of two different heat shields for infants under radiant warmers. *Journal of Pediatrics*, **100**, 787–790

Bejar, P, Curbelo, V, Davis, C and Gluck, L (1981) Premature labor II. Bacterial sources of phospholipase. *Obstetrics and Gynecology*, **57**, 479–482

Bennett, PR and Elder, MG (1988) Extreme prematurity: the aetiology of preterm delivery. *British Medical Bulletin*, **44**, 850–860

Besinger, RE, Compton, AA and Hayashi, RH (1987) The presence or absence of fetal breathing movements as a predictor of outcome in preterm labor. *American Journal of Obstetrics and Gynecology*, **157**, 753–757

Blake, A, Pollitzer, M and Reynolds, EOR (1979) Referral of mothers and infants for intensive care. *British Medical Journal*, **2**, 147–150

Blake, A, McIntosh, N, Reynolds, EOR and St Andrew, D (1975) Transport of newborn infants for intensive care. *British Medical Journal*, **4**, 13–17

Bowes, WA (1981) Delivery of the very low birthweight infant. *Clinics in Perinatology*, **8**, 183–195

Boyer, DM and Gotoff, SP (1986) Prevention of early onset neonatal group B streptococcal disease with selective intrapartum chemoprophylaxis. *New England Journal of Medicine*, **314**, 1665–1669

Boylan, P and O'Driscoll, K (1983) Improvement in perinatal mortality rate attributed to spontaneous preterm labor without the use of tocolytic agents. *American Journal of Obstetrics and Gynecology*, **145**, 781–783

Castle, BM and Turnbull, AC (1983) The presence or absence of fetal breathing movements predicts the outcome of preterm labour. *Lancet*, **ii**, 471–472

Catlin, EA, Carpenter, MW, Brann, BS *et al.* (1986) The Apgar score revisited: influence of gestational age. *Journal of Pediatrics*, **109**, 865–868

Chalmers, I (1984) Confronting Cochrane's challenge to obstetrics. *British Journal of Obstetrics and Gynaecology*, **91**, 721–723

Clyman, RI, Sniderman, SH, Ballard, RA *et al.* (1979) What pediatricians say to mothers of sick newborns: an indirect evaluation of the counselling process. *Pediatrics*, **63**, 719–723

Collaborative European Multicentre Group (1988) Surfactant replacement therapy for severe neonatal respiratory distress syndrome: an international randomized clinical trial. *Pediatrics*, **82**, 683–691

Collaborative Group on Antenatal Steroid Therapy (1981) Effect of antenatal dexamethasone adminis- tration on the prevention of respiratory distress syndrome. *American Journal of Obstetrics and Gynecology*, **151**, 276–286

Cordero, L, Backes, CR and Zuspan, FP (1982) Very low-birthweight infant. I: Influence of place of birth on survival. *American Journal of Obstetrics and Gynecology*, **143**, 533–537

Cox, C, Kendall, AC and Hommers, M (1982) Changed prognosis of breech presenting low birthweight infants. *British Journal of Obstetrics and Gynaecology*, **89**, 881–886

Creasy, RK and Herron, MA (1981) Prevention of preterm birth. *Seminars in Perinatology*, **5**, 295–302

Creasy, RK, Gummer, BA and Liggins, GC (1980) System for predicting spontaneous preterm birth. *Obstetrics and Gynecology*, **55**, 692–695

Cross, G, Becker, M and Congdon, P (1985) Prognosis for babies born with fused eyelids. *Archives of Disease in Childhood*, **60**, 479–480

Crowley, P (1989) Promoting pulmonary maturity. In *Effective Care in Pregnancy and Childbirth* (edited by M Enkin, MJNC Keirse and I Chalmers) chapter 45, pp. 746–764. Oxford: Oxford University Press

Daikoku, NH, Kaltreider, DF, Johnson, TRB *et al.* (1981) Premature rupture of membranes and preterm labor: neonatal infection and perinatal mortality risks. *Obstetrics and Gynecology*, **58**, 417–425

Deter, RL, Rossavik, IK, Harrist, RB *et al.* (1986) Mathematical modelling of fetal growth: development of individual growth curve standards. *Obstetrics and Gynecology*, **68**, 156–161

Dor, J, Shalev, J, Mashioch, S *et al.* (1982) Elective cervical suture of twin pregnancies diagnosed ultrasonically in the first trimester following induced ovulation. *Gynecologic and Obstetric Investi- gation*, **13**, 57–60

Dornan, JC and Halliday, HL (1988) Preterm birth. In *Perinatal Medicine* (edited by G McClure, HL Halliday and W Thompson) pp. 66–116. London: Baillière Tindall

Downey, LJ and Martin, AJ (1983) Ritodrine in the treatment of preterm labour: a study of 213 patients. *British Journal of Obstetrics and Gynaecology*, **90**, 1046–1053

Drew, JH (1982) Immediate intubation at birth of the very low-birth-weight infant. *American Journal of Diseases of Children*, **136**, 207–210

Drillien, C (1967) The long-term prospects of handicaps in babies of low birthweight. *British Journal of Hospital Medicine*, **1**, 937–944

Dubin, WH, Johnson, JWC, Calhoun, S *et al.* (1980) Plasma prostaglandin in pregnant women with term and preterm deliveries. *Obstetrics and Gynecology*, **57**, 203–206

Ducker, DA, Lyon, AJ, Russell, RR *et al.* (1985) Incubator temperature control: effects on the very low birthweight infant. *Archives of Disease in Childhood*, **60**, 902–907

Duenhoelter, JH, Wells, CE, Reisch, JS *et al.* (1979) A paired controlled study of vaginal and abdominal delivery of the low birthweight breech fetus. *Obstetrics and Gynecology*, **54**, 310–313

Dunn, PM (1976) Premature delivery and the preterm infant. *Irish Medical Journal*, **69**, 256–264

Enhorning, G, Shennan, A, Possmayer, F *et al.* (1985) Prevention of neonatal respiratory distress syndrome by tracheal installation of surfactant: a randomized clinical trial. *Pediatrics*, **76**, 145–153

Ericson, A, Eriksson, M, Westerholm, P and Zetterstrom, R (1984) Pregnancy outcome and social indicators in Sweden. *Acta Paediatrica Scandinavica*, **73**, 69–74

Escalona, SK (1982) Babies at double hazard: early development of infants at biologic and social risk. *Pediatrics*, **70**, 670–675

Evans, MI, Hajj, SN, Dovoe, LD *et al.* (1980) C-reactive protein as a predictor of infectious morbidity with premature rupture of membranes. *American Journal of Obstetrics and Gynecology*, **138**, 648–652

Fairweather, DVI (1981) Obstetric management and follow up of the very low birthweight infant. *Journal of Reproductive Medicine*, **26**, 387–392

Fisk, NM, Fysh, J, Child, AG *et al.* (1987) Is C-reactive protein really useful in preterm premature rupture of the membranes? *British Journal of Obstetrics and Gynaecology*, **94**, 1159–1164

Fitzhardinge, PM (1978) Follow-up studies of children treated by mechanical ventilation as neonates. *Clinics in Perinatology*, **5**, 451–461

Forman, A, Andersson, KE and Ulmsten, U (1981) Inhibition of myometrial activity by calcium antagonists. *Seminars in Perinatology*, **5**, 288–294

Fuchs, AR and Fuchs, F (1981) Ethanol for prevention of preterm birth. *Seminars in Perinatology*, **5**, 236–251

Garite, TJ, Freeman, RK, Linzey, EM and Braly, P (1979) The use of amniocentesis in patients with premature rupture of the membranes. *Obstetrics and Gynecology*, **54**, 226–230

Gibbs, RS (1977) Diagnosis of intra-amniotic infection. *Seminars in Perinatology*, **1**, 71–77

Goldenberg, RL, Nelson, KG, Dyer, RL *et al.* (1982) The variability of viability: the effect of physician's perceptions of viability on the survival of very low birth-weight infants. *American Journal of Obstetrics and Gynecology*, **143**, 678–684

Goldenberg, RL, Nelson, KG, Koski, JF *et al.* (1985) Neonatal mortality in infants born weighing 501–1000 grams. *American Journal of Obstetrics and Gynecology*, **151**, 608–611

Goldstein, AS, Mangurten, HH, Libretti, JV and Berman, AM (1980) Lecithin/sphingomyelin ratio in amniotic fluid obtained vaginally. *American Journal of Obstetrics and Gynecology*, **138**, 232–233

Grant, A, Chalmers, I and Enkin, M (1982) Physical intervention intended to prolong pregnancy and increase fetal growth. In *Effectiveness and Satisfaction in Antenatal Care* (edited by M Enkin and I Chalmers) pp. 198–208. London: Heinemann

Gummerus, M and Halonen, O (1987) Prophylactic long-term oral tocolysis of multiple pregnancies. *British Journal of Obstetrics and Gynaecology*, **94**, 249–251

Guzick, DS, Daikoku, NH and Kaltreider, DF (1984) Predictability of pregnancy outcome in preterm delivery. *Obstetrics and Gynecology*, **63**, 645–650

Hack, M and Breslau, N (1986) Very low birthweight infants: effects of brain growth during infancy on intelligence quotient at 3 years of age. *Pediatrics*, **77**, 196–202

Hack, M and Fanaroff, AA (1988) How small is too small? Considerations in evaluating the outcome of the tiny infant. *Clinics in Perinatology*, **15**, 773–788

Hadders-Algra, H, Touwen, B and Huisjes, HJ (1986) Follow-up of children exposed to ritodrine. *British Journal of Obstetrics and Gynaecology*, **93**, 156–161

Haesslein, HC and Goodlin, RC (1979) Delivery of the tiny newborn. *American Journal of Obstetrics and Gynecology*, **134**, 192–200

Hall, MH (1985) Incidence and distribution of preterm labour. In *Preterm Labour and its Consequences. Proceedings of the Thirteenth Study Group of the Royal College of Obstetricians and Gynaecologists* (edited by RW Beard and F Sharp) pp. 5–13. London: Royal College of Obstetricians and Gynaecologists

Hall, MH and Chang, PK (1982) Antenatal care in practice. In *Effectiveness and Satisfaction in Antenatal Care* (edited by M Enkin and I Chalmers) pp. 60–68. London: Heinemann

Hall, MH, Carr-Hill, RA, Fraser, C *et al.* (1985) The extent and antecedents of uncertain gestation. *British Journal of Obstetrics and Gynaecology*, **92**, 445–451

Halliday, HL (1988) Care of preterm babies in the first hour. *Care of the Critically Ill*, **4**, 7–12

Halliday, HL (1989) Clinical experience with exogenous natural surfactant. *Developmental Pharmacology and Therapeutics*, **13**, 173–181

Halliday, HL (1990) Hot topics '88 in Neonatology. Report of Ross Laboratory Special Conference. *Pediatric Reviews and Communications*, **4**, 173–181

Halliday, HL, Jones, PK and Jones, SL (1980) Method of screening obstetric patients to prevent reproductive wastage. *Obstetrics and Gynecology*, **55**, 656–661

Halliday, HL, McClure, G and Reid, M (1989) Asphyxia and resuscitation. In *Handbook of Neonatal Intensive Care*, 3rd edn, pp. 26–37. London: Baillière Tindall

Halliday, HL, Patterson, CC, McClure, BG and Reid, NMcC (1986) Where should low birthweight babies be born? *British Medical Journal*, **293**, 1437

Halperin, ME, Moore, DC and Hannah, WJ (1988) Classical versus low-segment transverse incision for preterm caesarean section: maternal complications and outcome of subsequent pregnancies. *British Journal of Obstetrics and Gynaecology*, **95**, 990–996

Harpin, VA and Rutter, N (1985) Humidification of incubators. *Archives of Disease in Childhood*, **60**, 219–224

Hartikainen-Sorri, AL and Jouppila, P (1984) Is routine hospitalization needed in antenatal care of twin pregnancy? *Journal of Perinatal Medicine*, **12**, 31–34

Healy, DL (1987) Obstetric management of preterm birth. In *Prematurity* (edited by VYH Yu and EC Wood) pp. 76–96. Edinburgh: Churchill Livingstone

Herron, MA, Katz, M and Creasy, RK (1982) Evaluation of a preterm birth prevention program: preliminary report. *Obstetrics and Gynecology*, **59**, 452–456

Herschel, M, Kennedy, JL, Kayne, HL *et al.* (1982) Survival of infants born at 24 to 28 weeks gestation. *Obstetrics and Gynecology*, **60**, 154–158

Hirata, T, Epcar, JT, Walsh, A *et al.* (1983) Survival and outcome of infants 501 to 750 g: a six-year experience. *Journal of Pediatrics*, **102**, 741–748

Hobel, CJ (1982) Identification of the patient at risk. In *Perinatal Medicine: Management of the High Risk Fetus and Newborn*, 2nd edn (edited by RJ Bolognese, RH Schwarz and J Schneider) pp. 3–28. Baltimore: Williams and Wilkins

Huddleston, JF (1982) Preterm labour. *Clinical Obstetrics and Gynecology*, **25**, 123–126

Hull, D and Chellappah, G (1983) On keeping babies warm. In *Recent Advances in Perinatal Medicine, Vol 1* (edited by ML Chiswick) pp. 153–168. Edinburgh: Churchill Livingstone

Iams, JD, Johnson, FF, O'Shaughnessy, RW and West, LC (1987) A prospective random trial of home uterine activity monitoring in pregnancies at increased risk of preterm labour. *American Journal of Obstetrics and Gynecology*, **157**, 638–643

Ingemarsson, I, Westgrin, M and Svenningsen, NW (1978) Long term follow-up of pre-term infants in breech presentation delivered by caesarean section. *Lancet*, **ii**, 172–175

Johnson, JWC, Daikoku, NH, Niebyl, JR *et al.* (1981) Premature rupture of the membranes and prolonged latency. *Obstetrics and Gynecology*, **57**, 547–556

Jones, JM, Sweetman, P and Hibbard, BM (1979) The outcome of pregnancy after cone biopsy, a case control study. *British Journal of Obstetrics and Gynaecology*, **86**, 913–916

Joseph, KS (1989) The Matthew effect in health development. *British Medical Journal*, **298**, 1497–1498

Kauppila, O, Gronroos, M, Aro, P *et al.* (1981) Management of low birthweight breech delivery: should caesarean section be routine? *Obstetrics and Gynecology*, **57**, 289–294

Keen, DV and Pearse, RG (1985) Birthweight between 14 and 42 weeks gestation. *Archives of Disease in Childhood*, **60**, 440–446

Keirse, MJNC (1984a) Betamimetic drugs in the prophylaxis of preterm labour: extent and rationale of their use. *British Journal of Obstetrics and Gynaecology*, **91**, 431–437

Keirse, MJNC (1984b) A survey of tocolytic drug treatment in preterm labour. *British Journal of Obstetrics and Gynaecology*, **91**, 424–430

King, JF, Keirse, MJNC, Grant, A and Chalmers, I (1985) Tocolysis – the case for and against. In *Preterm Labour and its Consequences. Proceedings of the Thirteenth Study Group of the RCOG* (edited by RW Beard and F Sharp) pp. 199–208. London: Royal College of Obstetricians and Gynaecologists

King, JF, Grant, A, Keirse, MJNC and Chalmers, I (1988) Beta-mimetics in preterm labour: an overview of the randomized controlled trials. *British Journal of Obstetrics and Gynaecology*, **95**, 211–222

Kitchen, WH, Ryan, MM, Richards, A *et al.* (1982) Changing outcome over 13 years of very low birthweight infants. *Seminars in Perinatology*, **6**, 373–389

Kitchen, WH, Ford, GW, Orgill, AA *et al.* (1984) Outcome of extremely low birthweight infants in relation to hospital of birth. *Australia and New Zealand Journal of Obstetrics and Gynaecology*, **24**, 1–5

Kitchen, WH, Ford, GW, Doyle, LW *et al.* (1985) Cesarean section or vaginal delivery at 24 to 28 weeks' gestation: comparison of survival and neonatal and two-year mortality. *Obstetrics and Gynecology*, **66**, 149–157

Konte, JM, Creasy, RK and Laros, RK (1988) California North Coast preterm birth prevention project. *Obstetrics and Gynecology*, **71**, 727–730

Lamont, RF, Rose, M and Elder, MG (1985) Effect of bacterial products on prostaglandin E production by amnion cells. *Lancet*, **ii**, 1331–1333

Lancaster, PAL (1986) High incidence of preterm births and early losses in pregnancy after in vitro fertilization. *British Medical Journal*, **229**, 1160–1163

Lancet Editorial (1980) The fate of the baby under 1500 g at birth. *Lancet*, **i**, 461–463

Lazar, P, Guegen, S, Dreyfus, J *et al.* (1984) Multicentred controlled trial of cervical cerclage in women at moderate risk of preterm delivery. *British Journal of Obstetrics and Gynaecology*, **91**, 731–735

Le Blanc, MH (1982) Relative efficacy of an incubator and an open warmer in producing thermoneutrality for the small premature infant. *Pediatrics*, **69**, 439–445

Leveno, KJ, Cox, K and Roark, ML (1986) Cervical dilatation and prematurity revisited. *Obstetrics and Gynecology*, **68**, 434–435

Liggins, GC and Howie, RN (1972) A controlled trial of antepartum glucocorticoid treatment for prevention of the respiratory distress syndrome in premature infants. *Pediatrics*, **50**, 515–525

Lubchenco, L, Horner, FA, Reed, LH *et al.* (1963) Sequelae of premature births: evaluations of premature infants of low birthweights at 10 years of age. *American Journal of Diseases of Children*, **106**, 101–115

Lucas, A, Cole, TJ and Gandy, GM (1986) Birthweight centiles in preterm infants reappraised. *Early Human Development*, **13**, 313–322

Lumley, J (1986) Very low birth-weight (less than 1500 g) and previous induced abortion: Victoria 1982–83. *Australian and New Zealand Journal of Obstetrics and Gynaecology*, **26**, 268–272

Lumley, J (1987) Prediction of preterm birth. In *Prematurity* (edited by VYH Yu and EC Wood) pp. 43–53. Edinburgh: Churchill Livingstone

McClure, G and Scott, M (1988) Why perinatal medicine? In *Perinatal Medicine* (edited by G McClure, HL Halliday and W Thompson) pp. 1–9. London: Baillière Tindall

Macfarlane, A, Cole, S, Johnson, A and Botting, B (1988) Epidemiology of birth before 28 weeks of gestation. *British Medical Bulletin*, **44**, 861–893

Main, DM and Gabbe, SG (1987) Risk scoring for preterm labor: where do we go from here? *American Journal of Obstetrics and Gynecology*, **157**, 789–793

Markestad, T and Fitzhardinge, PM (1981) Growth and development in children recovering from bronchopulmonary dysplasia. *Journal of Pediatrics*, **98**, 597–602

Marks, KH, Lee, CA, Bolan, CD and Maisels, MJ (1981) Oxygen consumption and temperature control of premature infants in a double-wall incubator. *Pediatrics*, **68**, 93–98

Mead, PB (1983) Premature rupture of the membranes. In *Recent Advances in Perinatal Medicine Vol 1* (edited by ML Chiswick) pp. 77–94. Edinburgh: Churchill Livingstone

Mead, PB and Clapp, JF (1977) The use of betamethasone and timed delivery in management of premature rupture of the membranes in the preterm pregnancy. *Journal of Reproductive Medicine*, **19**, 3–7

Merritt, TA, Hallman, M, Bloom, BT *et al.* (1986) Prophylactic treatment of very premature infants with human surfactant. *New England Journal of Medicine*, **315**, 785–790

Miller, JM, Hill, GB, Welt, SI and Pupkin, MJ (1980) Bacterial colonization of amniotic fluid in the presence of ruptured membranes. *American Journal of Obstetrics and Gynecology*, **137**, 451–458

Milligan, JE, Shennan, AT and Hoskins, EM (1984) Perinatal intensive care: where and how to draw the line. *American Journal of Obstetrics and Gynecology*, **148**, 499–503

Milner, RA, Enkin, M and Mohide, PT (1984) The importance of clinical trials of preterm labor. *Clinical Obstetrics and Gynecology*, **27**, 606–613

Minkoff, H (1983) Prematurity: infection as an etiologic factor. *Obstetrics and Gynecology*, **62**, 137–144

Mitchell, MD (1984) The mechanism(s) of human parturition. *Journal of Developmental Physiology*, **6**, 107–118

MRC/RCOG Working Party on Cervical Cerclage (1988) Interim report of the Medical Research Council/Royal College of Obstetricians and Gynaecologists multicentre randomized trial of cervical cerclage. *British Journal of Obstetrics and Gynaecology*, **95**, 437–445

Nelson, KB and Ellenberg, JH (1982) Children who outgrew cerebral palsy. *Pediatrics*, **69**, 529–536

Newman, KB, Gill, RJ, Campion, S and Katz, M (1987) Antepartum ambulatory tocodynamometry: the significance of low-amplitude, high-frequency contractions. *Obstetrics and Gynecology*, **70**, 701–705

Nickel, RE, Bennett, FC and Lawson, FN (1982) School performance of children with birthweights of 1000 g or less. *American Journal of Diseases of Children*, **136**, 105–110

Niebyl, JR, Blake, DA and White, RD (1980) The inhibition of premature labor with indomethacin. *American Journal of Obstetrics and Gynecology*, **136**, 1014–1019

Olds, DL, Henderson, CR, Tatelbaum, R and Chamberlin, R (1986) Improving the delivery of prenatal care and outcomes of pregnancy: a randomized trial of nurse home visitation. *Pediatrics*, **17**, 16–28

Ostheimer, GW (1982) Resuscitation of the newborn infant. *Clinics in Perinatology*, **9**, 177–190

Ozminkowski, RJ, Wortman, RM and Roloff, DW (1988) Inborn/outborn status and neonatal survival: a meta-analysis of non-randomized studies. *Statistics in Medicine*, **7**, 1207–1221

Papiernik, E (1984) Proposals for a programmed prevention policy of preterm birth. *Clinical Obstetrics and Gynecology*, **27**, 614–635

Papiernik, E, Bouyer, J and Dreyfus, J (1985) Risk factors for preterm births and results of a prevention policy. The Haguenau Perinatal Study 1971–1982. In *Preterm Labour and its Consequences. Proceedings of the Thirteenth Study Group of the Royal College of Obstetricians and Gynaecologists* (edited by RW Beard and F Sharp) pp. 15–20. London: Royal College of Obstetricians and Gynaecologists

Papiernik, E, Bouyer, J, Dreyfus, J *et al.* (1985) Prevention of preterm birth: a perinatal study in Haguenau, France. *Pediatrics*, **76**, 154–158

Papiernik, E, Bouyer, J, Collin, D *et al.* (1986) Precocious cervical ripening and preterm labour. *Obstetrics and Gynecology*, **67**, 238–242

Pasnick, MK, Mead, PB and Philip, AGS (1980) Selective maternal culturing to identify group B streptococcal infection. *American Journal of Obstetrics and Gynecology*, **138**, 480–484

Patterson, CC and Halliday, HL (1988) Prediction of outcome shortly after delivery for the very low birthweight (less than 1500 g) infant. *Paediatric and Perinatal Epidemiology*, **2**, 221–228

Peacock, WG and Hirata, T (1981) Outcome in low birthweight infants (750–1000 g). A report on 164 cases managed at Childrens Hospital, San Francisco, California. *American Journal of Obstetrics and Gynecology*, **140**, 165–172

Polowczyk, D, Tejani, N, Lauersen, N and Siddiq, F (1984) Evaluation of seven to nine year old children exposed to ritodrine in utero. *Obstetrics and Gynecology*, **64**, 485–488

Pomerance, JJ, Schifrin, BS and Meredith, JL (1980) Womb rent. *American Journal of Obstetrics and Gynecology*, **137**, 4866–490

Regan, JA, Chao, S and Jones, LS (1981) Premature rupture of membranes, preterm delivery, and group B streptococcal colonization of mothers. *American Journal of Obstetrics and Gynecology*, **141**, 184–186

Rice, GE, Jenkin, G and Thorburn, GD (1987) Physiology and endocrinology of preterm labour. In *Prematurity* (edited by VYH Yu and EC Wood) pp. 25–42. Edinburgh: Churchill Livingstone

Ritchie, K and McClure, G (1979) Prematurity. *Lancet*, **ii**, 1227–1229

Roberton, NRC (1983) The care of neonates with respiratory failure. In *Recent Advances in Perinatal Medicine. Vol 1* (edited by ML Chiswick) pp. 169–190. Edinburgh: Churchill Livingstone

Royal College of Physicians of London (1988) *Medical Care of the Newborn in England and Wales*, a report of the RCP, 1988. London: RCP

Rush, RW, Keirse, MJNC, Howat, P *et al.* (1976) Contribution of preterm delivery to perinatal mortality. *British Medical Journal*, **2**, 965–968

Rush, RW, Isaccs, S, McPherson, K *et al.* (1984) A randomized controlled trial of cervical cerclage in women at high risk of spontaneous preterm delivery. *British Journal of Obstetrics and Gynaecology*, **91**, 724–730

Saunders, MC, Dick, JS, Brown, IM *et al.* (1985) The effects of hospital admission for bed rest on the duration of twin pregnancy: a randomized trial. *Lancet*, **ii**, 793–795

Schreiber, J and Benedetti, T (1980) Conservative management of preterm rupture of the fetal membranes in a low socioeconomic population. *American Journal of Obstetrics and Gynecology*, **136**, 92–96

Shennan, AT, Milligan, JE and Hoskins, EM (1985) Perinatal factors associated with death or handicap in very preterm infants. *American Journal of Obstetrics and Gynecology*, **151**, 231–238

Smith, ML, Spencer, SA and Hull, D (1980) Mode of delivery and survival in babies weighing less than 2000 g at birth. *British Medical Journal*, **281**, 1118–1119

Spellacy, WN, Cruz, AC, Birk, SA et al. (1979) Treatment of premature labor with ritodrine: a randomized controlled study. Obstetrics and Gynecology, **54**, 220–223

Spira, N, Audras, F, Chapel, A et al. (1981) Surveillance domicile des grossesses pathologique par les sage-femmes. Essai comparatif controle sur 996 femmes. Journal de Gynécologie Obstétrique et Biologie de la Reproduction, **10**, 543–548

Spisso, KR, Harbert, GM and Thiagarajah, S (1982) The use of magnesium sulfate as the primary therapeutic agent to prevent preterm delivery. American Journal of Obstetrics and Gynecology, **142**, 840–845

Stedman, CM, Crawford, S, Staten, E and Cherry, WB (1981) Management of preterm premature rupture of membranes: assessing amniotic fluid in the vagina for phosphatidylglycerol. American Journal of Obstetrics and Gynecology, **140**, 34–38

Stewart, AL and Reynolds, EOR (1974) Improved prognosis for infants of very low birthweight. Pediatrics, **54**, 724–735

Stewart, AL, Turcan, DM and Rawlings, G (1977) Prognosis for infants weighing 1000 g or less at birth. Archives of Disease in Childhood, **52**, 97–104

Szymonowicz, W, Yu, VYH and Wilson, F (1984) Antecedents of periventricular haemorrhage in infants weighing 1250 g or less at birth. Archives of Disease in Childhood, **59**, 13–17

Taeusch, HW, Frigoletto, F, Kitzmiller, JA et al. (1979) Risk of respiratory distress syndrome after prenatal dexamethasone treatment. Pediatrics, **63**, 64–72

Tarnow-Mordi, W (1988) How to ventilate premature babies. Care of the Critically Ill, **4**, 26–30

Ten Centre Study Group (1987) Ten centre trial of artificial surfactant (artificial lung expanding compound) in very premature babies. British Medical Journal, **294**, 991–996

Thorburn, GD (1986) The orchestration of parturition: does the fetus play the tune? Proceedings of the International Union of Physiological Sciences. Vancouver: IUPS

Toth, M, Witkin, SS, Ledger, W and Thaler, H (1988) The role of infection in the etiology of preterm birth. Obstetrics and Gynecology, **71**, 723–726

Traub, AI, McClure, G and Reid, MMcC (1988) Malpresentation and multiple pregnancy. In Perinatal Medicine (edited by G McClure, HL Halliday and W Thompson) pp. 145–160. London: Bailliere Tindall

Vaalamo, IP and Kivikoski, A (1983) The incompetent cervix during pregnancy diagnosed by ultrasound. Acta Obstetrica Gynaecologica Scandinavica, **62**, 19–23

Valenzuela, G and Cline, S (1982) Use of magnesium sulfate in premature labor that fails to respond to beta-mimetic drugs. American Journal of Obstetrics and Gynecology, **143**, 718–719

van den Berg, BJ and Oechsli, F (1984) Prematurity. In Perinatal Epidemiology (edited by MB Bracken) pp. 69–85. Oxford: Oxford University Press

van Zeben-Van der Aa, TM, Verloove-Vanhorick, SP, Bond, R and Ruys, JH (1989) Morbidity of very low birthweight infants at corrected age of two years in a geographically defined population. Lancet, **i**, 253–255

Veille, JC (1988) Management of premature rupture of membranes. Clinics in Perinatology, **15**, 851–862

Verloove-Vanhorick, SP, Verwey, RA, Bland, R et al. (1986) Neonatal mortality risk in relation to gestational age and birthweight. Lancet, **i**, 55–57

Villar, J and Belizan, JM (1982) The relative contribution of prematurity and fetal growth retardation to low birthweight in developing and developed societies. American Journal of Obstetrics and Gynecology, **143**, 792–798

Wariyar, U, Richmond, S and Hey, E (1989) Pregnancy outcome at 24–31 weeks' gestation: mortality. Archives of Disease in Childhood, **64**, 670–677

Weldon, AE and Rutter, N (1982) The heat balance of small babies nursed in incubators and under radiant warmers. Early Human Development, **6**, 131–143

Wennergren, M, Krantz, M, Hjalmarson, O and Karlsson, K (1986) Interval from rupture of the membranes to delivery and neonatal respiratory adaptation. British Journal of Obstetrics and Gynaecology, **93**, 799–803

Wigglesworth, JS, Desai, R and Guerrini, P (1981) Fetal lung hypoplasia: biochemical and structural variations and their possible significance. Archives of Disease in Childhood, **56**, 606–615

Wilson, AL, Wellman, LR, Fenton, LJ and Wizke, DB (1983) What physicians know about the prognosis of preterm newborns. American Journal of Diseases of Children, **137**, 551–554

Wood, C, Downing, B, Trounson, A and Rogers, P (1984) Clinical implications of developments in in vitro fertilization. *British Medical Journal*, **289**, 978–980

World Health Organization (1977) *Manual of the International Classification of Diseases, Injuries and Causes of Death, Vol 1*. Geneva: World Health Organization

World Health Organization Division of Family Health (1980) The incidence of low birthweight. A critical review of available information. *World Health Statistics Quarterly*, **33**, 197–204

Worthington, D, Maloney, GH and Smith, BT (1977) Fetal lung maturation. I Mode of onset of premature labor: influence of premature rupture of the membranes. *Obstetrics and Gynecology*, **49**, 275–279

Young, BK, Klein, SA, Katz, M *et al.* (1980) Intravenous dexamethasone for prevention of neonatal respiratory distress: a prospective controlled study. *American Journal of Obstetrics and Gynecology*, **138**, 203–209

Yow, MD, Mason, EO, Leeds, LJ *et al.* (1979) Ampicillin prevents intrapartum transmission of Group B streptococcus. *Journal of the American Medical Association*, **241**, 1245–1247

Yu, VYH (1987) Survival and neurodevelopmental outcome of preterm infants. In *Prematurity* (edited by VYH Yu and EC Wood) pp. 223–245. Edinburgh: Churchill Livingstone

Yu, VYH and Wood, EC (1978) Perinatal asphyxia and outcome of very low birthweight infants. *Medical Journal of Australia*, **2**, 578–581

Yu, VYH, Zhao, SM and Bajuk, B (1982) Results of intensive care for 375 very low birthweight infants. *Australian Paediatric Journal*, **18**, 188–192

Yu, VYH, Bajuk, B, Cutting, D *et al.* (1984a) The effect of mode of delivery on outcome of very low birthweight infants. *British Journal of Obstetrics and Gynaecology*, **91**, 633–639

Yu, VYH, Orgill, AA, Bajuk, B and Astbury, J (1984b) Survival and 2-year outcome of extremely preterm infants. *British Journal of Obstetrics and Gynaecology*, **91**, 640–646

Yu, VYH, Loke, HL, Bajuk, B *et al.* (1986) Prognosis for infants born at 23 to 28 weeks' gestation. *British Medical Journal*, **293**, 1200–1203

Chapter 11

Abnormalities of fetal growth

JP Neilson

Introduction

Although the main emphasis of this chapter is firmly on the pathophysiology, significance and clinical management of fetuses that are born 'too small', the development of abnormal fetal proportions (in association with, for example, malformation and oligohydramnios) and the problems of the very large baby are also considered briefly. Babies born 'too small' should be distinguished clearly from those born 'too early' (preterm but normally grown) and the use of such collective terms as 'low birthweight' and 'very low birthweight' have little value now outside the developing world where medical facilities are scarce and gestational age is often uncertain. Babies 'too small' may be small for dates, or growth retarded, or both. These terms are frequently, but wrongly, used as synonyms and the resulting confusion has slowed progress in our understanding of abnormal fetal growth.

Small-for-dates is a statistical concept useful not only because it is easily determined, as long as gestational age and birthweight are known and appropriate criteria agreed to separate normal from abnormal, but also because it undoubtedly identifies a group of babies at increased perinatal risk. The major risks are of death (especially intrauterine), intrapartum asphyxia, neonatal hypoglycaemia and, possibly, long-term neurological and intellectual impairment. Large epidemiological studies have emphasized both the important contribution that this group of babies makes to perinatal mortality (McIlwaine et al., 1979; Northern RHA Co-ordinating Group, 1984) and also the frequent failure to identify such babies during routine antenatal care (Rosenberg, Grant and Hepburn, 1982). Disadvantages of the small-for-dates concept include the probability that charts of birthweight for gestational age (upon which the classification is based) do not accurately reflect intrauterine standards of size (MacGregor et al., 1988), and that the separation of normality from abnormality by arbitrary (and varying) criteria ensures a small-for-dates group of great heterogeneity: thus, included are babies that have major malformations, those malnourished through uteroplacental insufficiency and others that are small merely because of their genetic endowment. A large number of factors may operate to produce a small-for-dates baby and the perinatal risks applicable to the group as a whole are not equally applicable to individual fetuses.

Fetal growth retardation is more difficult to define than is the state of being small for dates. A reasonable working definition is the failure of a fetus to achieve its intrinsic growth potential through lack of nutritional support. Although it has proved difficult to apply a numerical definition to this concept, all obstetricians and neonatal paediatricians recognize the classic description by Clifford (1954), from his study of post-term pregnancies, of these babies as wasted, often associated with meconium staining of the amniotic fluid, and prone to become asphyxiated during labour. The important point to stress here is that, just as small-for-dates babies may not necessarily be growth retarded, so the genuinely growth retarded fetus that has stopped growing because of uteroplacental insufficiency, may not be small for dates. It is possible that many babies who experience growth retardation in late pregnancy, but who are not small for dates, have sufficient metabolic reserve to ensure that they are not put at substantial perinatal risk; on the other hand, the phenomenon may be responsible for some intrauterine deaths that at present are unexplained because the growth problem is unrecognized as the baby is not small for dates. Clarification is urgently required both for clinical reasons and also to allow better evaluation of established and new techniques of fetal assessment (e.g. Doppler ultrasound). This should be an important focus for perinatal research.

Determinants of fetal growth rate

The rate of fetal growth is determined by the interaction of the intrinsic drive of the baby to grow, and the extrinsic support it receives during pregnancy to ensure an adequate supply of nutrients such as glucose, lactate and amino acids, and of oxygen. This necessitates a satisfactory supply of blood to the intervillous space of the placenta and adequate exchange mechanisms.

The intrinsic drive

The principal determinant of the intrinsic growth potential of the fetus is probably genetic, although this may be modified by insults in early intrauterine life. It has long been recognized that larger mothers tend to have larger babies (Thomson, Billewicz and Hytten, 1968) and that the maternal genetic contribution has a much more important influence on intrauterine growth than does the paternal. In a famous experiment, Walton and Hammond (1938) found that foals born to (small) Shetland pony mares impregnated by (large) Shire stallions were of similar birthweight to pure Shetlands; foals born to Shire mares by Shetland stallions were closer in birthweight to pure Shires than to pure Shetlands. From these findings the existence of a 'maternal regulator' was proposed which determined fetal growth rate: this could have biological advantages if viewed from a teleological standpoint by ensuring that the female is not required to deliver excessively large offspring. A similar mechanism seems to exist in other mammalian species including humans: evidence includes a very much higher correlation between birthweights of maternal half-siblings than of paternal half-siblings (Ounsted, 1978). Although speculative, it may be that some recent interesting findings by biologists are relevant to 'maternal regulation' as they indicate that the origin of the genome (whether maternal or paternal) has an important influence on embryonic development. Thus, it is possible to manipulate, under experimental conditions, mouse eggs in order to insert (from different animals) either two male or two female pronuclei. Pregnancies resulting from eggs containing chromosomes only from females, develop embryos with very sparse trophoblast; those resulting from only male pronuclei show very poor embryonic development but good trophoblast formation (Surani, Barton and Norris, 1987). The implication that the female genome is primarily responsible for embryonic development whereas the male genome controls placental development may represent a more general feature of mammalian (including human) development. Certainly the presence of a double male chromosome complement in human triploidy is universally associated with trophoblastic proliferation (partial hydatidiform mole), whereas a double female complement among the 69 chromosomes is rarely associated with molar change (Jacobs *et al.*, 1982).

Fetal intrinsic growth potential is commonly diminished in association with chromosomal abnormalities including triploidy and trisomies 13, 18 and 21, and also with other types of malformation including renal agenesis, various forms of congenital dwarfism, and several uncommon inherited conditions including the de Lange and Neu–Laxova syndromes. As already stated, insults during the first trimester may modify the intrinsic drive: thus, early rubella infection results in a decreased number of cells in the embryo and reduced growth potential (Naeye and Blanc, 1965).

The influence of ethnic factors on growth potential is difficult to disentangle from socioeconomic factors. The lowest mean birthweight recorded in any community is that of the Lumi tribe of Papua New Guinea at 2.40 kg (Wark and Malcolm, 1969); the largest is that of the Cheyenne people of North America at 3.88 kg (Meredith, 1970). Ethnic influences are of relevance to the question of whether standard charts of birthweight for gestational age should be applied to the offspring of immigrant groups. This question remains unresolved, but evidence of rapid increases in mean birthweight in subsequent generations of immigrant groups suggests that apparent differences between racial groups may owe more to environment than to genes.

The role of fetal endocrine organs in influencing growth rate seems to be limited. Anencephaly, with associated absence of hypothalamic tissue and sometimes of the pituitary, produces only a modest decrease in growth rate (allowing for absence of the cranium and brain). Congenital pituitary hypoplasia (Liggins, 1974), familial growth hormone deficiency (Laron and Pertzelan, 1969) and congenital adrenal hypoplasia (Liggins, 1974) are all usually associated with normal birthweight. Thyroxine appears to be necessary for normal growth and development in the fetal sheep and rhesus monkey but growth retardation is not evident in the athyroid human fetus (Thorburn, 1974). The one fetal hormone that is important is insulin: insulin does not cross the human placenta and the hypoinsulinism of congenital diabetes mellitus leads to marked impairment of growth rate (Scott, 1966) while the chronic fetal hyperinsulinism of poorly controlled maternal diabetes is well recognized to be associated with excessive growth.

The general lack of endocrine influence however, suggests that the intrinsic drive to grow rests largely at the tissue level (Hill and Milner, 1985) and the effects of locally acting growth factors such as the insulin-like growth factors (Milner and Hill, 1987), and epidermal, transforming and nerve growth factors (Hill and Milner, 1985) are probably important and certainly require further study. Insulin-like growth factors 1 and 2 share >40 per cent amino acid homology with the A and B chains of insulin respectively. Insulin-like growth factor 1 is the more active but both are found in the fetus from early pregnancy. During postnatal life, nutrition and the action of growth hormone are important regulators of insulin-like growth factor 1; during intrauterine life, human placental lactogen (similar to growth hormone), insulin and nutrition may all influence activity of this growth factor (D'Ercole, 1987).

Extrinsic support

The support necessary to allow full expression of the intrinsic growth potential of the fetus may be less than optimal under certain circumstances.

Altitude
In the hypoxic environment of high altitude, as in the Andes, birthweight is markedly reduced although placental weight is increased (Kruger and Arias-Stella, 1970) suggesting a compensatory response that occurs when hypoxia is present although nutrition and placental blood flow are adequate. Similar findings have been noted in sheep raised at high altitude (Alexander, 1978).

Maternal nutrition
The relationship of maternal nutritional status to the rate of fetal growth has been studied extensively. There is little evidence, in 'developed' countries, of improved outcome by dietary supplementation (Rosa and Turshen, 1970) although improved birthweight has been reported in poor Guatemalan populations following calorific supplementation (Halbicht *et al.*, 1974). High-density protein supplementation may be associated with a *decrease* in birthweight (Rush, 1982).

Drugs and other agents
Exposure of the mother to various agents may be associated with impairment of fetal growth either by an effect on the fetus directly or on its supply line, or by concomitant socioeconomic deprivation (see also Chapter 8). Such agents include cigarettes, alcohol in excess (Jones *et al.*, 1974) and heroin (Stone *et al.*, 1971). Corticosteroids and β-blockers have been implicated inconsistently as possible causes of reduced growth rate.

Multiple pregnancy
The human uterus has difficulty in sustaining the normal growth of more than one fetus at a time and many babies born from multiple pregnancies are small-for-dates at birth. This is discussed in more detail below.

Uteroplacental insufficiency

The placenta
There is little evidence to suggest that primary impairment of placental exchange is an important cause of retarded fetal growth. Inadequacy of maternal blood flow to the intervillous space is much more important and this is addressed separately in the next section. When histological abnormalities are found in the trophoblast in cases of fetal growth retardation, they are non-specific in nature and probably occur in response to ischaemia (Fox and Jones, 1983). The placenta not only has a large functional reserve but it also has a considerable ability to effect repairs to areas of damage. Thus, although areas of necrosis may be identified in the syncytiotrophoblast in some cases, the number of villous cytotrophoblast cells increases (the 'stem cells' of the placenta) to allow production of more syncytiotrophoblast. Other features that may be seen include thickening of the basement membrane and loss of microvilli (Fox and Jones, 1983).

THE VASCULAR SUPPLY

Uteroplacental insufficiency may occur in association with maternal vascular diseases (pre-eclampsia, chronic hypertension, diabetes with vascular complications, systemic lupus erythematosus and other connective tissue disorders) or in women without obvious disease, including a few with lupus anticoagulant (Lubbe and Liggins, 1985). The main sites of pathology are, as stated, the maternal spiral arteries supplying the intervillous space. In early pregnancy, cytotrophoblast invades those parts of the arteries within the decidua to replace their muscular coats and make them flaccid and dilated. During the second trimester of normal pregnancies, a second wave of invasion occurs into the myometrial segments of the spiral arteries (Robertson, Brosens and Dixon, 1975). In pregnancies later to be complicated by pre-eclampsia, this process does not occur; in pregnancies later to be complicated by fetal growth retardation without associated maternal hypertension, similar findings may be seen, although less consistently (Khong et al., 1986). The issue has not, however, been completely elucidated, because some pregnancies that are associated with a failure of 'physiological change' have a completely normal outcome (McFadyen, Price and Geirsson, 1986). None the less, unaltered muscular arteries are more reactive to vasoactive stimuli and are more vulnerable to the later development of atheromatous lesions and to the laying down of fibrin and platelets. Both primary lack of change and secondary pathology are associated with diminished blood flow to the intervillous space.

Other unusual features may be identified. A balance between the actions of the eicosanoids prostacyclin and thromboxane A_2 has been proposed as an important physiological mechanism in the local control of regional, including uteroplacental, blood flow. Thromboxane A_2 stimulates platelet aggregation and causes vasoconstriction, and its production by activated platelets is enhanced in normo- and hypertensive pregnancies associated with impaired fetal growth (Wallenberg and Rotmans, 1982). Prostacyclin, in contrast, is a strong vasodilator and an extremely potent inhibitor of platelet aggregation; its production by trophoblast may be decreased in cases of fetal growth retardation (Jogee, Myatt and Elder, 1983).

The effects on the fetus of uteroplacental vascular insufficiency are becoming better understood. The use of cordocentesis in human pregnancy (Soothill, Nicolaides and Campbell, 1987; Cox et al., 1988) has allowed comparisons to be made with biochemical findings in growth-retarded fetuses in appropriate animal models (Owens and Robinson, 1988). Both hypoglycaemia and hypoxaemia may be found. When acidosis develops, this may represent acute decompensation (Cox et al., 1988) after a long period during which various compensatory mechanisms have operated to protect the fetus. These mechanisms include the following:

1. Increased extraction of oxygen by the fetoplacental unit from the diminished supply presented to it (Clapp, 1978).
2. Redistribution of blood flow to increase that to the brain, heart and adrenals and decrease flow to less important structures such as the lungs, gut and carcass (Peeters et al., 1979). This process is mediated by increased α-adrenergic activity, probably by both neural and catecholamine stimulation (Reuss et al., 1982).
3. Increase in haematocrit to increase oxygen content.
4. Preferential growth of the fetus compared with the placenta (Bonds et al., 1984; Owens, Owens and Robinson, 1989).

The clinical significance of being small for dates

Because of the heterogeneity of the small-for-dates group, the degree and nature of perinatal risk to the individual baby will vary greatly. Those at least risk are babies that are small merely because of their genetic inheritance; those at greatest risk are babies with major malformations and babies that are genuinely growth retarded because of uteroplacental insufficiency. Because the risks to the group as a whole are increased, antenatal detection is important.

Perinatal death

For the assessment of the risks of perinatal death and damage, the study of 500 consecutive small-for-dates babies by Dobson, Abell and Beischer (1981) in Melbourne is probably most useful: the perinatal mortality rates for babies with birth-weights above the 10th percentile, between 5th and 10th percentiles, and below the 5th percentile were respectively 12, 22 and 190 per thousand. This not only emphasizes the important risk of perinatal death but also the desirability of using the 5th rather than the 10th percentile to define 'small for dates'. Approximately 80 per cent of perinatal deaths of small-for-dates babies occur *in utero*, and almost one-half occur after 36 weeks (McIlwaine *et al.*, 1979); these are certainly potentially avoidable. It should also be noted that growth retardation is as important a cause of fetal loss during the late second trimester as during the third (Whitfield *et al.*, 1986).

Perinatal asphyxia

In the Melbourne study it was found that 13 per cent of small-for-dates babies had low Apgar scores. There are a number of reasons why intrapartum asphyxia is more common among growth-retarded babies: (1) pre-existing uteroplacental insufficiency is made worse by the effect of myometrial contractions; (2) because of intrauterine malnutrition, growth-retarded fetuses have less metabolic reserve to withstand the hypoxic effect of labour; (3) some growth-retarded fetuses are hypoxaemic before the onset of labour, and (4) the vessels in the umbilical cord are more vulnerable to compression due to reduction in both amniotic fluid and Wharton's jelly.

Lin and colleagues (1980) studied 37 small-for-dates babies during labour and 108 normally grown controls. In the absence of decelerations on continuous fetal heart-rate monitoring, there was no difference in acid–base status between the two groups. Late decelerations were, however, more common in the small-for-dates group (30 per cent versus 7 per cent) and the small-for-dates fetuses that did develop heart rate decelerations of any sort were more likely to develop lactic acidosis than were controls. The need for vigilance during labour is clear.

Neonatal problems

Morbidity among small-for-dates neonates may conveniently be divided into three categories (Oh, 1977): (1) fetal problems (e.g. chromosomal abnormalities, congenital infections and other malformations); (2) sequelae of intrapartum asphyxia (e.g. meconium aspiration syndrome, hyperviscosity and post-asphyxial encephalopathy), and (3) abnormalities of substrate transfer and aberrations of hormonal control (e.g. hypoglycaemia and hypocalcaemia). Hypoglycaemia may have accounted in part for the very high prevalence of long-term neurological impairment noted in early studies during the 1950s of the postnatal development of small-for-dates infants.

Fetal malformation

The increased incidence of major malformation among the small-for-dates group has already been stressed. Dobson, Abell and Beischer (1981) found the rate to be as high as 17 per cent in infants with birthweights less than the fifth percentile.

Long-term handicap

Although data about the risk of long term neurological and intellectual handicap are conflicting, overall risk is probably increased in small-for-dates babies (Breart and Poisson-Salomon, 1988) especially when growth retardation starts during the second trimester.

Clinical management

The preceding discussion has sought to emphasize the importance of optimizing the antenatal care of the small-for-dates fetus. Clinical management usually follows, to a greater or lesser extent, the sequence: (1) detection, by clinical examination, of the fetus as probably small for dates; (2) confirmation by fetal measurement using diagnostic ultrasound; (3) investigation of the probable cause, with special attention to fetal abnormality and uteroplacental insufficiency; (4) assessment of fetal well-being; (5) consideration of treatment; (6) decision about the optimal timing and mode of delivery. This scheme is used as a convenient framework for discussion in the next section.

Clinical detection of the small-for-dates fetus

Abdominal palpation remains the primary method for detecting small-for-dates fetuses. The size of the fetus may be observed and compared with that expected for the given gestational age, but reported detection rates by abdominal palpation during routine antenatal care are poor, ranging between 30 per cent and 50 per cent (Hall, Chng and MacGillivray, 1980; Rosenberg, Grant and Hepburn, 1982). In attempts to improve this, the simple tape measure is being increasingly used in antenatal clinics: measurement of abdominal girth is not helpful in detecting small-for-dates fetuses (Elder et al., 1970) but tape measurement of symphysis–fundal height allows detection rates of between 56 per cent (Rosenberg et al., 1982) and 86 per cent (Belizan et al., 1978). Measurement is best performed from the highest point of the uterus (whether or not in the midline) by minimally indenting the fundus and positioning the marked surface of the tape downwards (to ensure objectivity). Much of the success of tape measurement probably stems from the necessity of the examiner to record a numerical value in the case notes and therefore to consider further when this is at variance with that expected. As with virtually all techniques, an accurate knowledge of gestational age is needed to interpret clinical findings.

In attempts to achieve further improvement in detection rates during routine antenatal care, ultrasound screening of all pregnancies has been investigated. The ideal method for evaluating screening (as for other forms of fetal assessment) is randomized controlled trial to avoid selection biases and to control for unknown as well as known confounding variables. Four randomized controlled trials of routine late pregnancy ultrasonography with the main purpose of detecting the clinically unsuspected small-for-dates fetus, have been published (Bakkateig et al., 1984; Eik-Nes et al., 1984; Neilson, Munjanja and Whitfield, 1984; Secher et al., 1987). These studies took different forms, used different ultrasound techniques, and were associated with great variation in sensitivity in identifying small-for-gestational age fetuses – from 25 per cent (Bakkateig et al., 1984) to 94 per cent (Neilson, Munjanja and Whitfield, 1984). Combining the results of these trials to give a consensus view, by so-called 'meta-analysis', does not encourage the use of routine measurement of all fetuses by ultrasound in late pregnancy as no clear benefit has been demonstrated in improving fetal outcome or obstetric management (Neilson and Grant, 1989). Ultrasound is, therefore, best utilized when there are specific clinical indications, such as when the fetus is suspected of being small for dates, or where there is increased clinical risk of impaired growth.

Confirmation by diagnostic ultrasound

Diagnostic ultrasound is the technique that provides most information about fetal size and shape and, by repeated measurements, growth; because of its ability to image soft tissues, it also gives information about many more facets of fetal status than merely an estimate of size. Ultrasound is therefore given due prominence here. Descriptions of new fetal measurements have rapidly outstripped a critical assessment of their value in practice but it is useful to consider the large range now available. Some measurements are useful for confirming a clinical suspicion that the fetus is small for dates; others have different functions.

Fetal measurement
The biparietal diameter was the first fetal measurement to be performed using ultrasound, initially by a simple A-mode technique (Willocks et al., 1964), later by the combined A- and B-mode technique using static B-scanners, (Campbell, 1968), and now with real-time systems. It is best measured in the occipitofrontal plane in which the head circumference (or area) may also be measured. Head circumference measurements are of particular value when fetal head shape is unusual, as in dolichocephaly (very narrow) or brachycephaly (very broad). In these cases the biparietal diameter does not represent accurately overall head size. The 'cephalic index' (ratio of biparietal diameter to occipitofrontal diameter expressed as a percentage) allows a quantitative assessment of head shape. Dolichocephaly may be associated with breech presentation and with oligohydramnios and is not, in itself, a sinister finding; brachycephaly may be associated with Down's syndrome. As imaging has improved dramatically in recent years to allow more anatomical detail to be seen, more fetal head measurements have been described. These include distances from the lateral ventricles to the midline, the transverse dimensions of the cerebellum, the width of the cisterna magna, and the binocular distance (stretching from the outer margin of one orbit to the outer margin of the other).

Measurement of the fetal trunk started with measurement of the thorax but the main developmental thrust came with Campbell's description of the abdominal section at the level of the liver (Campbell and Wilkin, 1975), which is best identified by the confluence of the umbilical vein and the left portal vein. Normal values have also been published for the dimensions of a number of organs in the trunk. These include the heart (best studied by real-time B mode and M mode ultrasound), the liver (Vintzileos et al., 1985a), the spleen (Schmidt et al., 1985), the kidneys (Grannum et al., 1980) and even the adrenal gland (Lewis et al., 1982). The volume of urine in the fetal bladder may be estimated and the rate of urine production thus calculated from repeated observations (Wladimiroff and Campbell, 1974). The lumen of the large bowel may also be measured (Goldstein, Lockwood and Hobbins, 1987).

Fetal long bones are readily measured, although patience is required when the fetus is moving. Normal values have been described for femur, tibia, fibula, humerus, ulna and radius (Jeanty et al., 1984). The volume of the fetal limbs may be estimated (Jeanty, Romero and Hobbins, 1985) and the length of the feet measured (Mercer et al., 1987). Limb measurements have been performed not only for direct purposes but also as indices of fetal length (e.g. femoral length; Vintzileos et al., 1985b) or soft tissue mass (e.g. thigh circumference; Deter et al., 1987).

Other measurements
It is important to consider the fetus in the context of its environment, and study of the other contents of the gravid uterus, using ultrasound, has also proved fruitful.

The amount of amniotic fluid may be assessed subjectively or objectively. Subjective assessment, which is based on an overall impression with special attention paid to fluid between the limbs, is, because of the irregular distribution of fluid around the fetus, not unreasonable; it certainly seems to be a replicable examination by both the same and also by different observers (Halperin et al., 1985). However, attempts have been made to quantify the amount of amniotic fluid more objectively. Various approaches have been used, mainly concentrating on the largest visible pool of amniotic fluid. Calculation of an average diameter of the pool (from one vertical and two horizontal measurements) gives a more replicable result than does simply measuring the vertical diameter alone (Patterson, Prihoda and Pouliot, 1987). Despite this, the maximum vertical diameter of the largest pool is now a commonly used parameter. It has been suggested that a distance of <2 cm indicates oligohydramnios (Chamberlain et al., 1984a), whereas one of ≥8 cm indicates polyhydramnios (Chamberlain et al., 1984b).

Ultrasound measurement of the thickness of the placenta (Hoddick et al., 1985), has never become popular, nor has estimation of placental volume, which was an early focus of investigation by ultrasound (Hellmann et al., 1970) and which has also been studied more recently (Geirsson, 1986; Wolf, Oosting and Treffers, 1987). Of more interest to ultrasonographers than the physical dimensions of the placenta has been its appearance or 'texture'. This has been known for some time to change with increasing gestation and these features, which have been attributed to placental 'ageing', were classified by Grannum, Berkowitz and Hobbins (1979). Placental grading has remained as a method of assessment in potentially compromised pregnancies (Proud and Grant, 1987).

Measurement of total intrauterine volume, which was popular at one time in the United States, was prompted by the fact that small-for-dates fetuses tend to have small placentae and diminished amniotic fluid volume (Gohari, Berkowitz and Hobbins, 1977). However, even when measured using a complex and time-consuming planimetric technique, this method did not prove more sensitive than simple fetal measurements (Geirsson, 1986) and it fell into disfavour.

Ultrasound detection of small-for-dates fetuses
Despite the shortcomings of the small-for-dates concept already discussed, it remains the 'gold standard' against which most ultrasound measurements have been evaluated. Campbell and Dewhurst (1971) showed that up to 73 per cent of small-for-dates babies could be identified by repeated measurement of the biparietal diameter and for many years this was the standard ultrasound technique used in high risk pregnancies. However, it is relatively insensitive because of the 'brain sparing' effect. If the organ weights of small-for-dates babies are compared with those of controls, of either similar bodyweight or gestational age, it is found that the organs most diminished in weight are the thymus, spleen and liver (Gruenwald, 1974); in contrast, brain weight is very much less reduced. It was, therefore, predicted that measurement of the abdominal circumference (at the liver) would prove more sensitive (Campbell and Wilkin, 1975) and this was confirmed on prospective study. In a study of 474 unselected pregnancies at between 34 and 36 weeks of pregnancy, the abdominal circumference had a sensitivity of 81 per cent in predicting small-for-dates babies with a specificity of 89 per cent and the method was superior to others assessed (Neilson, Whitfield and Aitchison, 1980). Abdominal measurement remains the best single method for identifying small-for-dates fetuses, and, indeed, also for predicting macrosomia (Bochner *et al.*, 1987). We await the results of the newer measurements in large, broadly based populations to see if any will prove better.

In the investigation of the small-for-dates fetus, measurements are best compared with normal intrauterine standards rather than converted to an estimate of fetal weight and plotted on a chart of birthweight for gestational age. However, an estimate of fetal weight may be useful in managing women who have had a caesarean section previously, those with a fetus presenting by the breech and those in preterm labour, although gestational age gives better prognostic information (Verloove-Vanhorick *et al.*, 1986). Formulae exist for the estimation of fetal weight from abdominal measurement (Campbell and Wilkin, 1975), abdominal and head measurements (Shepard *et al.*, 1982), and abdominal, head and femur measurements (Hadlock *et al.*, 1985); other authors have reported minor variations of these. In general, estimates are only accurate to within 10–15 per cent of the actual weight and therefore may, at times, be misleading.

Investigation of cause of being small for dates

Having confirmed the clinical impression that a fetus is small for dates, an attempt should be made to establish aetiology, although this often proves unsuccessful. In particular, it is vital to identify fetal abnormality and uteroplacental insufficiency, as these causes carry important implications for subsequent management. It is, for example, usually inappropriate to deliver a fetus with a major malformation by caesarean section; diagnosis of uteroplacental insufficiency heightens anxiety about mortality and morbidity. Both abnormality and uteroplacental insufficiency may be identified by ultrasound, sometimes in combination with other techniques.

Ultrasound
Ultrasonography contributes to identification of malformations, both by imaging the defect and also by measuring the fetus. Thus, calculation of the ventricular–hemispheric ratio will assist the diagnosis of hydrocephalus (Nicolaides and Campbell, 1987) whereas measurements of the fetal head, thorax and long bones may identify,

respectively, microcephaly (Chervenak *et al.*, 1987), spondylothoracic dysplasia (Chitkara *et al.*, 1987), and other skeletal dysplasias (Fowlie, 1989). It has also been reported that trisomy 21 can be diagnosed by measurement of the soft-tissue thickness at the neck (Benacceraf and Frigoletto, 1987), although this has not been confirmed by other workers (Toi, Simpson and Filly, 1987). Amniocentesis, placental biopsy and cordocentesis may be used when chromosomal abnormality is suspected, such as when a small-for-dates fetus is found to have dysmorphic features or associated polyhydramnios on ultrasound study.

Uteroplacental insufficiency, on the other hand, can be assumed to be the cause when genuine growth retardation is demonstrated. Because diagnostic ultrasound provides the ideal tool for monitoring the rate of growth of individual fetuses, it is the definitive method for detecting cessation of growth. This approach has, however received less attention than it deserves. Deter and colleagues (1986) have proposed that the growth potential of individual fetuses could be assessed by two measurements during the second trimester separated by several weeks e.g. at 20 and 28 weeks. The rate of growth derived from these could then be projected into the third trimester and significant slowing could be detected by subsequent measurement. This approach, concentrating on growth rather than size, and using each fetus as its own control, is attractive; however, the fact that growth retardation may start in the second trimester poses obvious difficulties.

Using serial measurement of the biparietal diameter, attempts were made to establish pathogenesis by demonstrating different patterns of growth among small-for-dates fetuses (Campbell, 1974). Those that were genuinely growth retarded showed abrupt cessation of previously normal growth, whereas those with low growth potential showed early departure from normal rates but continued to grow until delivery. The calculation of head–abdomen circumference ratios was proposed as a useful method of further differentiating these two groups (Campbell and Thoms, 1977), based on the hypothesis that those babies that are genuinely growth retarded will show evidence of brain sparing and thus have disproportionately high head–abdomen ratios. This probably has a limited role in fetal assessment – the demonstration of asymmetry suggests, but does not prove, uteroplacental insufficiency; the demonstration of a symmetrically small-for-dates fetus emphasizes the need to exclude abnormality, but this pattern is also seen in some perfectly normal babies and some with genuine growth retardation (Davies *et al.*, 1979).

An alternative approach is to concentrate on wasting. The ponderal index which is calculated by the formula [birthweight $\times$ 100/(crown-heel length)^3], has been used by paediatricians to estimate the degree of intrauterine malnutrition experienced by the growth retarded neonate. Some regard this as an index of growth retardation superior to the state of being small for dates (Patterson and Pouliot, 1987). Although this requires further study, attempts to calculate the fetal ponderal index from ultrasound measurement are certainly of interest. The most popular technique is to calculate the ratio of femur length to abdominal circumference (Vintzileos *et al.*, 1985b; Divon *et al.*, 1986); the wasted fetus should have a high ratio. Ratios seem constant over different gestational ages in normally grown fetuses, so they may have a very useful role when growth retardation is suspected but gestational age is uncertain. Yagel and colleagues (1987) investigated a slightly different form of fetal ponderal index by dividing the estimated weight by the femur length cubed. This appeared to provide useful prognostic information after fetuses were identified as small for gestational age.

Estimation of amniotic fluid volume by ultrasonography also helps to separate the healthy from the unhealthy among the small-for-dates group (Chamberlain *et al.*, 1984a), the latter usually being associated with oligohydramnios. Oligohydramnios occurring in association with fetal growth retardation has to be distinguished from that resulting from fetal renal tract abnormalities and spontaneous rupture of the membranes which, if it occurs during the second trimester, may be associated with fetal pulmonary hypoplasia. Sustained absence of fetal breathing (on real-time ultrasonography) is, it has been suggested, highly predictive of lung hypoplasia (Blott *et al.*, 1987) although this is disputed by others (Moessinger *et al.*, 1987). Ultrasound measurement of the thoracic circumference (at the level of the lungs) may be useful (Nimrod *et al.*, 1986) although, because there is overlap in results between fetuses with pulmonary hypoplasia and those that are small for dates, the ratio of thoracic to abdominal circumferences should give better discrimination (Johnson *et al.*, 1987).

Doppler ultrasound
It is appropriate to consider here the relatively new technique of Doppler ultrasound and its probable role in the management of fetal growth retardation. As a clearer picture starts to emerge as to what its role may be in obstetric practice, Doppler ultrasound appears best at predicting serious compromise in high risk pregnancies, including those complicated by fetal growth retardation. It is thus potentially helpful in separating the pathological from the non-pathological in the small-for-dates group. Vessels on both sides of the placenta have been studied with Doppler ultrasound, starting with the work of Fitzgerald and Drumm (1977) on the umbilical artery, and now include the umbilical vein, the fetal aorta and internal carotid and anterior and middle cerebral arteries, and branches of the maternal uterine artery. The umbilical artery remains the most popular vessel for study. Both the utero-placental and fetoplacental circulations are usually low resistance systems in which downstream flow continues throughout the cardiac cycle. When vascular resistance increases, diastolic flow may decrease, stop or even become reversed and this is reflected in the blood-velocity waveform. Two different types of Doppler equipment may be used: continuous-wave systems which are relatively inexpensive and simple, and pulsed wave systems which have the advantage of allowing the blood vessel to be imaged and range gating performed.

Failure of the physiological invasion of myometrial spiral arteries by cytotropho-blast early in the second trimester and the later development of acute atherosis would both be expected to be associated with higher vascular resistance and these features are, as has been discussed, sometimes seen in fetal growth retardation. Thus, in theory, diminished diastolic blood-flow velocities in the uterine arterial system may not only identify uteroplacental insufficiency but might also give early warning of it long before the clinical features become obvious.

The impact of uteroplacental insufficiency on fetal umbilical artery waveforms is less easily predicted. However, in a study of pregnant sheep, embolization of the uterine circulation with microspheres produced a rapid increase in umbilical artery resistance if fetal growth retardation were to result later (Clapp *et al.*, 1980). Although direct extrapolation of these findings to human pregnancy must be avoided (Mellor, 1984), a similar phenomenon is recognized in the human fetus and probably results from vascular abnormalities in tertiary stem villi (Giles, Trudinger and Baird, 1985). Increased blood viscosity, which was once thought important, probably has relatively little influence on the umbilical artery waveform (Giles, Trudinger and Palmer, 1986).

Much of the work published on Doppler ultrasound has concentrated on predicting babies that are small for dates at birth. Comparison between reports is difficult because of varying diagnostic criteria, selection of patients and vessels studied but a comprehensive review of data then available (Neilson and Whittle, 1988) suggested that fetal measurement with diagnostic ultrasound gave better prediction; subsequent study has confirmed this (Divon *et al.*, 1988). Doppler study of the umbilical artery as a screening technique in unselected (rather than high risk) populations appears especially poor at predicting small-for-dates babies (Beattie and Dornan, 1989; Sijmons *et al.*, 1989; Hanretty *et al.*, 1989) although some authors have not found the method useful even in high risk populations (Dempster *et al.*, 1989). It had been hoped that Doppler study of maternal uteroplacental arteries during mid-pregnancy would prove a useful screening technique for predicting subsequent uteroplacental insufficiency (Campbell *et al.*, 1986), but this seems unlikely to be sufficiently sensitive. Steel and colleagues (Steel, Pearce and Chamberlain, 1988), in a study of 200 primigravidae found that only 10 of the 27 pregnancies that produced a small-for-dates baby had abnormal Doppler results.

Whether it is possible, using Doppler ultrasound, to separate anatomically normal small-for-dates fetuses into growth retarded and non-growth retarded sub-groups, seems a more fruitful area of investigation, the hypothesis being that those that are genuinely growth retarded would be associated with abnormal flow variables on the maternal side of the placenta. Studies that have been addressed to this question (Campbell *et al.*, 1983; Trudinger, Giles and Cook, 1985) have been difficult to interpret because of differing mean gestational age in the two sub-groups. More recent work has shown a wide range of Doppler results from the uteroplacental vessels in pregnancies complicated by fetal growth retardation without coexisting pre-eclampsia (McCowan *et al.*, 1988).

Doppler study of the umbilical artery waveform does, however, appear to help predict perinatal risk among small-for-dates fetuses. In a careful study, which not only assessed the value of umbilical artery velocimetry blind (i.e. the results were not reported to clinicians) but which also grappled with the difficult problem of defining appropriate endpoints, Reuwer and colleagues (1987) reported on 51 women admitted antenatally to hospital because of suspected fetal growth retardation. Following delivery, 16 of them (group 1) were classified as having had 'normal placental function' (birthweight greater than the fifth percentile, ponderal index normal, no perinatal problems); 30 were classified as having had 'manifest placental insufficiency' (birthweight less than fifth percentile and/or low ponderal index) and subdivided into those which died *in utero* or required delivery for fetal distress (group 2a, numbering 19) and those which did not require either obstetric intervention or paediatric resuscitation (group 2b, numbering 11); five were unclassifiable. Group 1 fetuses all had normal Doppler findings; group 2a fetuses all developed abnormal Doppler findings, usually with completely absent end-diastolic velocities; group 2b had variable results – some normal, some abnormal but none with the extreme abnormality of absent end-diastolic velocities.

The fact that adverse perinatal outcome among these small-for-dates babies was predicted by Doppler study does not necessarily mean that either outcome or management could have been improved by knowledge of the results. Established forms of assessment (clinical or non-clinical) could, for example, have provided the same prognostic information. In addition, although reversed end-diastolic flow appears to be associated with especially poor outcome (Brar and Platt, 1988), the significance of absent end-diastolic velocities is more variable as it can sometimes be seen for weeks in compromised pregnancies before a need to deliver (Johnstone *et al.*, 1988) and also in some normal pregnancies (Hanretty *et al.*, 1989). The necessity for randomized controlled study to determine whether benefit does result from Doppler study (Neilson, 1987) should require no further elaboration here. One randomized controlled trial has been reported (Trudinger *et al.*, 1987). Three hundred women who had been admitted to hospital for various antenatal complications (including suspected fetal growth retardation) were included. The results of umbilical artery Doppler study were reported for 133 and concealed for the rest: there was a lower incidence of caesarean section during labour among the reported group but, overall, caesarean section rates (and other indices of outcome) were not significantly different between the groups. Several other randomized controlled trials are now in progress and, at present, an unequivocal recommendation that Doppler ultrasound should be part of routine fetal assessment would not be appropriate.

The dynamics of regional blood flow to other organs of the fetus may also be studied. Examination of the cerebral arteries using pulsed Doppler equipment, although technically difficult (Mari *et al.*, 1989), raises exciting possibilities. Increased blood flow to the brain is one of the compensatory responses of the hypoxaemic fetus and this has already been discussed. In some cases of fetal growth retardation, increased end-diastolic velocities in the internal carotid artery are found which are consistent with this phenomenon (Wladimiroff *et al.*, 1986). Comparing the waveforms in umbilical artery and internal carotid artery in individual fetuses may prove useful (Wladimiroff, Tonge and Stewart, 1987), including the responses to maternal oxygen therapy (Arduini *et al.*, 1989). It may be that some of the compensatory mechanisms evoked in the fetus by hypoxaemia may ultimately prove harmful; hence, the suggestion that neonatal necrotizing enterocolitis may result, in part, from gut ischaemia secondary to diminished blood flow (Hackett *et al.*, 1987). This requires further study.

Assessment of fetal well-being

Apart from Doppler ultrasound (which has been discussed) and cordocentesis to assess fetal blood gases and acid–base balance (which is still experimental), other forms of fetal assessment such as cardiotocography, kick counts and the biophysical profile, have been available for sufficiently long for individual clinicians to reach individual conclusions about their value and role in monitoring the small-for-dates fetus. Although these tests will not be discussed further here, they do contribute a very important element in management. Most small-for-dates fetuses can be safely monitored on an outpatient basis at intervals of between 2 and 7 days, depending on individual circumstances. A specially designated and equipped day care unit is particularly valuable in managing these cases.

Consideration of treatment

At present there is no proven therapy for improving growth rate when a fetus is found to be growth retarded. This is not a problem in late pregnancy, when delivery can be effected safely but it would be desirable when the diagnosis is made at a time at which fetal immaturity pre-empts delivery. The rate of fetal growth is not improved by bed rest (Grant, Chalmers and Enkin, 1982) or by the administration of β-blockers to women with mild to moderate pregnancy-induced hypertension (Rubin *et al.*, 1983).

It has been suggested that pre-eclampsia may be prevented by the use of low-dose aspirin from mid-pregnancy in women at high risk (Beaufils *et al.*, 1985; Wallenberg *et al.*, 1986) and that similar prophylactic therapy may also be useful in women at high risk of producing growth-retarded babies (Elder *et al.*, 1988; Trudinger *et al.*, 1988). The possible advantages (and disadvantages) of low dose aspirin therapy in preventing both complications are now being assessed by a large multicentre randomized trial.

In sheep experiments it has proved possible to prevent growth retardation in fetal lambs, following maternal dietary restriction, by intragastric supplementation of the fetus with glucose and amino acids (Charlton and Johengen, 1985) and, following maternal uterine artery embolization, by intravenous infusion of glucose and amino acids into the fetus (Charlton and Johengen, 1987). In neither of these studies were the fetuses hypoxaemic. Fetal hypoxaemia is commonly found in growth retarded lamb fetuses following placental restriction experiments (Owens, Falconer and Robinson, 1987) and may be found in some human growth retarded fetuses (Soothill, Nicoloides and Campbell, 1987; Cox *et al.*, 1988); it is possible that nutritional supplementation might prove dangerous under these circumstances. Oxygen supplementation has been found to improve survival rates among growth retarded rat fetuses and to cause a modest improvement in growth rate (Vileisis, 1985). Experience of oxygen therapy in human pregnancy is limited. Nicolaides and colleagues (1987) described five pregnancies complicated by severe intrauterine growth retardation during the second trimester. There was no improvement in growth rate in response to maternal oxygen therapy but in four cases there was some apparent improvement in the state of fetal health.

Therapy to improve the health of growth retarded fetuses during the second trimester, to allow the pregnancy to continue until a stage at which fetal survival is likely, would be an important advance; further study is required. At present, the main management decision is when and how to deliver the growth-retarded fetus.

Decision about delivery

Identification of the best time for delivery will be based on several pieces of information, including gestational age, the severity of growth retardation, whether or not there is accompanying maternal disease such as pre-eclampsia, the results of tests of fetal well-being, past obstetric history, (possibly) the state of fetal lung maturation, and the ripeness of the mother's cervix. Individual cases require individual decisions.

It is better to effect planned delivery before severe oligohydramnios occurs, as this may prevent vaginal delivery through severe cord compression during labour.

An incompletely resolved question is whether it is better to deliver early an apparently healthy small-for-dates baby because of possible adverse effects on brain development. Ounsted and colleagues (Ounsted, Moar and Scott, 1989) suggest that prolongation of pregnancy beyond 38 weeks is not associated with improved long-term developmental prognosis in small-for-dates babies and this may be positively harmful in some cases (especially when associated with maternal hypertensive conditions). Perhaps the use of Doppler ultrasound study of cerebral arteries will provide fresh insights and allow greater individualization of management.

The best method of delivery will, like timing, depend on a number of factors. The hazards of intrapartum asphyxia have already been discussed. There is evidence that small-for-dates babies tend to tolerate vaginal breech delivery poorly.

Multiple pregnancy

The problems of abnormal fetal growth in multiple pregnancies are considered here separately because of both the high incidence of small-for-dates babies and also the unusual pathogenetic features that may exist. Unusual difficulties in fetal assessment may also occur.

A number of authors have recommended that separate standards of size, growth and birthweight should be applied to twin babies, and not conventional singleton standards. This is not logical: dizygotic twins, at least, will possess the same intrinsic growth potential as do singleton fetuses and similar slowing of growth will have similar prognostic significance. It is conceivable that the events that surround the splitting of the conceptus in monozygotic twinning could leave the babies with reduced growth potential. We have, however, found monozygotic and dizygotic twin fetuses to be of similar size from early/mid pregnancy (Neilson and Hastie, 1988) and, although acknowledging that others have reported different findings (Grennert *et al.*, 1980), conclude that conventional singleton standards are appropriate for both types of twins. Certainly the high rate of fetal loss from twin pregnancy attributable to impaired growth (Manlan and Scott, 1978) should discourage the use of less stringent definitions in assessing twin babies than singleton babies.

Because of the relative frequency of twin pregnancies compared with higher multiples, further discussion here concentrates on twins. The risks of fetal growth retardation, however increase with increasing number of babies.

The twin transfusion syndrome

There is a high rate of fetal loss from twin pregnancies generally (Patel *et al.*, 1984), with a higher loss rate from monozygotic than dizygotic pregnancies (Naeye *et al.*, 1978). This is because of more frequent fetal malformation among monozygotic twins (Fogel, Nitowsky and Gruenwald, 1965) and the adverse consequences of monochorionic placentation. Three-quarters of monozygotic pregnancies have monochorionic placentas and, almost always, these contain vascular anastomoses connecting the circulations of each twin (Robertson and Neer, 1983). Arteriovenous anastomoses enable the shunting of blood from one fetus to the other and thus the twin transfusion syndrome. In its most florid form, this is associated with anaemia and growth retardation in the donor twin and polycythaemia in the recipient, and with oligohydramnios in the amniotic sac of the donor and polyhydramnios in that of the recipient (Benirschke and Kim, 1973). Fetal ascites can occur in either fetus. These features, which are rare, may be identified on ultrasound examination (Wittmann, Baldwin and Nichol, 1981) to allow the possibility of treatment (Wittmann *et al.*, 1986).

Various (and conflicting) opinions have been expressed about Doppler findings in twin transfusion syndrome. Thus, Farmakides and colleagues (1985) described two cases, using unspecified diagnostic criteria, in which umbilical artery waveforms of the respective twins were discordant. In contrast, Giles, Trudinger and Cook (1985) provided evidence that *discordant* growth in association with *concordant* umbilical artery waveforms is highly suggestive of twin transfusion syndrome. Gerson and colleagues (1987) proposed, but did not test, the hypothesis that twin transfusion syndrome is associated with normal (and concordant) umbilical artery flow to the placenta but with discordant return flow in the umbilical veins. Erskine and colleagues (Erskine, Ritchie and Murnaghan, 1986) describe a case in which an artery–

artery anastomosis in a monochorionic placenta appeared to alter the umbilical artery flow of the smaller twin in a cyclical fashion; this was attributed to increased vascular resistance during systoles synchronous with those of the co-twin. Pretorius and colleagues (1988) found no consistent pattern in eight examples of twin transfusion syndrome.

These different reports probably reflect both the diverse nature of anastomotic links in monochorionic placentas and also a lack of satisfactory diagnostic criteria to confirm diagnosis of the twin transfusion syndrome (Danskin and Neilson, 1989).

We have been unable to show any consistent pattern of umbilical artery waveform resulting from vascular anastomoses in monochorionic placentas in pregnancies unaffected by the florid form of the twin transfusion syndrome. Similarly we have not found any consistent difference in fetal size or growth or discordancy of size in monozygotic pregnancies with monochorionic placentas compared with those with dichorionic placentas (Neilson, Danskin and Hastie, 1989). This indicates that vascular anastomoses do not, in the absence of florid twin transfusion syndrome, exert a strong influence on fetal growth.

Detection of the small-for-dates twin fetus

Small-for-dates twin fetuses are difficult to identify by abdominal palpation antenatally because of the presence of the other baby. Tape measurements of symphysis–fundal height will, by 34–36 weeks, allow the detection of between 55 and 65 per cent of pregnancies in which both twins are small for dates (Neilson, Verkuyl and Bannerman, 1988), but this simple technique is not helpful in identifying pregnancies in which only one of the twins is small for dates.

There is a need for a technique, such as ultrasound, that allows individual twin fetuses to be studied separately (Secher, Kaern and Hanson, 1985). As in singleton pregnancies, abdominal measurements are manifestly superior to head measurements (Neilson, 1981), although we have found abdominal circumference measurements to be less sensitive in twin than singleton pregnancies; this may be due to frequent mechanical flexion of twins in late gestation distorting transverse abdominal dimensions (Neilson, 1988).

Some workers have reported sensitive identification of small-for-dates twin fetuses by Doppler ultrasound study of umbilical arteries (Giles, Trudinger and Cook, 1985; Farmakides et al., 1985; Nimrod et al., 1987). Our own study of unselected twin pregnancies studied serially has not produced similar results, as most small-for-dates fetuses had quite normal Doppler results (Hastie et al., 1989). In our experience, only consistently absent end-diastolic velocities proved useful prognostically. Degani and colleagues (1988), likewise, did not find umbilical artery velocimetry helpful in predicting small-for-dates twin fetuses (sensitivity 33 per cent), although study of the internal carotid artery appeared better.

Conclusions

The next few years are likely to see a rapid advance in our understanding of the physiological regulation of fetal growth (and especially the role of tissue growth factors) and of the pathophysiological processes that may disrupt it. However, to maximize the influence of such advances, as well as to apply new techniques of fetal assessment sensibly, it is vital that a satisfactory system of defining and classifying growth-retarded babies be established. The limitations of the small-for-dates concept have been discussed.

Biophysical assessment remains a key element of managing the growth-retarded fetus. Abdominal circumference remains the most useful single ultrasound measurement. The place of Doppler ultrasound has yet to be definitively established. A number of randomized controlled trials are now in progress. Cordocentesis to assess fetal karyotype, blood gases and acid–base status in the growth-retarded fetus has generated interesting biochemical findings to allow comparison with the results of experiments in various animal models. This technique may not become widespread in use but it can, perhaps, provide a more objective standard against which to evaluate less invasive methods.

Therapy for fetal growth retardation is being actively researched in animal experiments at present; the rational use of therapy in human pregnancy is probably still some way off.

References

Alexander, G (1978) Factors regulating the growth of the placenta. In *Abnormal Fetal Growth: Biological Bases and Consequences, edited by F Naftolin* (pp. 149–164. Berlin: Dahlem Konferenzen

Arduini, D, Rizzo, G, Romanini, C and Mancuso, S (1989) Fetal haemodynamic response to acute maternal hyperoxygenation as predictor of fetal distress in intrauterine growth retardation. *British Medical Journal*, **298**, 1561–1562

Bakkateig, LS, Eik-Nes, SH, Jacobsen, G *et al.* (1984) Randomized controlled trial of ultrasonographic screening in pregnancy. *Lancet*, **ii**, 207–211

Beattie, RB and Dornan, JC (1989) Antenatal screening for intrauterine growth retardation with umbilical artery Doppler ultrasonography. *British Medical Journal*, **298**, 631–635

Beaufils, M, Uzan, S, Dousimoni, R and Colau, JC (1985) Prevention of pre-eclampsia by early antiplatelet therapy. *Lancet*, **i**, 840–842

Belizan, JM, Villar, J, Nardin, JC *et al.* (1978) Diagnosis of IUGR by a simple clinical method: measurement of fundal height. *American Journal of Obstetrics and Gynecology*, **131**, 643–646

Benacerraf, BR and Frigoletto, FD (1987) Soft tissue fold in the second-trimester fetus: standards for normal measurements compared with those in Down syndrome. *American Journal of Obstetrics and Gynecology*, **157**, 1146–1149

Benirschke, K and Kim, CK (1973) Multiple pregnancy. *New England Journal of Medicine*, 1276–1284

Blott, M, Greenough, A, Nicolaides, KH *et al.* (1987) Fetal breathing movements as predictor of favourable outcome after oligohydramnios due to membrane rupture in the second trimester. *Lancet*, **ii**, 129–131

Bochner, CJ, Medearis, AL, Williams, J *et al.* (1987) Early third-trimester ultrasound screening in gestational diabetes to determine the risk of macrosomia and labor dystocia at term. *American Journal of Obstetrics and Gynecology*, **157**, 703–708

Bonds, DR, Gabbe, SG, Kumar, S and Taylor, T (1984) Fetal weight/placental weight ratios and perinatal outcome. *American Journal of Obstetrics and Gynecology*, **149**, 195–200

Brar, HS and Platt, LD (1988) Reverse end-diastolic flow velocity on umbilical artery velocimetry in high-risk pregnancies: an ominous finding with adverse pregnancy outcome. *American Journal of Obstetrics and Gynecology*, **159**, 559–561

Breart, G and Poisson-Salomon, AS (1988) Intrauterine growth retardation and mental handicap: epidemiological evidence. *Baillière's Clinical Obstetrics and Gynaecology*, **2**, 91–100

Campbell, S (1968) An improved method of fetal cephalometry by ultrasound. *Journal of Obstetrics and Gynaecology of the British Commonwealth*, **75**, 568–576

Campbell, S (1974) Fetal growth. *Clinics in Obstetrics and Gynaecology*, **1**, 41–65

Campbell, S and Dewhurst, CJ (1971) Diagnosis of the small-for-dates fetus by serial ultrasonic cephalometry. *Lancet*, **ii**, 1002–1006

Campbell, S and Thoms, A (1977) Ultrasonic measurement of the fetal head to abdomen circumference ratio in the assessment of growth retardation. *British Journal of Obstetrics and Gynaecology*, **84**, 165–174

Campbell, S and Wilkin, D (1975) Ultrasonic measurement of fetal abdominal circumference in the estimation of fetal weight. *British Journal of Obstetrics and Gynaecology*, **82**, 689–697

Campbell, S, Diaz-Racasens, J, Griffin, D *et al.* (1983) New Doppler technique for assessing uteroplacental blood flow. *Lancet*, **i**, 675–679

Campbell, S, Pearce, JMF, Hackett, G *et al.* (1986) Qualitative assessment of uteroplacental blood flow: early screening test for high-risk pregnancies. *Obstetrics and Gynecology*, **68**, 649–653

Chamberlain, PF, Manning, FA, Morrison, I *et al.* (1984a) Ultrasound evaluation of amniotic fluid volume, 1. The relationship of marginal and decreased amniotic fluid volume to perinatal outcome. *American Journal of Obstetrics and Gynecology*, **150**, 245–249

Chamberlain, PF, Manning, FA, Morrison, I *et al.* (1984b) Ultrasound evaluation of amniotic fluid volume, 2. The relationship of increased amniotic fluid volume to perinatal outcome. *American Journal of Obstetrics and Gynecology*, **150**, 250–2540

Charlton, V and Johengen, M (1985) Effects of intrauterine supplementation on fetal growth retardation. *Biology of the Neonate*, **48**, 125–142

Charlton, V and Johengen, M (1987) Fetal intravenous nutritional supplementation ameliorates the development of embolization-induced growth retardation in sheep. *Pediatric Research*, **22**, 55–61

Chervenak, FA, Rosenberg, J, Brightman, RC *et al.* (1987) A prospective study of the accuracy of ultrasound in predicting microcephaly. *Obstetrics and Gynecology*, **69**, 908–910

Chitkara, U, Rosenberg, J, Chervenak, FA *et al.* (1987) Prenatal sonographic assessment of the fetal thorax: normal values. *American Journal of Obstetrics and Gynecology*, **156**, 1069–1074

Clapp, JF (1978) The relationship between blood flow and oxygen take up in the uterine and umbilical circulations. *American Journal of Obstetrics and Gynecology*, **132**, 410–413

Clapp, JF, Szeto, HH, Larrow, R *et al.* (1980) Umbilical blood flow response to embolization of the uterine circulation. *American Journal of Obstetrics and Gynecology*, **138**, 60–67

Clifford, SH (1954) Postmaturity with placental dysfunction. *Journal of Pediatrics*, **44**, 1–13

Cox, WL, Daffos, F, Forestier, F *et al.* (1988) Physiology and management of intrauterine growth retardation: a biologic approach with fetal blood sampling. *American Journal of Obstetrics and Gynecology*, **159**, 36–41

Danskin, FH and Neilson, JP (1989) The twin to twin transfusion syndrome: what are appropriate diagnostic criteria? *American Journal of Obstetrics and Gynecology*, **161**, 365–369

Davies, DP, Platts, P, Pritchard, JM and Wilkinson, PW (1979) Nutritional status of light-for-dates infants at birth and its influence on early postnatal growth. *Archives of Disease in Childhood*, **54**, 703–706

Degani, S, Paltiely, Y, Lewinsky, R *et al.* (1988) Fetal internal corotid artery velocity time waveforms in twin pregnancies. *Journal of Perinatal Medicine*, **16**, 405–409

Dempster, J, Mires, GJ, Patel, N and Taylor, DJ (1989) Umbilical artery velocity waveforms: poor association with small-for-gestational-age babies. *British Journal of Obstetrics and Gynaecology*, **96**, 692–696

D'Ercole, AJ (1987) Somatomedins/insulin-like growth factors and fetal growth. *Journal of Developmental Physiology*, **9**, 481–495

Deter, RL, Rossavik, IK, Harrist, RB and Hadlock, FP (1986) Mathematic modeling of fetal growth: development of individual growth curve standards. *Obstetrics and Gynecology*, **68**, 156–161

Deter, RL, Rossavik, IK, Harrist, RB and Hadlock, FP (1987) Longitudinal studies of thigh circumference growth in normal fetuses. *Journal of Clinical Ultrasound*, **15**, 388–393

Divon, MY, Chamberlain, PF, Sipos, L *et al.* (1986) Identification of the small for gestational age fetus with the use of gestational age-independent indices of fetal growth. *American Journal of Obstetrics and Gynecology*, **155**, 1197–1201

Divon, MY, Guidetti, DA, Bravermau, JJ *et al.* (1988) Intrauterine growth retardation – a prospective study of the diagnostic value of real-time sonography combined with umbilical artery flow velocimetry. *Obstetrics and Gynecology*, **72**, 611–614

Dobson, PC, Abell, DA and Beischer, NA (1981) Mortality and morbidity of fetal growth retardation. *Australian and New Zealand Journal of Obstetrics and Gynaecology*, **21**, 69–72

Eik-Nes, SH, Okland, O, Aure, JC and Ulstein, M (1984) Ultrasound screening in pregnancy: a randomized controlled trial. *Lancet*, **i**, 1347

Elder, MG, Burton, ER, Gordon, H *et al.* (1970) Maternal weight and girth changes in late pregnancy and the diagnosis of placental insufficiency. *Journal of Obstetrics and Gynaecology of the British Commonwealth*, **77**, 481–491

Elder, MG, De Swiet, M, Robertson, A *et al.* (1988) Low-dose aspirin in pregnancy. *Lancet*, **i**, 410

Erskine, RLA, Ritchie, JWK and Murnaghan, GA (1986) Antenatal diagnosis of placental anastomoses in a twin pregnancy using Doppler ultrasound. *British Journal of Obstetrics and Gynaecology*, **93**, 955–959

Farmakides, G, Schulman, H, Saldana, LR *et al.* (1985) Surveillance of twin pregnancy with umbilical artery velocimetry. *American Journal of Obstetrics and Gynecology*, **153**, 789–7920

Fitzgerald, DF, and Drumm, JE (1977) Non-invasive measurement of human fetal circulation using ultrasound: a new method. *British Medical Journal*, **2**, 1450–1451

Fogel, BJ, Nitowsky, HM and Gruenwald, P (1965) Discordant abnormalities in monozygotic twins. *Journal of Pediatrics*, **66**, 64–72

Fowlie, A (1989) Ultrasonic antenatal diagnosis of skeletal dysplasia. *Contemporary Reviews in Obstetrics and Gynaecology*, **1**, 111–112

Fox, H and Jones, CJP (1983) Pathology of trophoblast. In *Biology of Trophoblast* (edited by YW Loke and A White) pp. 137–185. Amsterdam: Elsevier

Geirsson, RT (1986) Intrauterine volume in pregnancy. *Acta Obstetrica Gynaecologica Scandinavica*, **Suppl 136**

Gerson, AG, Wallace, DM, Bridgens, NK *et al.* (1987) Duplex Doppler ultrasound in the evaluation of growth in twin pregnancies. *Obstetrics and Gynecology*, **70**, 419–423

Giles, WB, Trudinger, BJ and Baird, PJ (1985) Fetal umbilical artery flow velocity waveforms and placental resistance: pathological correlation. *British Journal of Obstetrics and Gynaecology*, **92**, 31–38

Giles, WB, Trudinger, BJ and Cook, CM (1985) Fetal umbilical artery flow velocity – time waveforms in twin pregnancies. *British Journal of Obstetrics and Gynaecology*, **92**, 490–497

Giles, WB, Trudinger, BJ and Palmer, AA (1986) Umbilical cord whole blood viscosity and the umbilical artery flow velocity waveforms: a correlation. *British Journal of Obstetrics and Gynaecology*, **93**, 466–470

Gohari, P, Berkowitz, RL and Hobbins, JC (1977) Prediction of intrauterine growth retardation by determination of total intrauterine volume. *American Journal of Obstetrics and Gynecology*, **127**, 255–260

Goldstein, I, Lockwood, C and Hobbins, JC (1987) Ultrasound assessment of fetal intestinal development in the evaluation of gestational age. *Obstetrics and Gynecology*, **70**, 682–686

Grannum, PAT, Berkowitz, RL and Hobbins, JC (1979) The ultrasonic changes in the maturing placenta and their relation to fetal pulmonic maturity. *American Journal of Obstetrics and Gynecology*, **133**, 915–922

Grannum, P, Bracken, M, Silverman, R and Hobbins, JC (1980) Assessment of fetal kidney size in normal gestation by comparison of ratio of kidney circumference to abdominal circumference. *American Journal of Obstetrics and Gynecology*, **136**, 249–254

Grant, A, Chalmers, I and Enkin, M (1982) Physical interventions intended to prolong pregnancy and increase fetal growth. In *Effectiveness and Satisfaction in Antenatal Care* (edited by M Enkin and I Chalmers) pp. 198–208. London: Spastics International Medical Publications

Grennert, L, Persson, PH, Gennser, G and Gullberg, B (1980) Zygosity and the intrauterine growth of twins. *Obstetrics and Gynecology*, **55**, 684–687

Gruenwald, P (1974) Pathology of the fetus and its supply line. In *Ciba Foundation Symposium 27: Size at Birth*, pp. 3–19. Amsterdam: Associated Scientific Publishers

Hackett, GA, Campbell, S, Gamsu, H *et al.* (1987) Doppler studies in the growth retarded fetus and prediction of neonatal necrotizing enterocolitis, haemorrhage and neonatal morbidity. *British Medical Journal*, **294**, 13–16

Hadlock, FP, Harrist, RB, Sharman, RS *et al.* (1985) Estimation of fetal weight with the use of head, body and femur measurements – a prospective study. *American Journal of Obstetrics and Gynecology*, **151**, 333–337

Halbicht, JP, Lechtig, A, Yarbrough, C and Klein, RE (1974) Maternal nutrition, birthweight and infant mortality. In *Ciba Foundation Symposium 27: Size at Birth*, pp. 353–370. Amsterdam: Associated Scientific Publishers

Hall, M, Chng, PK and MacGillivray, I (1980) Is routine antenatal care worthwhile? *Lancet*, **ii**, 78–80

Halperin, ME, Fong, KW, Zalev, AH and Goldsmith, CH (1985) Reliability of amniotic fluid volume estimation from ultrasonograms. Intraobserver and interobserver variation before and after the establishment of criteria. *American Journal of Obstetrics and Gynecology*, **153**, 264–267

Hanretty, KP, Primrose, MH, Neilson, JP and Whittle, MJ (1989) Pregnancy screening by Doppler uteroplacental and umbilical artery waveforms. *British Journal of Obstetrics and Gynaecology*, **96**, 960–963

Hastie, SJ, Danskin, F, Neilson, JP and Whittle, MJ (1989) Prediction of the small for gestational age twin fetus by Doppler umbilical artery waveform analysis. *Obstetrics and Gynecology*, **74**, 730–733

Hellman, LM, Kobayashi, M, Tolles, WE and Cromb, E (1970) Ultrasonic studies on the volumetric growth of the human placenta. *American Journal of Obstetrics and Gynecology*, **108**, 740–748

Hill, DJ and Milner, RDG (1985) The role of peptide growth factors and hormones in the control of fetal growth. In *Recent Advances in Perinatal Medicine 2* (edited by ML Chiswick) pp. 79–102. Edinburgh: Churchill Livingstone

Hoddick, WK, Mahoney, BS, Callen, PW and Filly, RA (1985) Placental thickness. *Journal of Ultrasound in Medicine*, **4**, 479–482

Jacobs, PA, Szulman, AE, Funkhauser, J *et al.* (1982) Human triploidy: relationship between parental origin of the additional haploid complement and development of partial hydatidiform mole. *Annals of Human Genetics*, **46**, 223–231

Jeanty, P, Romero, R and Hobbins, JC (1985) Fetal limb volume: a new parameter to assess fetal growth and nutrition. *Journal of Ultrasound in Medicine*, **4**, 273–282

Jeanty, P, Rodesch. F, Delbeke, D and Dumont, JE (1984) Estimation of gestational age by measurement of fetal long bones. *Journal of Ultrasound in Medicine*, **3**, 75–79

Jogee, M, Myatt, L and Elder, MG (1983) Decreased prostacyclin production by placental cells in culture from pregnancies complicated by fetal growth retardation. *British Journal of Obstetrics and Gynaecology*, **90**, 247–250

Johnson, A, Callan, NA, Bhutani, VK *et al.* (1987) Ultrasonic ratio of fetal thoracic to abdominal circumference: an association with fetal pulmonary hypoplasia. *American Journal of Obstetrics and Gynecology*, **157**, 764–769

Johnstone, FD, Haddad, NG, Hoskins, P *et al.* (1988) Umbilical artery doppler flow velocity waveform: the outcome of pregnancies with absent end-diastolic flow. *European Journal of Obstetrics and Gynecology and Reproductive Biology*, **28**, 171–178

Jones, KL, Smith, DW, Streissguth, AP and Myrianthopoulos, NC (1974) Outcome in offspring of chronic alcoholic women. *Lancet*, **i**, 1076–1078

Khong, TY, De Wolf, F, Robertson, WB and Brosens, I (1986) Inadequate vascular response to placentation in pregnancies complicated by pre-eclampsia and by small-for-gestational age infants. *British Journal of Obstetrics and Gynaecology*, **106**, 589–591

Kruger, H and Arias-Stella, J (1970) The placenta and the newborn infant at high altitudes. *American Journal of Obstetrics and Gynecology*, **106**, 586–591

Laron, Z and Pertzelan, A (1969) Somatotrophin in antenatal and postnatal growth and development. *Lancet*, **i**, 680–681

Lewis, E, Kurtz, AB, Dubbins, PA *et al.* (1982) Real-time ultrasonographic evaluation of normal fetal adrenal glands. *Journal of Ultrasound in Medicine*, **1**, 265–270

Liggins, GC (1974) The influence of the fetal hypothalamus and pituitary on growth. In *Ciba Foundation Symposium 27: Size at Birth*, pp. 165–183. Amsterdam: Associated Scientific Publishers

Lin, CC, Moawad, AH, Rosenow, PJ and Rivar, P (1980) Acid base characteristics of fetuses with intrauterine growth retardation during labor and delivery. *American Journal of Obstetrics and Gynecology*, **137**, 553–559

Lubbe, WF and Liggins, GC (1985) Lupus anticoagulant and pregnancy. *American Journal of Obstetrics and Gynecology*, **152**, 322

McCowan, LM, Ritchie, K, Mo, LY *et al.* (1988) Uterine artery flow velocity waveforms in normal and growth-retarded pregnancies. *American Journal of Obstetrics and Gynecology*, **158**, 499–504

McFadyen, IR, Price, AB and Geirsson, RT (1986) The relation of birthweight to histological appearances in vessels in the placental bed. *British Journal of Obstetrics and Gynaecology*, **93**, 476–481

MacGregor, SN, Sabbagha, RE, Tamura, RK *et al.* (1988) Differing fetal growth patterns in pregnancies complicated by preterm labor. *Obstetrics and Gynecology*, **72**, 834–837

McIlwaine, GM, Howat, RCL, Dunn, F and MacNaughton, MC (1979) The Scottish perinatal mortality survey. *British Medical Journal*, **2**, 1103–1106

Manlan, G and Scott, KE (1978) Contribution of twin pregnancy to perinatal mortality and fetal growth retardation: reversal of growth retardation after birth. *Canadian Medical Association Journal*, **118**, 365–368

Mari, G, Moise, KJ, Deter, RL *et al.* (1989) Doppler assessment of the pulsatility index in the cerebral circulation of the human fetus. *American Journal of Obstetrics and Gynecology*, **160**, 698–703

Mellor, DJ (1984) Investigation of fetal growth in sheep. In *Animal Models in Fetal Medicine*, (edited by PW Nathanielsz) pp. 149–173. Ithaca: Perinatology Press

Mercer, BM, Sikar, S, Shariatmadar, A *et al.* (1987) Fetal foot length as a predictor of gestational age. *American Journal of Obstetrics and Gynecology*, **156**, 350–355

Meredith, HV (1970) Body weight at birth of viable human infants: a worldwide comparative treatise. *Human Biology*, **42**, 217–264

Milner, RDG and Hill, DJ (1987) Interaction between endocrine and paracrine peptides in prenatal growth control. *European Journal of Pediatrics*, **146**, 113–122

Moessinger, AC, Fox, HE, Higgins, A *et al.* (1987) Fetal breathing movements are not a reliable predictor of continued lung development in pregnancies complicated by oligohydramnios. *Lancet*, **ii**, 1297–1300

Naeye, RL and Blanc, W (1965) Pathogenesis of congenital rubella. *Journal of the American Medical Association*, **194**, 109–115

Naeye, RL, Tafari, N, Judge, D and Marboe, CC (1978) Twins: causes of perinatal death in 12 United States cities and one African city. *American Journal of Obstetrics and Gynecology*, **131**, 257–272

Neilson, JP (1981) Detection of the small-for-dates twin fetus by ultrasound. *British Journal of Obstetrics and Gynaecology*, **88**, 27–32

Neilson, JP (1987) Doppler ultrasound. *British Journal of Obstetrics and Gynaecology*, **94**, 929–934

Neilson, JP (1988) Fetal growth in twin pregnancies. *Acta Geneticae Medicae Gemmelologiae*, **37**, 35–39

Neilson, JP and Grant, A (1989) Ultrasound in pregnancy. In *Effective Care in Pregnancy and Childbirth* (edited by I Chalmers, MW Enkin and M Keirse), pp. 419–439. Oxford: Oxford University Press

Neilson, JP and Hastie, SJ (1988) Ultrasound studies of monozygotic and dizygotic twin pregnancies. In *Fetal and Neonatal Development*, (ed by CT Jones) pp. 541–543. New York: Perinatology Press

Neilson, JP and Whittle, MJ (1988) Doppler blood flow studies in fetal growth retardation. In *Fetal and Neonatal Growth* (edited by F Cockburn) pp. 79–91. Chichester: John Wiley

Neilson, JP, Danskin, F and Hastie, SJ (1989) Monozygotic twin pregnancy: diagnostic and Doppler ultrasound studies. *British Journal of Obstetrics and Gynaecology*, **96**, 1413–1418

Neilson, JP, Munjanja, SP and Whitfield, CR (1984) Screening for the small-for-dates fetus: a controlled trial. *British Medical Journal*, **289**, 1179–1182

Neilson, JP, Verkuyl, DAA and Bannerman, C (1988) Tape measurement of symphysis–fundal height in twin pregnancies. *British Journal of Obstetrics and Gynaecology*, **95**, 1054–1059

Neilson, JP, Whitfield, CR and Aitchison, TC (1980) Screening for the small-for-dates fetus: a two-stage ultrasound examination schedule. *British Medical Journal*, **280**, 1203–1206

Nicolaides, KH and Campbell, S (1987) Diagnosis and management of fetal malformations. *Baillière's Clinics in Obstetrics and Gynaecology*, **1**, 591–622

Nicolaides, KH, Campbell, S, Bradley, RJ *et al.* (1987) Maternal oxygen therapy for intrauterine growth retardation. *Lancet*, **i**, 942–945

Nimrod, C, Davies, D, Iwanick, S *et al.* (1986) Ultrasound prediction of pulmonary hypoplasia. *Obstetrics and Gynecology*, **68**, 495–497

Nimrod, C, Davies, D, Harper, J *et al.* (1987) Doppler ultrasound prediction of fetal outcome in twin pregnancies. *American Journal of Obstetrics and Gynecology*, **156**, 402–406

Northern Regional Health Authority Co-ordinating Group (1984) Perinatal mortality: a continuing collaborative regional survey. *British Medical Journal*, **288**, 1717–1720

Oh, W (1977) Considerations in neonates with intrauterine growth retardation. *Clinical Obstetrics and Gynecology*, **20**, 991–1003

Ounsted, M (1978) Concepts and criteria of fetal growth. In *Abnormal Fetal Growth: Biological Bases and Consequences* (edited by F Naftolin) pp. 21–48. Berlin: Dahlem Konferenzen

Ounsted, M, Moar, VA and Scott, A (1989) Small-for-dates babies, gestational age and developmental ability at 7 years. *Early Human Development*, **19**, 77–86

Owens, JA and Robinson, JS (1988) The effect of experimental manipulation of placental growth and development. In *Fetal and Neonatal Growth* (edited by F Cockburn) pp. 49–77. Chichester: John Wiley

Owens, JA, Falconer, J and Robinson, JS (1987) Effect of restriction of placental growth on oxygen delivery to and consumption by the pregnant uterus and fetus. *Journal of Developmental Physiology*, **9**, 137–150

Owens, JA, Owens, PC and Robinson, JS (1989) Experimental fetal growth retardation: metabolic and endocrine aspects. In *The Liggins Symposium – Fetal Physiology and Medicine* (edited by P Gluckman, B Johnston and PW Nathanielsz) **in press**. New York: Perinatology Press

Patel, N, Barrie, W, Campbell, D *et al.* (1984) *Scottish twin study 1983: preliminary report*. Glasgow: University of Glasgow

Patterson, RM and Pouliot, MR (1987) Neonatal morphometrics and perinatal outcome: who is growth retarded? *American Journal of Obstetrics and Gynecology*, **157**, 1406–1410

Patterson, RM, Prihoda, TJ and Pouliot, MR (1987) Sonographic amniotic fluid measurement and fetal growth retardation: a reappraisal. *American Journal of Obstetrics and Gynecology*, **157**, 1406–1410

Peeters, LLH, Sheldon, RE, Jones, MD *et al.* (1979) Blood flow to fetal organs as a function of arterial oxygen content. *American Journal of Obstetrics and Gynecology*, **135**, 637–646

Pretorius, DH, Manchester, D, Barkin, S *et al.* (1988) Doppler ultrasound of twin transfusion syndrome. *Journal of Ultrasound in Medicine*, **7**, 117–124

Proud, J and Grant, A (1987) Third trimester placental grading by ultrasonography as a test of fetal wellbeing. *British Medical Journal*, **294**, 1641–1644

Reuss, ML, Parer, JT, Harris, JL and Kruger, TR (1982) Hemodynamic effects of alpha-adrenergic blockade during hypoxia in fetal sheep. *American Journal of Obstetrics and Gynecology*, **142**, 410–415

Reuwer, PJHM, Sijmons, EA, Rietman, GW *et al.* (1987) Intrauterine growth retardation: prediction of perinatal distress by Doppler ultrasound. *Lancet*, **ii**, 415–418

Robertson, EG and Neer, KJ (1983) Placental injection studies in twin gestation. *American Journal of Obstetrics and Gynecology*, **147**, 170–173

Robertson, WB, Brosens, I and Dixon, G (1975) Utero-placental vascular pathology. *European Journal of Obstetrics, Gynaecology and Reproductive Biology*, **5**, 47–65

Rosa, FW and Turshen, M (1970) Fetal nutrition. *Bulletin of the World Health Organization*, **43**, 785–795

Rosenberg, K, Grant, JM and Hepburn, M (1982) Antenatal detection of growth retardation: actual practice in a large maternity hospital. *British Journal of Obstetrics and Gynaecology*, **89**, 12–15

Rosenberg, K, Grant, JM, Tweedie, I *et al.* (1982) Measurement of fundal height as a screening test for fetal growth retardation. *British Journal of Obstetrics and Gynaecology*, **89**, 447–450

Rubin, PC, Butters, L, Clark, DM *et al.* (1983) Placebo-controlled trial of atenolol in treatment of pregnancy-associated hypertension. *Lancet*, **i**, 431–434

Rush, D (1982) Effects of changes in protein and calorie intake during pregnancy on the growth of the human fetus. In *Effectiveness and Satisfaction in Antenatal Care* (edited by M Enkin and I Chalmers) pp. 92–113. London: Spastics International Publications

Schmidt, W, Yarkoni, S, Jeanty, P *et al.* (1985) Sonographic measurements of the fetal spleen: clinical implications. *Journal of Ultrasound in Medicine*, **4**, 667–672

Scott, JS (1966) Immunological diseases and pregnancy. *British Medical Journal*, **1**, 1559–1567

Secher, NH, Kaern, J and Hansen, PK (1985) Intrauterine growth in twin pregnancies: prediction of fetal growth retardation. *Obstetrics and Gynecology*, **66**, 63–68

Secher, NJ, Hansen, PK, Lenstrup, C *et al.* (1987) A randomized study of fetal abdominal diameter and fetal weight estimation for detection of light-for-gestation infants in low-risk pregnancies. *British Journal of Obstetrics and Gynaecology*, **94**, 105–109

Shepard, MJ, Richards, VA, Berkowitz, RL *et al.* (1982) An evaluation of two equations for predicting fetal weight by ultrasound. *American Journal of Obstetrics and Gynecology*, **142**, 47–54

Sijmons, EA, Reuwer, PJHM, van Beek, E and Bruinse, HW (1989) The validity of screening for small-for-gestational-age and low-weight-for-length infants by Doppler ultrasound. *British Journal of Obstetrics and Gynaecology*, **96**, 557–561

Soothill, PW, Nicolaides, KH and Campbell, S (1987) Perinatal asphyxia, hyperlacticaemia, hypoglycaemia, and erythroblastosis in growth retarded fetuses. *British Medical Journal*, **294**, 1051–1053

Steel, SA, Pearce, JM and Chamberlain, GV (1988) Doppler ultrasound of the uteroplacental circulation as a screening test for severe pre-eclampsia with intra-uterine growth retardation. *European Journal of Obstetrics and Gynecology and Reproductive Biology*, **28**, 279–287

Stone, ML, Salerno, LJ, Green, M and Zelson, C (1971) Narcotic addiction in pregnancy. *American Journal of Obstetrics and Gynecology*, **109**, 716–720

Surani, MAH, Barton, SC and Norris, ML (1987) Experimental reconstruction of mouse eggs and embryos: an analysis of mammalian development. *Biology of Reproduction*, **36**, 1–16

Thomson, AM, Billewicz, WZ and Hytten, FE (1968) The assessment of fetal growth. *Journal of Obstetrics and Gynaecology of the British Commonwealth*, **75**, 903–916

Thorburn, GD (1974) The role of the thyroid gland and kidneys in fetal growth. In *Ciba Foundation Symposium 27: Size at Birth*, pp. 185–200. Amsterdam: Associated Scientific Publishers

Toi, A, Simpson, GF and Filly, RA (1987) Ultrasonically evident fetal nuchal thickening: is it specific for Down syndrome? *American Journal of Obstetrics and Gynecology*, **156**, 150–153

Trudinger, BJ, Giles, WB and Cook, CM (1985) Flow velocity waveforms in the maternal uteroplacental and fetal umbilical placental circulations. *American Journal of Obstetrics and Gynecology*, **152**, 155–160

Trudinger, BJ, Cook, CM, Giles, WB *et al.* (1987) Umbilical artery flow velocity waveforms in high risk pregnancy: randomized controlled trial. *Lancet*, **i**, 188–190

Trudinger, BJ, Cook, CM, Thompson, RS, *et al.* (1988) Low-dose aspirin therapy improves fetal weight in umbilical placental insufficiency. *American Journal of Obstetrics and Gynecology*, **159**, 681–685

Verloove-Vanhorick, SP, Verwey, RA, Braud, R *et al.* (1986) Neonatal mortality risk in relation to gestational age and birthweight. *Lancet*, **i**, 55–57

Vileisis, RA (1985) Effect of maternal oxygen inhalation on the fetus with growth retardation. *Pediatric Research*, **19**, 324–327

Vintzileos, AM, Neckles, S, Campbell, WA *et al.* (1985a) Fetal liver measurements during normal pregnancy. *Obstetrics and Gynecology*, **66**, 477–480

Vintzileos, AM, Neckles, S, Campbell, WA *et al.* (1985b) Three fetal ponderal indexes in normal pregnancy. *Obstetrics and Gynecology*, **65**, 807–811

Wallenberg, HCS and Rotmans, N (1982) Enhanced reactivity of the platelet thromboxane pathway in normotensive and hypertensive pregnancies with insufficient fetal growth. *American Journal of Obstetrics and Gynecology*, **144**, 523–528

Wallenberg, HCS, Dekker, GA, Makvitz, JW and Rotmans, P (1986) Low-dose aspirin prevents pregnancy induced hypertension and pre-eclampsia in angiotensin sensitive primigravidae. *Lancet*, **i**, 1–3

Walton, A and Hammond, J (1938) The maternal effects on growth and conformation in Shire horse–Shetland pony crosses. *Proceedings of the Royal Society*, **125B**, 311–335

Wark, L and Malcolm, LA (1969) Growth and development of the Lumi child in the Sepik district of New Guinea. *Medical Journal of Australia*, **2**, 129–136

Whitfield, CR, Smith, NC, Cockburn, F and Gibson, AAM (1986) Perinatally related wastage – a proposed classification of primary obstetric factors. *British Journal of Obstetrics and Gynaecology*, **93**, 694–703

Willocks, J, Donald, I, Duggan, TC and Day, N (1964) Foetal cephalometry by ultrasound. *Journal of Obstetrics and Gynaecology of the British Commonwealth*, **71**, 11–20

Wittman, BK, Baldwin, VJ and Nichol, B (1981) Antenatal diagnosis of twin transfusion syndrome. *Obstetrics and Gynecology*, **58**, 123–127

Wittmann, BK, Farquharson, DF, Thomas, NDS *et al.* (1986) The role of feticide in the management of severe twin transfusion syndrome. *American Journal of Obstetrics and Gynecology*, **155**, 1023–1026

Wladimiroff, JW and Campbell, S (1974) Fetal urine production rates in normal and complicated pregnancy. *Lancet*, **i**, 151–154

Wladimiroff, JW, Tonge, HM and Stewart, PA (1986) Doppler ultrasound assessment of cerebral blood flow in the human fetus. *British Journal of Obstetrics and Gynaecology*, **93**, 471–475

Wladimiroff, JW, Wijngaard, JAGW, Degani, S *et al.* (1987) Cerebral and umbilical arterial blood flow velocity waveforms in normal and growth-retarded pregnancies. *Obstetrics and Gynecology*, **69**, 705–709

Wolf, H, Oosting, H and Treffers, PE (1987) Placental volume measurement by ultrasonography: evaluation of the method. *American Journal of Obstetrics and Gynecology*, **156**, 1191–1194

Yagel, S, Zacut, D, Igelstein, S *et al.* (1987) In utero ponderal index as a prognostic factor in the evaluation of intrauterine growth retardation. *American Journal of Obstetrics and Gynecology*, **157**, 415–419

Chapter 12

Neurodevelopmental handicap: the obstetric perspective

David J Taylor

Introduction

Each child has a genetic potential for development. Whether he or she will achieve this potential will depend on the interplay of numerous biological and environment influences which occur during and after intrauterine life (Figure 12.1). Here we are interested in the relation between biological influences during prenatal and perinatal life and subsequent development, so that – it is hoped – we can attempt to modify any negative effects of the former. However, the area is very difficult to study. Some of the investigative difficulties are addressed here.

Biological influences

One of the difficulties in studying the relationship between pregnancy and subsequent development is that the antecedent or risk factor is almost always defined arbitrarily: the definition used will, therefore, include a range both of heterogeneous pathologies and of normal pregnancies. The former will have differing effects on development and any effect seen will be diluted by the latter. The problem is compounded by definitions varying from study to study, country to country, continent to continent. For example, a widely studied risk factor is that of intrauterine growth retardation. Almost all definitions of this problem are based on birthweight for gestation, i.e. small for dates. Three definitions are used: <10th centile, <5th centile and >2 standard deviation below the mean. Below the arbitrary cut-off there will be babies who are small owing to chromosomal abnormality, congenital

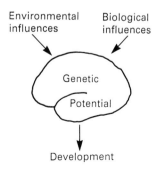

Figure 12.1   A simplified scheme of brain development

infection, maternal tobacco or alcohol consumption, severe pre-eclampsia and ante-partum haemorrhage, to name just a few conditions, but there are also babies who are perfectly normal and are small simply as a result of gene expression.

There will also be babies who have suffered severe late intrauterine growth retardation but whose birthweights will be above the arbitrary cut-off. It is not surprising that other ways of defining intrauterine growth retardation are being sought, e.g. skin-fold measurements (Hill, Verniaud and Deter, 1984; Villar *et al.*, 1984) and ponderal index (Walther and Raemaekers, 1982). Similar misclassification errors occur in the study of hypertension and antepartum haemorrhage (Taylor, 1988) and intrapartum hypoxia/acidosis. This last condition is very difficult to diagnose precisely: fetal heart rate changes correlate poorly with it; intermittent scalp or a single umbilical vein blood-gas analysis cannot determine the duration of the episode, and neonatal indices of respiratory depression (Apgar score, time to regular respiration, need for intermittent positive pressure ventilation) are only proxy variables of intrapartum hypoxia/acidosis and therefore inevitably imprecise.

Environmental influences

The environment has a very powerful effect on development, particularly cognitive development. Whenever a claim is made in the literature for a direct causative relationship between pregnancy and the child's subsequent development, it should be examined with cautious scepticism as a possible artefact from the child's psychosocial environment. Illsley (1967) reviewed in detail the theoretical and methodological problems inherent in the interpretation of simple correlations and gave examples of alternative models of explanation for such associations. When attempting to isolate a causal correlation, efforts must be made to allow for the long process of interacting influences of the environment on development. No study has been able to document precisely the composition of these influences but parenting is thought to be the most important. Proxy variables are used to measure this, such as father's occupation (social class), which is the most common, per capita income, area of residence, housing conditions, educational level, marital status, unemployment and social and geographical mobility, as well as more directly health-related factors, such as week of first attendance at the antenatal clinic. One or more of these variables can be entered into multiple regression analyses of the relationship between pregnancy and development. An alternative strategy is to recruit a control group matched for a variety of social factors at the time of pregnancy or birth, i.e. before environmental effects are possible. However, this presupposes that prenatal social matching ensures postnatal matching and it is apparent that this is not always the case, owing to social mobility (Illsley, 1980). The use of sibling comparisons can control for parental influences but the widely differing ages of the sibs can make comparative developmental assessment difficult. The obvious model that will match for environmental influences is the study of twins, but this can be used only in situations where one twin is affected by the risk factor under study: thus, it can be used to study growth retardation and intrapartum hypoxia/acidosis but cannot be used in maternal conditions such as hypertension.

Developmental assessment

When making comparisons between groups, it is imperative that errors in the measurement of the outcome variable (development in this case) are reduced to a minimum so that results can be interpreted with confidence. The quality of the developmental assessment is pivotal in this field. The assessment must be undertaken blind to the previous obstetric history, in order to reduce the possibility of observer bias. In prospective studies, therefore, the observer must not have contributed to the care of the child and in retrospective studies involving case notes, steps must be taken to blind the investigator to the outcome of the child. Intra-observer variation is recognized to fall exponentially with time and, therefore, a period of training in a pilot study is necessary before a study is initiated.

The tests to be applied must be standardized, previously validated and appropriate to the age of the child. As gestational age at birth has an inverse relationship with development, allowance must be made for this in the timing of the assessment. Investigators should take into account whether the test will measure outcome as a continuous variable (e.g. developmental or intelligence quotients) or as a dichotomous variable (e.g. the presence or absence of a handicap like cerebral palsy) as this will influence the sample size required. The former can be described as mean and standard deviation, entered into multiple regression analyses and can give statistically significant information on relatively small population samples. Although the latter can be analysed by discriminant or logistic regression it requires much larger samples for statistical analysis.

Definitions

Most obstetricians are unfamiliar with the terms used to define abnormalities of development. The most widely accepted is that of the WHO International Classification of Impairments, Disabilities and Handicap (1980) which is as follows:

Impairment: in the context of health experience, an impairment is any loss or abnormality of psychological, physiological or anatomical structure or function.

Disability: in the context of health experience, a disability is any restriction or lack (resulting from an impairment) of ability to perform an activity in the manner or within the range considered normal for a human being.

Handicap: in the context of health experience, a handicap is a disadvantage for a given individual, resulting from an impairment or a disability, that limits or prevents the fulfilment of a role that is normal (depending on age, sex and social and cultural factors) for that individual.

In relation to neurodevelopment, the handicapping condition of motor function is cerebral palsy and that of cognitive function is mental retardation.

Cerebral palsy

Pathology

Cerebral palsy is not a single entity nor does it have a single aetiology. From an obstetric perspective, cerebral palsy secondary to cerebral haemorrhagic and cerebral ischaemic lesions are the most relevant. Before the advent of modern imaging techniques, investigation of these conditions was limited to postmortem studies and, therefore, was confined to more severe cases. During the last decade the use of

Table 12.1.   Change in the proportion of intracranial haemorrhage found at autopsy over a 40-year period (Levene, 1985)

	Type of intracranial haemorrhage			
Source	*Subdural*	*Intraparenchymal*	*Intraventricular*	*Subcranial*
Craig (1938)	62 (49[a])	6 (5)	22 (17)	36 (29)
Hammersmith Hospital (1978–1979)	14 (16)	8 (9)	47 (55)	16 (19)

[a] Percentages in parentheses

neonatal cerebral ultrasound has allowed the visualization of the whole spectrum of these lesions and with it is coming a gradual understanding of the aetiology of cerebral haemorrhage and infarction.

Cerebral haemorrhage

Before the development of intensive intrapartum care, subdural haemorrhage accounted for about one-half of the cases of neonatal cerebral haemorrhage (Levene, 1985) and this was presumably a reflection of traumatic forceps and vaginal breech delivery. Although these still do occur, the commonest type of haemorrhage seen in present practice is periventricular haemorrhage in very-low-birthweight infants (Table 12.1).

Subdural haemorrhage

Subdural haemorrhage may be secondary to dural tears, occipital osteodiastasis or rupture of the superior cerebral bridging veins. The dura mater divides the brain into three compartments, the two cerebral hemispheres and the cerebellum. Tearing of the dura results in bleeding from venous sinuses contained within its folds and this usually results from excessive and rapid elongation of the fetal skull during traumatic delivery. Tearing of the tentorium cerebelli is the most common. Occipital osteodiastasis, i.e. separation of the squamous and lateral portions of the occipital bone, can lead to haemorrhage into the posterior fossa. This condition has been associated with excessive extension of the neck during vaginal breech delivery (Wigglesworth and Husemeyer, 1977). The commonest cause of subdural haemorrhage is rupture of the superior cerebral bridging veins associated with tentorial tears but without rupture of the venous sinuses. This type does not appear to be related to obstetric factors, being seen in infants with coagulation defects or those undergoing exchange transfusion.

Subdural haemorrhage in the neonatal period is associated with a very poor prognosis, with only one-half of the children being neurologically normal at follow-up.

Subarachnoid haemorrhage

Subarachnoid haemorrhage can be primary or secondary. Primary subarachnoid haemorrhage can arise from rupture either of the fine vessels of the leptomeningeal plexus or of the bridging veins within the subarachnoid space, and is characteristically seen in infants with bleeding disorders, although rapid compression and decompression of the fetal skull during uncontrolled delivery has been incriminated (Philip and Allan, 1985). Secondary haemorrhage is due to blood from intraventricular haemorrhage (see below) tracking down through the ventricular system and exiting through the foramina of Luska and Magendie into the subarachnoid space. Prognosis is generally thought to be good (Rose and Lombroso, 1970), but recent analysis of a small group of 10 children with a computerized tomography diagnosis of subarachnoid haemorrhage showed a 50 per cent rate of sequelae (Fenichel, Webster and Wong, 1984).

Intraparenchymal haemorrhage

This type of haemorrhage, like subarachnoid haemorrhage, can be secondary to extension of an intraventricular haemorrhage (see below). Primary haemorrhages are usually seen in infants with bleeding tendencies (e.g. thrombocytopenia, vitamin K deficiency) and can occur prenatally in infants of women taking anti-convulsants (Bleyer and Skinner, 1976) and women with immune thrombocytopenia (Zalneraitis, Young and Krishnamoorthy, 1979). Haemorrhage can occur into the cerebrum, the thalamus and the cerebellum.

Periventricular haemorrhage

This type of haemorrhage, which arises from the germinal matrix, is the commonest type of neonatal cerebral haemorrhage and is characteristically seen in very low birthweight babies. The germinal matrix is closely related to the caudate nucleus and is the site of glial cell formation. During the time period 24–34 weeks this area is supported by a fragile matrix of capillaries with thin immature walls, supplied in turn by Heubner's artery, a branch from the origin of the anterior cerebral artery, and by branches of the choroidal and lateral striate arteries. Drainage is through the terminal vein to the vein of Galen. Hambleton and Wigglesworth (1976) have demonstrated that bleeding occurs from multiple sites in the capillary bed, most commonly over the head of the caudate nucleus but bleeding may arise more posteriorly over the temporal pole of the lateral ventricle. Rupture of the germinal matrix capillaries causes haemorrhage through the ependyma into the lateral ventricles in 80 per cent of cases. More rarely (17 per cent), but more seriously, bleeding can extend into the cerebral parenchyma. The bleeding usually occurs during the first week of life. Some groups have reported up to two-thirds of haemorrhages within a few hours of birth (Bejar et al., 1980; de Crespigny et al., 1982; McDonald et al., 1984), whereas others have reported occurrences equally distributed between the first, second and third days of life (Levene, Fawer and Lamont, 1982; Thorburn et al., 1982; Szymonowicz and Yu, 1984). Approximately one-half of infants of birthweight <1500 g develop some degree of periventricular haemorrhage, with the rate rising to >60 per cent in infants of <28 weeks' gestation, but it is much rarer after 34 weeks' gestation. It does occur in term infants, one report quoting a 4 per cent incidence (Hayden et al., 1985), but it is usually confined to the germinal matrix in these cases.

There have been numerous studies of factors predisposing to periventricular haemorrhage and a consensus appears to be emerging that respiratory distress syndrome and associated abnormalities of metabolic acidosis, cerebral blood pressure and coagulation are important. It is well recognized that the better the condition of the baby at birth, the less the risk and severity of respiratory distress syndrome and there is some evidence that fetal acidosis, whether measured as Apgar score (Sinha et al., 1985), late decelerations during labour (Westgren, Malcus and Svenningsen,

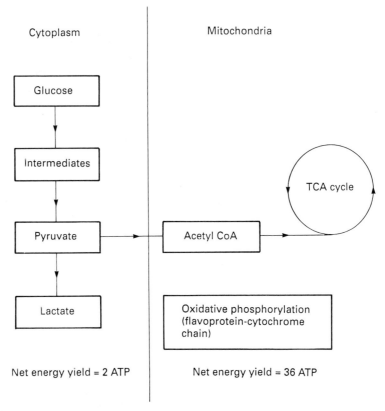

Figure 12.2   Anaerobic and aerobic metabolism in the brain.

1986) or base excess (Agustsson and Patel, 1988), increases the risk of periventricular haemorrhage.

The prognosis associated with periventricular haemorrhage depends on the extent of the lesion. Infants with mild haemorrhages confined to the germinal matrix have the same outcome as similar infants without haemorrhage – about a 10 per cent mortality and a 10 per cent neurological abnormality rate in survivors. Where there is intraventricular haemorrhage there is very little increased risk of death but the neurological abnormality rate increases to 20 per cent. The most severe type of periventricular haemorrhage where there is parenchymal extension, which may represent haemorrhage into an area of cerebral infarction, is associated with a disastrous prognosis – a 60 per cent mortality rate and only 0–15 per cent of the survivors neurologically intact.

Cerebral infarction

Cerebral infarction is caused by relative lack of substrate metabolism in brain cells. Although ketone bodies can be used as a source of energy, the main substrate for energy production in the brain is glucose. This is degraded initially in the cytoplasm to pyruvate (Embden–Meyerhof pathway) with the production of 2 moles of ATP per mole of glucose (Figure 12.2). In the presence of oxygen, pyruvate is metabolized within the mitochondria in the tricarboxylic acid cycle, resulting in the production of a further 36 moles of ATP per mole of glucose and thereby providing energy to maintain the function (approximately 40 per cent) and the integrity (60 per cent) of the cell. Under anaerobic conditions only lactate can be produced from pyruvate, with no further increase in ATP production. Anaerobic metabolism is unable to satisfy the energy requirements of cerebral cells and thus a constant supply of glucose and oxygen is required to maintain cellular function and integrity.

Supply through the cerebral circulation is autoregulated. Cerebral blood flow remains constant when cerebral perfusion pressure (mean arterial pressure minus intracranial pressure) is between 60 and 120 mmHg. When cerebral perfusion pressure falls below 60 mmHg, autoregulation ceases and cerebral blood flow falls. When oxygen supply fails in a normal circulation there is a compensatory increase in cerebral blood flow. Although lactic acidosis may occur, the total amount of energy remains adequate to maintain cellular integrity. However, if the ability of the cerebral circulation to dilate is impaired, either globally or focally, then ischaemic changes will occur. In complete ischaemia, e.g. total asphyxia, oxidative phosphorylation ceases within 15 s. Anaerobic metabolism continues until the cellular stores of glucose and glycogen have been exhausted. Intracellular lactate increases, pH falls and, after 2–3 min, intracellular ATP concentration approaches zero and all energy-requiring reactions, including the sodium pump, stop. This leads to neuronal, glial and endothelial cell oedema and death.

This picture is very rare in human fetal experience. The characteristic pathology here is partial asphyxia, usually of gradual onset. The present hypothesis of events is as follows. At first there is a reactive increase in cerebral blood flow to maintain substrate provision. As cerebral blood flow begins to fail, lactic acid builds up, causing cytotoxic oedema and further vasospasm. The release of free oxygen radicals causes further mitochondrial damage and then neuronal death. If blood flow is re-established, further damage can occur as, in addition to lactic acid, there is accumulation of arachidonic acid in the cell. On reperfusion this is metabolized to thromboxane, causing intense local vasospasm and ischaemia. The vasospasm and associated erythrocyte aggregation cause secondary depletion of cellular energy and a downward spiral of cerebral injury.

Pathology

The brain is vulnerable to ischaemia in areas of anastomosing arterial supply where perfusion is most precarious and this leads to the commonly seen patterns of infarction. The commonest type is periventricular infarction.

Periventricular leukomalacia

Banker and Larroche (1962) described a postmortem appearance of white spots usually <2 mm in diameter and usually bilateral (although not symmetrical) in the periventricular region. These white spots are masses of microglial cells containing lipid and represent a microglial reaction around a necrotic area. Some lesions cavitate and form pseudo-cysts. If reperfusion is established, haemorrhage into the infarcted area can occur. Leukomalacia can occur anterior to the anterior horn of the lateral ventricle, in the corona radiata adjacent to the body of the lateral ventricle or posteriorly adjacent and lateral to the occipital horns of the lateral ventricles.

There is debate as to whether infarction in the periventricular area occurs as a result of hypoperfusion either of the vascular watersheds of the anterior, middle and posterior cerebral arteries or of the border zones between the ventriculo-fungal branches of the cerebral arteries and the ventriculopedal deep medullary arteries.

This type of infarction is most commonly seen in preterm infants of <34 weeks' gestation, although it occasionally occurs in term babies. In a prospective study of very low birthweight infants there was a 13.5 per cent incidence of periventricular leukomalacia and a further 12.5 per cent of infants developed a periventricular flare which is believed to represent non-cystic gliosis (Trounce, Rutter and Levene, 1986).

The important predisposing factors include antepartum haemorrhage, birth as-phyxia (Sinha *et al.*, 1985; Weindling *et al.*, 1985), respiratory distress syndrome, patent ductus arteriosus and causes of neonatal shock such as bacterial infection.

Periventricular infarction destroys the pyramidal tracts descending from the motor cortex. Small lesions are found close to the lateral ventricles, affecting the tracts supplying the legs, and result in the clinical condition of spastic diplegia. More extensive lesions involve the more lateral motor tracts which supply the arms and this results in spastic quadriplegia. When the optic radiations are involved this causes cortical blindness or severe visual impairment.

Subcortical leukomalacia

As the fetus develops, the blood supply to the periventricular area improves with an increasing number of branches from the deep medullary artery. Concurrently, however, the leptomeningeal supply to the subcortical region decreases and pre-disposes this region to ischaemic injury. Numerous cystic spaces develop approxi-mately 7–14 days after an ischaemic event and the outcome is very poor, the children being severely handicapped.

Other types of cerebral infarction

Parasaggital area
This type of infarction involves the motor cortex supplying the upper limbs causing weakness with normal or increased leg tone.

Cortex
Discrete or diffuse areas of the cortex may be infarcted causing ulegyria. The visual cortex and the hippocampus are particularly vulnerable. These children are charac-teristically profoundly physically and mentally handicapped.

Basal nuclei/brain stem
Very occasionally the basal nuclei, the thalamus, the inferior coeliculus and reticular formation are damaged.

Epidemiology

Definitions of cerebral palsy differ but that used by Nelson and Ellenberg (1979) is 'a chronic disability, characterized by aberrant control of movement and posture, appearing in early life, and not the result of recognized progressive disease'. There have been many studies of prevalence rates of cerebral palsy and most report rates of 2–3/1000, no matter whether live births or school age populations are used as denominators.

Birthweight and gestational age

Before the concept of weight for gestational age was recognized, relationships between birthweight and different types of cerebral palsy had been reported, initially during the last century by Little (1862) and Freud (1897), and then in this century by Evans (1948), Childs and Evans (1954), Plum (1956), Fuldner (1957), Churchill (1958) and Russell (1960). From these studies it could be concluded that: (1) the birth prevalence of cerebral palsy increases with decreasing birthweight; (2) there is a bimodal distribution of birthweight with cerebral palsy from which (a) the low birthweight group tend to have simple spastic diplegia with little other handicap, and (b) the normal birthweight group tend to have other types of cerebral palsy often associated with other handicaps including mental retardation and choreo-athetosis.

Subsequent studies, particularly the cohort studies of McDonald (1967) and the US National Collaborative Perinatal Project (Niswander, Friedman and Berendes, 1969; Ellenberg and Nelson, 1979; Nelson and Ellenberg, 1979, 1981, 1986) and the population studies of Stanley and her colleagues in Western Australia (Dale and Stanley, 1980; Stanley, 1981) and Hagberg and colleagues in Sweden (Hagberg, Hagberg and Olow, 1976; Hagberg and Hagberg, 1984), have confirmed these findings and have emphasized particularly that the striking increase in birth prevalence of spastic diplegia with decreasing birthweight is a reflection of decreasing gestation. For example, in the unselected population study of 681 cases of cerebral palsy born in Sweden from 1959 to 1976, 224 (33 per cent) were preterm and, of the 226 cases of spastic diplegia, 55 per cent were preterm; in contrast, the preterm delivery rate in the general Swedish population was 6 per cent. Although these figures stress the importance of preterm delivery as a major risk factor in the genesis of cerebral palsy, it must not be forgotten that the majority of cerebral palsy occurs in children born at term.

At the time when intrauterine growth retardation was becoming recognized as a clinical entity, Alberman (1963) studied 242 cases of cerebral palsy in London and reported that birthweight for gestational age was low in spastic diplegia, spastic quadriplegia and athetosis but was normal in spastic paraplegia. Shortly after this report McDonald (1964) described a 15.4 per cent incidence of infants whose birthweight for gestation was ≤2 standard deviations from the mean among children who had spastic diplegia and had been born after 34 weeks' gestation. These findings could have been explained by inaccuracies in gestational age assessment (that these infants were, in fact, very preterm and not growth retarded) but contemporary studies, whether case-control studies or case series with a population comparison group, have demonstrated an excess of small-for-gestational-age infants among cases of cerebral palsy (Durkin *et al.*, 1976; Hagberg, Hagberg and Olow, 1976; Dale and Stanley, 1980; Stanley, 1981; Bennett *et al.*, 1981; Veelken, Hagberg and Olow, 1983). Dale and Stanley (1980) reported a 17.8 per cent incidence of small-for-gestational-age infants in cerebral palsy cases compared with 2.9 per cent in controls, a pattern similar to that found by Veelken, Hagberg and Olow, (1983) (14 per cent in cerebral palsy cases compared with an expected 2.3 per cent were small for gestational age). Other data from the Swedish group, using 5th and 10th centiles to define small-for-gestational-age infants, show the importance of both preterm delivery and growth restriction in the genesis of cerebral palsy.

Most cohort studies have recruited infants of low birthweight or very low birthweight from neonatal intensive care units and therefore have been biased against infants at particularly high risk of cerebral palsy. Sabel, Olegard and Victorin (1976), however, undertook a follow-up study of an unselected population of 6700 3-year-old Swedish children and found that two-thirds of the children with handicap (cerebral palsy, psychomotor retardation, sensorineural deafness and acquired hydrocephaly) came from the 16 per cent of children with a birthweight >1 standard deviation below the mean.

Hypoxia/acidosis

Despite the pathological evidence above, implicating ischaemic lesions of the brain in cerebral palsy, and the epidemiological evidence showing that preterm and growth-retarded infants are the groups at risk of cerebral palsy (groups known to be at increased risk of birth asphyxia), birth asphyxia appears to be a rare cause of cerebral palsy. The Western Australian group could implicate birth asphyxia in only 8 per cent of cases of cerebral palsy (Blair and Stanley, 1988), and Nelson and Ellenberg (1986) reported birth asphyxia in only 9 per cent of their cases. The main problem in interpreting these data is that asphyxia is a nebulous term for which there is no agreed definition. It is a clinical concept comprising hypoxia, hypercapnia and ischaemia and covering a very large spectrum. Attempts to define this condition using, variously, intrapartum fetal heart rate changes, passage of meconium, fetal scalp or cord umbilical vessel pH or blood gas analyses, Apgar score and delayed onset of respiration, have all failed. Furthermore, profound abnormalities of these indices are not closely associated with cerebral palsy. The Dublin randomized controlled trial of intrapartum electronic fetal heart rate monitoring (Grant et al., 1989) showed that abnormalities of the fetal heart rate failed to predict cerebral palsy, and the Finnish study (Ruth and Raivio, 1988) reported a positive predictive value for perinatal brain damage of 8 per cent for a low pH value and 5 per cent for a high lactate value. An extremely low Apgar score performs a little better: the American collaborative perinatal project reported that 27 per cent of children with cerebral palsy had an Apgar score of <7 at 5 min (Nelson and Ellenberg, 1981) and Ruth and Raivio (1988) reported that a low 5-min Apgar score had a positive predictive value of 19 per cent. Neonatal hypoxic–ischaemic encephalopathy is a more reliable predictor of adverse outcome than the above. Three grades of encephalopathy are described (Table 12.2): grade I is associated with a favourable outcome but Grades II and III are associated with increasing risk of death and handicap (Levene et al., 1986). We must, therefore, strive to understand better which factors are implicated in the genesis of hypoxic ischaemic encephalopathy so that better methods of prevention can be developed. In the meantime we must continue to use the techniques of electronic fetal heart-rate monitoring, fetal scalp sampling and early recourse to delivery in the presence of fetal acidosis. The powerful effects of hypoxia/acidosis are reflected in the data of Stewart and Reynolds (1974), which showed that 23 infants without neonatal complications developed normally, that only one out of 44 children with neonatal complications other than hypoxia developed a serious handicap but that eight of the nine children who were handicapped had suffered from hypoxia.

Table 12.2. Characteristics of hypoxic–ischaemic encephalopathy

Grade I (mild)	Grade II (moderate)	Grade III (severe)
Irritability	Lethargy	Comatose
Mild hypotonia	Marked abnormalities of tone	Severe hypotonia
Poor sucking	Requires tube feeding	Failure to maintain respiration
No seizures	Seizures	Prolonged seizures

Mode of delivery

Birth trauma in the infant associated with prolonged and precipitate labour, cephalo–pelvic disproportion, abnormal presentation and instrumental delivery should now be of historical interest only. The preterm infant, in particular when presenting by the breech, is at risk from trauma, from footling presentation, from cord prolapse, from entrapment of the after-coming head in the incompletely dilated cervix causing tentorial rupture and from occipital osteodiastasis due to hyperextension of the head beneath the symphysis pubis. Delivery by caesarean section of infants ≤1500 g birthweight and presenting by the breech can result in a significant reduction in mortality (Goldenberg and Nelson, 1977; Ingemarsson, Westgren and Svenningsen, 1978; Bowes *et al.*, 1979; Duenholter *et al.*, 1979; Karp *et al.*, 1979; Mann and Gallant, 1979; Woods, 1979; Kauppila *et al.*, 1981; Nisell, Bistoletti and Palme, 1981; Geirsson *et al.*, 1982), but there have been few studies of whether handicap is reduced. Ingemarsson, Westgren and Svenningsen (1978) showed a fourfold reduction in Apgar scores <7 at 10 min, and a tenfold reduction in developmental and neurological abnormality in preterm infants, presenting by the breech, routinely delivered by caesarean section. The authors agreed that their study was open to criticism because results from two different time periods were compared, so that other factors, particularly neonatal intensive care, could have contributed to the improvement in outcome. However, autopsy examination of the neonatal deaths that occurred revealed a much higher incidence of tentorial rupture, subdural haematoma and spinal cord injury in the infants delivered vaginally, suggesting that delivery by caesarean section did prevent birth trauma. Cox, Kendall and Hommers (1982), although confirming a reduction in neonatal mortality from 29 per cent to 15 per cent associated with delivery by caesarean section, found an increase in handicap from 4.7 per cent to 21.9 per cent. It should be pointed out that in this study, unlike the Ingemarsson study, caesarean section was carried out only for associated obstetric pathology; the associated obstetric pathology, and not iatrogenic factors, could have been the cause of much of the handicap found. Evidence that intracerebral damage can be prevented by delivery of the preterm breech by caesarean section is supported by the report of Lamont *et al.* (1983), demonstrating a 55 per cent incidence of periventricular haemorrhage in those infants delivered vaginally compared with 13 per cent in those delivered by caesarean section.

Selection of mode of delivery for the very low birthweight infant presenting by the vertex is perhaps more contentious than that of breech presentation. It is recognized that the preterm cranium offers less resistance to compression than the term cranium (Kriewall and McPherson, 1981) and that the preterm brain is more liable to damage (Pape and Wigglesworth, 1979). To avoid trauma, low-outlet forceps and episiotomy

Table 12.3.   Origin of severe mental retardation according to five epidemiological studies with slightly different criteria for their groupings

Origin	Percentage in study [a]				
	A	B	C	D	E
Prenatal	56	44	73	68	62
(Genetic)	(36)	(44)	(43)	(52)	(48)
(Other)	(20)		(30)	(16)	(14)
Untraceable	20	30–37	12	22	14
Perinatal	13	7–11	10	8	12
Postnatal	9	9–12	3	1	9
Infantile psychosis and mental retatdation	2	2	2	1	3

[a] A: Drillien, Jameson and Wilkinson (1966); Edinburgh; n, 218; IQ <54; born 1950–1956.
  B: McDonald (1973); Quebec; n, 507; IQ <50; born 1958.
  C: Gustavson et al. (1977); Uppsala; n, 122; IQ <50; born 1959–1970.
  D: Gustavson et al. (1977); Vasterbotten; n, 161; IQ <50; born 1959–1970.
  E: Fryers and MacKay (1979); Salford; n, 401; IQ <50; born 1961–1975.

was advocated in the past (Bishop, Israel and Briscoe, 1965; Bowes, Halgrimson and Simmons, 1979) but this may not be the safest way of delivering these very small babies: a number of studies have demonstrated improved survival in very-low-birthweight babies delivered by caesarean section. The greatest improvement in survival appears to be among babies of birthweight $\leqslant$1000 g (Bowes, Halgrimson and Simmons, 1979; Haesslein and Goodlin, 1979; Paul, Koh and Monfared, 1979; Smith, Spencer and Hull, 1980; Bennett Britton, Fitzhardinge and Ashby, 1981; Dillon and Egan, 1981; Fairweather, 1981). Evidence regarding the long-term morbidity following vaginal delivery of very-low-birthweight infants presenting by the vertex is limited at present because of the small numbers studied and the difficulty in dissociating the effect of hypoxia on long-term morbidity.

Mental retardation

Global cognitive function is usually based on the results of developmental quotient (DQ) or intelligence quotient (IQ) tests. Retardation is severe if IQ is <50, mild if IQ is 51–70 and borderline if 71–85. The reported prevalence rate of severe retardation is 3–4/1000 and of mild retardation is 20–30/1000. Chromosomal and developmental defects dominate the causes of severe mental retardation (Table 12.3). Down's syndrome is the most common chromosomal cause of severe mental retardation, with an incidence at birth of about 1.3 per 1000. Most obstetricians offer prenatal diagnosis, either by amniocentesis or chorionic villus sampling, to women aged 35 or over, with a view to subsequent termination of pregnancy. If every woman accepted, 7.5 per cent of all pregnancies would be screened and 30 per cent of all Down's syndrome pregnancies would be detected. However, only one-half of the women at risk have prenatal diagnosis. Recently, Wald et al. (1988) described an antenatal screening strategy that combines measuring serum human chorionic gonadotrophin, unconjugated oestriol, alphafetoprotein and maternal age and claimed that 60 per cent of affected pregnancies would be detected with 5 per cent of women undergoing amniocentesis. Other groups are investigating this strategy, and its place in relation to chorionic villus sampling with first trimester termination of affected pregnancies still has to be elucidated.

The strategy for reducing the incidence of neural tube defects also relies on mid-trimester investigation (serum α-fetoprotein, α-fetoprotein and acetylcholinesterase in amniotic fluid, and ultrasonography) with a view to subsequent termination of affected pregnancies. Primary prevention of infants with neural tube defects has been reported by the administration of extra folic acid (Laurence *et al.*, 1981) or other vitamins (Smithells *et al.*, 1981a, b) before and after conception. Both of these studies were non-randomized; a randomized double-blind study of folic acid and vitamins in women with previously affected pregnancies is, therefore, under way. Prenatal conditions, including intrauterine growth retardation, and perinatal conditions do, however, contribute to this pool of unfortunate children. Unlike severe mental retardation, which does not vary with social class, mild mental retardation is much more common in socially deprived children. This over-representation of mild mental retardation in socially disadvantaged groups has been widely accepted to be the result of lack of environmental/educational stimulation within the home, which is a prerequisite to normal mental development. Stimulation in socially advantaged circumstances appears to be able to overcome mental deficits, whereas psychosocial deprivation in adverse circumstances can add significantly to an established deficit. The recently reported low level of mild mental retardation in Sweden (Hagberg *et al.*, 1981) at 4/1000 school children may be related to the relatively high socioeconomic and educational status of the population.

Pathology

The mature brain contains enormous numbers of cells and is incredibly complex. For example the rat's brain, which weighs only 2 g, is said to contain 150×10^6 neurones, eight times as many glial cells, and each single neurone in the cerebral cortex has >20 000 synapses. The human brain is about 700 times the size of the rat brain and is much more complex. The rapid growth and the dynamic developmental processes that integrate during fetal life to form the brain are just two of the factors that make the brain vulnerable to insult. Another characteristic that makes the brain vulnerable is that many developmental events within the brain have only one opportunity to occur (Dobbing and Sands, 1971): if conditions are unfavourable for a particular development then the opportunity for that event to occur will be lost for ever. The brain will be permanently deficient in that area and the relationship of that area with normally developed brain will be permanently distorted.

Much of our understanding of the normal cellular growth of the fetal brain comes from the work of Dobbing and his group (Dobbing and Sands, 1973). They examined 139 complete human brains from 10 weeks' gestation to 7 postnatal years, together with nine mature brains that represented adult growth achievement. Brains were examined from infants before 22 weeks' gestation from pregnancies terminated for non-pathological reasons, from infants of 25 weeks' gestation to term whose birth-weight for gestation was within 1 standard deviation of the mean and who had no specific neuropathology, and from children who suffered accidental death or died acutely from non-neurological disease between birth and 7 years of age. Brain cell numbers were estimated from DNA content and the extent of myelination from cholesterol content of the brains. After the period of embryogenesis, when the gross shape of the brain is formed, there is a rapid increase in cell numbers in the forebrain between 10 and 18 weeks' gestation, which represents neuroblast multiplication with differentiation into non-dividing neurones occurring towards the end of this time. Neuroblast multiplication is followed by dendritic growth and synaptic connection, a developmental process that is probably very important in determining intelligence achieved.

With the exception of the granular cells of the cerebellum and some parts of the forebrain, the number of neurones characteristic of the adult is achieved during the first half of pregnancy; thereafter, the enormous proliferation occurs mainly in glial cells. This phase, which initiates myelination from oligodendroglial cells, continues well into the second year of postnatal life. Thus, the major structural events that occur during the second half of fetal life, when growth restriction is characteristic, are dendrite formation, synaptic connectivity, glial cell multiplication and myelination.

It is important to comment on the different growth pattern of the cerebellum. The rate of cellular growth in the cerebellum is much more rapid than that in other parts of the brain, adult characteristics and dimensions being achieved by 15 months of age. In contrast, the remainder of the brain has achieved only 65 per cent of its adult dimensions by this age. This extremely rapid growth of the cerebellum makes it particularly vulnerable to insult.

The insult that has been most widely studied is growth restriction. In experimental studies of growth restriction the brain is small, with the cerebellum being retarded more than other parts of the brain (Dobbing, Hopewell and Lynch, 1971); this occurs even in the presence of 'brain sparing'. Postmortem studies (Gruenwald, 1963; Naeye and Kelly, 1966; Larroche and Korn, 1977) show brain weight to be reduced by a similar proportion in both symmetric and asymmetric growth retardation, i.e. 18 and 19–21 per cent, respectively. It is the relatively more severe retardation of growth of other organs in the asymmetric type that gives the characteristic anthropomorphy. Liver and spleen weights are reduced by 53 and 57 per cent, respectively, in asymmetric growth retardation compared with liver and spleen weight reductions of 28 and 23 per cent in symmetric growth retardation. Occipitofrontal head circumference measurements, which are linearly related to brain weight (Cooke et al., 1977), confirm a reduction in brain size in growth retardation (Crane and Kopta, 1980; Brooke, Wood and Butters, 1984). Head circumference does have a statistical relationship with intelligence (Dobbing, 1970; Fedrick, 1971), particularly at the extremes of the population, where children with mental handicap have smaller heads than children of normal intelligence (Brandon, Kirman and Williams, 1959; Davies and Kirman, 1962; Allen, 1964) and gifted children tend to have larger heads (Terman, 1926).

The smaller brains of growth retardation have fewer cells especially in some areas of the cortex and the cerebellum where the granular neurones are disproportionately reduced (Dobbing, Hopewell and Lynch, 1971). However, most of the deficit is in glial cells, as would be expected because it is these that which are rapidly multiplying during the latter part of pregnancy. Brain cholesterol, which is a marker of brain myelination, is also permanently reduced in fetal growth restriction (Dobbing, 1968). It has been established that certain lipids are more closely associated with myelin: these are the glycolipids, proteolipid proteins and plasmalogens, which are all reduced in growth retardation (Benton et al., 1966; Culley and Lindberg, 1968). Fishman, Madyastha and Prensky (1971) have directly isolated myelin and reported retarded myelination in undernourished animals.

If placental transfer is sufficiently impaired to cause hypoxia/ischaemia, then cerebral infarction (see above) can occur. More minor degrees of damage may occur if findings from ovine pregnancy can be extrapolated to the human. Mann et al. (1978) and Clapp et al. (1981) developed an ovine model of intrauterine growth retardation where the placental vascular bed was repetitively embolized with 15 μm microspheres. They demonstrated microscopic multifocal infarctions confined to the white matter but primarily involving non-myelinated axonal elements. These findings may explain some of the deficits seen in children who have suffered intrauterine growth retardation.

Epidemiology

Prior to the recognition of the concept of infants being small for gestational age, premature infants had been recognized to be at a disadvantage in terms of later functioning. Impairment of perceptual–motor skills, abstract reasoning, comprehension, motor coordination, speech articulation, intelligence, reading ability and arithmetic were all found to be increased by the controlled longitudinal studies of low birthweight infants born in Baltimore in 1952. These studies, which controlled for the effects on development of race, infant sex, social class, maternal child rearing attitudes and personality, demonstrated increasing impairment with decreasing birthweight (Knobloch et al., 1956; Harper, Fischer and Rider, 1959; Weiner et al., 1968; Weiner, 1968, 1970). Similar findings have been reported recently from Aberdeen (Illsley and Mitchell, 1984) and Vancouver (Dunn, 1986). The outcome at 6.5 years in the Vancouver children was very disturbing in that 140 of the 335 (41.8 per cent) low-birthweight children had neurological or ophthalmic disorders including mental retardation, IQ <70 (n = 30), cerebral palsy (n = 27), visual defects (n = 16), minimal brain dysfunction (n = 61), epilepsy (n = 14), sensorineural deafness (n = 12) and miscellaneous disorders (n = 21). There were 181 disorders in 140 children, but the present-day picture may be somewhat better than this, as the Vancouver children were born before the introduction of neonatal intensive care; we await the data.

Effect of the environment

Drillien's study reported in 1970, which was one of the earliest investigations of the effect of being small for gestational age on development, demonstrated how powerful environmental influences can be: she found a seven point deficit in IQ in children from average and working class families whose birthweight for gestation had been more than the 25th centile for gestational age; however, no deficit in IQ was apparent between similar-birthweight groups in children from middle-class and 'superior' working-class families. The National Child Development Study (Davie, Butler and Goldstein, 1972) controlled for social class and birth order, and found increased incidences of educational backwardness (i.e. severely subnormal; in special schools for the educationally subnormal; in need of such schooling; judged by doctors as needing special schooling) and poor copying designs scores in light-for-dates children. Interestingly, although the proportion of recognized handicaps was higher in light-for-dates children, there was no social-class effect on this outcome. The Toronto group have made important contributions to this field. In 1972, Fitzhardinge and Steven reported very tragic outcome results for a group of 96 term infants whose birthweights had been <2 standard deviations below the mean for gestation: there was a 6 per cent incidence of convulsions, 25 per cent had minimal brain damage and there were more than twice as many EEG abnormalities and five times as many speech defects as among the controls.

One way of examining the effect of impaired fetal growth on development without the need to control for social factors is to study the development of twins of

Table 12.4.   IQ differences in like-sex twins of differing birthweight

Author	n	Weight difference	IQ differences	p value
Babson et al. (1964), US	12	> 25[a]	6.5 ± 2.4	<0.02
Churchill (1965), USA	17	>300[b]	5.8 ± 2.2	<0.02
Kaelber and Pugh (1969), USA	16	>300[b]	−1.9 ± 3.3	N.S.
Dizygous Monozygous	17	>300[b]	5.8 ± 2.5	<0.05
Hohenauer (1971) Austria	16	>300[b]	7.7	<0.001
Henrichsen, Skinhj and Anderson (1986)	14	>25[a]	3.6	<0.05

[a] Per cent; [b] g

significantly different birthweights. Five studies of intelligence in like-sex twins of significantly different birthweights have been reported (Babson et al., 1964; Churchill, 1965; Kaelber and Pugh, 1969; Hohenauer, 1971; Henrichsen, Skinhj and Anderson, 1986). Three studies used a 300 g difference in birthweight between the smaller and larger twin and two studies used a 25 per cent difference in weight (Table 12.4). All showed a detriment to the smaller twin in terms of IQ of the order of 6–7 points.

Degree of growth retardation

Suboptimal development in small-for-gestational-age infants has also been reported by Francis-Williams and Davies (1974) and Neligan et al. (1976). The latter was an elegant and intensive study of intelligence in children born in Newcastle upon Tyne in 1960–1962 and showed that the degree of growth retardation was related to development. Measures of performance at 5, 6 and 7 years of age, adjusted for the mother's age and care of the child, child's sex and ordinal position in the family, antepartum haemorrhage and mode of delivery, demonstrated poorer growth, IQ and language and increased incidences of visuomotor and neurological abnormalities in children who were born small for dates compared with children who were appropriately grown or preterm. The degree of impairment was related to the presumed severity of growth retardation (Table 12.5).

Hypoxia/acidosis

In 1978, Fitzhardinge and her colleagues examined the outcome of infants of very low birthweight. After intraventricular haemorrhage, low birthweight for gestation was the second most important association with handicap. Of 40 infants with birthweights <2 standard deviations below the mean for gestation, 21 (52 per cent) had major handicaps. To try to examine the effect of prenatal growth achievement on development, they compared the outcome of 28 growth-retarded infants with that of a group of appropriately grown infants controlled for weight, sex and similar neonatal course: the growth-retarded infants had significantly more neurological defects and much poorer development (Table 12.6). Their results suggest that, even if hypoxic/ischaemic and biochemical insults are prevented during birth and early neonatal life, intrauterine growth retardation does impair brain development. However, the Hospital for Sick Children, Toronto (where this study was performed) is a referral centre with no maternity unit, so that the intrapartum care of the children studied was very varied and the sequelae of hospital transfer in the early hours of life (e.g. hypothermia, hypoglycaemia and acidosis) were also common. Even though an

Table 12.5.   Performance of the children from the Newcastle survey of child development

Measures of performance	Control group	Short gestation	Intrauterine growth retardation		
			5th–10th centile	<5th centile	Significance of F ratio
Height at 7 years (cm)	121.9	119.7	120.5	117.8	$p < 0.001$
Weight increment to 7 years (kg)	20.3	20.4	19.9	18.8	$p < 0.01$
Verbal IQ at 6 years (Wechsler)	100.5	96.9	97.0	94.7	$p < 0.05$
Language quotient at 7 years (Illinois)	98.6	93.5	94.2	91.8	$p < 0.01$
Reading quotient at 7 years (Holborn)	93.1	92.3	94.3	91.3	N.S.
Visuomotor errors (Bender–Gestalt)	5.0	5.5	5.1	6.6	$p < 0.05$
Motor impairment (Ozeretsky–Stott)	2.0	3.0	2.6	3.4	$p < 0.058$
Behaviour abnormalities (mother's observations)	37.1	38.0	36.4	39.2	N.S.
Neurological abnormalities (teacher's observations)	4.6	4.5	5.0	5.2	N.S.
Neurological abnormalities (mother's observations)	12.6	13.8	12.8	14.2	$p < 0.05$
Neurological abnormalities ('soft')	12.7	13.8	13.4	14.3	$p < 0.001$
Neurological abnormalities (gesture)	29.1	33.3	29.3	34.4	$p < 0.001$

[a] From Neligan et al. (1976)

attempt was made to control for these perinatal events, these superimposed insults may have caused a proportion of the increased number of handicaps. Nevertheless, the Toronto results may be more representative of the norm than the good results reported from other centres of excellence (Stewart, Reynolds and Lipscomb, 1981).

In contrast to the results from Toronto, a small study from Montreal (Westwood *et al.*, 1983) reported normal function in 33 13–19-year-olds who were full term non-asphyxiated small-for-dates infants at birth. They, therefore, suggested that poor function in small-for-dates infants is related to asphyxia and management should be directed to prevent the latter. However, the children were born during 1960–1966, when dating by ultrasound was not available and, therefore, the evidence that these children were truly small for dates must be insecure.

Duration of growth retardation

The duration, as well as the degree, of growth retardation appears to be negatively related to development. Ounsted, Moar and Scott, (1984) reported that development at 7 years of age was positively associated with gestational age at birth if the child had been appropriate to weight at birth; in contrast, however, development in small-for-dates infants was negatively related to gestational age. This is particularly so when a small for dates infant is born to a woman of average size who has previously had heavier birthweight infants (Ounsted, Moar and Scott, 1989), a group more likely to have maternal or fetal pathology (Bakketeig, Bjerkedal and Hoffman, 1986; Ounsted, Scott and Moar, 1988). Their data suggest that prolongation of pregnancy in growth-retarded infants may be detrimental (Ounsted, Moar and Scott, 1989) and that ways of determining optimal time for delivery of these infants must be sought.

Complicated growth retardation

Our own studies (Taylor *et al.*, 1985; Taylor and Howie, 1989) suggest that it is intrauterine growth retardation associated with severe hypertension, antepartum haemorrhage or preterm uterine activity that is particularly implicated in poor subsequent function.

Although the evidence above shows that there is a general relationship between poor intrauterine growth and abnormal neurological development, and that the risk of the latter is increased if the retardation is severe, prolonged or complicated by prenatal complications, we have as yet no way of identifying which infants in these groups are specifically at risk and what are the mechanisms underlying the poor development. Recommendations regarding management must await this knowledge but in the mean time it is important to prevent superimposed hypoxia/acidosis, which can lead ultimately to death or cerebral palsy.

Table 12.6.   Outcome of small-for-gestational-age infants (<33 weeks' gestation) compared with weight-matched appropriate-weight-for-gestation infants with a similar neonatal course

	Small for gestational age	*Appropriate for gestational age*	*P value*
Number (total)	28	28	<0.001
CNS defect (*n*)	10	0	<0.005
Bayley – mental score	85.5	97.4	<0.01
Bayley – motor score	76.5	89.9	<0.01
Handicap (*n*)	12	3	

References

Agustsson, P and Patel, N (1988) Intrapartum asphyxia and subsequent disability. In *Antenatal and Perinatal Causes of Handicap, Clinical Obstetrics and Gynaecology* (edited by N Patel) Vol 2, No 1, pp. 167–186, London: Baillière Tindall

Alberman, ED (1963) Birthweight and length of gestation in cerebral palsy. *Developmental Medicine and Child Neurology*, **5**, 388–394

Allen, N (1964) Developmental and degenerative diseases of the brain. In *Paediatric Neurology*, (edited by TW Farmer) p. 176. New York: Harper and Row

Babson, SG, Kangas, J, Young, N and Bramhall, JL (1964) Growth and development of twins of dissimilar size at birth. *Pediatrics*, **33**, 327–333

Bakketeig, LS, Bjerkedal, T and Hoffman, HJ (1986) Small for gestational age births in successive pregnancy outcomes: results from a longitudinal study of births in Norway. *Early Human Development*, **14**, 187–200

Banker, BQ and Larroche, J-C (1962) Periventricular leukomalacia of infancy. *Archives of Neurology*, **7**, 386–410

Bejar, R, Curbelo, V, Coen, RW *et al.* (1980) Diagnosis and follow up of intraventricular and intracerebral haemorrhages by ultrasound studies of infant's brain through the fontanelles and sutures. *Pediatrics*, **66**, 661–673

Bennett, FL, Chandler, LS, Robinson, NM and Sells, CJ (1981) Spastic diplegia in premature infants – aetiologic and diagnostic considerations. *American Journal of Diseases of Children*, **135**, 732–737

Bennett Britton, S, Fitzhardinge, PM and Ashby, S (1981) Is intensive care justified for infants weighing less than 801 g at birth? *Journal of Pediatrics*, **99**, 937–943

Benton, JW, Moser, NW, Dodge, PR and Carr, S (1966) Modification of the schedule of myelination in the rat by early nutritional deprivation. *Pediatrics*, **38**, 801–807

Bishop, EH, Israel, L and Briscoe, CC (1965) Obstetric influences on the premature infant's first year of development. *Obstetrics and Gynecology*, **26**, 628–635

Blair, E and Stanley, FJ (1988) Intrapartum asphyxia: a rare cause of cerebral palsy. *Journal of Pediatrics*, **112**, 515–519

Bleyer, WA and Skinner, AL (1976) Fatal neonatal hemorrhage after maternal anticonvulsant therapy. *Journal of the American Medical Association*, **235**, 626–627

Bowes, WA, Halgrimson, M and Simmons, MA (1979) Results of the intensive perinatal management of very low birthweight infants (501–1500 g). *Journal of Reproductive Medicine*, **23**, 245–250

Bowes, WA, Taylor, ES, O'Brien, M and Bowes, C (1979) Breech delivery: evaluation of the method of delivery on perinatal results and maternal morbidity. *American Journal of Obstetrics and Gynecology*, **135**, 965–973

Brandon, MWG, Kirman, BH and Williams, CE (1959) Microcephaly. *Journal of Mental Science*, **105**, 721

Brooke, OG, Wood, C and Butters, F (1984) The body proportions for small for dates infants. *Early Human Development*, **10**, 85–94

Childs, B and Evans, PR (1954) Birthweights of children with cerebral palsy. *Lancet*, **i**, 642–645

Churchill, JA (1958) The relationship of Little's disease to premature births. *American Journal of Diseases of Children*, **96**, 32–39

Churchill, JA (1965) Relationship between intelligence and birthweight in twins. *Neurology*, **15**, 341–347

Clapp, JF III, Mann, LI, Peress, NS and Szeto, HH (1981) Neuropathology in the chronic fetal lamb preparation: structure–function correlates under different environmental conditions. *American Journal of Obstetrics and Gynecology*, **141**, 973–986

Cooke, RWI, Lucas, A, Yudkin, PLN and Pryse-Davies, J (1977) Head circumference as an index of brain weight in the fetus and newborn. *Early Human Development*, **1/2**, 145–149

Cox, C, Kendall, AC and Hommers, M (1982) Changed prognosis of breech presenting low birthweight infants. *British Journal of Obstetrics and Gynaecology*, **89**, 881–886

Crane, JP and Kopta, MM (1980) Comparative newborn anthropometric data in symmetric versus asymmetric intrauterine growth retardation. *American Journal of Obstetrics and Gynecology*, **138**, 518–522

Craig, WS (1938) Intracranial haemorrhage in the newborn. *Archives of Disease in Childhood*, **13**, 89–124

Culley, WJ and Lindberg, RO (1968) Effect of undernutrition on the size and composition of the rat brain. *Journal of Nutrition*, **96**, 375–381

Dale, A and Stanley, FJ (1980) An epidemiological study of cerebral palsy in Western Australia, 1956–1970. II: Spastic cerebral palsy and perinatal factors. *Developmental Medicine and Child Neurology*, **22**, 13–25

Davie, R, Butler, N and Goldstein, H (1972) The effect of birthweight, gestation and other obstetric factors on disabilities at the age of seven. In *From Birth to Seven. A Report of the National Child Development Study*, pp. 165–174, Longman in association with The National Children's Bureau

Davies, W and Kirman, BH (1962) Microcephaly. *Archives of Disease in Childhood*, **37**, 623

de Crespigny, L, Mackay, R, Muston, LJ *et al.* (1982) Timing of neonatal cerebro-ventricular haemorrhage with ultrasound. *Archives of Disease in Childhood*, **57**, 231–233

Dillon, WP and Egan, EA (1981) Aggressive obstetric management in late second-trimester deliveries. *Obstetrics and Gynecology*, **58**, 685–690

Dobbing, J (1968) Vulnerable periods in developing brain. In *Applied Neuro-Chemistry* (edited by AN Davison and J Dobbing) pp. 287–316, Oxford: Blackwell

Dobbing, J (1970) The kinetics of growth. *Lancet*, **ii**, 1358

Dobbing, J and Sands, J (1971) Vulnerability of developing brain IX. The effect of nutritional growth retardation on the timing of the brain growth spurt. *Biological Neonatology*, **19**, 363–378

Dobbing, J and Sands, J (1973) Quantitative growth and development of human brain. *Archives of Disease in Childhood*, **48**, 757–767

Dobbing, J, Hopewell, JW and Lynch, A (1971) Vulnerability of developing brain III. Permanent deficit of neurons in cerebral and cerebellar cortex following early mild undernutrition. *Experimental Neurology*, **32**, 439–447

Drillien, CM (1970) The small for date infant: etiology and prognosis. *Pediatric Clinics of North America*, **17**, 9–24

Drillien, CM, Jameson, S and Wilkinson, EM (1966) Studies in mental handicap I. Prevalence and distribution by clinical type and severity of defect. *Archives of Disease in Childhood*, **41**, 528–538

Duenholter, JH, Wells, CE, Reisch, JS *et al.* (1979) A paired controlled study of vaginal and abdominal delivery of the low birthweight breech fetus. *Obstetrics and Gynecology*, **54**, 310–313

Dunn, HG (1986) Sequelae of low birthweight: the Vancouver study. *Clinics in Developmental Medicine, No 95/96*. MacKeith Press; Oxford: Blackwell Scientific Publications Ltd; Philadelphia: JB Lippincott Co

Durkin, MV, Kaveggia, EG, Pendleton, E, Neuhauser, G and Opitz, JM (1976) Analysis of etiologic factors in cerebral palsy with severe mental retardation; analysis of gestational, parturitional and neonatal data. *European Journal of Pediatrics*, **123**, 67

Ellenberg, JH and Nelson, KB (1979) Birthweight and gestational age in children with cerebral palsy or seizure disorders. *American Journal of Diseases of Children*, **133**, 1044–1048

Evans, PR (1948) Antecedents of infantile cerebral palsy. *Archives of Disease in Childhood*, **23**, 213–219

Fairweather, DVI (1981) Obstetric management and follow up of the very low birthweight infant. *Journal of Reproductive Medicine*, **26**, 387–392

Fedrick, J (1971) The kinetics of growth. *Lancet*, **i**, 133

Fenichel, GM, Webster, DL and Wong, WKT (1984) Intracranial haemorrhage in the term newborn. *Archives of Neurology*, **41**, 30–34

Fishman, MA, Madyastha, P and Prensky, AL (1971) The effect of undernutrition on the development of myelin in the rat central nervous system. *Lipids*, **6**, 458–465

Fitzhardinge, PM and Steven, EM (1972) The small for date infant II. Neurological and intellectual sequelae. *Pediatrics*, **50**, 50–57

Fitzhardinge, PM, Kalman, E, Ashby, S and Pape, K (1978) Present status of the infant of very low birthweight treated in a referred neonatal intensive care unit in 1974. In *Major Mental Handicap: Methods and Costs of Prevention* (edited by K Elliott and M O'Connor), pp. 139–150, North-Holland: Elsevier Excerpta Medica

Francis-Williams, J and Davies, PA (1974) Very low birthweight and later intelligence. *Developmental Medicine and Child Neurology*, **16**, 709–728

Freud, S (1897) *Infantile Cerebral Paralysis* (translation by Russin, LA (1968)). *Die Infantile Cerebrallahmung.* Vienna: Alfred Hoder, Coral Gables, Florida: University of Miami Press

Fryers, T and Mackay, RI (1979) The epidemiology of severe mental handicap. *Early Human Development*, **3**, 277–294

Fuldner, RV (1957) Labor complications and cerebral palsy. *American Journal of Obstetrics and Gynecology*, **74**, 159–166

Geirsson, RT, Namunkangula, R, Calder, AA and Lunan, CB (1982) Preterm singleton presentation: the impact of traumatic intracranial haemorrhage on neonatal mortality. *Journal of Obstetrics and Gynaecology*, **2**, 219–223

Goldenberg, RL and Nelson, KG (1977) The premature breech. *American Journal of Obstetrics and Gynecology*, **127**, 240–244

Grant, A, O'Brian, N, Joy, M-T *et al.* (1989) Cerebral palsy among children born during the Dublin randomized trial of intrapartum monitoring. *Lancet*, **ii**, 1233–1235

Gruenwald, P (1963) Chronic fetal distress and placental insufficiency. *Biological Neonatology*, **5**, 215–265

Gustavson, K-H, Hagberg, B, Hagberg, G and Sars, K (1977) Severe mental retardation in a Swedish country: etiologic and pathogenetic aspects of children born 1959–1970. *Neuropediatrics*, **8**, 293–304

Haesslein, HC and Goodlin, RC (1979) Delivery of the tiny newborn. *American Journal of Obstetrics and Gynecology*, **134**, 192–200

Hagberg, B and Hagberg, G (1984) Prenatal and perinatal risk factors in a survey of 681 Swedish cases. The epidemiology of the cerebral palsies. In *Clinics in Developmental Medicine No. 87* (edited by F Stanley and E Alberman) pp. 116–134. Oxford: Blackwell Scientific Publications

Hagberg, G, Hagberg, B and Olow, I (1976) The changing panorama of cerebral palsy in Sweden 1954–1970 III. The importance of fetal deprivation of supply. *Acta Paediatrica Scandinavica*, **65**, 403–408

Hagberg, B, Hagberg, G, Lewerth, A and Lindberg, U (1981) Mild mental retardation in Swedish school children II. Etiologic and pathogenic aspects. *Acta Paediatrica Scandinavica*, **70**, 445–452

Hambleton, G and Wigglesworth, JS (1976) Origin of intraventricular haemorrhage in the preterm infant. *Archives of Disease in Childhood*, **51**, 651–659

Harper, PA, Fischer, LK and Rider, RV (1959) Neurological and intellectual status of prematures at three to five years of age. *Journal of Pediatrics*, **55**, 679–690

Hayden, CK, Sharruck, KE, Richardson, CJ *et al.* (1985) Subependymal germinal matrix haemorrhage in full term neonates. *Pediatrics*, **75**, 714–718

Henrichsen, L, Skinhj, K and Andersen, GE (1986) Delayed growth and reduced intelligence in 9–17 year old intrauterine growth retarded children compared with their monozygous co-twins. *Acta Paediatrica Scandinavica*, **75**, 31–35

Hill, RM, Verniaud, WM and Deter, RL (1984) The effect of intrauterine malnutrition on the term infant. *Acta Paediatrica Scandinavica*, **173**, 482–487

Hohenauer, L (1971) Prenatal nutrition and subsequent development. *Lancet*, **i**, 644–645

Illsley, R (1967) Family growth and its effects on the relationship between obstetric factors and child functioning. In *Social and Genetic Influences on Life and Death* (edited by Lord Platt and AS Parker) pp. 29–422. Edinburgh: Oliver and Boyd

Illsley, R (1980) *Professional and Public Health: Sociology in Health and Medicine*, pp. 11–44. London: Nuffield Provincial Hospitals Trust

Illsley, R and Mitchell, RG (1984) *Low Birthweight: a Medical, Psychological and Social Study.* Chichester: J Wiley and Sons

Ingemarsson, I, Westgren, M and Svenningsen, NW (1978) Long-term follow up of preterm infants in breech presentation delivered by Caesarean section – a prospective study. *Lancet*, **ii**, 172–175

Kaelber, CT and Pugh, TF (1969) Influence of intrauterine relations on the intelligence of twins. *New England Journal of Medicine*, **19**, 1030–1034

Karp, LE, Doney, JR, McCarthy, T *et al.* (1979) The premature breech: trial of labor or Cesarean section? *Obstetrics and Gynecology*, **53**, 8–92

Kauppila, O, Gronros, M, Aro, P *et al.* (1981) Management of low birthweight breech delivery: should Cesarean section be routine? *Obstetrics and Gynecology*, **57**, 289–294

Knobloch, H, Rider, RV, Harper, PA and Pasamanick, B (1956) Neuropsychiatric sequelae of prematurity. *Journal of the American Medical Association*, **161**, 581–585

Kriewall, T and McPherson, GK (1981) Effects of uterine contractility on the fetal cranium. In *Advances in Perinatal Medicine, Volume 1* (edited by A Milunsky, E Friedman and L Gluck) pp. 295–356, New York: Plenum Publishing Corp

Lamont, RF, Dunlop, PDM, Crowley, P and Elder, MG (1983) Spontaneous pre-term labour and delivery at under 34 weeks gestation. *British Medical Journal*, **286**, 454–457

Larroche, JC and Korn, G (1977) Brain damage in intrauterine growth retardation. In *Intrauterine Asphyxia and the Developing Fetal Brain* (edited by L Gluck) pp. 25–35, Chicago, London: Year Book Medical Publishers Inc

Laurence, KM, James, N, Miller, MH *et al.* (1981) Double blind randomised controlled trial of folate treatment before conception to prevent recurrence of neural tube defects. *British Medical Journal*, **282**, 1509–1511

Levene, MI (1985) Diagnosis and management of intraventricular haemorrhage in the neonate. *World Paediatrics and Childcare*, **1**, 7–12

Levene, MI, Fawer, C-L and Lamont, LF (1982) Risk factors in the development of intraventricular haemorrhage in the preterm neonate. *Archives of Disease in Childhood*, **57**, 410–417

Levene, MI, Kornberg, J and Williams, THC (1985) The incidence and severity of post-asphyxial encephalopathy in full term infants. *Early Human Development*, **1**, 21–28

Levene, MI, Sands, C Grindulis, H and Moore, JR (1986) Comparison of two methods of predicting outcome in perinatal asphyxia. *Lancet*, **i**, 67–69

Little, WJ (1862) On the influence of abnormal parturition, difficult labour, premature birth and asphyxia neonatorum on the mental and physical condition of the child especially in relation to deformities. *Transactions of the Obstetrical Society of London*, **3**, 239 (Reprinted: *Cerebral Palsy Bulletin* (1958), **1, (i)**, 5)

McDonald, AD (1964) The aetiology of spastic diplegia. *Developmental Medicine and Child Neurology*, **6**, 277–285

McDonald, AD (1967) Children of very low birthweight. *MEIU Research Monograph No 1*, London: SIMP with Heinemann

McDonald, AD (1973) Severely retarded children in Quebec: prevalence, causes and care. *American Journal of Mental Deficiency*, **78**, 205–215

McDonald, MM, Koops, BL, Johnson, ML *et al.* (1984) Timing of antecedents of intracranial haemorrhage in the newborn. *Pediatrics*, **74**, 32–36

Mann, LI and Gallant, JM (1979) Modern management of the breech delivery. *American Journal of Obstetrics and Gynecology*, **134**, 611–614

Mann, LI, Bhakthavathsalan, A, Peress, N *et al.* (1978) Fetal brain function, metabolism and neuropathology following acute hypoxia. In *Fetal and Newborn Cardiovascular Physiology, Vol. 2* (edited by LD Longo and DD Renean) pp. 313–335, New York: Garland Press

Naeye, RL and Kelly, JA (1966) Judgement of fetal age III. The pathologist's evaluation. *Pediatric Clinics of North America*, **13**, 849

Neligan, GA, Kolvin, I, Scott, DMcI and Garside, RF (1976) *Born too Soon or Born too Small. A Follow Up Study to Seven Years of Age.* Spastic International Medical Publications, London: William Heinemann Medical Books Ltd; Philadelphia: JB Lippincott Co

Nelson, KB and Ellenberg, JH (1979) Epidemiology of cerebral palsy. In *Advances in Neurology Vol. 19*, (edited by BS Schoenberg) pp. 421–436. New York: Raven Press

Nelson, K and Ellenberg, J (1981) Apgar scores as predictors of chronic neurologic disability. *Pediatrics*, **68**, 36–44

Nelson, KB and Ellenberg, JH (1986) Antecedents of cerebral palsy. Multivariate analysis of risk. *New England Journal of Medicine*, **315**, 81–86

Nisell, H, Bistoletti, P and Palme, C (1981) Preterm breech delivery, early and late complications. *Acta Obstetrica et Gynaecologica Scandinavica*, **60**, 363–366

Niswander, KR, Friedman, EA and Berendes, H (1969) Do placenta praevia, abruptio placentae and prolapsed cord cause neurological damage to the infant who survives? In *Studies in Infancy. Clinics in Developmental Medicine, No. 27* (edited by R MacKeith and R Bar) pp. 78–83. London: SIMP with Heinemann

Ounstead, M, Moar, VA and Scott, A (1984) Children of deviant birthweight at age seven years: health, handicap, size and developmental status. *Early Human Development*, **9**, 323–340

Ounstead, M, Moar, VA and Scott, A (1989) Small-for-dates babies, gestational age and developmental ability at 7 years. *Early Human Development*, **19**, 77–86

Ounstead, M, Scott, A and Moar, VA (1988) Constrained and unconstrained fetal growth associated with some biological and pathological factors. *Annals of Human Biology*, **15**, 119–129

Pape, KE and Wigglesworth, JS (1979) *Haemorrhage, Ischaemia and the Perinatal Brain*. Spastics International Medical Publications, London: William Heinemann Medical Books, Philadelphia: JB Lippincott Co

Paul, RH, Koh, KS and Monfared, H (1979) Obstetric factors influencing outcome in infants weighing from 1001–1500 grams. *American Journal of Obstetrics and Gynecology*, **133**, 503–508

Philip, AGS and Allan, WC (1985) Neonatal intracranial haemorrhage and cerebral oedema. In *Risks of Labour* (edited by JW Crawford) pp. 95–117, Chichester: John Wiley

Plum, P (1956) Cerebral palsy: a clinical survey of 543 cases. *Danish Medical Bulletin*, **3**, 99–108

Rose, AC and Lombroso, CT (1970) Neonatal seizure states. A study of clinical, pathological and electroencephalographic features in 137 full term babies with a long term follow up. *Pediatrics*, **45**, 404–425

Russell, EM (1960) Correlation between birthweight and clinical findings in diplegia. *Archives of Disease in Childhood*, **35**, 548–551

Ruth, VJ and Raivio, KO (1988) Perinatal brain damage: predictive value of metabolic acidosis and Apgar score. *British Medical Journal*, **297**, 24–27

Sabel, K-G, Olegard, R and Victorin, L (1976) Remaining sequelae with modern perinatal care. *Pediatrics*, **57**, 652–658

Sinha, SK, Davies, JM, Sims, DG and Chiswick, ML (1985) Relation between periventricular haemorrhage and ischaemic brain lesions diagnosed by ultrasound in very pre-term infants. *Lancet*, **ii**, 1154–1155

Smith, ML, Spencer, SA and Hull, D (1980) Mode of delivery and survival in babies weighing less than 2000 g at birth. *British Medical Journal*, **281**, 1118–1119

Smithells, RW, Shepherd, S, Schorah, CJ *et al.* (1981a) Apparent prevention of neural tube defects by vitamin supplementation. *Archives of Disease in Childhood*, **56**, 911–918

Smithells, RW, Shepherd, S, Schorah, CJ *et al.* (1981b) Vitamin supplementation and neural tube defects. *Lancet*, **ii**, 1424–1425

Stanley, FJ (1981) Spastic cerebral palsy: changes in birthweight and gestational age. *Early Human Development*, **5**, 167–178

Stewart, AL and Reynolds, EOR (1974) Improved prognosis for infants of very low birthweight. *Pediatrics*, **54**, 724–735

Stewart, AL, Reynolds, EOR and Lipscomb, AP (1981) Outcome for infants of very low birthweight: survey of world literature. *Archives of Disease in Childhood*, **59**, 7–12

Szymonowicz, W and Yu, VYH (1984) Timing and evolution of periventricular haemorrhage in infants weighing 12150 g or less at birth. *Archives of Disease in Childhood*, **59**, 7–12

Szymonowicz, W and Yu, VYH (1987) Severe pre-eclampsia and infants of very low birthweight. *Archives of Disease in Childhood*, **62**, 712–716

Taylor, DJ (1988) Prenatal complications, handicap and disability. In *Clinical Obstetrics and Gynaecology, Vol. 2 No. 1* (edited by N Patel) pp. 73–90, London: Baillière Tindall

Taylor, DJ and Howie, PW (1989) Fetal growth achievement and neurodevelopmental disability. *British Journal of Obstetrics and Gynaecology*, **96**, 789–794

Taylor, DJ, Howie, PW, Davidson, J *et al.* (1985) Do pregnancy complications contribute to neurodevelopmental disability? *Lancet*, **i**, 713–716

Terman, LM (1926) *Genetic Studies of Genius, Vol 1. Mental and Physical Traits of a Thousand Gifted Children*, 2nd ed. Stanford, California: Stanford University Press

Thorburn, RJ, Lipscomb, AP, Stewart *et al.* (1982) Timing and antecedents of periventricular haemorrhage of cerebral atrophy in very preterm infants. *Early Human Development*, **7**, 221–238

Trounce, JQ, Rutter, N and Levene, MI (1986) Periventricular leukomalacia and intraventricular haemorrhage in the preterm neonate. *Archives of Disease in Childhood*, **61**, 1196–1202

Veelken, N, Hagberg, G and Olow, I (1983) Diplegic cerebral palsy in Swedish term and preterm children. Differences in reduced optimality, relations to neurologic and pathogenic factors. *Neuropediatrics*, **14**, 20–28

Villar, J, Smeriglio, V, Martorell, R *et al.* (1984) Heterogeneous growth and mental development of intrauterine growth retarded infants during the first 3 years of life. *Pediatrics*, **74**, 783–791

Wald, NJH, Cuckle, HS, Densem, JW *et al.* (1988) Maternal serum screening for Down's Syndrome in early pregnancy. *British Medical Journal*, **297**, 883–887

Walther, FJ and Raemaekers, LHJ (1982) Neonatal morbidity of SGA infants in relation to their nutritional status at birth. *Acta Paediatrica Scandinavica*, **71**, 437–440

Weindling, AM, Wilkinson, AR, Cook, J *et al.* (1985) Perinatal events which precede periventricular haemorrhage and leukomalacia in the newborn. *British Journal of Obstetrics and Gynaecology*, **92**, 1218–1223

Weiner, G (1968) Scholastic achievement at age 12–13 of prematurely born infants. *Journal of Special Education*, **2**, 237–250

Weiner, G (1970) The relationship of birthweight and length of gestation to intellectual development at ages 8 to 10 years. *Journal of Pediatrics*, **76**, 694–699

Weiner, G, Rider, RV, Oppel, WC and Harper, PA (1968) Correlates of low birthweight. Psychological status at eight to ten years of age. *Pediatric Research*, **2**, 110–118

Westgren, CMR, Malcus, P and Svenningsen, NW (1986) Intrauterine asphyxia and long term outcome in preterm fetuses. *Obstetrics and Gynecology*, **67**, 512–561

Westwood, M, Kaamer, MS, Munz, D *et al.* (1983) Growth and development of full term non-asphyxiated small-for-gestational age newborns: follow up through adolescence. *Pediatrics*, **71**, 376–383

Wigglesworth, JS and Husemeyer, RP (1977) Intracranial birth trauma in vaginal breech delivery: the continued importance of injury to the occipital zone. *British Journal of Obstetrics and Gynaecology*, **84**, 684–691

Woods, JR (1979) Effects of low-birth-weight breech delivery on neonatal mortality. *Obstetrics and Gynecology*, **53**, 735–740

World Health Organization (1980) *International Classification of Impairments, Disabilities and Handicap*. Geneva: WHO

Zalneraitis, EL, Young, RSK and Krishnamoorthy, KS (1979) Intracranial haemorrhage in utero as a complication of isoimmune thrombocytopaenia. *Journal of Pediatrics*, **95**, 611–614

Chapter 13

Fetal haemolytic disease

SL Barron and MM Reid

Introduction

Haemolytic disease of the newborn (HDN) was, until the 1970s, an important cause of perinatal death but even though the condition is now much less frequent, as a result of anti-D prophylaxis and demographic change, it is still an important problem, especially for those families who are affected by it.

Jaundice affecting the newborn was described in the seventeenth century and hydrops fetalis was recognized long before the aetiology was understood. Diamond, Blackfan and Batey (1932) recognized that HDN, icterus gravis and hydrops were linked. Parsons proposed that erythroblastosis fetalis was also a feature of the haemolytic process, but was still defending this hypothesis in 1938 (Parsons, 1938) against the prevailing view that it was an abnormality in the same class as Cooley's anaemia and other erythroblastoses. During the following three years a remarkable series of papers not only clarified the pathogenesis of haemolytic disease of the newborn but also resulted in a great advance in the understanding of human blood groups; it was the foundation of transfusion immunology as we now know it.

In 1938, Ruth Darrow (Darrow, 1938) made a detailed analysis of icterus gravis neonatorum, with particular emphasis on the familial pattern of the disease, and concluded that the disease was due to maternal sensitization to an unknown fetal antigen. A year later, Levine and Stetson (1939) proposed that the process was due to a form of immunization of the fetus by some sort of blood group incompatibility. In 1940, Landsteiner and Wiener (1940) described the rhesus factor in human erythrocytes and it was not long before Levine and his co-workers (Levine *et al.*, 1941) described the role of isoimmunization in the pathogenesis of erythroblastosis fetalis.

Early attempts to treat the affected children by transfusion were partially successful, but were hampered by the lack of knowledge of the rhesus factors. The great step came with the description of exchange transfusion by Wiener and Wexler (1946) and, finally, in the only controlled trial of pre- or postnatal management of this disease, exchange transfusion was shown to be superior to simple transfusion in preventing neonatal death (Mollison and Walker, 1952).

The prevention of immunization to the D antigen was proposed by the Liverpool group (Finn, 1960) and shortly afterwards in New York (Freda, Gorman and Pollack, 1964). As a result of international collaboration, an immunization programme is now in operation throughout the world. Although alloimmunization by the Rh(D) antigen is still the most important cause of haemolytic disease of the

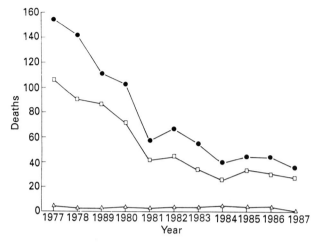

Figure 13.1   Deaths from haemolytic disease of the fetus and newborn in England and Wales, 1977–1987 (Clarke and Mollison, 1989): ●, due to haemolytic disease, probable true numbers; □, due to anti-D; △, due to anti-c̄ etc.

newborn, other blood group antigens, such as c̄ and Kell, are assuming a greater importance as cases of HDN due to Rh(D) decline. There are, however, other causes of fetal haemolytic disease and they are mentioned below.

Epidemiology and mortality

In Britain, about 15 per cent of the population are Rh(D) negative (dd) and about 13 per cent of all marital partnerships will be between a rhesus positive man and a rhesus negative woman. As about 40 per cent of the men are heterozygous for D, only 67 per cent of those children are Rh(D) positive. The risk of a mother developing anti-D is, however, very much less than the predicted number. Knox (1968) examined the case records of 24 000 births to Rh(D) negative women in Birmingham. Apart from ABO incompatibility, which is known to protect against rhesus immunization, Knox identified a number of factors during pregnancy which increased the risks. These were toxaemia, breech delivery, caesarean section and a short interval between pregnancies.

In 1961, the perinatal mortality from HDN was 1.5/1000 births and following the introduction of anti-D immunoprophylaxis in about 1970, the incidence and the

Table 13.1.   Deaths from haemolytic disease of the newborn due to Rh(D) in England and Wales[a]

Relation to prevention	1977–1980		1981–1987	
	(no.)	(%)	(no.)	(%)
Unavailable[b] in first pregnancy	164	46.5	50	21.4
Failure[c] to give anti-D	107	30.3	80	34.1
Immunized during first pregnancy	39	11.0	46	19.7
True failure of prophylaxis[d]	39	11.0	56	23.9
Due to blood transfusion	4	1.1	2	0.9

[a] From Clarke and Mollison, 1989; [b] Immunizing pregnancy occurred before 1970; [c] Immunizing pregnancy occurred after 1970; [d] Immunized in spite of receiving anti-Rh Ig.

mortality from HDN has declined to 0.39/1000 births in 1987 (Figure 13.1) (Clarke and Mollison, 1989). The fall in mortality is due to a number of factors, which include an improvement in neonatal care, a dilution of the rhesus-negative population by non-European immigrants, an increased use of induced abortion and a reduction in the number of highly parous women. This trend, in turn, was magnified by the selective use of sterilization in women with previously affected infants (Knox, 1968).

The effect of the prevention programme on mortality has been followed in a series of reports by Clarke and Mollison and others based on the examination of death or stillbirth certificates (Table 13.1). Deaths due to non-D remained fairly constant but low, whereas there has been a steady decline in the cases caused by failure to administer anti-D.

Pathology of haemolytic disease

In Western countries, where approximately 15 per cent of the population are Rh negative, the most common cause of haemolytic disease of the newborn (HDN) is immunization to the D antigen.

Destruction of fetal erythrocytes

Fetal red cells coated with IgG antibody are rapidly destroyed in the spleen: the greater the quantity of antibody, the more rapid the destruction, the rate of destruction being limited by the ability of the reticulo-endothelial system to cope with the sensitized cells. Splenic macrophages bear Fc receptors which bind to the IgG on the red cells. Destruction occurs both on the macrophage surface and by ingestion of the red cells. Very occasionally, intravascular haemolysis can occur, in which case free haemoglobin may be found. The liberated haemoglobin is digested by lysosomal enzymes that destroy the globin chains and release haem, which is further degraded by haem oxidase to produce bile pigments.

The fetal response to the haemolytic process

The chronic haemolytic anaemia in the fetus results in increased production of erythropoietin and a massive increase in erythropoiesis in the liver, marrow and spleen. The peripheral blood is full of immature erythroblasts and for that reason, the condition in the neonate was described as erythroblastosis fetalis. As the placental circulation deals with the products of haemolysis, the affected babies are pale but not jaundiced at birth. Jaundice develops rapidly (icterus gravis neonatorum) and may cause kernicterus with permanent brain damage.

Hydrops fetalis

Eventually, the fetus develops high output cardiac failure, tissue hypoxia and acidosis. The ultimate condition is hydrops fetalis, in which the baby is grossly oedematous with a large abdomen due to a combination of ascites and massive hepatosplenomegaly. The placenta is equally oedematous and shows persistence of the cytotrophoblast; it can weigh more than one half of the fetal weight, with an oedematous cord which is sometimes stained yellow. There is often fluid in the pleural cavities and few of these babies survive, even if born alive. Not all of the findings are explained on the basis of fetal anaemia and high output failure: for example, there is marked hypoproteinaemia which may be due to interference with normal liver function by the haemopoietic tissue. New light on the pathogenesis is provided by the findings of cordocentesis. Although the degree of anaemia is not always correlated with the appearance of ascites, the changes of hydrops can often be reversed by an intravascular transfusion, supporting the idea that anaemia is the prime cause (Grannum et al., 1988). Hydrops fetalis is also found in association with haemolytic anaemia due to haemoglobinopathy, and the subject of non-immune hydrops is discussed below.

Alloimmunization by blood group antigens

The rhesus groups

Although much has been learned since the original description by Levine and Stetson (1939) and Landsteiner and Wiener (1940), the exact nature and genetic control of the rhesus antigens is still uncertain and from the outset there have been two main methods of classifying the Rh genotypes.

Wiener, who was the first to classify the antigens, has always argued that the Rh antigen complex is under the control of a single pair of allelic genes, which are named as variants of Rh (D positive) and Hr (D negative). Expression of the gene results in the production of an agglutinogen which can be composed of an almost infinite number of blood 'factors' (Wiener and Wexler, 1956). Each 'factor' is immunogenic in its own right and can stimulate a specific antibody. It is, therefore, possible for a single agglutinogen to stimulate production of a range of specific antibodies. The Wiener system describes the phenotype and makes no assumptions about the genotype (Wiener, 1948).

It was a geneticist, RA Fisher, who after examining the antibody patterns, proposed that there were three pairs of alleles, which he called C c̄; D d; E e (Fisher cited by Race, 1944; Race, 1948, Race et al., 1948). Fisher's theory was well received because it made the subject understandable but the concept was bitterly attacked by Wiener (Wiener, 1948). At the time of Fisher's proposal, anti-e had not yet been demonstrated, and at the time when this chapter was written, no one had yet proved the existence of 'd'.

A third terminology was introduced by Rosenfield et al. (1962) in which each of the known antigens or factors was given a number. As each new unique antigen was discovered it was assigned a number in sequence. The major advantage of this scheme is, like Wiener's, that it makes no attempt at genetic interpretation and is very suitable for computer storage and analysis; the major disadvantage of Rosenfield's scheme is that clinicians and serologists are very familiar with the established nomenclatures of Wiener and Fisher. The routine clinical management of Rh alloimmunization requires a simple and practical scheme that allows for genetic prediction, and the numerical one is too cumbersome for such use.

Table 13.2 shows the most common rhesus genotypes with their equivalents in the Fisher and Wiener classifications.

If the phenotype of each parent is known, it is possible to predict the blood group of the fetus, but the accuracy of prediction is based on the assumed frequency of the genotypes in the population. For example, if a mother is rr (c̄de/c̄de) and the father R_1/R_2 (CDe/c̄DE) then all of the children should possess D and will therefore be

Table 13.2. Rh gene complex frequencies (English population)[a]

Fisher–Race	Wiener	(shorthand symbol)	Frequency[a] (%)
CDe	Rh_1	R_1	41
c̄de	rh	r	39
c̄DE	Rh_2	R_2	14
c̄De	Rh_0	R_0	3
cde	rh'	r'	1
c̄dE	rh''	r''	1
all others			1
			100

[a] Source: Mourant, Kopec and Domaniewska–Sobczak, 1976

Rh(D) positive. It is, however, possible (although unlikely) that the father is hetero-zygous for D, i.e. phenotype, C,c̄,D,e,E; probable genotype, CDe/c̄DE; rarer alternative, Cde/c̄DE.

The accuracy of the prediction can be improved if the blood groups of other children are known, but it is not possible to test for the presence of 'd' (if, indeed, it exists).

There is considerable variation in the distribution of phenotypes between popu-lations; c̄de/c̄de declines in frequency from west to east across Asia and is virtually unknown east of Burma.

Antigen structure

The complicated nature of each antigen site is illustrated by considering that of the 'D' antigen. The first variation of D was recognized when it was found that the cells of some apparently D-positive individuals failed to react with a number of anti-D sera. This 'weak' form of D was named D^u (Stratton, 1946). It became clear that the cells of some individuals, who were D-negative but D^u-positive, could induce an immune anti-D response in recipients, whereas other D^u-positive individuals could be immu-nized by receiving a transfusion of D-positive cells. It is now known that the 'D' antigen consists of at least seven epitopes, each of which is antigenically different from the others (Tippett and Sanger, 1977). In some c̄de/c̄de (rr) individuals who have been exposed to either C or D, antibodies have been detected that appear to react to *both* D and C. It is now clear that most individuals who possess the C or the D antigen also possess the antigen 'G' (Allen and Tippett, 1958) and that rr individuals who do not possess the G antigen will, when immunized by C- or D-positive cells, produce anti-G as well as anti-C or anti-D. This anti-G will be detected by panels of cells that are either C or D positive, thus giving a false impression of cross-reactivity. The nature of C, c̄, E and e antigens is at least as complex and Issitt (1985) has reviewed this difficult subject in detail.

Variations in immunogenicity of D

In general, cells of individuals who are homozygous for D express about twice the number of D antigen sites as those who are heterozygous. The severity of haemolytic disease of the newborn in first-affected infants whose genotype is c̄DE/c̄de (R_2/r) is greater than those whose genotype is CDe/c̄de (R_1r) (Murray, Knox and Walker, 1965). This variation is said to be due to a 'cis' effect of C on D, i.e. a modulatory effect of one gene on another on the same chromosome, and is manifest by a lower D antigen density on R_1r cells than on R_2r cells. Variation in D density associated with the presence of C on the opposite chromosome is said to be the result of a 'trans' effect.

Pathogenesis of haemolytic disease of the newborn

Maternal sensitization

The source of immunizing antigen is usually transplacental haemorrhage, which may occur at any time in pregnancy but is especially frequent following an episode of antepartum haemorrhage and in the presence of hypertension (Jones, McNay and Walker (1969). It is now rare for a woman to be immunized to D as the result of an incompatible transfusion, although cases are reported in which women have injected themselves with blood as part of some ritual associated with drug abuse (Wong, Smith and Jensen, 1983). The most important time for transplacental haemorrhage to occur is with the delivery of the placenta, and alloimmunization is therefore found in only 1 per cent of Rh(D)-negative primigravidae (Tovey and Maroni, 1976).

Once the fetal red cell crosses into the maternal circulation it is capable of inducing an immune response to any antigen not already present in the mother. Both IgM (19S) and the smaller IgG (7S) molecules may be produced. IgM antibodies induce agglutination of red cells suspended in saline and are therefore known as 'complete' antibodies, whereas IgG does not produce agglutination unless the surface charge on the red cell is modified by the addition of albumin or by treatment with an enzyme – hence the term 'albumin', 'incomplete' or 'immune' antibody.

Only IgG antibodies can cross the placenta to enter the fetal circulation, being actively transported by a mechanism involving the Fc fragment; this is part of the placenta's normal function in transferring passive immunity to the fetus. It is important to realize that only about 20 per cent of Rh-negative women develop antibodies in response to a challenge by Rh (D) cells (Woodrow and Donohoe, 1968). The fact that not all Rh(D) women are sensitized by a challenge with D is partly due to the small dose of red cells, but is also because one-third of Rh(D) negative individuals are non-responders and will never produce antibodies. The larger the dose of fetal cells, the greater the risk of immunization. The risk is also increased in the presence of hypertension and manual removal of the placenta, probably because both are associated with an increased transplacental haemorrhage.

Non-D (c̄ and E) haemolytic disease

The great majority of cases of haemolytic disease of the newborn, severe enough to require treatment, are due to anti-D and >90 per cent of women immunized by pregnancy during the 1950s had anti-D, alone or in combination with anti-C. With the decline in the incidence of Rh(D) haemolytic disease, other causes of HDN are becoming relatively more important. Immunization due to c̄, often in combination with E, may be attributable to a previous transfusion of an R_1/R_1(CDe/CDe) woman with blood from a donor with R_2 (c̄DE). 'Paradoxical' immunization describes the situation in which a rhesus-positive mother can have a child with HDN and is shown in Figure 13.2; the antigen concerned is c̄, with or without E. As a rule, disease attributable to these irregular antibodies is milder than that with anti-D.

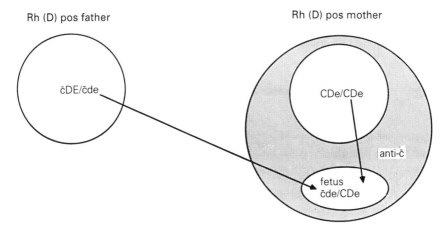

Figure 13.2 'Paradoxical' rhesus haemolytic disease with both parents Rh(D) positive

Influence of the ABO group

If the fetal cells that enter the maternal circulation are ABO incompatible with the mother, they will be destroyed by the natural anti-A or anti-B antibodies in the maternal blood. The rapid removal of these intruders greatly reduces the possibility that they will also induce the production of anti-D. It is not clear whether this affects the overall rate of immunization to D, but the production of high-titre anti-D is certainly reduced. The severity of HDN is also diminished, a phenomenon described over 40 years ago by Levine (1943).

HDN due to ABO incompatibility

A similar mechanism exists for immunization to the ABO groups but unlike rhesus haemolytic disease, the immune antibodies produced by Group B or Group A mothers contain substantial amounts of IgM, which does not cross the placenta, whereas in Group O women the immune antibody is much more likely to contain high titres of IgG. The IgG component of anti-A or anti-B produced by such women will cross the placenta and attach to fetal red cells. The resulting disease in the infants is of slow onset and usually mild; subclinical disease is hard to detect and there is considerable doubt as to the clinical importance of ABO incompatibility in European women (Quinn, Weindling and Davidson, 1988; Brouwers *et al*, 1988).

HDN caused by other antibodies

The list of antibodies that are associated with HDN continues to grow but many such as anti-Kidd, Duffy, MN are comparatively uncommon and rarely cause significant disease. Anti-Kell is the most common of the non-Rh, non-ABO system antibodies that cause haemolytic disease of the newborn and, although intervention may be necessary, intrauterine death is not common (Leggat *et al.*, 1991). The pathogenesis in these cases appears to be similar to that with anti-D, although there is frequently a previous history of blood transfusion, presumably with Kell-positive blood. There is also a suggestion that anaemia in infants affected by anti-Kell may be due, in part, to a depression of haematopoiesis rather than solely to haemolysis (Mollison,

Engelfriet and Contreras, 1987) and that the criteria used to measure bilirubin products in classic HDN may not be appropriate for alloimmunization due to Kell (Rodeck and Letsky, 1989).

Non-immune causes of fetal haemolysis

Among the hereditary disorders that may cause fetal haemolysis, spherocytosis, elliptocytosis and deficiency of glucose-6-phosphate dehydrogenase (G6PD) or pyruvate kinase cause significant disease in the neonate but hardly ever affect obstetric management. Hereditary pyropoikilocytosis may cause more severe disease but is very rare.

In β-thalassaemia the fetus is able to produce normal quantities of fetal haemoglobin and fetal problems do not, therefore, occur, but in the most severe form of α-thalassaemia deletion of all four α-chain genes leads to severe anaemia and hydrops ('Bart's hydrops') because the fetus can make only embryonic haemoglobins. Prenatal diagnosis of these haemoglobinopathies is now possible by means of fetal blood sampling.

Transplacental haemorrhage (TPH)

There is evidence of some TPH in >75 per cent of women during or after delivery, although in 60 per cent of them the amount of fetal blood in the maternal circulation is <0.1 ml. The frequency and amount of TPH increases with gestation, and by the third trimester, 45 per cent of pregnant women have had a TPH; by that time the volume of fetal blood can be quite large (Bowman, Pollock and Penston, 1986). Among the obstetric complications that carry an increased risk of TPH (Jones, McNay and Walker, 1969), are antepartum haemorrhage, hypertension and manual removal of placenta and external version of the fetus.

The detection of TPH depends on the property of fetal haemoglobin to resist elution when the red cell is treated with a suitable acid buffer (Kleihauer, Braun and Betke, 1957). The amount of fetal blood is estimated by the ratio of fetal to maternal cells: 1 fetal cell to 20 000 maternal cells is equivalent to a fetal bleed of 0.25 ml (Woodrow and Donohoe, 1968). This test is not of value if the mother has a condition associated with a raised level of fetal haemoglobin, such as sickle cell disease, some thalassaemias or hereditary persistence of fetal haemoglobin.

Both amniocentesis and cordocentesis can cause a TPH and, as both procedures are performed in cases of suspected fetal haemolytic disease, there is a real risk of exacerbating the degree of alloimmunization (Nicolini et al, 1988).

In first trimester abortion, whether spontaneous or induced, the amount of TPH is limited by the fetal blood volume. As the D antigen can be demonstrated in fetal blood cells 35 days after conception, alloimmunization can result from TPH even though the amount of fetal blood is small (Murray and Barron, 1971). The risk of sensitization varies with the amount of the TPH and rises from 3 per cent with a TPH of 0–0.1 ml to 65 per cent when the TPH is >5 ml (Harmon and Manning, 1988).

Antibody screening

Routine testing for Rh groups was introduced in Britain in 1944 once HDN was recognized as being attributable to rhesus immunization. Having identified rhesus-negative women as being susceptible, the next problem was the detection and identification of the antibodies. Simple incubation of serum with known rhesus positive cells was not effective as a screening test because it usually failed to detect the presence of the 'incomplete' antibody. This was partly overcome by the addition of albumin, which reduces the charge on the red cell allowing it to be agglutinated. The way forward came with the description by Coombs, Mourant and Race (1945) of the anti-human globulin test, an advance which must rank in importance alongside the discovery of the blood groups.

The *direct* Coombs test is used to test cells suspected of being affected by antibody and in the investigation of HDN is normally applied to cord blood. The red cells are first separated and washed in saline to remove any free antibody present in the plasma. The washed red cells are then incubated with an antiglobulin serum (produced by immunizing rabbits with human globulin). If antibodies have been bound to the cells under test, agglutination occurs.

In order to detect maternal antibodies, the *indirect* Coombs test is used. The maternal serum is first incubated at 37°C with a series of red cells from a panel of known genotypes. The red cells are then removed, washed and submitted to the *direct* test. Those which react indicate the presence in the maternal serum of the corresponding antibody. If the red cells used in the screening panel are first treated with an enzyme, such as papain or trypsin (Morton and Pickles, 1947), very low levels of antibody can be detected.

The indirect Coombs test, although without equal in the investigation of individual sera, is too cumbersome for the large scale automated programmes now employed by many blood laboratories. Autoanalysers commonly use a single-step agglutination of enzyme-treated cells, or cells suspended in saline of low ionic strength. Detection of an irregular antibody by these techniques is followed by a standard bench test, such as the indirect Coombs test, to identify its specificity. Autoanalysers therefore detect a higher incidence of so-called 'non-specific' antibodies and over-reporting can be confusing to obstetricians. It is important to maintain close collaboration between laboratory and clinician in order to make the best use of these techniques.

Modifications of the autoanalyser techniques have been applied to the quantitative measurement of anti-D by calibrating the machines against international standards. Anti-D is usually expressed as international units per ml (i.u./ml) and this allows more accurate comparison of results between different patients and laboratories than with the older method using titres obtained by serial dilution, which is still widely used for measuring all other antibodies. Anti-D levels quoted as µg protein per ml can be confusing because there may be marked variation in activity between samples containing the same amount of protein.

Predicting the severity of HDN

Without treatment, about 15 per cent of all Rh(D)-immunized pregnancies result in stillbirth. The most important task is, therefore, to identify those pregnancies most likely to end in fetal death and to change the natural history by intervening. Unfortunately, there is no proven way of distinguishing a fetus that will require up to two neonatal exchange transfusions from one that will simply be Coombs positive but will need no treatment. The section which follows is concerned with Rh(D) immunization; the natural history of other forms of HDN is less clear.

Table 13.3.   Rh(D) antibody titre in relation to
outcome in 185 first affected pregnancies[a]

Outcome	Antibody titre (i.u./ml)	
	<4	≥4
Rhesus negative infant	13	7
Mildly affected	53	18
Moderately affected	23	54
Severely affected	0	4
Stillbirth	1	12
Total	90	95

[a] From Walker (1971)

Antibody levels

The degree to which a fetus is affected by HDN is a function of: (1) the affinity of the antibody for the fetal antigen; (2) the level of antibody in maternal blood, and (3) the length of time during which the fetus is exposed.

There is a great deal of variation in the fetal response to antibody, but anti-D is more potent than either c̄, E or Kell.

When the anti-D level stays <4 i.u./ml (roughly equivalent to a titre of 1/16) throughout pregnancy, it is uncommon for a fetus to require treatment: Bowell et al., (1982) reported that only 3 out of 78 (3.8 per cent) of such babies required an exchange transfusion. In such cases there is no indication for amniocentesis, nor for interfering with the course of a normal pregnancy. It is wise, however, to arrange for the delivery to take place in a unit where facilities are available for immediate exchange transfusion should tests on the cord blood prove it to be necessary. When the antibody level rises to >4 i.u./ml, the chances of needing an exchange transfusion increase (Table 13.3) and so does the risk of stillbirth.

A rising antibody titre can occasionally be misleading. A mother who has already been immunized may respond during the subsequent pregnancy by increasing the level of the antibody, even in the absence of a new stimulus (the 'anamnestic reaction'). It cannot be assumed that, because the titre rises, the baby will necessarily be affected by HDN, and other evidence must be sought before taking action.

Antenatal screening of all women at booking is essential, whatever their rhesus groups (*Lancet* Editorial, 1986). Even if no antibodies are found, rhesus negative women should be retested at 28 and 36 weeks. More frequent testing is not necessary, as antibodies appearing for the first time after 28 weeks rarely cause severe HDN.

In women who are already immunized at booking, the tests need to be repeated more often but the frequency will depend on the past history of HDN and the level of antibody. Antibody levels decline after the birth of an affected infant but they can rise rapidly in the subsequent pregnancy, especially when the fetal red cells are antigenic.

Value of the previous history

Walker (1971) reviewed >3500 cases in the North East of England and found that the previous history of severity of HDN was a valuable guide to outcome. With the fall in the number of cases, such data are hard to come by, and although the outcome for the severely affected fetus has been improved by the use of cordocentesis, the history is still invaluable in clinical management.

First affected pregnancy
The risk of stillbirth was 8 per cent, but 37 per cent of livebirths were only mildly affected.

Previous mild disease (not requiring exchange transfusion)
The stillbirth rate was 2 per cent, 64 per cent had a mildly affected infant and 34 per cent needed exchange transfusion.

Previous severely or very severely affected infant
The risk of stillbirth was about 20 per cent and about 80 per cent needed exchange transfusion.

Previous baby stillborn
The risk of another stillbirth was 63 per cent. Management of the current pregnancy is therefore aimed at intervening to prevent hydrops. A very high antibody level (>30 i.u./ml) occurring before 16 weeks of pregnancy in a woman with a history of previous stillbirth is an indication for early intervention. With present-day management it may be possible to save a fetus if hydrops is diagnosed during the second trimester.

Amniocentesis

The orange colour of amniotic fluid associated with HDN has been recognized for a century, but the source of the pigment is not at all obvious. As the placental circulation effectively removes the bilirubin as it is produced, the newborn is not noticeably jaundiced at the time of birth, although the cord is frequently stained yellow. The most likely explanation is that there is transudation of bile pigments from the lungs and through the cord.

The amount of pigment present in mild cases is too low to be measured reliably by conventional biochemical methods; furthermore, the specimen obtained by amniocentesis may be blood-stained. The systematic measurement of bile pigment in the amniotic fluid is based on the work of Bevis (1952). The method used employs spectrophotometry, which measures the absorption of light at different wavelengths in the visible range; the results are plotted on a logarithmic scale, when normal fluid gives a straight line. Bilirubin produces peak absorption at 450 nm and this is the basis of a number of different methods for estimating bilirubin. Liley (1961) plotted the optical density at 450 nm at different gestations and drew two diagonal parallel lines to separate values into those indicating mild disease from those in the upper zone, which predict severe disease and a risk of stillbirth. Whitfield, Neely and Telford, (1968) produced a modification in the form of a curved 'action' line which falls steeply towards term (Figure 13.3a).

Contamination by blood confuses the interpretation of the curves, and Knox, Fairweather and Walker (1965), advocated the use of a transmission ratio: (percentage transmittance at 520 nm)/(percentage transmittance at 490 nm). Savage *et al.* (1966) showed that this approach is significantly better at predicting the severity of HDN, particularly stillbirth rates, than either the peak absorption at 450 nm or the calculated bilirubin content of amniotic fluid obtained after 33 weeks' gestation.

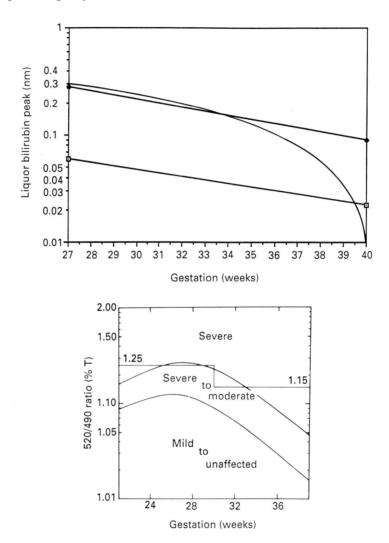

Figure 13.3 Interpretation of liquor bilirubin: (a) parallel lines represent Liley's zones and the super-imposed curve is the 'action line' of Whitfield; (b) prediction chart from liquor ratios (Fairweather, Whyley and Millar, 1976)

Fairweather, Whyley and Millar (1976) came to a similar conclusion and the prediction chart that they published (Figure 13.3b), a modification of earlier schemes developed in Newcastle upon Tyne, is the one used by the authors.

The amount of bilirubin in amniotic fluid tends to fall with advancing gestation and an abnormally high ratio should be confirmed by a repeat estimation after 10 days. The only exception is where there is clear evidence, from ultrasound, that immediate intervention is necessary. Before 33 weeks of pregnancy there are no significant differences between the three methods in their ability to predict hydrops or stillbirth (Savage *et al.*, 1966). Rodeck and Letsky (1989) have drawn attention to the unreliability of amniocentesis performed very early in pregnancy.

In summary, it is usually possible by combining the past history, the antibody level and the paternal genotype to select those patients in whom amniocentesis or fetal blood sampling is appropriate.

Technique of amniocentesis
About 10 ml of amniotic fluid is necessary for the test and the specimen must be protected from light, which degrades bilirubin. The fluid is therefore placed in a brown bottle or one that is covered in some way.

Wherever possible, the procedure should be performed under direct ultrasound control, but in any case the site of the puncture is determined by previous ultrasound examination, which can localize a pool of amniotic fluid and help to avoid puncturing the placenta.

After emptying her bladder, the woman lies comfortably on a couch. The site is identified and the skin is sterilized with a suitable antiseptic. A small skin bleb is raised with 1 per cent lignocaine and about 2 ml of the local anaesthetic is injected into the abdominal wall down to the peritoneum. A 20 or 22 gauge spinal needle is then passed into the uterus at a predetermined depth or under direct ultrasound control and 10–15 ml of amniotic fluid is collected with the minimum of suction. If there is significant blood staining, the first few millilitres should be discarded.

Properly conducted, amniocentesis carries a minimal risk of injury to the fetus, although needle injuries were more common before the use of ultrasound. More important is the risk of damage to the placenta, which may result in a retroplacental haemorrhage and premature onset of labour. Placental puncture can also result in transplacental bleeding and a rise in the maternal antibody level.

Sources of error
The most frequent cause of erroneous measurement is recent bleeding, methaemal-bumin resulting from a previous amniocentesis or the presence of other pigments, such as meconium. Other sources of error result from inadvertent puncture of the maternal bladder or of the ascitic fetal abdomen. A false reading will also occur if the sample has been exposed to light. Maternal urine is normally clear and unlike the slightly turbid liquor which contains fetal squames, whereas fetal ascitic fluid is deep yellow and will give an exceptionally high reading on spectrophotometry.

Timing of amniocentesis
The purpose of amniocentesis is to prevent hydrops and stillbirth by identifying the fetus suffering from haemolytic disease that is sufficiently severe to warrant inter-vention. There is, therefore, no justification for the procedure when other indi-cations suggest that the fetus is not at risk or that intervention is already required on other grounds, e.g. there is ultrasonic evidence of hydrops.

In cases where a severely affected fetus is possible, the most appropriate time is at 31 weeks with the possibility of a repeat about 10 days later. Where there is a risk of early hydrops as in a woman with a previous stillbirth, cordocentesis (if available) is the most reliable method of assessment.

The case for amniocentesis in pregnancies affected by antibodies other than anti-D is by no means clear. Certainly, prediction is less certain (see below).

Ultrasound

The ultrasound appearances of hydrops fetalis are easy to see: oedema of the scalp and abdominal wall, fluid in the fetal peritoneum, pericardial effusion, enlargement of the liver, dilatation of the umbilical vein and ductus venosus, and the very large placenta with a loss of structure. Unfortunately, the changes of hydrops develop quite quickly and there is no warning of impending deterioration.

Serial measurements of placental thickness, umbilical vein diameter, abdominal circumference and intraperitoneal volume were measured by Nicolaides *et al.*, (1988a) in a series of >400 cases but did not predict the onset of severe haemolytic disease. A thin film of fluid under the diaphragm is not uncommon and is unreliable as a warning sign. The ultrasound changes of hydrops are not confined to cases of haemolytic disease and the differential diagnosis is discussed below.

Non-immune hydrops

The routine use of real-time diagnostic sonar in pregnancy has brought to light previously undiagnosed cases of hydrops fetalis, as the characteristic oedema of the skin is easily seen. There has been a spate of published cases and the list of causes is very large; in at least one-half of cases, however, no cause was found (Romero *et al.*, 1988). Some of among the more important causes are given below.

CONGENITAL HEART DISEASE

This accounts for 40 per cent of cases of non-immune hydrops. Congestive cardiac failure, which may be due to structural anomalies or to arrhythmias, produces all the features of hydrops.

CHROMOSOMAL ANOMALIES

The mechanism is obscure but in Turner's syndrome (45, XO), lymphatic abnormalities result in localized cystic areas in the neck (cystic hygroma) or more general changes which give sonar appearances similar to those of hydrops.

OBSTRUCTIVE TUMOURS OF THE CHEST OR ABDOMEN

These include abnormalities of the gut, pulmonary tumours and portal hypertension.

ANGIOMATOUS MALFORMATIONS OF THE PLACENTA

These lead to massive transplacental haemorrhage and fetal anaemia, with the same consequences as haemolytic disease.

For a full list of known causes, the reader is referred to the review by Romero *et al.* (1988).

Biophysical profile

The fetal biophysical profile, as described by Vintzileos *et al.* (1983) and Manning *et al.* (1984), uses a series of observations involving real-time ultrasound and cardiotocography. The score is intended to identify early evidence of fetal compromise, particularly in relation to growth retardation and chronic hypoxia. Frigoletto *et al.* (1986) used the concept to monitor the fetus in a series of cases in which intrauterine transfusion would have been indicated. They claimed to have postponed intervention by careful surveillance but the experience of others is less reassuring. SA Walkinshaw and colleagues (personal communication) found normal biophysical profiles in fetuses that were known to be severely compromised. One characteristic sign is the appearance of a sinusoidal fetal heart trace (Figure 13.4) which denotes severe fetal anaemia.

Fetal blood sampling

The first fetal blood samples were taken in the course of the early attempts at direct open fetal transfusion by hysterotomy (Freda and Adamsons, 1964). More recently, fetoscopy was used to guide a needle into the umbilical vessels (Rodeck and Campbell, 1978), but the technique is difficult and has been replaced by ultrasound guidance known variously as cordocentesis or percutaneous umbilical blood sampling (PUBS). Modern high-resolution ultrasound has made it relatively easy to take fetal blood samples, either from umbilical vessels or from the ductus venosus and the procedure has been suggested as an alternative to amniocentesis (Mackenzie *et al.*, 1988). The advantages are obvious: a fetal sample provides a direct and reliable assessment of the fetal blood group, Coombs test, haematocrit and bilirubin level. Fetal blood sampling has also provided a great deal of information, not previously available, about fetal haematology, especially during the second trimester of pregnancy. The technique is described below in the section on intrauterine transfusion.

Risks of fetal blood sampling

Enthusiasm for cordocentesis must be tempered by the realization that the procedure has risks for mother and fetus. The complications include haemorrhage from the umbilical vessels, tamponade and thrombosis of the umbilical artery, infection, fetal bradycardia and unexplained stillbirth. After removal of the needle, there is often bleeding into the amniotic sac, which can be seen on ultrasound to last up to a minute. Transplacental haemorrhage also occurs and may considerably enhance the maternal antibody level (Bowell *et al.*, 1988).

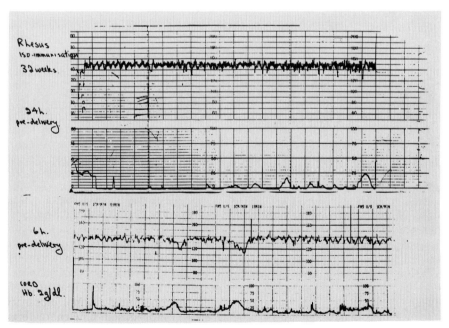

Figure 13.4 Cardiotocographic record from a fetus with severe haemolytic anaemia, showing a sinusoidal-pattern fetal heart rate

In a review of 64 attempts at the procedure, Pielet *et al.* (1988) reported a 9.4 per cent complication rate with a mortality of 4.7 per cent. Other authors are less pessimistic but the technique requires constant practice and is appropriate only for specialist referral centres (Whittle, 1989).

Clinical management

Reducing the effect of the antibody

Once the body has learned to produce antibodies, there seems to be no proven way of reducing the amount, nor of preventing them from crossing the placenta. Treatments that have been advocated for reducing the effect of the antibody include the injection of steroids or the administration of oral promethazine throughout pregnancy, but neither has been found to be very successful (Walker, 1971). Another approach has been to attempt to absorb the antibody by the use of haptens or of exogenous D antigen and by the oral administration of extract of red cell membrane derived from D-positive cells.

Intensive plasma exchange (plasmapheresis) has been used to reduce the concentration of anti-D. Blood is removed from the immunized mother and, by means of an automated process, the antibody-rich plasma is separated and the red cells resuspended in fresh frozen plasma in which they are returned to the mother. The procedure is time-consuming, tedious and distressing, as it may require the removal of up to 20 litres per week. Furthermore, the results are unimpressive and possibly harmful (Barclay, Greiss and Urbaniak, 1980).

In the absence of any method of reducing the effect of Rh antibodies, clinical management is directed to the prevention of stillbirth so that a live baby can undergo exchange transfusion.

Premature delivery

Delivery at about 34 weeks reduces the risk of stillbirth, half of which occur after 35 weeks (Walker, 1971). In the very severe cases, the risk of early hydrops can be avoided only by delivery as early as 32 weeks. Improvements in the care of the premature newborn, particularly the techniques for artificial ventilation and respiratory support have reduced the mortality of infants weighing >1.5 kg at birth, making delivery at about 34 weeks a realistic option. By that time, the fetal liver should be able to cope with the continued production of bile pigments resulting from previous haemolysis, and lung development will have reached a point where, with modern ventilatory support, the chances of survival exceed 90 per cent. Bowman (1989) advocates a cautious approach, with measurement of surfactant activity in the amniotic fluid and the administration of dexamethazone for 48 h before delivery.

Delivery at 30 weeks or less is an unattractive option. The liver is immature and the combination of poor lung function, clotting deficiency and profound jaundice leads to a cascade of neonatal complications and poor outcome.

Maternal rhesus syndrome

Women carrying a hydropic fetus are prone to a condition known as 'pseudotoxaemia' (Nicolay and Gainey, 1964) or 'maternal syndrome' (Goodlin, 1957), characterized by marked oedema (especially of the abdominal wall), malaise, hypertension and proteinuria. The condition is often of sudden onset and its development usually means that the fetus has become hydropic.

The cause is uncertain although Scott (1958) showed that pre-eclampsia occurred in pregnancies associated with excessive placental tissue, such as erythroblastosis, diabetes, twins and hydatidiform mole. As with pre-eclampsia, the signs and symptoms of maternal rhesus syndrome disappear rapidly with the death or delivery of the fetus.

Assessment of risk

There has always been a case for centralizing the management of HDN (Walker and Mollison, 1957) but, as the number of obstetricians with direct experience of alloimmunization diminishes, it is becoming increasingly important to establish regional or even national centres where expert advice and special technical skills are available.

The first step in assessment is a careful clinical history, followed by the investigation of the blood group genotype of both partners and the nature and strength of the antibody. Anti-D causes the most serious disease and, of the non-D antibodies, anti-c̄ and anti-Kell can also cause significant HDN. Antibodies such as anti-Lu, anti-Fy^a and anti-Wr^a, rarely cause HDN and, unless the titre is very high, action during pregnancy is not indicated. Even so, it is better to seek advice from a centre with the requisite experience. In the discussion below, it is assumed that the fetus is affected by anti-D alloimmunization.

The moderately affected fetus
In a first affected pregnancy, an antibody level of ⩾4 i.u./ml occurring before 28 weeks of pregnancy is an indication for amniocentesis at about 31 weeks. The antibody levels should be checked at 28 weeks and repeated following the amniocentesis. Severity is assessed by use of either the Liley zones, the Whitfield action lines or the ratio chart (Figure 13.3).

If the amniotic fluid ratio is <1.04, the risk of stillbirth or of a severely affected fetus is very low and pregnancy may be allowed to go to term. With ratio values in the 'affected' range, the amniocentesis is repeated after about 10 days at 32–33 weeks and the antibody level is also re-estimated. A rising bilirubin ratio or a rapidly rising antibody titre indicates an affected infant who requires monitoring by ultrasound and, provided that there is no suggestion of placental thickening or fetal ascites, labour should be induced at 35 weeks.

The potentially severely affected fetus
If there is a history of a previous baby with severe disease or if the antibody level in early pregnancy is >20 i.u/ml, early intervention is indicated. Amniocentesis in early pregnancy is difficult to interpret and fetal blood sampling offers more reliable information. Where a family has suffered stillbirth from HDN and the father is known to be heterozygous for D, attempts have been made to detect fetal blood cells in chorionic villus samples (Kanhai *et al.*, 1987), the purpose being to offer the mother an induced abortion if the fetus is Rh(D) positive. The technique is difficult and fetal blood sampling can provide more reliable information, although not before 16 weeks.

Once it has been established that the fetus is in danger of developing hydrops, some form of intrauterine transfusion will be needed. If, however, the diagnosis is not made until after 28 weeks then there is the alternative strategy of delivery by caesarean section at 30 weeks.

Transfusion *in utero*

Intraperitoneal transfusion (IPT)
The idea of transfusing the fetus came from Liley (1963) who argued that if children were able to absorb red cells from the peritoneal cavity then the fetus should also be able to do so. The technique of IPT involved the use of radiological screening and the identification of the peritoneal cavity by means of a radio-opaque dye. Visualization of the fetus is now carried out by means of ultrasound but the method does have one disadvantage, namely the inability to identify with certainty the placement of the needle.

The procedure can be performed on an outpatient basis but as it takes many hours to complete, it is sometimes more humane to keep the patient in hospital overnight. The woman should empty her bladder (a full bladder is not necessary to visualize the fetus). A high resolution, linear array ultrasound transducer is preferable to a sector scanner, as the narrow beam helps to localize the plane of the needle. A site is selected that will give access to the fetal abdomen without penetrating the placenta, although that is not always possible. The ideal point of entry to the fetal abdomen is on the left side, about 5 cm below the costal margin.

A solution of 1 per cent lignocaine is injected to anaesthetize the maternal skin and abdominal wall at the selected site. While the local anaesthetic is taking effect, an intravenous injection of 10 mg diazepam is given to the mother in order to act as a sedative and to reduce fetal activity. An alternative to sedation, used by some obstetricians for intravascular transfusion, is to administer a muscle relaxant such as pancuronium directly into the fetus (Weiner and Anderson, 1989).

Preliminary assessment by ultrasound is essential. If the placenta is anterior, the procedure is both difficult and hazardous and should be reconsidered. Where possible, facilities for simultaneous radiography are very helpful for accurate localization of the catheter in the peritoneal cavity, because the needle can easily enter an abdominal viscus or fail to penetrate the abdominal wall.

A 16 gauge Tuohy needle is inserted through the wall of the mother's abdomen and, under ultrasound guidance, the fetal abdominal wall is punctured. Placement of the needle-tip can be judged by observing the turbulence caused by injecting a small volume of normal saline. Harmon and Manning (1988) consider that radiographic confirmation is essential, but if this means moving the patient, uncertain placement may be preferable to the possibility of disturbing the catheter. Once the needle has been correctly sited, about 2 ml of saline is injected to displace any bowel and a fine plastic epidural canula is threaded through the needle until at least 5 cm is beyond the needle tip, using the distance marks on the catheter as a guide. If there is any fetal ascites, as much fluid as possible is aspirated.

The donor blood, which is first irradiated, must be ABO compatible, rhesus negative, and screened for CMV, hepatitis and HIV. The authors now use plasma reduced blood with a haematocrit of ≈60%. With this degree of concentration the blood passes freely down the needle and can be introduced over a period of ≈10 min. The passage of blood into the fetal abdomen is monitored by ultrasound and on occasions the blood can be seen to enter the pleural cavity, from which it also appears to be absorbed.

The amount of blood infused depends upon gestation. A useful formula is Volume = (Weeks of pregnancy − 20) × 10 ml: e.g. 28 weeks = 80 ml; 30 weeks = 100 ml; 32 weeks = 120 ml.

During the infusion, the fetal heart rate is monitored and particular attention is

paid to bradycardia, which suggests overload. If blood is entering the fetal peritoneum, a rim of fluid becomes visible on sonar.

IPT in the presence of hydrops

The presence of ascites is usually obvious on preliminary sonar and bodes ill for the
fetus. Even if the fluid is aspirated, the addition of blood to the peritoneal cavity in a
fetus which already has circulatory failure may be the *coup de grâce*. Furthermore,
there is evidence that blood in the presence of ascites is poorly absorbed. For these
reasons, intravascular transfusion, with an attempt at exchange may offer a better
outcome.

Complications of IPT include failure to catheterize the peritoneum, puncture of an
abdominal organ, such as the gut or urinary bladder, and premature onset of labour.
Some authors advocate the routine use of a tocolytic such as ritodrine during and
after an IPT. Infection is rare.

Intravascular transfusion (IVT)

The early attempts at IVT involved hysterotomy and exteriorization of a fetal limb
(Freda and Adamsons, 1964). The results were poor and the method did not
re-emerge until the development of the fetoscope enabled a needle to be directed
into an umbilical vessel on the placental surface. Direct injection of the umbilical
vein and ductus venosus, using ultrasound guidance, was reported by Bang, Bock
and Trolle (1982), and this method has largely replaced the use of the fetoscope.

High resolution real-time ultrasound allows the needle to be guided with some
accuracy, so that blood can be transfused into the cord insertion of the umbilical
vessels, into a free loop of cord (Barss *et al.*, 1988), perumbilically into the hepatic
vein or even directly into the fetal heart (Westgren, Selbing and Stangenberg, 1988).
Gaining direct access to the fetal circulation has led to an important therapeutic
advance in the management of HDN. Not only is the transfusion direct but it can also
be given in the second trimester, before the onset of hydrops.

The technique is still relatively new and although numerous reports on the use of
cordocentesis and IVT continue to appear, it is still too soon to be certain of its value.
Twelve American and British reports have been reviewed and have provided details
of 194 cases up to 1989: in the 174 for whom the outcome was stated, there were 39
perinatal deaths, a mortality of 22.4 per cent (Table 13.4).

There is little doubt that IVT can reverse fetal hydrops (Grannum *et al.*, 1988) and
that, in experienced hands, the method is relatively safe. When successful, the baby
is born with a high proportion of donor, Rh(D)-negative, blood and a negative
Coombs test. Such an infant is spared the risks of very early gestation and of
immediate exchange transfusion with its attendant risks, including that of necrotizing
enterocolitis.

The danger lies in the overenthusiastic use of an invasive technique with a fetal
mortality rate of 2 per cent per transfusion (Rodeck and Letsky, 1989), when some
cases would be better managed conservatively or at the most by amniocentesis. The
selection of cases for IVT is therefore of great importance. From their large experience of fetal blood sampling, Nicolaides *et al.*, (1988b) concluded that the most
important criterion was the degree to which the fetal cord haemoglobin fell below the
normal for gestation, which they described. They recommended that IVT should be
performed when the cord haemoglobin was 7g/dl below the norm, whereas for the
fetus with a deficit of <2g/dl, no treatment was required. For intermediate values,

they suggested that repeated amniocentesis and ultrasound should be used to monitor the fetus until there was evidence of severe haemolysis. Reece *et al.* (1988) used a similar approach, although they advocated cordocentesis more readily than would be accepted in Britain.

Techniques of cordocentesis and IVT

The procedure is best done in a tertiary referral centre and although the principles are similar, there are differences of detail in the various accounts (see list in Table 13.4). The target site, usually the insertion of the cord into the placenta, is first identified using high resolution ultrasound equipment with a linear transducer. At least one assistant is needed to manipulate the syringe so that the operator can concentrate on watching the needle. Most operators prefer to hold the transducer in the left hand in such a way as to show the target vessel and the needle in the same narrow beam of ultrasound. The transducer is enclosed in a sterile bag containing some coupling gel and if a solution of povidone–iodine is painted on the abdominal wall, it not only sterilizes the skin, but also acts a coupling medium. The maternal entry site is first anaesthetized with 1 per cent lignocaine and a 20 gauge spinal needle of appropriate length is guided to the target vessel. The operator needs to hold the transducer absolutely still or there is a loss of three dimensional sense. An assistant connects a fine 1 ml syringe and aspirates the blood which is immediately tested to confirm that it is fetal. This is done either by a rapid alkaline denaturation technique or by measuring red cell size in a Coulter counter and comparing the mean corpuscular volume (MCV) with that in a maternal blood sample.

The haematocrit or haemoglobin is then measured while the operator holds the needle rigid in case transfusion proves necessary. Three methods of transfusion are described – bolus injection, slow infusion or exchange transfusion. A direct transfusion takes about 30 min, considerably less time than an exchange transfusion (Rodeck and Letsky, 1989; Tannirandorn and Rodeck, 1990).

Intraperitoneal versus intravascular transfusion

IVT has clear advantages over IPT in cases of hydrops fetalis but, as experience

Table 13.4.   Published experience of IVT

Author and year	Approach	n	Reported deaths
Bang, Bock and Trolle, 1982	Hepatic vein	1	0
Barss et al., 1988	Cord insertion	23	3
Berkowitz et al., 1988	Cord insertion/liver	17	4
Bowman, 1989	Cord insertion	15	3
Grannum et al., 1988	Cord insertion (XT)	26	5
Mackenzie et al., 1987	Cord insertion	10	9
Nicolini et al., 1988[a]	Various	20	(n.s.)
Parer, 1988	Not stated	45	9
Pielet et al., 1988	Cord insertion	19	4
Ronkin et al., 1989	Cord insertion	8	0
Seeds and Bowes, 1986	Umbilical vein	1	0
Socol et al., 1987	Cord insertion	3	0
Westgren, Selbing and Stangenberg, 1988	Intracardiac	6	2
TOTAL		174	39 (22.4%)

[a] Excluded from total because outcome was not stated (n.s.)

accumulates, IVT is seen increasingly to be the treatment of choice in all cases of severe fetal anaemia (Harman *et al.*, 1990).

Management of non-D HDN

Disease attributable to anti-c̄, anti-Kell and anti-E accounts for the vast majority of cases.

ANTI-c̄
Some authors have suggested that the behaviour of anti-c̄ is very similar to that of anti-D (Astrup and Kornstad, 1977). Bowell *et al.* (1986) in a study of 177 affected pregnancies, pointed out that significant rises in the titre of anti-c̄ were rare. They found only three severely affected infants, one of whom died, and there were no intrauterine deaths. As 84 per cent of the population is c̄ positive, the rate of severe HDN is well below that expected for anti-D. The indications for amniocentesis are much the same as for anti-D, using a titre of 1/16 as the equivalent to 4 i.u./ml of anti-D.

ANTI-E
This even less common as a cause of HDN.

ANTI-KELL
This is by far the most potent non-rhesus antibody causing HDN. Most women with anti-Kell have acquired the antibody through blood transfusion but, as 91 per cent of the population is Kell-negative, only 9 per cent of women with anti-Kell are likely to have a Kell-positive husband and most of them will be heterozygous for 'K'. The size of the population at risk is, therefore, small and information about the natural history of HDN in this situation is sparse. Most reports deal with fewer than ten affected cases and do not provide denominator information about pregnancies with Kell antibodies in which there was an unaffected infant. It is clear from individual case reports that anti-Kell can cause severe HDN and some authors (Pepperell, Barrie and Flieguer, 1977; Caine and Meuller–Heubach, 1986) report cases of severely affected infants. There is insufficient information, however, to estimate the risk of stillbirth or hydrops fetalis.

Clinical management
In the absence of specific information, it is usual to extrapolate from the experience with anti-D to the management of HDN due to the 'minor' antibodies, an approach strongly supported by Bowman (1989). Even if it were true that history, antibody levels and amniotic fluid pigment levels provide good predictors of severity, there is no proven basis from which to select those patients who are likely to benefit from a diagnostic amniocentesis in the first place. In the end, the management of these 'minor' antibodies is governed by personal experience.

Cordocentesis offers a more direct approach because it provides reliable information on the fetal blood group, haematocrit and Coombs test. For other 'minor' groups, the risk of HDN is not sufficient to warrant such invasive procedures.

Where a woman has suffered a previous stillbirth from an affected fetus, Rodesch *et al.* (1987) have reported the value of chorionic villus sampling for the determination of the Kell group and a similar approach might be appropriate for c̄.

This technique makes it possible to offer an early termination of pregnancy in appropriate cases.

Prevention of rhesus immunization

The idea of preventing Rh immunization stems from the observation that in Rh(D) negative mothers, ABO incompatibility between maternal and fetal blood protects the mother against the development of Rh(D) antibodies (Nevanlinna and Vainio, 1956). The idea was developed in Liverpool by Finn and his colleagues (Finn *et al.*, 1961), who suggested that the adminstration of anti-D would cause Rh(D)-positive fetal cells to be removed from the circulation as if they were ABO incompatible. Experimental work in the USA (Stern, Goodman and Berger,1961) showed that the idea would work and extensive clinical trials were conducted in Britain, Canada and USA. By 1968, preparations of anti-D were licensed for use in USA and the material became generally available in Britain by 1970. The question of dosage was of particular importance because supplies were limited by the ability to recruit plasma donors from among affected women. The other source was from the deliberate immunization of volunteers, either men or post-menopausal women but there were doubts in Britain about the propriety of using such a source.

To be effective, the anti-D immunoglobulin must be injected within 72 h of the antigenic challenge and the dose must be sufficient to mop up all the fetal cells in the maternal circulation. It was estimated that 20 mcg of anti-D (25 mcg to be safe) would protect against 1ml of fetal red cells. From the known distribution of TPH it was calculated that 100 mcg would protect 99.3 per cent of the population at risk. A system was therefore devised to screen, immediately after birth, all Rh(D)-negative women who were not already known to be sensitized. A post-delivery blood sample was examined for the presence of anti-D antibodies and submitted to a Kleihauer test for evidence of TPH. Women who still had no detectable anti-D were deemed 'suitable' for prophylaxis and were given 100 mcg (500 i.u.) of anti-D immunoglobulin. If the Kleihauer test showed a TPH of 4 ml, additional anti-D was advised so as to make up the total dose to 25 mcg of anti-D for every 1 ml of fetal cells (Mollison, Engelfriet and Contreras, 1987). This rather complicated system was required to make the best use of the relatively small supplies of therapeutic anti-D, but it is prone to error because it involves the transfer of information between laboratory and ward. We advocated that *all* Rh(D)-negative women (not already known to be immunized) should be offered anti-D immediately after delivery. The Kleihauer test should be performed on the post-delivery blood sample to identify those women who will need a higher dose.

A single pregnancy with an Rh(D) positive, ABO-compatible infant will produce immunization in about 17 per cent of Rh(D), negative women; the use of prophylactic anti-D reduces the immunization rate to about 1.5 per cent (Mollison, Engelfriet and Contreras, 1987). In USA and continental Europe, the standard dose of commercially produced anti-D is 300 mcg, which will protect against a TPH of up to 12 ml fetal cells.

Spontaneous and induced abortion

The occurrence of immunization is related to the size of the TPH, but even when the TPH is undetectable, there is still a 3 per cent risk of immunization (Woodrow and Donohoe, 1968). The issue is important in relation to abortion before 20 weeks when the size of the TPH is small but where about 3 per cent of patients are likely to become immunized (Murray, Barron and McNay, 1970; Murray and Barron, 1971). It is therefore the policy in Britain to give 50 µg (250 i.u) anti-D after an abortion of <20 weeks.

Failure of prophylaxis

There are no reliable data on the incidence of immunization in the population, but some indication of the scale of the problem and of secular trends is provided by the regular reports, based on death certification, by Clarke, Mollison and others (see Clarke and Mollison, 1989). From inspection of the case records, the antecedents of perinatal deaths attributable to HDN have been analysed, and the results are summarized in Table 13.1. As the proportion of deaths due to non-administration has fallen from 46 per cent in 1977–1980 to 21.4 per cent in 1981–1987, so the cases of immunization during a first pregnancy have assumed a relatively greater importance, rising from 11 per cent to 19.7 per cent in the same time period.

Antenatal prophylaxis

The use of anti-D during a first pregnancy has long been advocated by Bowman *et al.* (1978), but there has been resistance to such a policy in Britain for two reasons: the first was the expense of providing the additional immunoglobulin and the difficulty of obtaining supplies and the second was the fear that anti-D given during pregnancy might harm the fetus. A full-scale trial has now been completed in Yorkshire (Thornton *et al.*, 1989), which demonstrated the practicability and suggested the efficacy of giving anti-D during the antenatal period. A dose of 100 µg was given to mothers in their first pregnancies at 28 weeks and again at 34 weeks. The outcome of the next three pregnancies was compared with a control group of mothers who had been delivered 2 years earlier and who had received postnatal prophylaxis with 100 µg of anti-D. Not only was the incidence of immunization reduced in the index group, but the protection appeared to last into subsequent pregnancies. A randomized controlled trial of the administration of anti-D during pregnancy is currently under way in Britain. There is a strong case for giving 100 µg of anti-D after any episode of bleeding or after amniocentesis in a Rh(D)-negative woman at risk.

Neonatal problems

The combination of anaemia and hyperbilirubinaemia produces the major problems in HDN. Controlled trials by Mollison and Walker (1952) comparing exchange transfusion with simple transfusion established that exchange transfusion was very much preferable because it not only corrected the anaemia but also reduced the hyperbilirubinaemia. Walker and Neligan (1955) established criteria for early exchange transfusion based on the cord levels of haemoglobin and bilirubin. These were later revised in the light of experience (Walker, 1971) and exchange transfusion was recommended if the haemoglobin was <13.2 g/dl or the bilirubin >4 mg/dl (68 µmol/); this is still the guideline used by the authors.

The danger of hyperbilirubinaemia is that the unconjugated bilirubin can cross the blood–brain barrier and cause staining and damage to the mitochondria in the basal ganglia (kernicterus), leading to severe neural damage which, if not fatal, causes choreo-athetosis, spasticity, mental retardation and deafness. The bilirubin level can rise sharply and various graphs are available on which serial measurements can be plotted. This helps to predict the likelihood of the bilirubin reaching levels at which kernicterus will occur. Kernicterus can develop with a peak bilirubin level as low as 15 mg/dl (255 μmol/l) and repeated exchange transfusions may be necessary, particularly if the baby is premature.

Exposure of the skin to blue light causes the decomposition of bilirubin and phototherapy is useful as an adjunct in the treatment of mild hyperbilirubinaemia (Ebbeson, 1979). Phototherapy is not a substitute for exchange transfusion although it does reduce the frequency of repeat transfusion.

A wide range of clinical problems afflict affected infants. In a review of the causes of death among 4000 affected babies in Newcastle upon Tyne (Ellis, Hey and Walker, 1979), the major causes were cerebral and/or pulmonary haemorrhage, hydrops fetalis, hyaline membrane disease and sudden collapse during exchange transfusion. Sudden collapse during transfusion is now very rare, but later complications, such as coagulation defects (Hey and Jones, 1979) and necrotizing enterocolitis, are now important causes of morbidity and death.

As with the obstetric management of the mother, the experience of the paediatrician with exchange transfusion is decreasing. The treatment of babies with HDN therefore needs to be concentrated in centres with the experience and facilities to deal with all the complications.

Acknowledgement

The authors are grateful to Professor W Walker for his advice over many years and for access to his unpublished work.

References

Allen, FH and Tippett, PA (1958) A new Rh blood type which reveals the Rh antigen G. *Vox Sanguinis*, **3**, 321–330

Astrup, J and Kornstad, L (1977) Presence of anti-c̄ in the serum of 42 women giving birth to c̄ positive babies: serological and clinical findings. *Acta Obstetrica et Gynecologica Scandinavia*, **56**, 185–188

Bang, J, Bock, JE and Trolle, D (1982) Ultrasound-guided fetal intravenous transfusion for severe rhesus haemolytic disease. *British Medical Journal* **284**, 373–374

Barclay, GR, Greiss, MA and Urbaniak, SJ (1980) Adverse effect of plasma exchange on anti-D production in rhesus immunisation owing to removal of inhibitory factors. *British Medical Journal*, **1**, 1569–1571

Barss, VA, Benacerraf, BR, Frigoletto, FD *et al.* (1988) Management of isoimmunized pregnancy by use of intravascular techniques. *American Journal of Obstetrics and Gynecology*, **159**, 932–937

Berkowitz, RL, Chitkara, MD, Wilkins, IA *et al.* (1988) Intravascular monitoring and management of erythroblastosis fetalis. *American Journal of Obstetrics and Gynecology*, **158**, 783–795

Bevis, DCA (1952) The antenatal prediction of haemolytic disease of the newborn. *Lancet*, **i**, 395–398

Bowell, P, Wainscoat, JS, Peto, TEA and Gunson, HH (1982) Maternal anti-D concentrations and outcome in rhesus haemolytic disease of the newborn. *British Medical Journal*, **285**, 327–329

Bowell, PJ, Brown, SE, Dike, AE and Inskip, MJ (1986) The significance of anti-c alloimmunization in pregnancy. *British Journal of Obstetrics and Gynaecology*, **93**, 1044–1048

Bowell, PJ, Selinger, M, Ferguson, J *et al.* (1988) Antenatal fetal blood sampling for alloimmunized pregnancies: effect upon maternal anti-D potency levels. *British Journal of Obstetrics and Gynaecology*, **95**, 759–764

Bowman, JM (1989) Maternal blood group immunization. In *Maternal–Fetal Medicine*, 2nd edn (edited by RK Creasy and R Resnik) pp. 613–655. Philadephia: WB Saunders

Bowman, JM, Pollock, JM and Penston, LE (1986) Fetomaternal transplacental haemorrhage during pregnancy and after delivery. *Vox Sanguinis*, **51**, 117

Bowman, JM, Chown, B, Lewis, M and Pollock, JM (1978) Rh isoimmunization during pregnancy: antenatal prophylaxis. *Canadian Medical Association Journal*, **118**, 626–627

Brouwers, HAA, Overbeeke, MAM, van Ertbruggen, I *et al.* (1988) What is the best predictor of the severity of ABO-haemolytic disease of the newborn? *Lancet*, **ii**, 641–644

Caine, ME and Meuller-Heubach, E (1986) Kell sensitization in pregnancy. *American Journal of Obstetrics and Gynecology,* **154**, 85–90

Clarke, CA and Mollison, PL (1989) Deaths from Rh haemolytic disease of the fetus and newborn, 1977–87. *Journal of the Royal College of Physicians of London*, **23**, 181–184

Coombs, RRA, Mourant, AE and Race, RR (1945) A new test for the detection of weak and 'incomplete' Rh agglutinins. *British Journal of Experimental Pathology,* **26**, 15–16

Darrow, RR (1938) Icterus gravis (erythroblastosis) neonatorum; examination of etiological considerations. *Archives of Pathology*, **25**, 378–417

Diamond, LK, Blackfan, KD and Baley, JM (1932) Erythroblastosis fetalis and its association with universal edema of the fetus, icterus gravis neonatorum and anemia of the newborn. *Journal of Pediatrics*, **1**, 269–309

Ebbeson, F (1979) Superiority of intensive phototherapy – blue double light – in rhesus haemolytic disease. *European Journal of Paediatrics*, **130**, 279–284

Ellis, MI, Hey, EN and Walker, W (1979) Neonatal death in babies with rhesus isoimmunization. *Quarterly Journal of Medicine*, **48**, 211–225

Fairweather, DVI, Whyley, GA and Millar, MD (1976) Six years' experience of the prediction of severity in rhesus haemolytic disease. *British Journal of Obstetrics and Gynaecology*, **83**, 698–706

Finn, R (1960) Erythroblastosis. *Lancet*, **i**, 526

Finn, R, Clarke, CA, Donohoe, WTA *et al.* (1961) Experimental studies on the prevention of Rh haemolytic disease. *British Medical Journal*, **1**, 1486–1490

Freda, VJ and Adamsons, K (1964) Exchange transfusion in utero. *American Journal Obstetrics and Gynecology*, **89**, 817–821

Freda, VJ, Gorman, JG and Pollack, W (1964) Successful prevention of experimental Rh sensitization in man with an anti-Rh gamma$_2$-globulin antibody preparation. *Transfusion*, **4**, 26–32

Frigoletto, FD, Greene, MF, Benacerraf, BR *et al.* (1986) Ultrasonic fetal surveillance in the management of the isoimmunized pregnancy. *New England Journal* of Medicine, **315**, 430–432

Goodlin, EC (1957) Impending fetal death in utero due to isoimmunization. *Obstetrics and Gynecology*, **10**, 299–302

Grannum, PAT, Copel, JA, Moya, FR, *et al.* (1988) The reversal of hydrops fetalis by intravenous intrauterine transfusion in severe isoimmune fetal anemia. *American Journal of Obstetrics and Gynecology*, **158**, 914–919

Harman, CR, Bowman, JM, Manning, FA and Menticoglou, SM (1990) Intrauterine transfusion– intraperitoneal versus intravascular approach: a case-control comparison. *American Journal of Obstetrics and Gynecology*, **162**, 1053–1059

Harmon, CR and Manning, FA (1988) Alloimmune disease. In *Clinical Obstetrics* (edited by CJ Pauerstein) pp. 441–469. New York: Churchill Livingstone

Hey, E and Jones, P (1979) Coagulation failure in babies with rhesus isoimmunization. *British Journal of Haematology*, **42**, 441–454

Issitt, PD (1985) *Applied Blood Group Serology*, 3rd edn. Miami: Montgomery

Jones, P, McNay, A and Walker, W (1969) Association between foeto–maternal bleeding and hypertension in pregnancy. *British Medical Journal*, **2**, 738–742

Kanhai, HH, Gravenhorst, JB, Gemke, RJ *et al.* (1987) Fetal blood group determination for the management of severe immunization. *American Journal of Obstetrics and Gynecology*, **156**, 120–123

Kleihauer, E, Braun, H and Betke, K (1957) Demonstration von fetalem Hamoglobin in den Erythrocyten eines Blutausstrichs. *Klinische Wochenschrift*, **35**, 637–638

Knox, EG (1968) Obstetric determinants of Rhesus sensitisation. *Lancet*, **i**, 433–437

Knox, EG, Fairweather, DVI and Walker, W (1965) Spectrophotometric measurements on liquor amnii in relation to the severity of haemolytic disease of the newborn. *Clinical Science*, **28**, 147–156

Lancet Editorial (1986). Prenatal screening for irregular blood group antibodies. *Lancet*, **ii**, 1369–1370

Landsteiner, K and Wiener, AS (1940) Agglutinable factor in human blood recognised by human sera for rhesus blood. *Proceedings of the Society for Experimental Biology and Medicine*, **43**, 223

Leggat, HM, Gibson, JM, Barron, SL and Reid, MM (1991) Anti-Kell in pregnancy. *British Journal of Obstetrics and Gynaecology*, **98**, 162–165

Levine, P (1943) Serological factors as possible causes in spontaneous abortions. *Journal of Heredity*, **34**, 71–80

Levine, P and Stetson, RE (1939) An unusual case of intra-group agglutination. *Journal of the American Medical Association*, **113**, 126–127

Levine, P, Burnham, L, Katzin, EM and Vogel, P (1941) The role of isoimmunization in the pathogenesis of erythroblastosis fetalis. *American Journal of Obstetrics and Gynecology*, **42**, 925–937

Liley, AW (1961) Liquor amnii analysis in the management of the pregnancy complicated by rhesus sensitisation. *American Journal of Obstetrics and Gynecology*, **82**, 1359–1370

Liley, AW (1963) Intrauterine transfusion of foetus in haemolytic disease. *British Medical Journal*, **2**, 1107–1109

Mackenzie, IZ, Bowell, PJ, Ferguson, J *et al*. (1987) In-utero intravascular transfusion of the fetus for the management of severe Rhesus isoimmunisation: a reappraisal. *British Journal of Obstetrics and Gynaecology*, **94**, 1068–1073

Mackenzie, IZ, Bowell, PJ, Castle, BM *et al*. (1988) Serial fetal sampling for the management of pregnancies complicated by severe rhesus (D) isoimmunization. *British Journal of Obstetrics and Gynaecology*, **95**, 753–758

Manning, FA, Lange, IR, Morrison, IM and Harman, CR (1984) Fetal biophysical profile score and the nonstress test: a comparative trial. *Obstetrics and Gynecology*, **64**, 326–331

Mollison, P and Walker, W (1952) Controlled trials of the treatment of haemolytic disease of the newborn. *Lancet* , **i**, 429–433

Mollison, PL, Engelfriet, CR and Contreras, M (1987) *Transfusion in Clinical Medicine*, 8th edn, pp. 637–687. Oxford: Blackwell

Morton, JA and Pickles, MM (1947) Use of trypsin in the detection of incomplete anti-rh antibodies. *Nature*, **159**, 779–780

Mourant, AE, Kopec, AC and Domaniewska-Sobczak, K (1976) *The Distribution of Human Blood Groups and other polymorphisms*, 2nd edn. London: Oxford University Press

Murray, S and Barron, SL (1971) Rhesus isoimmunization after abortion. *British Medical Journal*, **3**, 90–92

Murray, S, Barron, SL and McNay, RA (1970) Transplacental haemorrhage after abortion. *Lancet*, **i**, 631–634

Murray, S, Knox, G and Walker, W (1965) Haemolytic disease and the rhesus genotypes. *Vox Sanguinis*, **10**, 257–268

Nevanlinna, HR and Vainio, T (1956) The influence of mother–child ABO compatibility on Rh immunisation. *Vox Sanguinis*, **1**, 26

Nicolaides, KH, Clewell, WH, Mibashan, RS *et al*. (1988a) Fetal haemoglobin measurement in the assessment of red cell isoimmunisation. *Lancet*, **i**, 1073–1075

Nicolaides, KH, Fontanarosa, M, Gabbe, SG and Rodeck, CH (1988b) Failure of ultrasonographic parameters to predict the severity of fetal anemia in rhesus isoimmunization. *American Journal of Obstetrics and Gynecology*, **158**, 920–926

Nicolay, KS and Gainey, HL (1964) Pseudotoxemic state associated with severe Rh isoimmunization. *American Journal of Obstetrics and Gynecology*, **89**, 41–45

Nicolini, U, Kochenour, NK, Greco, P *et al*. (1988) Consequences of fetomaternal haemorrhage after intrauterine transfusion. *British Medical Journal*, **297**, 1379–1381

Parer, JT (1988) Severe Rh isoimmunisation – current methods of in utero diagnosis and treatment. *American Journal of Obstetrics and Gynecology*, **158**, 1323–1329

Parsons, LG (1938) The haemolytic anaemias of childhood. *Lancet*, **ii**, 1395–1401

Pepperell, RJ, Barrie, JU and Fliegner, JR (1977) Significance of red cell irregular antibodies in the obstetric patient. *Medical Journal of Australia*, **2**, 453–456

Pielet, BW, Socol, M, Macgregor, SN *et al*. (1988) Cordocentesis: an appraisal of risks. *American Journal of Obstetrics and Gynecology*, **159**, 1497–1500

Quinn, MW, Weindling, AM and Davidson, DC (1988) Does ABO incompatibility matter? *Archives of Disease in Childhood*, **63**, 1258–1260

Race, RR (1944) An 'incomplete' antibody in human serum. *Nature*, **153**, 771–772

Race, RR (1948) Rh genotypes and Fisher's theory. *Blood*, Special issue **No.2**, 27–42

Race, RR, Mourant, AE, Lawler, SD and Sanger, R (1948) The Rh chromosome frequencies in England. *Blood*, **3**, 689–695

Reece, EA, Copel, JA, Scioscia, AL *et al.* (1988) Diagnostic fetal umbilical blood sampling in the management of isoimmunisation. *American Journal of Obstetrics and Gynecology*, **159**, 1057–1065

Rodeck, CH and Campbell, S (1978) Sampling pure fetal blood by fetoscopy in the second trimester of pregnancy. *British Medical Journal*, **2**, 728–730

Rodeck, CH and Letsky, E (1989) How the management of erythroblastosis has changed. *British Journal of Obstetrics and Gynaecology*, **96**, 759–763

Rodesch, F, Lambermont, M, Donner, C *et al.*, (1987) Chorionic biopsy in management of severe Kell alloimmunization. *American Journal of Obstetrics and Gynecology*, **156**, 124–125

Romero, R, Pilu, G, Jeanty, P, Ghindi, A and Hobbins, JC (1988) In *Diagnosis of Congenital Anomalies*, pp. 414–426. Norwalk: Appleton

Ronkin, S, Chayen, B, Wapner, RJ *et al.* (1989) Intravascular exchange and bolus transfusion in the severely isoimmunized fetus. *American Journal of Obstetrics and Gynecology*, **160**, 407–426

Rosenfield, RE, Allen, FH, Swisher, SN and Kochwa, S (1962) A review of Rh serology and presentation of a new terminology. *Transfusion*, **2**, 287–312

Savage, RD, Walker, W, Fairweather, DVI and Knox, EG (1966) Quantitative estimation of bilirubin in liquor amnii. *Lancet*, **ii**, 816–819

Scott, JS (1958) Pregnancy toxaemia associated with hydrops foetalis, hydatidiform mole and hydramnios. *Journal of Obstetrics and Gynaecology of the British Empire*, **65**, 689–701

Seeds, JW and Bowes, WA (1986) Ultrasound-guided fetal intravascular transfusion in severe rhesus immunization. *American Journal of Obstetrics and Gynecology*, **154**, 1105–1107

Socol, ML, Macgregor, DO, Pielet, BW *et al.* (1987) Percutaneous umbilical transfusion in severe rhesus isoimmunization: resolution of fetal hydrops. *American Journal of Obstetrics and Gynecology*, **157**, 1370–1375

Stern, K, Goodman, HS and Berger, M (1961) Experimental isoimmunisation to haemo antigens in Man. *Journal of Immunology*, **87**, 189–198

Stratton, F (1946) New Rh allelomorph. *Nature*, **54**, 25–28

Tannirandorn, Y and Rodeck, CH (1990) New approaches in the treatment of haemolytic disease of the fetus. *Baillière's Clinical Haematology*, **3**, 289–320

Thornton, JG, Page, C, Foote, G *et al.* (1989) Efficacy and long term effects of antenatal prophylaxis with anti-D immunoglobulin. *British Medical Journal*, **298**, 1671–1673

Tippett, PA and Sanger, R (1977) Further observations of the Rh antigen D. *Arztliche Laboratorium*, **23**, 476–480

Tovey, LAD and Maroni, ES (1976) Rhesus isoimmunisation. In *Immunology of Human Reproduction* (edited by JS Scott and WR Jones) pp. 187–227. London: Academic Press

Vintzileos, AM, Campbell, WA, Ingardia, CJ and Nochimson, DJ (1983) The fetal biophysical profile and its predictive value. *Obstetrics and Gynecology*, **62**, 271–178

Walker, W (1971) Haemolytic disease of the newborn. In *Recent Advances in Paediatrics* (edited by D Gairdner and D Hull) pp. 119–170. London: Churchill

Walker, W and Mollison, PL (1957) Haemolytic disease of the newborn. Deaths in England and Wales during 1953 and 1955. *Lancet*, **i**, 1309–1314

Walker, W and Neligan, GA (1955) Exchange transfusion in haemolytic disease of the newborn. *British Medical Journal*, **1**, 681–691

Weiner, CP and Anderson, TL (1989) The acute effects of cordocentesis with or without fetal curarization and of intravascular transfusion upon umbilical waveform indices. *Obstetrics and Gynecology*, **73**, 219–224

Westgren, M, Selbing, A and Stangenberg, M (1988) Fetal intracardiac transfusions in patients with severe rhesus isoimmunisation. *British Medical Journal*, **296**, 885–886

Whitfield, CR, Neely, RA and Telford, ME (1968) Amniotic fluid analysis in rhesus iso immunization. *Journal of Obstetrics and Gynaecology of the British Commonwealth*, **75**, 121–127

Whittle, MJ (1989) Cordocentesis. *British Journal of Obstetrics and Gynaecology*, **96,** 262–264

Wiener, AS (1948) Anti-Rh Serum Nomenclature (letter). *British Medical Journal*, **1,** 805

Wiener, AS and Wexler, IB (1946) The use of heparin when performing exchange transfusions in newborn infants. *Journal of Laboratory and Clinical Medicine*, **31,** 1016–1019

Wiener, AS and Wexler, IB (1956) The Rh-Hr types; a complex problem in serology, genetics and nomenclature. *Annals of Internal Medicine*, **45,** 725–729

Wong, LK, Smith, LH and Jensen, HM (1983) Hemolytic disease of the newborn following maternal self-injection of blood. *Transfusion*, **23,** 348–349

Woodrow, JC and Donohoe, WT (1968) Rh-immunization by pregnancy: results of a survey and their relevance to prophylactic therapy. *British Medical Journal*, **4,** 139–144

Index